Tubes with BD Hemogard™ Closure	Tubes with Conventional Stopper	Additive		
Gold	Red/Black	• Clot activator a_ for serum separa_		...determinations in chemistry. May be used for routine blood donor screening and diagnostic testing of serum for infectious disease.** Tube inversions ensure mixing of clot activator with blood. Blood clotting time: 30 minutes.
Light Green	Green/Gray	• Lithium heparin and gel for plasma separation	8	BD Vacutainer® PST™ Tube for plasma determinations in chemistry. Tube inversions prevent clotting.
Red		• None (glass) • Clot activator (plastic)	0 5	For serum determinations in chemistry. May be used for routine blood donor screening and diagnostic testing of serum for infectious disease.** Tube inversions ensure mixing of clot activator with blood. Blood clotting time: 60 minutes.
Orange	Gray/Yellow	• Thrombin	8	For stat serum determinations in chemistry. Tube inversions ensure complete clotting, which usually occurs in less than 5 minutes.
Royal Blue		• Clot activator (plastic serum) • K_2EDTA (plastic)	8 8 0 5 8	For trace-element, toxicology, and nutritional chemistry determinations. Special stopper formulation provides low levels of trace elements (see package insert).
Green		• Sodium heparin • Lithium heparin	8 8	For plasma determinations in chemistry. Tube inversions prevent clotting.
Gray		• Potassium oxalate/ sodium fluoride • Sodium fluoride/ Na_2 EDTA • Sodium fluoride (serum tube)	8 8 8	For glucose determinations. Oxalate and EDTA anticoagulants will give plasma samples. Sodium fluoride is the antiglycolytic agent. Tube inversions ensure proper mixing of additive and blood.
Tan		• K_2EDTA (plastic)	8 8	For lead determinations. This tube is certified to contain less than .01 µg/mL (ppm) lead. Tube inversions prevent clotting.
	Yellow	• Sodium polyanethol sulfonate (SPS) • Acid citrate dextrose additives (ACD): **Solution A -** 22.0 g/L trisodium citrate, 8.0 g/L citric acid, 24.5 g/L dextrose **Solution B -** 13.2 g/L trisodium citrate, 4.8 g/L citric acid, 14.7 g/L dextrose	8 8 8	SPS for blood culture specimen collections in microbiology. Tube inversions prevent clotting. ACD for use in blood bank studies, HLA phenotyping, and DNA and paternity testing.

Tubes with BD Hemogard™ Closure	Tubes with Conventional Stopper	Additive	Inversions at Blood Collection*	Laboratory Use
Lavender		• Liquid K₃EDTA (glass) • Spray-coated K₂EDTA (plastic)	8 8	K₂EDTA and K₃EDTA for whole blood hematology determinations. K₂EDTA may be used for routine immunohematology testing and blood donor screening.*** Tube inversions prevent clotting.
White		• K₂EDTA with gel	8	For use in molecular diagnostic test methods (such as but not limited to polymerase chain reaction [PCR] and/or branched DNA [bDNA] amplification techniques).
Pink		• Spray-coated K₂EDTA	8	For whole blood hematology determinations. May be used for routine immunohematology testing and blood donor screening.*** Designed with special cross-match label for patient information required by the AABB. Tube inversions prevent clotting.
Light Blue Clear		• Buffered sodium citrate 0.105 M (≈3.2%) glass 0.109 M (≈3.2%) plastic • Citrate, theophylline, adenosine, dipyridamole (CTAD)	3-4 3-4	For coagulation determinations. CTAD for platelet function assays and routine coagulation determination. Tube inversions prevent clotting.
Clear Red/Gray		• None (plastic)	0	For use as a discard tube or secondary specimen collection tube.

Partial-draw Tubes (2 ml and 3 mL: 13 x 75 mm)	Additive	Inversions at Blood Collection*	Laboratory Use
Red	• None	0	For serum determinations in chemistry. May be used for routine blood donor screening, immunohematology testing,*** and diagnostic testing of serum for infectious disease.** Tube inversions ensure mixing of clot activator with blood. Blood clotting time: 60 minutes.
Green	• Sodium heparin • Lithium heparin	8 8	For plasma determinations in chemistry. Tube inversions prevent clotting.
Lavender	• Spray-coated K₂EDTA (plastic)	8 8	For whole blood hematology determinations. May be used for routine immunohematology testing and blood donor screening.*** Tube inversions prevent clotting.

Small-volume Pediatric Tubes (2 mL: 10.25 x 47 mm, 3 mL: 10.25 x 64 mm)	Additive	Inversions at Blood Collection*	Laboratory Use
Light Blue	• 0.105 M sodium citrate (≈3.2%)	3-4	For coagulation determinations. Tube inversions prevent clotting.

* Invert gently, do not shake

** The performance characteristics of these tubes have not been established for infectious disease testing in general; therefore, users must validate the use of these tubes for their specific assay-instrument/reagent system combinations and specimen storage conditions.

*** The performance characteristics of these tubes have not been established for immunohematology testing in general; therefore, users must validate the use of these tubes for their specific assay-instrument/reagent system combinations and specimen storage conditions.

MANUAL OF I.V.
Therapeutics

Evidence-Based Practice
for Infusion Therapy

6th EDITION

Lynn Dianne Phillips, MSN, RN, CRNI®
Professor Emeritus
Butte College
Butte Valley, California
Nursing Education Consultant
President
Infusion Nurses Society 2009–2010

Lisa Gorski, MS, HHCNS-BC, CRNI®, FAAN
Clinical Nurse Specialist
Wheaton Franciscan Home Health & Hospice
Milwaukee, Wisconsin
President
Infusion Nurses Society 2007–2008

F.A. Davis Company • Philadelphia

F. A. Davis Company
1915 Arch Street
Philadelphia, PA 19103
www.fadavis.com

Printed in the United States of America

Last digit indicates print number: 10 9 8 7 6 5 4 3 2 1

Acquisitions Editor: Thomas A. Ciavarella
Director of Content Development: Darlene D. Pedersen
Project Editor: Echo K. Gerhart
Electronic Project Editor: Sandra Glennie
Cover Design: Carolyn O'Brien

As new scientific information becomes available through basic and clinical research, recommended treatments and drug therapies undergo changes. The author(s) and publisher have done everything possible to make this book accurate, up to date, and in accord with accepted standards at the time of publication. The author(s), editors, and publisher are not responsible for errors or omissions or for consequences from application of the book, and make no warranty, expressed or implied, in regard to the contents of the book. Any practice described in this book should be applied by the reader in accordance with professional standards of care used in regard to the unique circumstances that may apply in each situation. The reader is advised always to check product information (package inserts) for changes and new information regarding dose and contraindications before administering any drug. Caution is especially urged when using new or infrequently ordered drugs.

Library of Congress Cataloging-in-Publication Data

Phillips, Lynn Dianne, 1947- author.
  Manual of I.V. therapeutics : evidence-based practice for infusion therapy / Lynn Dianne Phillips, Lisa Gorski. — Sixth edition.
    p. ; cm.
  Manual of I.V. therapeutics
  Manual of intravenous therapeutics
  Includes bibliographical references and index.
  ISBN 978-0-8036-3846-4
  I. Gorski, Lisa A., author. II. Title. III. Title: Manual of I.V. therapeutics. IV. Title: Manual of intravenous therapeutics.
  [DNLM: 1. Infusions, Intravenous—methods—Examination Questions. 2. Infusions, Intravenous—methods—Handbooks. 3. Infusions, Intravenous—nursing—Examination Questions. 4. Infusions, Intravenous—nursing—Handbooks. WB 39]
  RM170
  615'.6—dc23
                                                                                          2013045751

I want to dedicate this edition of the Manual to the supportive, loving friends I have had the good fortune to know through the Infusion Nurses Society: Mary Alexander, Michelle Berreth, Ann Corrigan, Beth Fabian, Lisa Gorski, Roxanne Perucca, Ofelia Santiago, Marvin Siegel, and Mary Walsh. I am truly blessed. To Lisa, it has been a pleasure having you co-author this edition. You have been an excellent author, and this edition is better than ever because of you!
Additionally, as always, to nursing students—you are our future!

Lynn Phillips

First of all, I want to thank Lynn for asking me to co-author this edition of the Manual—it was a joy to work together! I dedicate this book to my husband John, my parents John and Audrey Morrill, and my children Ben and Amanda Gorski, who have loved me and have supported me in all my professional endeavors. And also to my colleagues in the Infusion Nurses Society, who make a difference every day by supporting our Standards of Practice to ensure that our patients receive the best possible care.

Lisa Gorski

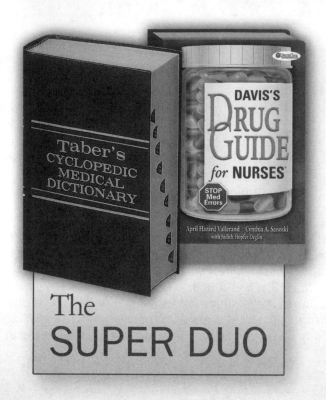
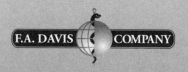

PREFACE

Manual of I.V. Therapeutics: Evidence-Based Practice for Infusion Therapy, Sixth Edition, provides comprehensive information on infusion therapy for the nursing student and practicing nurse. Continuing with this edition is the focus on evidence-based practice (EBP), defined as the conscientious use of current best evidence in making decisions about patient care. Evidence-based practice includes research evidence in the form of systematic reviews and clinical practice guidelines to a clinician's knowledge, judgment, and experience and de-emphasizes practice based on tradition and ritual. EBP is important to any nurse performing infusion therapy because of the rapidly expanding dimensions of the nurse's role, the ongoing introduction of new infusion devices and techniques, and the evolving research supporting the importance of nursing interventions in improving patient safety and reducing the risk of infusion-related complications. The sixth edition continues to address pediatric and the older adult patients in a separate section in each chapter. This textbook incorporates the 2011 Infusion Nurses Society Standards of Practice and the 2011 Centers of Disease Control and Prevention (CDC) guidelines for prevention of intravascular catheter-related infections.

This self-paced, comprehensive text presents information ranging from a simple to a complex format, incorporating theory into clinical application. The skills of recall, nursing process, critical thinking, and patient education are covered, along with detailed summaries, providing the foundation one needs to become a knowledgeable practitioner. The psychomotor skills associated with infusion therapy are presented in step-by-step procedures with rationales based on standards of practice at the end of the chapters.

Each chapter includes accompanying objectives, defined glossary terms that are bolded within the text, a post-test, a summary of chapter highlights, and a critical thinking case study. Icons and special boxes are used throughout each chapter to key the reader to websites, patient education, home care issues, cultural considerations, and standards of practice. Skill Checks, 100 test questions, PowerPoint presentations, and math calculations tests are included in the Davis*Plus* faculty ancillaries and can be used in the educational setting, as well as in agencies, for validating competencies of nurses in infusion skills. **The icons used in this sixth edition are as follows:**

NOTE > Identifies key points of theory content

⬤▷ **Identifies Nursing Fast Facts,** which are set in italics and shaded within the chapter for important nursing practice information

EBP **Identifies relevant studies in Evidence-Based Practice (EBP)**

⊕ **Identifies Websites**

⊠ **Identifies Nursing Points of Care**

▣ **Identifies Home Care Issues**

● **Identifies Patient Education information**

◉ **Identifies a media link,** which refers to Davis*Plus*, and is located in the critical thinking case study and post-test sections at the end of each chapter

INS Standard **Identifies Infusion Nurses Society (INS), Standards of Practice**

The sixth edition of this textbook is organized from foundations of practice followed by basic practices for all nurses and concludes with specialty infusion practices. The first three foundations chapters are designed to provide information to the reader on nursing practice related to infusion therapy (nursing process applied to infusion therapy, legal and ethical responsibilities, evidence-based practice background, and performance improvement), infection prevention and occupational hazards, and fundamentals of fluid and electrolyte balance.

The subsequent seven chapters provide the essential solid foundation in infusion therapy practices, including parenteral solutions, infusion equipment, peripheral and central vascular access techniques and management, complications, medication infusion, and infusion calculations. This sixth edition has incorporated recurring displays for cultural and ethnic-related issues. Key concepts for nursing practice are identified as "**Nursing Fast Facts**," and "**Note>**" identifies an important theory concept.

The last two chapters encompass the additional topics of transfusion therapy and parenteral nutrition. The Davis*Plus* website contains questions based on standards of practice and follows the guidelines of the INS Core Curriculum for certification. It includes guidelines for discussion and answers to the case studies, and additional math calculations problems and answers. It also provides the learner with web-based ancillaries, an additional 50 interactive flash cards for learning terminology, interactive case studies, and web links for further research.

We hope this new edition provides you, whether you are a practicing healthcare professional or a student, with valuable insights into the safe practice of infusion therapy and a reference for this rapidly advancing field.

Lynn Phillips and Lisa Gorski

CONSULTANTS

Michelle Gricar, MS, RN, RMA
Clinical Nurse Specialist–Wheaton
   Franciscan Healthcare St. Francis
Milwaukee, Wisconsin

Mark Hunter, RN, CRNI®
Senior Product Manager
Peripheral Vascular Access
CareFusion
Vernon Hills, Illinois

Elizabeth Krzywda, MSN, APNP, NP-C
Nurse Practitioner–Medical College of
  Wisconsin
Milwaukee, Wisconsin

Mary McGoldrick, MS, RN, CRNI®
Home Care and Hospice Consultant–
   Home Health Systems, Inc.
Saint Simons Island, Georgia

Heather Moore, RN, BSN
Manager, Maternal/Child Program
   Wheaton Franciscan Home Health
   & Hospice
Milwaukee, Wisconsin

Deb Richardson, RN, MS, CNS
Owner/President–Deb Richardson &
   Associates
Houston, Texas

REVIEWERS

Sharon L. Bateson, MSN, RN, B-C
Professor of Nursing
Sierra College
Rocklin, California

Laura L. Benton, RN, MSN, Ed
Faculty, Nursing Skills Lab Manager
Hondros College Nursing Programs
Fairborn, Ohio

Faith Chennette,
   MSN, OCN, CNE, CPHN, RN-BC
Nursing Faculty
College of Western Idaho
Nampa, Idaho

Susan M. Hampson,
   MS, RN, APN, FNP-BC, CNE
Assistant Professor
School of Nursing
Saint Xavier University
Chicago, Illinois

Diane Madsen, BSN, MA, PhD, RN
Nursing Faculty
Pueblo Community College–Fremont
   Campus
Canon City, Colorado

Judy Mahan, RN, MS
Director, Allied Health
Feather River College
Quincy, California

Rox Ann Sparks,
   RN, MSN, MICN, LNC
Professor, Assistant Director
   Vocational Nursing
Merced College
Merced, California

ACKNOWLEDGMENTS

The authors would like to acknowledge the following:
The nurses in the specialty practice of infusion therapy

At F. A. Davis:

Tom Ciavarella, Nursing Acquisitions Editor, who assisted in the final development of this manual.

Echo Gerhart, Project Editor, Nursing, who as project consultant helped bring this vision to reality.

Sam Rondinelli, Production Manager, for guiding this manuscript through the production process.

Robert G. Martone, Publisher, Nursing, whose foresight brought the project to F. A. Davis.

And....

Cassie Carey, Senior Production Editor at Graphic World Inc

Appreciation is also expressed to the following companies who provided product information, pictures, and illustrations:

3M Medical Division, St. Paul, MN
AngioDynamics, Marlborough, MA
Baxter Healthcare Corporation, Round Lake, IL
B. Braun Medical Inc., Bethlehem, PA
BD Medical, Sandy, UT
CareFusion, San Diego, CA
Catheter Connections, Salt Lake City, UT
Cenorin, Kent, WA
Centurion, Williamston, MI
Cook Medical, Bloomington, IN
C. R. Bard Inc., Salt Lake City, UT
Infusion Nurses Society, Norwood, MA
Interrad Medical, Plymouth, MN
I.V. House, Inc., Chesterfield, MO
Ivera Medical Corporation, San Diego, CA
J&J Wound Management, Division of Ethicon, Inc., Somerville, NJ
Lippincott Williams & Wilkins, Philadelphia, PA
MediVisuals, Inc., Dallas, TX
Moog Medical Devices Corp., Salt Lake City, UT
Norfolk Medical Products, Inc., Skokie, IL
Pall Medical, Port Washington, NY
RGB Medical Imagery, Delaware, OH

Smiths-Medical Critical Care, Inc., Carlsbad, CA
Tangent Medical, Ann Arbor, MI
TransLite LLC, Sugar Land, TX
Vidacare, San Antonio, TX
VueTek Scientific, Gray, ME

TABLES

CONTENTS IN BRIEF

CONTENTS

Chapter **1**

Professional Practice Concepts for Infusion Therapy

In dwelling upon the vital importance of sound observation, it must never be lost sight of what observation is for. It is not for the sake of piling up miscellaneous information or curious facts, but for the sake of saving life and increasing health and comfort.
—Florence Nightingale, 1873

Chapter Contents

1

■ LEARNING OBJECTIVES

On completion of this chapter, the reader will be able to:

1. Define the terminology related to infusion-related professional practice.
2. Identify the elements of infusion nurse competency.
3. Discuss the use of competency-based education programs in the practice of infusion therapy.
4. Discuss the value of nursing certification.
5. Discuss evidence-based practice.
6. Identify five steps used in developing an evidence-based protocol.
7. Identify the components of the nursing process and how they are applied to infusion practice.
8. Apply quality management strategies to infusion practice.
9. Identify risk management and risk assessment strategies.
10. Differentiate between standards of care and standards of practice.
11. Identify the sources of laws.
12. Identify the areas of breach of duty for the specialty of infusion nursing.
13. Identify the role of the nurse as an expert witness.
14. Identify the principles used in ethical decision making.

⌇ GLOSSARY

Assessment   The systematic and continuous collection, organization, validation, and documentation of data; the first step of the nursing process

Barcoding system   System that encodes data electronically into a series of bars and spaces, which is scanned by lasers into a computer to identify the object being labeled

Benchmarking Process of measuring and comparing the results of processes with those of the best performers

Civil law Laws that affect the legal rights of private persons or corporations

Competency Includes aspects of performance such as skills, knowledge, ability, and judgment

Criminal law Offense against the general public; affects welfare of society as a whole

Data collection Gathering information through interviewing, observing, and inspecting

Documentation A recording, in written or electronic form, containing original, official, or legal information

Evaluation Measuring the degree to which goals/outcomes have been achieved and identifying factors that positively or negatively influence goal achievement

Evidence-based practice (EBP) Conscientious use of current best evidence (e.g., research) in making decisions about patient care; it deemphasizes practice based on tradition and ritual.

Expert testimony Witness from the same professional specialty who examines evidence, reviews pertinent nursing literature, gives depositions, and potentially testifies in court. An expert nurse gives advice and consultation throughout the litigation process.

Goal Broad statement of a desired outcome

Implementation Carrying out planned nursing interventions; the fifth step of the nursing process

Liable Legally responsible for damages, answerable

Malpractice Negligent conduct of a professional person

Negligence Not acting in a reasonable or prudent manner

Nursing diagnosis A clinical judgment about actual or potential individual, family, or community experiences/responses to health problems; identification of nursing diagnoses is the second step of the nursing process

Nursing standard Specific statement about the quality of a facet of nursing care

Outcome Result of the performance (or nonperformance) of a function or process(es)

Performance improvement (PI) Continuous study and adaptation of functions and processes of a health-care organization to increase the probability of achieving desired outcomes and to better meet the needs of patients and other users of services

Planning Determining how to prevent, reduce, or resolve identified patient problems; how to support client strengths; and how to implement nursing interventions in an organized, individualized, and goal-directed manner; the fourth step of the nursing process

Process   A goal-directed, interrelated series of actions, events, mechanisms, or steps

Quality assessment (QA)   Process including data collection and data analysis in evaluating a problem

Quality improvement (QI)   Builds on the data identified in quality assessment to identify action steps including monitoring, evaluating, and problem solving.

Quality management (QM)   An organizational culture committed to achieving excellence

Risk management   Process that centers on identification, analysis, treatment, and evaluation of real and potential hazards

Standard of care   Focuses on the recipient of care consistent with minimum safe professional conduct and describes outcomes of care that patients can expect to receive

Standards of nursing practice   Focuses on the provider and defines competent care along with the activities and behavior needed to achieve positive patient outcomes

Statutes   Written laws enacted by the legislature

Structure   Standard that refers to conditions and mechanisms that provide support for the delivery of care (e.g., policy and resources)

Tort   Private wrong, by act or omission, that can result in a civil action by the harmed person

Total quality management (TQM)   Management system fostering continuously improving performance at every level of every function by focusing on maximization of customer satisfaction; focuses on process

■ Introduction

Infusion nursing is a recognized nursing specialty. Infusion nursing includes placement of an access device such as peripheral I.V. catheter, administration of a wide variety of infusion solutions and medications, interventions aimed at prevention of complications, and assessment and monitoring for patient response. The intravenous (I.V.) route is the most commonly used infusion route; however, other infusion routes include intraosseous, subcutaneous, and intraspinal. Non-I.V. infusions may be appropriate for administration in certain situations and with selected fluids and medications. The practice of infusion nursing encompasses nursing management and coordination of care (Corrigan, 2010) to the patient in accordance with:

1. State statutes
2. Infusion Nurses Society (INS) Standards of Practice

3. Established institutional policy
4. Accreditation requirements

Infusion therapy is administered in all health-care settings, including hospitals, long-term care facilities, outpatient settings, physician offices, and patients' homes. Most nurses at some point of, or throughout, their career will be involved in infusion care. The patient populations served by this specialty practice range from neonates to elderly patients. Because vascular access device (VAD) care and infusion administration have become such common areas of nursing practice, nurses may consider these practices very routine. However, there are risks, and some complications are serious and life threatening. Regardless of the setting, the nurse must have a thorough understanding and knowledge of the appropriate type of access device being utilized, the appropriateness of the selected device for the prescribed therapy, care and maintenance of the device, potential complications related to the device and infusion solutions, and safe infusion administration.

▪ Delivery of Quality Care

Clinical Competency

Competency Standards

The American Nurses Association (ANA, 2010a) asserts that the public has a right to expect the registered nurse to demonstrate professional competence. In their recommendations about the future of nursing, the Institute of Medicine (2011) states that nurses must be engaged in lifelong learning to gain the competencies needed to provide care for diverse populations across their patients' life spans. The ANA Standards of Professional Nursing Practice (2010a, p. 49) include the Standard of Education, which states that the registered nurse attain knowledge and competence reflective of current nursing practice.

Competence and **competency** are two frequently used terms that sound similar and may be used interchangeably; however, they do have different meanings. Nursing competence refers to the *potential* ability to perform at an expected level of practice, whereas competency focuses on *actual* performance. Competence is required before one can expect competency (National Board for Certification of Hospice and Palliative Nurses, 2011). Competency integrates the following aspects of performance related to patient care:

1. Skills: Psychomotor, communication, interpersonal, diagnostic
2. Knowledge: Examples include thinking, understanding, professional standards of practice, insights from personal experience

3. Ability: Capacity to act effectively
4. Judgment: Critical thinking, problem solving, ethical reasoning, decision making (ANA, 2010a, pp. 12-13)

Health-care organizations identify and measure competence, based on the needs of the organization (INS, 2011). Competency may be reviewed through information obtained from past and current employers, peer recommendations, validating specialty certifications, testing, ongoing performance data collection, and/or skills observation, either separately on in partnership with customers. Competency validation should occur on orientation to the organization, on an ongoing basis, with changes in scope of practice, and when new equipment, new technology, or a new practice is introduced (INS, 2011, p. S11). The need to validate competency may be identified through clinical outcome data (e.g., increase in infection rates), occurrence or sentinel event reports, implementation of new equipment or technology, evaluation of patient satisfaction (e.g., problems with peripheral I.V. placement), or changes in patient populations. When the health-care organization chooses to measure or validate specific competencies, it should do so in a thorough and ongoing fashion, including looking at new, significant, and/or high-risk practices, interventions, or activities that are unfamiliar to staff members.

Competence is assessed using different methods, yet there is no single tool or method that "guarantees" competence (ANA, 2010a). A variety of methods are used, including written tests and direct observation of a skill, whether in the work setting, in a skills laboratory, or through use of simulation. Observing performance of a skill in the work environment is the preferred method for evaluating invasive infusion therapy skills (INS, 2011, p. S11) (Table 1-1). Competence assessment requires a checklist that includes objective, measureable assessment of the actual performance,

> Table 1-1	ASSESSING COMPETENCY

Acceptable Methods of Assessing Competency

- Direct observation by a supervisor, designated evaluator, instructor, or preceptor while the employee/student demonstrates the skill in the work setting
- Observation by a supervisor, designated evaluator, instructor, or preceptor while the employee/student demonstrates the skills in simulated settings, such as skill laboratories and mock drills
- Direct observation and return demonstration may be supplemented with other forms of assessment, such as tests. The testing should not be the primary means of assessment.

Documentation of Competency

Competency assessments should be documented.
- Competency checklist
- Department job/specific competency

such as specific criteria or critical behaviors, and the criteria for achieving success in the performance.

Competency-Based Educational Programs

Competency-based educational programs establish specific **goals,** accountability, individualization, and behaviors for practitioners by defining clear expectations for levels of performance. The health-care organization has the responsibility of ensuring a competent staff. A framework for developing staff competencies and ensuring that the institution is delivering safe care includes:

- Development of standards
- Development of criteria for performance of skills
- Assessment of learning needs
- Establishment of a plan of educational programs
- Presentation of educational programs
- Evaluation of learning outcomes

Three-Part Competency Model

A three-part competency model includes:

1. Competency statement: Statement that reflects a measurable goal
2. Domains of learning criteria: Cognitive criteria (knowledge base) and performance criteria (psychomotor skills: observed behaviors)
3. Evaluation and learning outcomes: Written tests, return demonstrations, and clinical demonstration of skill to nurse preceptor

All professional nurses are accountable and responsible for all parts of the tasks associated with infusion therapy and for tasks that are delegated to the licensed practical nurse or technician for care rendered to the patient while under care. The three-part competency model is an effective tool for ensuring competent practice.

INS Standard The nurse shall be competent in the safe delivery of infusion therapy within his/her scope of practice and shall be responsible and accountable for attaining and maintaining competence with infusion therapy within her or his scope of practice (INS, 2011, p. S11).

Clinical Competency Validation Program

The INS provides a clinical competency validation program for infusion therapy; the latest version was published in 2012. The Clinical Competency Validation Program (CCVP) is a helpful tool for organizations to use when validating infusion-related nursing skills. There are 33 specific nursing competencies in the program, which can be used for procedural validation skills.

Value of Certification

Professional nursing certification programs have long established their value and importance to health-care organizations and to patients and their families. The American Board of Nursing Specialties (ABNS) was formed in 1991 with a mission to "promote the value of specialty nursing certification to all stake holders" (ABNS, 2006). Certification, as defined by the ABNS (2006), is the formal recognition of specialized knowledge, skills, and experience demonstrated by achievement of standards identified by a nursing specialty to promote optimal health outcomes.

Basic nursing licensure indicates a minimal professional practice standard. Certification is a mark of excellence, validates nursing knowledge and skills, and protects the public (Altman, 2011). There is a growing body of evidence supporting the impact of nursing certification on nursing knowledge, value to the organization, and patient outcomes (INS/Infusion Nursing Certification Corporation, 2009). The INS provides certification specific to infusion therapy with the designation of CRNI® (certified registered nurse, infusion). Other certifications that include components of infusion therapy are as follows:

1. Oncology Nursing Certification Corporation (OCN®): www.oncc.org
2. Pediatric Nursing Certification Board (CPN®): www.pncb.org
3. American Society for Parenteral and Enteral Nutrition (CNSC): www.nutritioncare.org
4. Association for Vascular Access (VA-BC): www.avainfo.org

Increasingly, health-care organizations are placing a high value on nursing certification. Based on initiatives for certification from across the country, the American Association of Critical Care Nurses identified five themes of best practices in creating a culture for nursing certification: commitment to excellence, a supportive and encouraging environment, goal-directed evaluations, availability of educational resources, and celebrations for rewarding excellence (Fleischman, Meyer, & Watson, 2011).

Evidence-Based Practice

Evidence-based practice (EBP) is an essential characteristic of an effective health-care system. It is expected that the nurse utilize evidence-based interventions and treatments (ANA, 2010a).

The ANA (2010a, p. 65) defines EBP as a scholarly and systematic problem-solving paradigm that results in the delivery of high-quality health care. A classic definition of EBP is the conscientious use of current best evidence in making decisions about patient care (Sackett et al., 2000).

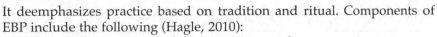

It deemphasizes practice based on tradition and ritual. Components of EBP include the following (Hagle, 2010):

- Evidence from research/evidence-based theories, and opinion leaders/expert panels
- Evidence from assessment of the patient's history and physical examination, and availability of health-care resources
- Clinical expertise
- Information about patient preferences and values

Consider the following simple example of EBP implementation: *You are a home care nurse who has been caring for a patient for several years. He has an implanted port that you access for a monthly infusion. You have used povidone iodine (Betadine) for skin antisepsis prior to port access. This patient has never had a catheter-related infection. There is now strong evidence that chlorhexidine/alcohol solution is a superior agent and is preferred for skin antisepsis; you also know that povidone iodine is still considered an acceptable agent. This patient does not want to switch antiseptic agents because he has never had a problem. You understand the research supporting the use of chlorhexidine, but you also use your clinical judgment based on the patient's history and take into account your patient's preferences, and you do not change his protocol.*

EBP is important to the infusion nurse because of the rapidly expanding dimensions of the nurse's role, the ongoing introduction of new infusion products and technology, and the growing base of research addressing complication prevention. Each time a new device or technique is introduced, new practices must be considered. Questions must be asked when new technology is introduced, such as:

- Are there studies supporting the benefits of the technology?
- In what health-care settings has the technology been evaluated?

Between the ongoing safety initiatives being introduced into health-care settings and the increasing presence of practice guidelines, it is imperative that the infusion nurse use evidence to support infusion practice. The 2011 INS Standards for Infusion Nursing were developed as an evidence-based document. There are 68 Standards, which are broad statements that describe expectations of practice applicable to infusion therapy in all settings. The Standards address areas such as the need for organizational policies and nurse competency. The Practice Criteria provide specific guidance on the implementation of each Standard. New to the 2011 document, each Practice Criterion is rated as reflecting the strength of the body of evidence. Although evidence that is research based is preferred, evidence may come from a variety of sources (Table 1-2).

The following is an example of a Standard and a Practice Criterion from *Standard 35: Vascular access site preparation and placement.*

Standard: The nurse shall prepare the intended VAD insertion site with antiseptic solution using aseptic technique.

> Table 1-2   SOURCES OF EVIDENCE

Published research
Published research utilization report
Published quality improvement report
Published meta-analysis
Published systematic or integrative literature review
Published review of the literature
Policies, procedures, protocols
Published guidelines
Practice exemplars, stories, opinions
General or background information/texts/reports
Unpublished research, reviews, poster presentations, similar materials
Conference proceedings, abstracts, presentations

Practice Criterion: Chlorhexidine solutions is preferred for skin antisepsis. One percent to two percent tincture of iodine, iodophor, and 70% alcohol may also be used. Chlorhexidine is not recommended for infants under 2 months of age.

This Practice Criterion is rated as Level I evidence. According to the INS table of the Strength of the Body of Evidence, this is the highest level of evidence, based on meta-analysis, systematic literature review, guideline based on randomized controlled trials (RCTs), or at least three well-designed RCTs.

Using the 2011 INS Standards to develop changes in procedure or policy is one way to apply EBP to infusion practice. As with many areas of nursing practice, there are unanswered questions, there often is limited research, and there is a constant influx of newly published studies to read and review. Although nurses may apply EBP through application of evidence-based guidelines, policies, or protocols, nurses also may be actively involved in EBP when the answers are not so easily found. Numerous evidence-based models are available; however, all share certain steps as follows:

1. Select a topic or ask the question.
2. Search and critique the evidence.
3. Adapt the evidence for use in a specific practice environment.
4. Implement the EBP.
5. Evaluate the effect on patient care processes and outcomes (Titler, 2007).

There are a variety of scales used to rate the evidence. Table 1-3 lists the rating scale used by the Centers for Disease Control and Prevention (CDC, 2011) in their guidelines addressing infection prevention related to intravascular devices, as well as excerpts from the INS (2011) rating scale. Of note, INS does not rate the strength of the recommendation; rather, it only rates the strength of the evidence used to support each Practice Criterion.

> Table 1-3	TWO EXAMPLES OF EVIDENCE RATING SCALES

From the Guidelines for the Prevention of Intravascular Catheter-Related Infections, 2011 (CDC, 2011)

Category IA: Strongly recommended for implementation and strongly supported by well-designed experimental, clinical, or epidemiological studies.
Category IB: Strongly recommended for implementation and supported by some experimental, clinical, or epidemiological studies and a strong theoretical rationale; or an accepted practice (e.g., aseptic technique) supported by limited evidence.
Category IC: Required by state or federal regulations, rules, or standards.
Category II: Suggested for implementation and supported by suggestive clinical or epidemiological studies or a theoretical rationale.
Unresolved issue: Represents an unresolved issue for which evidence is insufficient or no consensus regarding efficacy exists.

Excerpts from the Strength of the Body of Evidence Rating in the INS Standards of Infusion Nursing (INS, 2011)

Level 1: Evidence description: Meta-analysis, systematic literature review, guideline based on randomized controlled trials (RCTs), or at least three well-designed RCTs
Level I A/P: Includes evidence from anatomy, physiology, and pathophysiology as understood at the time of the writing
Level III: One well-designed RCT, several well-designed clinical trials without randomization, or several studies from quasi-experimental designs focused on the same question; includes two or more well-designed laboratory studies
Level V: Clinical article, clinical/professional book, consensus report, case report, guideline based on consensus, descriptive study, well-designed QI project, theoretical basis, recommendations by accrediting bodies and professional organizations, or manufacturer recommendations for products or services

Infusion Nurses Society (2011). Reprinted with permission.

 ## Websites

Center for Evidence-Based Nursing: www.york.ac.uk.healthsciences/centres/evidence/celon.htm
Agency for Healthcare Research and Quality: www.ahrq.gov/downloads/pub/advances/vol2
Additional websites on web-based Ancillary—Student/General

NOTE > Throughout this textbook, examples of evidence are noted in EBP Boxes threaded within the chapters in italic type.

Nursing Process Related to Infusion Therapy

The six steps of the nursing process are identified as the Standards of Professional Practice by the ANA (2010a). These Standards provide each nurse with a framework to utilize when working with a patient. For the patient who receives infusion therapy, the process begins with good basic assessment skills and continues until the patient no longer requires a VAD or infusions to meet health-care maintenance. The INS supports the ANA Standards and publishes its own specialty standards of practice approximately every 5 years. Relevant INS Standards will be highlighted throughout this text.

Assessment

According to ANA Standards of Practice (2010a), **assessment** consists of the comprehensive collection of data, including and addressing physiological, functional, emotional, cognitive, sexual, cultural, age-related, environmental, spiritual, and economic issues. Assessment includes both subjective and objective information. The following are examples of areas to assess in relation to infusion therapy:

Subjective

- Patient's related fears of infusion therapy
- Patient's experiences with prior infusion therapy
- Patient's needs and stated preferences for venipuncture site, if applicable
- Patient's best learning method, health literacy, language barriers, and readiness to learn

Objective

- Review of patient's past and present medical histories
- Physical assessment
- Review of laboratory data and radiographic studies
- Assessment of level of growth and development for neonate and pediatric clients
- Potential factors affecting readiness to learn, such as weakness, fatigue, anxiety, and/or functional limitations
- Factors that guide decision making in placing the most appropriate VAD for the patient: characteristics of the prescribed infusate, anticipated duration of therapy, physical assessment, health history, support systems and resources, patient preference
- Peripheral vein assessment and selection based on age, vein condition, activity level, and needs

Diagnosis

The **nursing diagnosis** is used to describe and label patient problems based on the assessment data. Defined by NANDA International (NANDA-I, n.d.), a nursing diagnosis is a clinical judgment about actual or potential individual, family, or community experiences/responses to health problems/life processes. The nursing diagnosis provides the basis for selecting nursing interventions to achieve outcomes for which the nurse has accountability. Nursing diagnoses are validated with the patient, family, and other health-care providers.

The ANA recognizes 12 terminology sets that support nursing practice. The following examples of terminologies include nursing diagnoses, interventions, and/or outcomes:

- NANDA-I Nursing diagnoses: www.nanda.org
- Nursing Interventions Classification (NIC): www.nursing.uiowa.edu/excellence/nursing_knowledge/clinical_effectiveness/index.htm
- Nursing Outcomes Classification (NOC): Same as above
- Omaha System: www.omahasystem.org
- Clinical Care Classification System (CCC): www.sabacare.com
- Perioperative Nursing Data Set: www.aorn.org

Use of a standard terminology or language in the electronic health record (EHR) allows for clear communication among members of the health-care team and for data collection that can be used in quality improvement. Standardized terminology is also critical in increasing visibility of nursing interventions and greater adherence to the standards of practice. In this textbook, nursing diagnoses developed by NANDA-I will be used. Nursing diagnoses related to infusion therapy are included in each chapter of this textbook. Some examples include:

1. Fluid volume deficit related to failure of regulatory mechanisms
2. Risk for infection related to compromised host defenses
3. Ineffective protection related to inadequate nutrition

Collaborative problems are physiological complications that nurses monitor to detect onset or changes in status. Nurses manage collaborative problems using physician-prescribed as well as nursing-prescribed interventions (Ackley & Ladwig, 2011).

Outcomes Identification

The third step in the nursing process is the identification of expected **outcomes** for a plan of care that is individualized to the patient (ANA, 2010a). It is important that time frames for attaining the outcomes be identified. It is also an essential step that the nurse collaborate with the patient, family, and other health-care providers (including the physician and other health-care disciplines) in developing expected outcomes. Patient values and ethical and cultural considerations should be incorporated into the process of identifying expected outcomes. Outcomes can be developed in one of two ways: by using the standardized terminology of the NOC list or by developing an appropriate outcome statement. General suggested outcome statements are provided in this textbook.

NOTE > In each of the subsequent chapters of this textbook, NOC is presented in a table with nursing diagnoses appropriate for the topic and along with NIC. A comprehensive list of NOC is listed in the book by Moorhead, Johnson, Maas, and Swanson (2013). All care plans must be individualized; the tables in the chapters are suggestions for use with the patient who receives infusion therapy.

Planning

Planning involves the prescription of strategies and alternative strategies to attain the identified expected outcomes (ANA, 2010a). Planning sets the stage for writing nursing actions by establishing the plan of care. Planning also includes development of strategies to attain the outcomes, validation of physician's or authorized prescriber's order(s), coordination and communication with the appropriate ancillary departments, and use of techniques to prevent complications.

Implementation of Interventions/Nursing Actions

Implementation is the "action plan" and the fifth step of the nursing process. The interventions are the concepts that link specific nursing activities and actions to expected outcomes. The nurse is expected to implement the plan in a safe and timely manner, utilize evidence-based interventions and treatments, coordinate the plan with all members of the health-care team, and use all appropriate resources (ANA, 2010a).

Nursing actions include both independent and collaborative activities. Independent activities are actions performed by the nurse, using his/her own discretionary judgment. Collaborative activities are actions that involve mutual decision making between two or more health-care practitioners. Implementation of infusion therapy includes administration of medications and solutions, care and maintenance of the VAD, and patient and family education. The care must be coordinated within and across all types of health-care settings for patients who transition to another setting (e.g., home care or long-term care). Specific examples of implementation of infusion therapy related nursing actions include:

1. Adherence to established infection prevention practices and maintenance of aseptic techniques
2. Preparation of infusate solutions with medication additives
3. Initiation of appropriate actions in the event of adverse reactions or complications

4. Provision of infusion therapy-related education that is culture and age appropriate
5. Documentation of all care delivered

NIC is a comprehensive, standardized classification of treatments that nurses perform. A comprehensive list of NIC interventions is provided in an NIC text by Bulecheck, Butcher, Dochterman & Wagner (2013).

NOTE > In each of the subsequent chapters of this textbook, NIC is presented in a table with nursing diagnoses appropriate for the topic along with NOC. All care plans must be individualized; therefore, the tables in the chapters present suggestions for direction of nursing actions related to the nursing diagnosis.

Evaluation

The **evaluation** phase of the nursing process is often the most ignored phase of the nursing process. Outcomes must be evaluated in relation to the structures and processes of the plan of care and the timelines for attainment (ANA, 2010a). The evaluation phase is the feedback and control part of the nursing process. Evaluation loops back to assessment, which was begun in the initial phase. As new data are collected, a nursing judgment must be made as to whether diagnoses, outcomes, the plan, and/or implementation need to be revised. Three judgments are possible:

1. The evaluation data indicate that the health-care problem has been resolved.
2. The plan of care should be revised.
3. The plan of care should be continued based on the conclusion that the outcome has not been met at this time.

Quality Management

Quality management is defined by an organizational culture committed to achieving excellence (Sierchio, 2010). It is not a single activity, and it does not occur only in the nursing department. An effective quality management program happens at all organizational levels. A quality management program seeks to improve the outcomes of care by focusing on processes and structures. There are a variety of quality models and approaches used in health care. "Quality assurance" is an old, outdated term that may still be used. Quality assurance focused mainly on documentation of certain aspects of care. For example, medical records could be reviewed to determine if there was documentation that the peripheral I.V. catheter site was assessed every 4 hours. Documentation is being assessed rather than patient care. The reality is that quality "cannot be assured, it can only be assessed, managed, or improved" (Sierchio, 2010, p. 28).

Quality Assessment/Quality Improvement

Quality assessment (QA) and **quality improvement** (QI) are components of a two-step process. QA includes data collection and data analysis. It may include a retrospective and/or a concurrent review of care and may include review of medical records as well as other data or observation of care. Outcomes of care and patient satisfaction are monitored. Consider the following example:

> On a hospital medical unit, the nurses identified what they believed were too many cases of phlebitis for their patients with peripheral I.V. catheters. Working with the QI director, the decision is made to collect data on the prevalence of phlebitis, to use a standardized tool in identifying phlebitis, and to define a time frame for data collection. Two certified infusion nurses on the unit both would evaluate the I.V. sites.

QI is the second step of the process. It builds on the data obtained in the QA process and identifies the action steps needed to improve the care. In the previous example, based on the literature, the prevalence of phlebitis on the medical unit was determined to be high. Potential causes of the high rate are discussed among the nursing team and the QI department, and plans to improve the rate are identified and implemented. To evaluate the effects of the changes, the QA process would be implemented again, using the same data collection strategy to assess whether changes in care lowered the phlebitis rate.

Performance Improvement

The term **performance improvement (PI)** was originally introduced by The Joint Commission (TJC) at the beginning of the millennium. It represents another shift in quality management philosophy. Although it has been acknowledged that quality is difficult to define, "performance" is more easily defined, described, and measured. Performance is described by what is done and how well it is done in providing health care. The accountability measures required by TJC are examples of PI measures. The measures include evidence-based processes that can be associated with positive patient outcomes. Care measured since 2002 by TJC (2012a) includes heart attack, heart failure, and pneumonia. Examples of other added PI measures include surgical care, venous thromboembolism, and stroke care. Hospitals that are accredited by TJC must select four measure sets for reporting. For example, the core measures for pneumonia that are measured and reported are:

- Pneumonia vaccine
- Blood cultures in the intensive care unit (ICU)
- Blood cultures in the emergency room

■ Antibiotics in the ICU
■ Antibiotics in the non-ICU

These measures are calculated individually for each evidence-based process as well as a composite measure reflected as adherence to all the measures collectively.

Total Quality Management

Total quality management (TQM) is an outgrowth of several health-care organizations that adopted a management system fostering continuous improvement at all levels and for all functions by focusing on maximizing customer satisfaction. This proactive approach emphasizes "doing the right thing" for customers.

Characteristics of what is done and how well it is done are called dimensions of performance.

Doing the right thing includes:

■ The *efficacy* of the procedure or treatment in relation to the client's condition
■ The *appropriateness* of a specific test, procedure, or service in meeting the client's need

Doing the right thing well includes:

■ The *availability* of a needed test, procedure, treatment, or service to the client who needs it
■ The *timeliness* with which a needed test, procedure, treatment, or service is provided to the client
■ The *effectiveness* with which tests, procedures, treatments, and services are provided
■ The *continuity* of the services provided to the client with respect to other services, practitioners, and providers over time
■ The *safety* of the client and others to whom the care and services are provided
■ The *efficiency* with which care and services are provided
■ The *respect and caring* with which care and services are provided

Examples of TQM models are six sigma and lean manufacturing. Six sigma focuses on eliminating variations so that there are no defects. An example cited by Sierchio (2010) is the use of a written standard for an insertion tray for peripherally inserted central catheter (PICC) placement, which reduces the risk for breaks in aseptic technique during the procedure. Lean manufacturing focuses on reduction of waste of supplies, for example, ensuring that all items on the PICC tray are used and not wasted.

Standards

Effective quality management is based on defined statements of quality (Sierchio, 2010). Standards are statements of quality that integrate technical features, behavioral aspects, and desired outcomes of health care.

Standards are developed by expert groups and represent acceptable levels of achievement.

Structure Standards

Structure standards consist of the conditions and mechanisms that provide support for the actual provision of care. Examples of organizational structure standards include mission, philosophy, and organizational goals. Another example is policies, which are not considered negotiable. An example of an infusion policy is that only nurses who have completed and demonstrated competence through attendance at a formal chemotherapy course are allowed to administer chemotherapy medications.

Process Standards

Process standards focus on the functions of what is actually done in giving and receiving care. Process is a goal-directed, interrelated series of actions, events, mechanisms, or steps. It includes a patient's activities in seeking care, **data collection**, and a practitioner's activities in making a nursing diagnosis, along with evaluation of actual performance of procedures. This link sets the standards by which evaluation can take place. Process standards include job descriptions, clinical procedures, practice guidelines, protocols, and clinical pathways.

Outcome Standards

Outcome standards are statements of the result of the performance (or nonperformance) of a function or process. Outcomes may be stated in negative terms, such as infection or mortality rates, but are more often stated in positive terms, such as pain control or prevented hospitalizations. Certain outcomes in health care are publicly reported as discussed below in a subsequent section.

Nursing-Sensitive Indicators

The National Database of Nursing Quality Indicators (NDNQI®) includes nursing-sensitive indicators that are reflective of the structure, process, and outcomes of nursing care. The impetus for health-care organizations to focus and report on nursing care and quality is increasing (NDNQI, 2012). Consider the following:

- The Centers for Medicare and Medicaid Services (CMS) as of 2010 require hospitals to report on whether or not they participate in a systematic clinical database regarding nursing-sensitive care.
- The American Nurses Credentialing Center (ANCC) Magnet Recognition Program requires data collection and benchmarking on nursing-sensitive measures.

Examples of structure indicators include staffing level, skills, and certification of nurses. Process indicators measure various aspects of care, including interventions and job satisfaction. Nursing-sensitive outcome measures for the acute care setting include pediatric I.V. infiltrations, patient fall rates, nosocomial infection rates, prevalence of pressure sores, physical restraint use, and patient satisfaction rates. These outcomes will improve based on quality and quantity of nursing care.

Standards as Domains of Organizational Structure

Quality of health care is also viewed in domains of structure. Sierchio (2010) identifies three domains: the organizational leadership, the health-care professional, and the patient/consumer of health care.

Standards of Care

The recipient of care, the patient, is the focus of standards of care. Standards of care can be voluntary, such as those promulgated by professional groups, or they may be mandated legislatively. TJC expects that an individual organization will develop standards of care that reflect the missions, values, and philosophy of that agency. **Standards of care** describe the results or outcomes of care and focus on the patient. An example of a **nursing standard** of care is: "The patient is free of infection related to infusion therapy" (Sierchio, 2010, p. 33).

Standards of Practice

Standards of practice focus on the provider of care and represent acceptable levels of practice in patient care delivery. Like the standards of care, practice standards address the clinical aspects of patient care services and imply patient outcomes. **Standards of nursing practice** define nursing accountability and provide a framework for evaluating professional competency. Standards of practice are consistent with research findings, national norms, and legal guidelines, and they complement the expectations of regulatory agencies. These standards reflect commitment to quality patient care and include generic and specialty standards of practice (Sierchio, 2010). A correlating standard of practice to the standard of care stated above is: "The peripheral insertion site is aseptically cleansed with antimicrobial solution before catheter insertion" (Sierchio, 2010, p. 33).

There are two types of nursing practice standards: internal and external. Internal standards are those developed within the profession of nursing for the purpose of establishing the minimum level of nursing care. These documents guide nursing care and can be used as a yardstick to measure the practice of individual nurses. An example of internal standards is the ANA (2012a) Standards of Nursing Practice.

The ANA Standards of Nursing Practice are universal to nursing practice in all settings. Specialty standards are applicable to specific areas of practice, such as the INS (2011) Standards of Practice.

External standards are guides for nursing developed by non-nurses, the government, or institutions. These standards describe the specific expectations of agencies or groups that utilize the services of nurses. Examples of external standards include nurse practice acts of each state, guidelines by TJC, and formal policies and procedures for individual agencies.

Staying Current with Standards of Care for Infusion Therapy

Whenever nurses administer infusion therapy, they must know and conform to acceptable nursing standards established by the facility, by the infusion specialty, and by state and federal guidelines. The following list presents guidelines for safeguarding practice:

- Collect assessment data before beginning infusion therapy.
- Apply knowledge of venous anatomy and physiology in selecting appropriate vein sites.
- Clarify unclear orders and refuse to follow orders you know are not within the scope of safe nursing practice.
- Identify adverse responses to medications and follow special precautions.
- Use infusion equipment appropriately.
- Administer the medications or infusions at the proper or prescribed rate and within the ordered intervals.
- Monitor the patient receiving an infusion for complications and implement interventions appropriate for those complications.
- Provide proper patient education.
- Document all aspects of infusion therapy, including patient teaching.
- Follow your institution's policies and procedures.
- Abide by your state's nurse practice act and national standards of I.V. practice, such as the INS Standards of Practice and guidelines for the CDC and the Occupational Safety and Health Administration.
- Use appropriate EBP in delivery of infusion therapy.

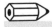 NURSING FAST FACT!

In relation to PI, hospitals accredited by TJC must select four sets of measures for reporting. The measures include heart attack, heart failure, pneumonia, surgical care, children's asthma, venous thromboembolism, stroke, perinatal care, and inpatient psychiatric care.

INS Standard The nurse shall participate in quality improvement activities that advance patient care, quality, and safety (INS, 2011, p. S12).

Additional Strategies in Quality Management

Benchmarking

Benchmarking is the process of measuring and comparing the results of processes with those of the best performers. For example, the NDNQI allows an individual hospital to benchmark nursing-sensitive indicators against those of other hospitals, down to the unit level. It is important to be able to compare outcomes or processes at the same level. For example, the patient fall rate is expected to be higher in a rehabilitation unit versus an ambulatory care unit. The goal of benchmarking is to identify the best practices so that an organization can improve its performance.

Problem-based benchmarking targets efforts toward improving specific concerns, such as lowering medication error rates or decreasing patient waiting times. More recently, facilities are turning to process-based benchmarking, which entails targeting continuous improvement of key processes.

Managers can benchmark to help decide a variety of factors, such as where to allocate resources more efficiently, when to seek outside assistance, how to quickly improve current operations, and whether customer requirements are being adequately met.

Benchmarking can be used in infusion therapy to validate infusion therapy teams. For example, the rate of I.V. infiltrations could be compared between hospitals that use an infusion therapy team and hospitals that do not.

National Patient Safety Goals

TJC has developed standards to guide critical activities performed by health-care organizations. Each year, TJC (2012b) identifies National Patient Safety Goals. The 2013 National Patient Safety Goals for hospitals include:
- Identify patients correctly.
- Use medicines safely.
- Prevent infection; this specifically includes infections related to central lines.
- Improve staff communication.
- Identify patient safety risks related to suicide.
- Prevent mistakes in surgery.

The 2013 National Patient Safety Goals for home care include:
- Identify patients correctly.
- Use medicines safely.
- Prevent infection.
- Prevent falls.
- Identify patient safety risks related to oxygen use in the home.

Publicly Reported Outcomes

A variety of health-care outcomes can be accessed by the public and may be used by health-care customers in choosing an organization. Organizations certified by CMS must provide data on outcomes. These data affect health-care reimbursement. The organizations with better outcomes will receive higher reimbursements, whereas those with poor performance will face financial penalties. The purpose of this data collection is to encourage organizations to improve quality. Examples of publicly reported hospital outcomes include timely treatment of certain conditions (e.g., heart failure), readmission rates, mortality rates, and patient satisfaction. Examples of publicly reported home care measures include hospitalization rates for home care patients, improvement in the symptom of dyspnea, improvement in pain, and patient satisfaction. Examples of publicly reported outcomes for long-term care facilities include health inspection results and deficiencies, and quality of care measures such as percentage of patients with pressure ulcers.

 ## Websites

Hospital Compare: www.hospitalcompare.hhs.gov
Home Health Care Compare: www.medicare.gov/homehealthcompare
Nursing Home Compare: www.medicare.gov/NursingHomeCompare

Patient Satisfaction Data

Patient satisfaction is now a publicly reported outcome for health-care organizations that has the potential to affect reimbursement, either positively or negatively, based on the results. The ability to compare or benchmark patient satisfaction data with data from other organizations can be helpful in improving quality. Specific questions must be asked during the patient satisfaction process. Organizations may also choose to perform other methods of patient data collection beyond standardized surveys, such as making follow-up phone calls after patient discharge or obtaining patient satisfaction information via a focus group or postcare interview.

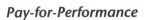

Pay-for-Performance

Pay-for-performance (P4P) sets differing payment levels for providers of care based on their performance on measures of quality and efficiency; in essence, P4P rewards better performance with better reimbursement. P4P has become a reality in part because of persistent deficiencies in quality in the U.S. health-care system. Value-Based Purchasing (VBP) is a CMS P4P program that was established by the Affordable Care Act. It is an approach to payment that is based on high-quality care. Beginning in October 2012, hospitals will be rewarded financially for both achievement and improvement in care. It will affect 1% of payments beginning in 2012 for all admissions and will increase to 2% in October 2017. Over time, VBP will affect other sectors of the health-care system beyond hospitals, such as home care.

▪ Risk Management and Risk Assessment

The INS (2011, p. S107) Standards of Practice define **risk management** as "a process that centers on identification, analysis, treatment, and evaluation of real and potential hazards." Risk assessment is the scientific process of collecting and analyzing scientific data "to describe the form, dimension, and characteristics of risk." Risk assessment and risk management are equally important but different processes, with disparate objectives, information content, and results.

Risk management concepts include the concerns that organizations face with exposure to losses. Organizations handle the chances of losses or risks by financing, purchasing insurance, or practicing loss control. Loss control consists of preventive and protective activities that are performed before, during, and after losses are incurred. Risk management involves all medical and facility staff. It provides for the review and analysis of risk and liability sources involving patients, visitors, staff, and facility property. Risk management consists of the following components:

- Identification and management of clinical areas of actual and high risk
- Identification and management of nonclinical (e.g., visitor, staff) areas of actual and high risk
- Identification and management of probable claims events
- Management of property loss occurrences
- Review and analysis of customer surveys and patient complaints
- Review and analysis of risk assessment surveys
- Operational linkages with hospital quality management, safety, and PI programs
- Provision of risk management education
- Compliance with state risk management and applicable federal statutes

Risk assessment is performed by government agencies such as the U.S. Environmental Protection Agency (EPA). Risk assessment takes different approaches depending on available information. Some assessments look back to evaluate effects after an event. They also may look ahead before a new product is approved for use.

An example of a risk assessment and management program from the U.S. Food and Drug Administration (FDA) is the Risk Evaluation and Mitigation Strategy (REMS) program. REMS is a strategy for managing the risks associated with certain high-risk drugs. The FDA can require a REMS:

- Before approval of the drug if the FDA determines a REMS is necessary to ensure the benefits of the drug outweigh the risks
- Postapproval if the FDA becomes aware of new safety information and determines that a REMS is necessary to ensure the benefits of the drug outweigh the risks

Nurses may be involved in REMS programs in the following ways:

- Possibly enrolling patients in specific REMS programs required for some high-risk drugs
- Assessing patients' understanding of the information they have been given, and providing and reinforcing patient education
- Explaining to patients why it is important to promptly report symptoms such as adverse reactions
- Assessing and monitoring patients for adverse events; in many cases, nurses have most of the primary contact with outpatients who are reporting symptoms
- Administering the drug in some cases

A listing of drugs that have a REMS in place can be found on the following website: www.fda.gov/Drugs/DrugSafety/PostmarketDrugSafety InformationforPatientsandProviders/ucm111350.htm#Current. There are a number of infusion drugs on the REMS list, including some monoclonal antibodies used in cancer care.

Risk management strategies combine the elements of both loss reduction and loss prevention. Risk management strategies that may decrease the risk of potential liability are as follows:

- Informed consent
- Analysis of unusual occurrence reports
- Root cause analysis (RCA) of sentinel events
- Documentation

Informed Consent

One of the most effective proactive strategies taken in risk management is informed consent (Alexander & Webster, 2010). Health-care professionals have a legal duty to provide a patient with ample information regarding the health treatment or procedure that will be performed and to obtain an informed consent before proceeding. The purpose of informed consent is to provide patients with the information they need to make a rational and knowledgeable decision regarding whether to undergo treatment. The focus is on the patient's understanding of the procedure and not just procurement of the patient's signed consent to undergo the procedure.

The right of self-determination provides the basis for informed consent and is grounded in the bioethical principles of autonomy. A competent adult (competence to consent) is aware of the consequences of a decision and has the ability to make reasonable choices about health care, including the right to refuse health care.

There are categories of necessary elements for informed consent and informed refusal. The first category comprises the information elements. This involves the disclosure of appropriate information. Generally, this disclosure must include benefits and risks of the procedure, alternative procedures, benefits and risks of the alternatives, and qualifications of the provider.

The second category consists of the consent elements. The consent must be voluntary, not coerced. Consent can be manifested by conduct. For example, the infusion specialist states, "I am going to restart your I.V. now," and the patient holds out his/her arm.

There may be limits to consent, such as waiver of consent. The patient must know that options and risks exist, even if he/she does not want to know what they are. Other limits to consent include verbal limits; for example, the patient may tell the infusion nurse, "Okay, I will let you try to restart my I.V., but only once."

Of note, although a minor child cannot grant consent, the concept of "assent," or agreement, to treatment is recommended for children age 7 years and older. Information regarding the treatment should be given to the child in a manner that considers the child's readiness for knowledge and developmental level (INS, 2011, p. S17).

The duty to obtain informed consent belongs to the person who will perform the procedure, but it also may belong to the licensed person who is aware that the patient has not been informed, does not understand, or did not consent (Table 1-4).

> **INS Standard:** The nurse shall confirm that the patient's informed consent was obtained for the defined procedure as identified in organizational policies, procedures, and/or practice guidelines and in accordance with local, state, and federal regulations. Consent shall be obtained by the health-care provider who will provide the procedure. The nurse shall advocate for the patient's or legally authorized representative's right to accept or refuse treatment (INS, 2011, p. S17).

> Table 1-4   **ELEMENTS OF INFORMED CONSENT**

Criteria

Patient must be mentally competent and capable of granting consent.
Patient must be of legal age, or the parent of a minor.
A legally designated health-care surrogate may act for the patient.
Patient must be able to understand the language.

Information Elements

Clear and sufficient information about the procedure
Information must include:
  Benefits and risks of the procedure
  Alternative procedures
  Benefits and risks of the alternatives
  Potential complications
  Risks of refusing the procedure
  Qualifications of the provider

Consent Elements

Consent form on chart or waiver of consent
Signature on an informed consent is a formality and not always required; typically used
  with special procedures such as central line placement

Adapted from Alexander & Webster, 2010; INS, 2011.

 NURSING FAST FACT!

Informed consents can become invalid if a change in the patient's medical status alters the risks and benefits of the treatment.

Unusual Occurrence Reports

Unusual occurrence reports, also called incident reports, are documented when there is a deviation in care. In fact, hospitals must track and analyze instances of patient harm as a condition of participation in the Medicare program; unusual occurrence reports are a common means for satisfying this requirement. In a 2010 report, 13.5% of hospitalized Medicare beneficiaries experienced an adverse event during their hospitalization that resulted in extra hospital days, life-sustaining intervention, or permanent disability, or resulted in death (U.S. Department of Health and Human Services [USDHHS], 2012). An additional 13.5% experienced temporary events that required treatment. In this report, failure to report events as incidents or occurrences was common. For example, symptomatic I.V. infiltration was reported only 20% of the time, and I.V. fluid overload was not reported at all.

Less is known about adverse events in other health-care settings. For example, a "line-related" problem (e.g., catheter occlusion, infection) was identified as one of eight categories of adverse events in a review of the home care literature (Masotti, McColl, & Green, 2010). The authors suggest that measurement of adverse events in home care should be considered a priority health-care issue.

Unusual occurrence reports are simple records of an event and are considered an internal and confidential reporting mechanism for QI. They should be reported to the superior staff member and the episode must be objectively charted, but reference to the report should not appear in the legal patient record.

The occurrence report should contain the following points:

1. Patient's admitting diagnosis
2. Date when the incident occurred
3. Patient's room number (hospitalized patient)
4. Age of the patient
5. Location of the incident
6. Type of incident
7. Nature of incident (e.g., medication error, mislabeling, misreading, policy and procedure not followed, overlooked order on chart, patient identification not checked). It should be noted (on the unusual occurrence report) if a physician's order was needed after the occurrence.
8. Factual description of the incident, including other people involved (witnesses)
9. Patient's condition before the incident
10. Results of the incident or injury
11. Actions taken (e.g., physician notification, interventions)

 NURSING FAST FACT!

> *Unusual occurrence reports are meant to be nonjudgmental, factual reports of the problem and its consequences.*

Patterns of unusual occurrences are monitored and analyzed for trends. Nursing staff members must feel free to file reports; a report is not an admission of **negligence.** These reports have the potential to save lives by identifying unsafe practices. More than ever before, risk may be managed by prevention.

INS Standard The nurse shall report and document unusual occurrences or sentinel events in practice as a result of infusion therapy according to organizational policies, procedures, and/or practice guidelines. The report should be shared with appropriate organizational levels and departments, such as risk management, nursing management, and quality improvement teams (INS, 2011, pp. S21-22).

Sentinel Events

TJC (2011) defines a sentinel event as an unexpected occurrence involving death or serious physical or psychological injury, or the risk thereof. Serious injury specifically includes loss of limb or function. Other outcomes of sentinel events might include unexpected, additional care. Sentinel events require *immediate* investigation and response. The RCA is an interdisciplinary approach that focuses on system issues, procedures, human resources, products/equipment, processes, and training gaps (INS, 2011). Through the RCA process, causes and event analysis and strategies for prevention are identified. It is important to recognize that not all sentinel events occur because of an error, and not all errors result in sentinel events. Information regarding sentinel event reporting to TJC is voluntary. The vast majority of events are reported from hospital settings; however, other accredited organizations also report sentinel events, including long-term care, home care, and ambulatory care facilities (TJC, 2012c). The most commonly reported sentinel event categories from 2012 are listed in Table 1-5.

Documentation

Documentation is an essential requirement for nurses across all health-care settings. Although documentation is often viewed as a burdensome process that detracts from patient care, it is a professional responsibility. Nursing documentation is used for a variety of purposes:

1. Communication within the health-care team: Includes assessments, medication records, orders and implementation, patient responses and outcomes, and plans of care to ensure that health-care team members make informed patient care decisions and provide quality care.

> Table 1-5	MOST FREQUENTLY REVIEWED SENTINEL EVENT CATEGORIES IN 2012
Unintended retention of a foreign body Delay in treatment Wrong patient, site, or procedure Suicide Operative/postoperative complications Patient fall Criminal event Medication error	

Source: The Joint Commission (2012).

2. Communication with other professionals not directly involved in patient care:
   - Credentialing of health-care practitioners within the organization
   - Legal matters: When a lawsuit is filed, the patient record becomes the major source of information about the care the patient received.
   - Regulation and legislation: Clinical documentation is used in evaluating and quantifying quality, such as the information seen in public reports of clinical outcomes.
   - Reimbursement: Documentation provides evidence of illness severity, service intensity, and outcomes of care on which reimbursement is based.
   - Research: Documentation may be used in research studies evaluating patient characteristics and outcomes of care.
   - Quality and PI: Documentation is the primary source of evidence for measuring performance outcomes, including nursing-sensitive measures such as data from the NDNQI (ANA, 2010b).

Use of the EHR instead of paper medical records to maintain health information is a national priority and a federal mandate and has made paper documentation a thing of the past. The advantages of an EHR include:
   - Availability of complete information about a patient's health, which allows better care and better coordination of care
   - A way to securely share information over the Internet with patients and their family caregivers (for those who opt for this convenience), which allows them to participate more fully in decisions about the patients' health care
   - Information to aid in diagnosing health problems sooner, reduce medical errors, and provide safer care at lower costs

 Website

The Office of the National Coordinator for Health Information Technology: http://healthit.hhs.gov/portal/server.pt/community/healthit_hhs_gov __home/1204

Documentation should be an accurate, timely, and complete account of the care rendered to the patient. The health-care record charts the patient's history, health status, and goal achievement. The record should be objective and completed promptly. Documentation should include only standard abbreviations according to the organization's policy and procedures. Nurses and other health-care providers should keep charts free of criticisms or complaints. There should be no vacant lines in charts, and every entry should be signed. In an office or home care environment, dates of return visit, canceled or failed appointments, all telephone conversations, and all follow-up instructions should be recorded on the chart.

Since the 1990s, the emphasis has been on QI, with a focus on evaluating organizational and clinical performance outcomes. Documentation is one way of evaluating outcomes. The many formats for charting include the problem-oriented medical record, pie charting, focus charting, narrative charting, and charting by exception. Regardless of the format developed for documenting infusion therapy, basic requirements of the plan of care exist, including goals, nursing diagnoses, and nursing interventions and outcomes. As discussed earlier in the chapter, use of standard nursing terminologies in the EHR allows for clear communication among the health-care team members and data collection that can be used in QI. Standardized terminology is also critical for increasing visibility of nursing interventions and greater adherence to the standards of practice.

The INS Standards of Practice (2011, p. S20) provides some specific recommendations related to infusion-related documentation. Documentation should include:

- Patient education
- Site preparation, infection prevention, safety precautions taken during insertion (e.g., standardized checklist to ensure all steps were followed)
- Type, length, and gauge of VAD
- Date and time of insertion, number and location of attempts, identification of site, type of dressing, identification of person inserting the device, use of visualization technology (e.g., ultrasound)
- For midline (ML) catheters and PICCs: External catheter length, midarm circumference, effective length of catheter inserted, radiographic confirmation of catheter tip location
- Confirmation of anatomic tip location (central vascular access devices [CVADs])
- Condition of site, dressing, site care/dressing changes
- Infusion drug/solution: Dose, rate, time, route, method of administration, VAD patency
- When multiple catheter devices or catheter lumens are being used, documentation should clearly indicate what fluids and medications are being infused through each pathway.
- Assessment of ongoing need for VAD
- Patient's symptoms, response to therapy, and/or laboratory test results

INS Standard Documentation shall be legible, accessible to qualified personnel, and readily retrievable. The protocol for documentation should be established in organizational policies and procedures
(INS, 2011, p. S20).

Infusion Medication Safety

There is a great potential for patient harm and death from errors related
to I.V. medications. The effects of medications given via the I.V. route are
immediate and systemic, and it is difficult to reverse the pharmacological effects after administration (American Society of Health-System
Pharmacists [ASHP], 2008a). Furthermore, many I.V. medications are
considered high-alert medications as identified by the Institute for Safe
Medication Practices (ISMP, 2012). High-risk medications are drugs that
bear a heightened risk of causing significant patient harm when they are
used in error. Some examples include chemotherapy medications, opioid
analgesics, insulin, and parenteral nutrition. Medication errors may not
occur more often with high-alert medications; however, the consequences of an error may be severe. Some measures that may be taken to
reduce risk include easy availability to drug information, limiting access
to high-alert medications, use of automated alerts, and standardizing the
ordering, storage, preparation, and administration of these products
(ISMP, 2012). A double-check of the high-risk medication prescription
prior to administration by two independent nurses is a common strategy
utilized by many organizations.

The use of "smart pumps" in administration of I.V. medications is
becoming the standard of care across all settings. Smart pumps incorporate technology that reduces the risk of errors during administration.
Some features include a drug library, clinical alert (i.e., prompts the
nurse to use a filter), dosing limit, and stop alert, which notifies the
nurse that a drug dosage is outside of the expected range. As with any
technology, errors can still occur. Nurses may bypass the drug library
and enter information manually or override alerts (ISMP, 2009). In a
published QI study, an assessment of practice found that nurses were
using the drug library only 37% of the time (Harding, 2012). Through
involvement of a QI team, interventions resulted in a doubling of drug
library use by the end of the study period. The use of smart pumps
is just a single, albeit important, component in infusion medication
administration safety.

Barcodes were implemented in 2004 as a response to the alarming
number of patient deaths resulting from medication errors uncovered by
the Institute of Medicine. A **barcoding system** encodes data electronically into a series of bars and spaces, which is scanned by lasers into
a computer to identify the object being labeled. Barcode medication

administration (BCMA) technology generates standard reports from recorded errors made, errors prevented, and reasons why nurses overrode warning messages. BCMA should be integrated into smart pump technology (Harding, 2012; ISMP, 2009). Use of BCMA is an additional important strategy in medication safety, but it is not failsafe. Computerized prescriber order entry (CPOE) is another medication safety strategy used in automating and standardizing medication orders.

Medication errors are possible at various times: during prescribing, storage, preparation, dispensing, administration, and monitoring. In 2008, a summit addressing prevention of harm from I.V. medications was convened and attended by the ASHP, TJC, INS, ISMP, and other organizations.

The following are some key recommendations in relation to prescribing and orders from both ASHP (2008a) and the INS Standards (2011):

1. Verify the completeness of the order. Orders should include:
   a. I.V. fluid type, volume, infusion rate
   b. I.V. medication dosage, route, frequency or time of administration, special considerations
   c. Use of standardized dosing protocols for emergency drugs and high-alert medications
2. Use verbal orders only when medically necessary.
3. Use a standardized "read-back" of the order when accepting a verbal or telephone order. Telephone orders are regularly taken by nurses who work at alternate sites (e.g., home care and long-term care facilities) because physicians are generally not available on site.
4. Accept only abbreviations approved by the organization.
5. Review the order for appropriateness of the prescribed therapy in relation to patient age, condition, type of VAD, dose, rate, and route of administration.

EBP In a systematic review of the literature related to BCMA and whether use of BCMA reduced medication administration errors, only six studies met the study criteria (Young, Slebodnik, & Sands, 2010). Although the researchers found limited evidence to evaluate BCMA effectiveness, they found additional medication error categories beyond the classic five rights of medication administration (right patient, right medication, right time, right dose, right route). These included omitted doses, wrong rate, doses administered without an order, extra doses given, expired dose, incorrect dilution, patient wristband not scanned or missing, allergies not documented, and incorrect dosage form.

Preparation and Verification of Parenteral Medications and Solutions

Intravenous drugs and solutions should be prepared in a pharmacy where standards for accuracy and sterility are best met. In some cases, and often in alternate sites, certain medications may need to be reconstituted by the nurse. Although the pharmacy in a hospital can mix the drug and transport it to the nursing unit, this is not always possible in the home care setting. This type of medication is referred to as an "immediate-use" compounded sterile preparation (CSP) by the United States Pharmacopeia (USP) Chapter <797> (ASHP, 2008b), which provides standards to ensure that CSPs are of high quality. Once mixed, administration of an immediate-use medication must start within 1 hour of preparation or the medication must be discarded (ASHP, 2008b). Clearly, it is important for all nurses to understand their role in medication preparation and to understand their organization's procedures. Staff education should focus on new medications used in all practice settings, high-alert medications, medication errors that have occurred both internally and externally, and protocols, policies, and procedures related to medication use.

> **INS Standard** The nurse should advocate for the use of engineering controls, protocols, and technologies that are intended and have been shown to reduce medication errors, including, but not limited to, electronic order entry, smart pumps with drug libraries, barcoding, procedures for distraction-free medication administration, establishment of protocols for high-risk intravenous drugs, and standardized drug concentrations or standard order sets (INS, 2011, p. S86).

 NURSING FAST FACT!

Always "read back" the order when accepting a verbal or telephone order.

Legal and Ethical Issues in Infusion Therapy

Sources of Law

In the United States, there are four primary sources of law: (1) constitutional law, (2) statutory law, (3) administrative law, and (4) common law. In addition, law can be divided into two main branches: private law and public law. Constitutional law is a formal set of rules and principles that describe the powers of a government and the rights of the people. Rights guaranteed in the Bill of Rights are consistent with the ethical principles of autonomy, confidentiality, respect for persons, and veracity. As participants in the health-care system, nurses cannot be forced to forfeit any constitutionally guaranteed rights.

Formal laws written and enacted by federal, state, or local legislatures are known as statutory or legislative laws. Only a minimal number of **statutes** dealing with malpractice existed before the malpractice crisis of the mid-1970s. Changes in Medicare and Medicaid laws, statutory recognition of nurses in advanced practice, and health-care reform legislation all are examples of statutory or legislative law.

Administrative law is a form of law set by administrative agencies, such as the FDA or CMS. State boards of nursing are another example of this type of legislative body. These boards are empowered to revoke or annul a nurse's license where there is evidence of incompetence, negligence, or fraud. The final source of law is common law, which is court-made law. The courts are responsible for interpreting the statutes. Most malpractice law is not addressed by statute but is established by the courts.

Legal Terms

Legal terms that nurses should become familiar with are *criminal law, civil law, tort, malpractice,* and the *rule of personal liability.* **Criminal law** relates to an offense against the general public caused by the potential harmful effect to society as a whole. A government authority prosecutes criminal actions, and punishment includes imprisonment, fine, or both. Violation of the Nurse Practice Act or the Medical Practice Act by an unlicensed person is considered a criminal offense.

Civil law or private law affects the legal rights of private persons and corporations. The branches of private law that are most applicable to nursing practice are contract law and tort law. Noncompliance with private law generally leads to a granting of monetary compensation to the injured party.

A private wrong, by act or omission, is referred to as a **tort.** Most tort law is founded in common law. Torts may be classified as intentional, quasi-intentional, or unintentional (Alexander & Webster, 2010). Intentional torts involve the purposeful invasion of a person's legal rights. Examples include assault, battery, false imprisonment, and restraints as a form of false imprisonment. The terms *assault* and *battery*, although usually used together, have different legal meanings. Both are intentional torts. Assault is defined as the unjustifiable attempt or threat to touch a person without consent that results in fear of immediately harmful or threatening contact. Touching need not actually occur. Battery is the unlawful, harmful, or unwarranted touching of another or the carrying out of threatened physical harm. Regardless of intent or outcome, touching without consent is considered battery. Even when the intention is beneficent and the outcome is positive, if the act is committed without permission, the nurse can be charged with battery. When dealing with a rational patient who refuses treatment, it is best to explain the treatment, verbally reassure the patient, and then notify the physician of refusal.

Quasi-intentional torts are civil wrongs that involve a person's reputation or peace of mind. They include slander (written statements that are false and malicious) and libel (spoken statements) (Alexander & Webster, 2010). Another example is breach of confidentiality, which may affect a person's peace of mind. Nurses have a legal duty and professional responsibility to ensure the right to privacy and confidentiality.

Negligence is an example of an unintentional tort, defined as "an inadvertent act or failure to act that results in injury or harm" (Alexander & Webster, 2010, p. 53).

Malpractice is a type or subset of negligence, committed by a person in a professional capacity. Above simple negligence, malpractice is the form of negligence in which any professional misconduct, unreasonable lack of professional skill, or nonadherence to the accepted standard of care causes injury to a patient.

There are four elements of a malpractice claim, all of which must be met to substantiate a claim:

1. It must be established that the nurse *had a duty to the patient*.
   - Simply put, the nurse is responsible in some way to the patient. For example, when a nurse is assigned to care for a specific patient, there is duty.
2. A *breach of care* or failure to carry out that duty must be proven.
   - Breach of duty may include an omission of care (e.g., failure to assess or provide an intervention) or a commission of care (e.g., administering an I.V. medication through a catheter despite patient complaints of pain). The nurse violates the duty of care by not adhering to an appropriate standard of care. Sources for the standard of care may include the state nurse practice act, organizational policies and procedures, published standards, and/or testimony of a nurse expert.
3. The patient must *suffer actual harm* or injury.
4. There must be *a causal relationship between the breach of duty and the injury suffered*.
   - The injury is a result of negligence on the part of the nurse. It must be proved that if the nurse had not been negligent, it is more likely than not that the patient would not have suffered harm (Reising, 2012).

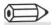 **NURSING FAST FACT!**

If an act of malpractice does not create harm, legal action cannot be initiated. Coercion of a rational adult patient to place an intravenous catheter constitutes assault and battery.

Legal Causes of Action Related to Nursing Practice

Malpractice suits against nurses have risen significantly over the past 10 years (Reising, 2012). In a review of the literature, Painter et al. (2011) assert that most malpractice cases involving nurses occur in hospital settings and involve nonspecialized nurses. More than 8000 closed claims involving registered or licensed practical nurses that resulted in a payment of greater than $10,000 were analyzed by a large professional liability insurance provider (CNA/NSO, 2009). Closed claims were defined as financial compensation sought and matter resolved through judgment, settlement, or verdict, with or without payment. Allegations of malpractice were divided into the categories of treatment and care (highest percentage), scope of practice, assessment, monitoring, medication administration, and patient rights. Of note, poor documentation was a contributing factor in many malpractice claims. Nurses must be aware at all times that failure to observe, failure to intervene, and verbal rather than written orders are potential risks for all nursing areas. Nurses must assess each patient and formulate a plan of care to meet the specific patient's needs.

Because of its invasive nature and risk for complications, infusion therapy is one area that carries a high risk for malpractice. When serious mistakes are made, patients can "lose limbs, their livelihoods or their lives" (Alexander, 2012, p. 75). For example, permanent nerve damage may occur when a peripheral I.V. catheter is placed in an inappropriate location or when an infiltration goes undetected, and the patient may die from a catheter-related bloodstream infection.

The rule of personal liability is "every person is **liable** for his own tortuous conduct" (his own wrongdoing). In years past, nurses were considered custodians who played a limited role in patient care and treatment, but today nurses are held responsible for using professional judgment (CNA/NSO, 2009). A physician cannot protect a nurse from an act of negligence by bypassing this rule with verbal assurance. Nurses are liable for their own wrongdoings in carrying out physicians' orders. This rule is relevant to nurses in the areas of medication errors and administration of I.V. fluids. Nurses have a legal and professional responsibility to be knowledgeable about administration of the I.V. fluids and medications, techniques for initiating and maintaining infusion devices, and identification of and interventions in the event of a complication.

When a nurse is named as a defendant in a malpractice suit, it is reported to the National Practitioner Data Bank (NPDB). This information clearinghouse, created in 1990 under Title V of Public Law 99-660, collects and releases all licensure actions taken against all health-care practitioners and health-care entities. The intent is to provide health-care quality, protect the public, and reduce health-care fraud and abuse (USDHHS, 2012). Information is submitted to the NPDB by medical mal-practice players, state boards of nursing, and hospitals. The NPDB reports are reviewed regularly by state boards of nursing and credentialing committees, allowing licensing bodies and employers to make informed decisions (Brooke, 2012). The NPDB identifies five distinct categories for registered nurses.

1. Nonspecialized RNs
2. Nurse anesthetists
3. Nurse midwives
4. Nurse practitioners
5. Clinical nurse specialists/advance practice nurses

The Infusion Nurse's Role as Expert Witness

The role of expert witness is relatively new to the nursing profession. The nurse acting as an expert witness strengthens the argument that nursing is an autonomous profession in that no other profession can appropriately judge the practice of nurses.

Expert testimony is required when the case is dependent on scientific and technical information that is more than common knowledge. Serving as an expert witness involves a complex and extensive process of examining evidence, reviewing pertinent nursing literature, giving depositions, and potentially testifying in court. An expert nurse gives advice and consultation throughout the litigation process. The nurse acting as an expert witness may testify either on behalf of the plaintiff, providing an opinion as to whether there was a deviation in the standard of care, or on behalf of the defendant, testifying that the actions represented reasonable nursing care. The role of the expert is *NOT* to establish standards of care; rather, the expert's role is to educate the judge and jury regarding the standards already established by the profession (Alexander & Webster, 2010). Extensive experience and certification, such as national I.V. certification, are important characteristics possessed by the nurse acting as an expert witness.

 NURSING FAST FACT!

Infusion nurses use multiple types of medical devices on a daily basis. Adherence to standards of practice, working within the scope of practice, and obtaining necessary competencies by the infusion nurse reduces the risk of being named in a malpractice suit.

Reducing the Risk for Malpractice

Maintain Clinical Competency

The nurse should understand the state's scope of practice and comply with organizational policies and procedures. It is important that the nurse not accept patient care assignments where competence has not been established, for example, accessing an implanted port without prior education. It is a nursing and professional responsibility to stay current in practice, to attend relevant educational classes and in-service programs, and to ensure that necessary competencies have been completed.

Assess and Monitor

Ongoing assessment of the patient receiving infusion therapy is critical. This includes assessment of the catheter site and the surrounding area for any signs of complications, such as infection, flow rate of medications/solutions, and patient's response to the infusion, and for evidence of potential side effects or adverse reactions. When laboratory work is ordered, the results should be reviewed for abnormalities. Changes in the patient's condition and abnormal laboratory test results should be communicated promptly to the physician. Examples of failure to monitor include not assessing the I.V. site with appropriate frequency and not addressing patient complaints about the I.V. site.

Prevent Infections

An infection is the result of an invasion of a pathogen in a host by various modes of transmission. The presence of an infusion device puts a patient at risk for infection. Considerable attention is placed on infusion-related infections because they are considered preventable events in all settings. Factors contributing to infection risk include inadequate or ill-timed site care, failure to adhere to aseptic technique during catheter insertion and during infusion administration, failure to remove an unnecessary catheter, and failure to recognize and report early signs of infection.

Use Equipment Properly

Failure to use equipment properly may lead to an adverse patient event, specifically the improper use of add-on devices, arm boards, and restraint devices. Incorrect use of filters or electronic infusion devices (EIDs) also has the potential to result in rapid or inadequate rates of infusion. Lack of immediate response to an audible alarm of an EID can compromise patient safety and place the patient at risk.

Protect the Patient from Harm

Protecting the patient from avoidable injury is an important practice issue. TJC's National Patient Safety Goals emphasize protection of the patient with adherence to the following 2012 standards:

- Identify the patient correctly.
- Improve staff communication.
- Use medicines safely.
- Prevent infection.
- Prevent errors in surgery.

Ethical Issues Related to Infusion Therapy

Code of Ethics

It is expected that all nurses practice in an ethical manner. Both the ANA (2010) and the INS (2011) reference the ANA's Code of Ethics for Nurses with Interpretive Statements (ANA, 2001) as the guide for practice. An ethical nurse acts as a patient advocate, maintains patient confidentiality, safety, and security, and respects, promotes, and preserves human autonomy, dignity, rights, and diversity (INS, 2011). A code of ethics acknowledges the acceptance by a profession of the responsibilities and trust that society has conferred and recognizes the duties and obligations inherent in that trust.

The Infusion Nursing Code of Ethics is based on the premise that infusion nurses both individually and collectively practice with awareness, and that there are principles that guide the infusion nurse's actions. It is the purpose of the code to offer the infusion nurse a model for ethical decision making (INS, 2001). The principles used in ethical and moral decision making are based on the following:

- Autonomy (right to self-determination, independence)
- Beneficence (doing good for patients)
- Nonmaleficence (doing no harm to patients)
- Veracity (truthfulness)
- Fidelity (obligation to be faithful)
- Justice (obligation to be fair to all people)

The infusion nurse should follow the ethical principles as stated in the Infusion Nursing Code of Ethics and the ANA Code of Ethics (INS, 2011). These codes are designed to serve as a helpful guide to assist the infusion nurse's practice. The codes includes duties to the patient, duties to society, duties to the profession, and limitations of the infusion nurse's duties and obligations, while ensuring compassionate patient care (ANA, 2001; INS, 2001).

Health Insurance Portability and Accountability Act of 1996 Privacy Rule

The USDHHS (n.d.) issued the Standards for Privacy of Individually Identifiable Health Information (the Privacy Rule) under the Health Insurance Portability and Accountability Act of 1996 (HIPAA) to provide the first comprehensive federal protection for the privacy of personal health information. The final rule went into effect in April 2003. The Privacy Rule requires health-care providers to take reasonable actions to safeguard protected health information (PHI) and to discipline individuals who violate privacy policies. The USDHHS is charged with enforcing the HIPAA legislation. External consequences can consist of fines levied on the organization and the individual(s) involved and can include jail time for disclosing PHI maliciously or for personal gain. This rule has affected professional malpractice and has ethical as well as legal ramifications for infusion nurses.

 Website

U.S. Department of Health and Human Services: www.hhs.gov/ocr/privacy/hipaa/understanding/index.html

 Home Care Issues

The home infusion nurse must deliver safe, effective quality care in the home. Safe and effective care is ensured when the nurse is educated and competent in infusion therapy, when the patient is assessed for appropriateness of home care, and when the intended infusion therapy is appropriate for home administration (Gorski, Miller, & Mortlock, 2010). The home care nurse must have a variety of well-developed skills, which include the following:
- Excellent assessment skills
- Ability to effectively teach patients and caregivers
- Ability to effectively communicate with patients, caregivers, and other health-care–related professionals, including physicians, pharmacists, insurance case managers, and other members of the agency health-care team
- In-depth knowledge of infusion access devices and infusion equipment including
  - Knowledge of community resources and reimbursement
  - Good organizational skills with the ability to function independently

A successful home infusion program ensures patient safety when the following processes and structures are in place:
- Written agency policies and procedures for home infusion therapy
- Discharge planning and/or agency intake processes, which include evaluation of the patient's status and the appropriateness and safety of administering the prescribed infusion drug or fluid in the home

Home Care Issues—cont'd

- Nurses are educated in agency protocols with validated competency in administration of home infusion therapies provided by the agency.
- Tools and educational resources are available to support home infusion nurses, patients, and caregivers.

Health-care providers deliver a variety of services in the home care setting. The following interventions may be provided:

1. Administration of I.V. medications (e.g., antimicrobials, chemotherapy, opioid analgesics), solutions, and parenteral nutrition
2. Peripheral I.V. catheter placement, care, and maintenance
3. ML catheter placement, care, and maintenance
4. Evaluation of infusion therapy-related equipment
5. CVAD care and management
   a. Routine site care and dressing changes
   b. Implanted port access
   c. Declotting
   d. Blood withdrawal from CVADs
6. Administration of intraspinal medications
7. Maintenance of intraspinal catheters
8. Data collection for infusion-related statistics

NURSING FAST FACT!

The HIPAA privacy rule pertains to all health-care settings; therefore, confidentiality has the same legal boundaries in the home care setting as in the hospital.

NOTE > Each subsequent chapter addresses home care issues related to the chapter topic.

Patient Education

Teaching is a major component of clinical infusion practice and is an independent nursing function. In many states, the requirement to teach is included as part of the Nurse Practice Act. According to the ANA Code of Ethics for Nurses (2001), nurses are responsible for promoting and protecting the health, safety, and rights of patients. The INS Standards (2011) address the development of teaching

Continued

Patient Education—cont'd

methods, assessment of health literacy, and evaluation of learning. When planning patient teaching, factors such as age, developmental and cognitive level, culture, and language preferences must be taken into account. Depending on the circumstances, patient family members and/or caregivers should also be involved in the education process.

Health literacy is a critical component of patient education (INS, 2011; Walker & Gerard, 2010). When providing patient education, nurses often use many written materials without consistently assessing the patient's or family member's ability, or even desire, to read multiple handouts. The assessment should address how the patient best learns. Many patients will prefer to learn skills through observation and supervised practice. Whether the nurse uses written materials or verbal presentation of concepts, simplicity is best. Medical jargon should be avoided, which often is difficult because health-care providers tend to speak using acronyms (e.g., CVAD) and terminology not always familiar to the lay person (e.g., "hand hygiene" instead of "wash your hands"). For patients who have limited literacy skills or those who speak English as a second language, the use of pictures, diagrams, and audiovisual aids should be considered.

It is critical that learning be evaluated and reevaluated. Patients or their family members who are learning to self-administer their infusions or to care for their VAD must adhere to the same level of aseptic technique for infusion administration as practiced by the nurse.

NOTE > Each subsequent chapter will present key patient education points related to the content of that chapter.

Chapter Highlights

- Clinical competency is the determination of an individual's capability to perform expectations. It is evidenced by clinical skills checklists/competency assessments; continuing education; documentation of training and education.
- Evidence-based practice (EBP) is the conscientious use of current best evidence in making decisions about patient care.
- Components of EBNP include evidence from research/evidence-based theories and opinions of leaders; evidence from assessment

of the patient's history, physical examination, and availability of health resources; clinical expertise; information about patient preferences and values.

- Clinical competencies incorporate the nursing process, which includes the six steps of assessment, diagnosis, outcomes identification, planning, implementation, and evaluation.
- Quality management is a systematic process to ensure desired patient outcomes. Standards of care focus on the recipient of care.
- Standards of practice focus on the provider of care and represent acceptable levels of practice.
- Benchmarking is the continual and collaborative discipline of measuring and comparing the results of key work processes with those of the best performers.
- Risk management is a process that centers on identification, analysis, treatment, and evaluation of real and potential hazards.
- Risk management strategies include informed consent, reporting unusual occurrences, review of sentinel events, thorough documentation, and safe medication administration strategies.
- Legal issues for the infusion nurse require that the practitioner be aware of the four primary sources of law and understand legal terms, especially *malpractice* and the *rule of personal liability* and *negligence*. In infusion therapy, once a nurse accepts a patient assignment, breaches in duty to the patient include a deficiency in performing that duty or failing to initiate, care, and maintain infusion therapy according to reasonable and prudent standards of care.
- Codes of ethics dictate the responsibilities, trust, and obligations inherent in that trust. The Infusion Nursing Code of Ethics and the ANA Code of Ethics guide the ethical practice of infusion therapy.

■■ Thinking Critically: Case Study

You are the supervisor of an outpatient infusion center. The chief executive officer has requested that you chair a newly established quality management (QM) committee because you had some experience in developing audit criteria in your previous position. A review of the patient population indicates that a high percentage of your patients receive infusion therapies through PICC lines. The committee has decided to review this patient population first. They have chosen to develop a tool for a *prospective audit* that would be appropriate for monitoring the quantity of complications of the PICC lines. The goal of QM is to improve the system.

Case Study Questions
1. *Identify process criteria for the tool.*
2. *Who should be included on this committee?*
3. *Design an audit tool that would be appropriate and convenient to use to collect data.*

Media Link: Answers to the case study questions and more critical thinking activities are provided on Davis*Plus*.

Post-Test

1. The three parts of a competency-based program include:
   a. Competency statement, goal, and return demonstration
   b. Competency statement, criteria for learning, and evaluation
   c. Goal, evaluation, and feedback
   d. Assessment, problem statement, and implementation

2. Which of the following describes the benchmarking process?
   a. Comparing your medical unit's data on phlebitis rate with that of the ICU.
   b. Collecting data on all patients with peripheral I.V.s.
   c. Collecting evidence-based practice to change policy and procedure on care and maintenance of peripheral I.V. sites.
   d. Comparing your unit's data on phlebitis rates to that of other organizations to identify improvement opportunities.

3. The process used to evaluate sentinel events is:
   a. Performance improvement
   b. Unusual occurrence reporting
   c. Competency validation
   d. Root cause analysis

4. To differentiate between standard of care and standard of practice, the standard of practice would be defined as:
   a. Activities and behaviors of the practitioner needed to achieve patient outcomes
   b. Focus on the recipient of care and description of outcomes that the patient can expect to receive
   c. An ongoing systematic process for monitoring and problem solving
   d. Conditions and mechanisms that provide support for the delivery of care

5. A nurse walks into a patient's room and finds the I.V. solution container is dry. The bag of 1000 mL of 5% dextrose and 0.9% sodium chloride had been hung 1 hour earlier. The nurse informs the charge nurse and the physician of this occurrence. The nurse is instructed to complete an unusual occurrence report. The report allows the analysis of adverse patient events by:
   a. Evaluating quality care and the potential risks for injury to the patient

  b. Determining the effectiveness of nursing interventions
  c. Providing a method for reporting injuries to local, state, and federal agencies
  d. Providing clients with necessary stabilizing treatments

6. Characteristics of performance improvement (doing the right thing well) include which of the following? (*Select all that apply.*)

  a. Availability of a needed test
  b. Documenting the quality of care received
  c. Timeliness with which the test, procedure, and treatment are provided
  d. Continuity of the services provided

7. The definition of a tort is:

  a. A written law enacted by the legislature
  b. A private wrong, by act or omission, that can result in a civil action by the harmed person
  c. An offense against the general public
  d. Being capable or able; knowing how to function

8. Components of evidence-based practice include: (*Select all that apply.*)

  a. Evidence from research and published guidelines
  b. Clinical expertise
  c. Physician's orders
  d. Information about patient preferences

9. Which of the following organizations develops clinical practice guidelines? (*Select all that apply.*)

  a. The Agency for Healthcare Research and Design
  b. The Joint Commission
  c. Infusion Nurses Society
  d. American Nurses Association

10. The assessment phase of the nursing process related to infusion therapy would include which of the following? (*Select all that apply.*)

  a. Physical assessment
  b. Review of laboratory data
  c. Teaching the patient and family about central line care
  d. Applying a nursing diagnosis of risk of infection related to tunneled catheter placement

 Media Link: Answers to the Chapter 1 Post-Test and more test questions together with rationales are provided on Davis*Plus*.

■ References

ABNS. (2006). *Definition of certification.* Retrieved from www.nursingcertification.org (Accessed March 4, 2008).

Ackley, B. J., & Ladwig, G. B. (2011). *Nursing diagnosis handbook: An evidence-based guide to planning care* (9th ed). St. Louis, MO: Mosby Elsevier.

Alexander, M. (2012). Editorial: Take care of yourself. *Journal of Infusion Nursing* 5 (2), 75-76.

Alexander, M., & Webster, H. K. (2010). Legal issues of infusion nursing. In M. Alexander, A. Corrigan, L. Gorski, J. Hankins, & R. Perucca (Eds.), *Infusion nursing: An evidence-based approach* (pp. 49-59). St. Louis, MO: Saunders Elsevier.

Altman, M. (2011). Let's get certified: Best practices for nurse leaders to create a culture of certification. *AACN Advanced Critical Care, 22*(1), 68-75.

American Nurses Association (ANA). (2001). *Code of ethics for nurses with interpretive statements.* Kansas City, MO: Author.

ANA. (2010a). *Nursing: Scope and standards of practice.* Kansas City, MO: Author.

ANA. (2010b). *ANA's principles for nursing documentation.* Kansas City, MO: Author.

American Society for Health-System Pharmacists (ASHP). (2008a). Proceedings of a summit on preventing patient harm and death from IV medication errors. *American Journal of Health-System Pharmacists, 65,* 2367-2379.

ASHP. (2008b). *The ASHP Discussion Guide on USP Chapter <797>.* Retrieved from www.ashp.org/s_ashp/docs/files/discguide797-2008.pdf (Accessed October 30, 2012).

Brooke, P. S. (2012). Legal questions. *Nursing,* April, 12.

Bulecheck, G. M., Butcher, H. K., Dochterman, J. M., & Wagner, C. M. (2013). *Nursing interventions classification (NIC)* (6th ed.). St. Louis: MO: Mosby Elsevier.

Centers for Disease Control and Prevention (CDC). (2011). *Guidelines for the prevention of intravascular catheter-related infections.* Atlanta, GA: Author.

CNA/NSO. (2009). *CNA HealthPro nurse claims study: An analysis of claims with risk management recommendations 1997-2007.* Retrieved from www.nso.com/pdfs/db/rnclaimstudy.pdf?fileName=rnclaimstudy.pdf&folder=pdfs/db&isLiveStr=Y&refID=rnclaim (Accessed September 26, 2012).

Corrigan, A. (2010). Infusion nursing as a specialty. In M. Alexander, A. Corrigan, L. Gorski, J. Hankins, & R. Perucca (Eds.), *Infusion nursing: An evidence-based approach* (pp. 1-9). St. Louis, MO: Saunders Elsevier.

Fleischman, R. K., Meyer, L., & Watson, C. (2011). Best practices in creating a culture of certification. *AACN Advanced Critical Care, 22*(1), 33-49.

Gorski, L., Miller, C., & Mortlock, N. (2010). Infusion therapy across the continuum. In M. Alexander, A. Corrigan, L. Gorski, J. Hankins, & R. Perucca (Eds.), *Infusion nursing: An evidence-based approach* (pp. 109-126). St. Louis, MO: Saunders Elsevier.

Hagle, M. E. (2010). Evidence-based practice. In M. Alexander, A. Corrigan, L. Gorski, J. Hankins, & R. Perucca (Eds.), *Infusion nursing: An evidence-based approach* (p. 10). St. Louis, MO: Saunders Elsevier.

Harding, A. D. (2012). Increasing the use of smart pump drug libraries by nurses: A continuous quality improvement project. *American Journal of Nursing, 112*(1), 26-35.

Infusion Nurses Society (INS). (2001). Infusion nursing code of ethics. *Journal of Infusion Nursing, 24*(4), 242-243.

INS. (2011). Infusion nursing standards of practice. *Journal of Infusion Nursing, 34*(1S), S1-S110.

INS/Infusion Nursing Certification Corporation. (2009). *The value of certification in infusion nursing.* Retrieved from www.ins1.org/files/public/06_09_Position_Paper.pdf (Accessed October 29, 2012).

Institute for Safe Medication Practices (ISMP). (2009). *Proceedings from the ISMP summit on the use of smart infusion pumps: Guidelines for safe implementation and use.* Retrieved from www.ismp.org/Tools/guidelines/smartpumps/default.asp (Accessed October 27, 2012).

ISMP. (2012). *ISMP's list of high alert medications.* Retrieved from www.ismp.org/Tools/institutionalhighAlert.asp (Accessed October 25, 2012).

Institute of Medicine. (2011). *The future of nursing: Leading change, advancing health.* Retrieved from www.thefutureofnursing.org/IOM-Report (Accessed October 29, 2012).

Masotti, P., McColl, M.A., Green, M. (2010). Adverse events experienced by homecare patients: a scoping review of the literature. *International Journal for Quality in Health Care, 22*(2), 115-125.

Moorhead, S., Johnson, M., Maas, M., & Swanson E. (2013). *Nursing outcomes classification* (NOC) (5th ed.). St. Louis, MO: Mosby Elsevier.

NANDA-I. (n.d.). *Frequently asked questions.* Retrieved from www.nanda.org/NursingDiagnosisFAQ.aspx. (Accessed September 2, 2013).

National Board for Certification of Hospice and Palliative Nurses. (2011). *Statement of continuing competence for nursing: A call to action.* Retrieved from www.nbchpn.org (Accessed October 13, 2012).

National Database of Nursing Quality Indicators. (2012). *NDNQI indicators.* Retrieved from www.nursingquality.org/data.aspx (Accessed October 29, 2012).

Painter, L. M., Dudjak, L. A., Kidwell, K. M., Simmons, R. L., & Kidwell, R. P. (2011). The nurse's role in causation of compensable injury. *Journal of Nursing Care Quality, 26*(4), 311-319.

Reising, D. L. (2012). Make your nursing care malpractice-proof. *American Nurse Today, 7*(1), 24-28.

Sackett, D. I., Straus, S. E., Richardson, W. E., et al. (2000). *Evidence-based medicine: How to practice and teach.* London: Churchill Livingstone.

Sierchio, G. P. (2010). Quality management. In J. Hankins, R. A. Lonsway, C. Hedrick, & M. Perdue (Eds.), *Infusion Nurses Society: The infusion therapy in clinical practice* (2nd ed.) (pp. 26-49). St. Louis, MO: WB Saunders.

The Joint Commission (TJC). (2011). *Sentinel event policies and procedures.* Retrieved from www.jointcommission.org/Sentinel_Event_Policy_and_Procedures (Accessed September 26, 2012).

TJC. (2012a). *Improving America's hospitals: The Joint Commission's annual report on quality and safety 2012.* Retrieved from www.jointcommission.org/assets/1/18/TJC_Annual_Report_2012.pdf (Accessed October 29, 2012).

TJC. (2012b). *National patient safety goals.* Retrieved from www.jointcommission.org/standards_information/npsgs.aspx (Accessed October 29, 2012).

TJC. (2012c). *Sentinel event data general information 1995-2012.* Retrieved from http://www.jointcommission.org/assets/1/18/SE_General_Info_1995_4Q2 012.pdf (Accessed September 2, 2013).

Titler, M. (2007). Translating research into practice. *American Journal of Nursing, 107*(6 Suppl), 26-33.

U.S. Department of Health and Human Services (USDHHS). (2012). *Hospital incident reporting systems do not capture most patient harm.* Retrieved from https://oig.hhs.gov/oei/reports/oei-06-09-00091.pdf (Accessed September 26, 2012).

USDHHS. (n.d.). *Data bank 101 for nurses: A guide to the data bank and how it affects you.* Retrieved from www.npdb-hipdb.hrsa.gov/resources/factsheets/Nurses.pdf (Accessed September 24, 2012).

USDHHS. (n.d.). *Understanding health information privacy.* Retrieved from www.hhs.gov/ocr/privacy/hipaa/understanding/index.html (Accessed September 25, 2012).

Walker, J., & Gerard, P. S. (2010). Assessing the health literacy levels of patients using selected hospital services. *Clinical Nurse Specialist, 24*(1), 31-37.

Young, J., Slebodnik, M., & Sands, L. (2010). Bar code technology and medication administration error. *Journal of Patient Safety, 6*(2), 115-120.

Chapter 2

Infection Prevention and Occupational Risks

True nursing ignores infection, except to prevent it.
—Florence Nightingale, 1859

─────────────── Chapter Contents ───────────────

Thinking Critically: Case Study   References
Post-Test   Procedures Display 2-1

■ **LEARNING**   *On completion of this chapter, the reader will be able to:*
OBJECTIVES
1. Define terminology related to the immune system, infections and infection prevention, and occupational hazards.
2. Describe the function of the immune system.
3. Identify the organs involved in the immune system.
4. Identify five mechanisms of transmission of microorganisms.
5. Identify the four potential routes for microorganisms to gain access to the bloodstream.
6. Describe potential intrinsic and extrinsic causes of bloodstream infection.
7. Describe standard and transmission-based precautions.
8. Identify the importance of aseptic technique in reducing infection risk.
9. State key interventions of the central line bundle.
10. Describe postinsertion vascular access device care and maintenance interventions important to infection prevention.
11. Discuss the importance of safe practices in relation to needlestick injury.
12. Discuss the occupational risks of hazardous drugs and latex allergy for the infusion nurse.

⟩ GLOSSARY

Airborne precautions   Methods used to prevent transmission of infectious agents (e.g., tuberculosis, rubeola) that remain infectious over long distances when suspended in the air

Antibody   A protective substance produced by B lymphocytes in response to an antigen. Antibodies identify and neutralize or destroy antigens.

Antigen   A foreign substance that induces an immune system response. Examples of antigens include disease-causing organisms and toxic substances (e.g., insect venom)

Aseptic technique   A set of specific practices and procedures performed in a manner that minimizes the risk of transmission of pathogenic microorganisms to patients

Bloodborne pathogens   Microorganisms carried in blood and body fluids that are capable of infecting other persons

Bloodstream infection (BSI)   The presence of bacteria in the blood

Chain of infection   The process by which infections spread

Colonization   Growth of microorganisms in a host without the production of overt clinical symptoms or detected immune reaction

Contact precautions   Methods used to prevent transmission of infectious agents by direct contact (person-to-person) or indirect contact (no direct person-to-contact; contact occurs from a reservoir on contaminated surfaces or objects or from vectors)

Dissemination   Shedding of microorganisms from an individual into the immediate environment or movement of microorganisms from a confined site (skin to bloodstream to other parts of the body)

Droplet precautions   Methods used to prevent transmission of infectious agents from the respiratory tract

Endogenous   Caused by factors within the body

Epidemiology   Branch of science concerned with the study of factors determining the occurrence of diseases in a defined human population; used in establishing programs to prevent and control development of disease and its spread

Exogenous   Originating outside of the organism

Extrinsic contamination   Contamination with microorganisms during preparation or administration

Hand hygiene   A general term that applies to hand washing, antiseptic hand wash, antiseptic hand rub, or surgical hand antisepsis

Health-care–associated infections (HAIs)   Infections that patients acquire during the course of receiving treatment for other conditions or that health-care workers (HCWs) acquire while performing their duties within a health-care setting

Hematogenous   Produced by or derived from the blood; disseminated through the bloodstream or by the circulation

Host   The organism from which a microorganism obtains its nourishment

Immunosuppression   Interference with the development of immunological responses; may be artificially induced by chemical, biological, or physical agents or may be caused by disease

Intrinsic contamination   Contamination that originates prior to use (e.g., during manufacturing)

Leukopenia   Any condition in which the number of leukocytes in the circulating blood is lower than normal

Pathogenicity   The state of producing or being able to produce pathological changes and disease

Reservoir   Living or nonliving material in or on which an infectious agent multiplies and develops and is dependent on for its survival in nature

Resident flora Microorganisms that are indigenous to each individual and are present mainly on the skin and in the respiratory, gastrointestinal, and reproductive systems

Septicemia The presence of pathogenic microorganisms or their toxins in the blood or other tissues; the condition associated with such a presence

Standard precautions Strategies to reduce the risk of exposure to blood and body fluids and to reduce the spread of infection; requires consistent use for all patients regardless of their infection status

Susceptible host Person with inadequate defenses against an invading pathogen. Host is the organism from which a parasite obtains its nourishment.

Transient flora Microorganisms that may be present in or on the body under certain conditions and for certain lengths of time; they are easier to remove by mechanical friction than are resident flora.

Transmission Movement of an organism from the source to the host

Vehicle-borne transmission Any substance that serves as an intermediate means to transport and introduce an infectious agent into a susceptible host through a suitable portal of entry (e.g., usually an insect or other animal, which transmits the causative organisms of disease from infected to noninfected individuals)

Virulence Relative power and degree of pathogenicity possessed by organisms to produce disease

■ Introduction

The presence of a vascular access device (VAD) allows microorganisms direct access to the circulatory system, thus providing risk for the development of a **bloodstream infection (BSI)**. In fact, the presence of a central vascular access device (CVAD) is the most common cause of BSIs. However, today such infections are considered preventable. An understanding of infection concepts and terminology, the immune system, common causative organisms, and evidence-based practices shown to decrease infection risk is essential for the nurse providing infusion therapy.

There are also occupational hazards for the nurse who provides infusion therapy, such as exposure to **bloodborne pathogens** and needlestick injury, chemical exposure to hazardous drugs, and latex allergy. In addition to protecting the patient from infection, nurses must be aware of such risks and protect themselves by adhering to important safety practices addressed in this chapter. In the United States, the following organizations set standards or guidelines for infection prevention and health-care worker (HCW) safety:

■ Association for Professionals in Infection Control and Epidemiology, Inc. (APIC), which emphasizes prevention and promotion of zero tolerance for health-care–associated infections (HAIs) and adverse events. APIC: www.apic.org

- Centers for Disease Control and Prevention (CDC), which is a division of the U.S. Department of Health and Human Services and establishes guidelines for infection control practices. CDC: www.cdc.org
- Centers for Medicare & Medicaid Services (CMS), whose goal is to achieve a transformed and modernized health-care system. CMS: www.cms.hhs.gov
- Infusion Nurses Society (INS), which sets national and global standards for infusion practice and provides a framework for the development of infusion policies and procedures in all practice settings. INS: www.ins1.org
- Institute for Healthcare Improvement (IHI), which is an independent not-for-profit organization that focuses on helping health-care organizations innovate and improve safety and quality. IHI: www.ihi.org
- National Institute for Occupational Safety and Health (NIOSH), which is the federal agency that provides research, information, education, and training in the field of occupational safety and health. NIOSH is part of the CDC in the Department of Health and Human Services. NIOSH: www.cdc.gov/niosh
- The Joint Commission (TJC), which oversees and establishes standards of quality and performance measurement in health care. TJC: www.jointcommission.org
- U.S. Occupational Safety and Health Administration (OSHA), which is the agency responsible for developing and enforcing workplace safety and health regulations. OSHA is located within the U.S. Department of Labor. OSHA: www.osha.gov

Immune System Function

The goal of the immune system is to prevent or limit invasion of the body by **antigens.** Antigens are defined as any foreign substances that induce an immune system response. They include pathogenic microorganisms such as bacteria, viruses, fungi, parasites, and cancer cells. The immune system consists of organs, the innate (or nonspecific) immune system, and the adaptive immune system, which recognizes and remembers antigens. The organs and cells involved in the immune system form a complex system in which antigens and immune system cells are constantly moving through the lymphatic and circulatory system and associated immune organs. Immune system organs include the thymus, bone marrow, lymph nodes, spleen, liver, Peyer's patches, appendix, tonsils and adenoids, and lungs. The location and functions of these organs are listed in Table 2-1.

> Table 2-1   ORGANS OF THE IMMUNE SYSTEM

Organs	Location	Function
Primary		
Thymus (part of lymphatic system)	Superior and anterior mediastinum	Largest and most active from neonate to puberty, then atrophies Involved in T-cell development
Bone marrow	Hollow interior of long bones	Major hematopoietic organ producing red and white blood cells (WBCs), and platelets
Secondary		
Lymphatic vessels and nodes	Interconnected system of vessels throughout body Lymph nodes are located in clusters in various parts of the body, such as the neck, armpit, groin, center of chest, and abdomen	Lymph fluid is filtered at the lymph nodes, removing foreign material such as bacteria and cancer cells. Involved in WBC production when bacteria are recognized, causing lymph node swelling
Spleen (part of lymphatic system)	Left upper abdominal quadrant beneath diaphragm	Filters antigens Removes old red blood cells and stores red cells, leukocytes, platelets, lymphocytes; serves as hematopoietic organ
Liver	Right upper abdominal quadrant, small intestine	Kupffer cells filter out antigens
Peyer's patches, appendix	Right lower abdominal quadrant	Areas of lymphoid tissue that contain B cells and T cells
Tonsils and adenoids	Pharynx	Tonsils and adenoids are part of lymphatic system
Lungs	Thoracic cavity	Filter antigenic material and cellular debris

The appropriate immune response occurs when the immune system recognizes and destroys invading antigens.

Mechanisms of Defense

There are two types of immunity: innate (also called nonspecific) and adaptive. Innate immunity is the first line of defense against antigens. Innate immunity is present before exposure to an antigen and is not enhanced by successive exposures (Levinson, 2012).

First Line of Defense/Nonspecific or Innate Defenses

The first line of defense of the innate system is the presence of physical and chemical barriers that limit entry of microorganisms into the body. These include:

- Intact skin and epithelial surfaces that act as mechanical barriers
- Presence of normal microflora on the skin that compete with pathogens for nutrients and inhibit pathogen growth through lactic acid production
- Normal flora of the throat, colon, and vagina occupy receptors that prevent **colonization** by pathogens
- Secretions, all of which (e.g., gastrointestinal [GI], respiratory, urogenital tracts, tear glands, breast milk) contain **antibodies**
- Hydrochloric acid production in the stomach and low pH in the vagina maintain an acidic pH that rapidly destroys microorganisms
- Lysosomes in tears and other secretions involved in degradation of bacterial cell walls (Levinson, 2012; Storey & Jordan, 2008)

Additional physiological mechanisms include the nares, trachea, and bronchi, which are covered with mucous membranes that trap and then expel pathogens. The nose contains hairs that filter the upper airway, and the nasal passages, sinuses, trachea, and larger bronchi are lined with cilia that elevate mucous-containing trapped organisms and sweep microorganisms upward from the lower airways. Coughing and sneezing forcefully expel organisms from the respiratory tract. Through mechanical action, peristalsis in the GI tract and urinary tract expels organisms from the internal environment of the **host.**

 NURSING FAST FACT!

Recognize that when a venipuncture is performed, the body's first line of defense—intact skin—is broken, thus presenting a potential portal of entry for microorganisms.

Second Line of Defense/Nonspecific or Innate Defenses

When the first line of defense fails, the innate immune system includes other components, which act as a second line of defense that limits growth of microorganisms in the body. These include:

- Natural killer (NK) cells, which kill cells infected by viruses
- Neutrophils, which ingest and destroy microbes
- Macrophages and dendritic cells, which ingest and destroy microbes and present antigens to helper T cells (these cells are involved not only in the innate immune system defense but also in activating the adaptive immune response)
- Interferons, which inhibit replication of viruses

- The complement cascade, which is activated by contact with bacterial cell walls, viruses, fungi, cancer cells, endotoxins, and antigen/antibody complexes.
  - This is a system of plasma proteins (complement) that trigger a cascade of reactions resulting in the coating of pathogens and attacking of cell membranes, causing the pathogens to rupture. Complement also signals basophils to release the chemical histamine, which prompts inflammation.
- Inflammation, which limits the spread of microorganisms
- Fever, which slows down bacterial growth
- Transferrin and lactoferrin sequester iron, which is required for bacterial proliferation (Levinson, 2012)

Although innate immunity eliminates microbes and prevents infectious diseases, it is not enough. For example, children who have intact innate immunity but no adaptive immunity suffer from repeated and life-threatening infections (Levinson, 2012).

Tertiary Defenses/Adaptive or Specific Immunity

Adaptive immunity develops after exposure to an antigen, improves on repeated exposures, and is specific (Levinson, 2012). Memory is formed so that the next time the same infection is encountered, there is immunity and there is no inflammatory response. Adaptive immunity is mediated by antibodies that are produced by B lymphocytes and two types of T lymphocytes: helper T cells and cytotoxic T cells. Cells accountable for adaptive immunity have a long memory for specific antigens and exhibit diversity in that they can respond to millions of different antigens (Levinson, 2012).

Adaptive immunity can be active or passive. Active immunity is resistance after contact with a foreign antigen such as a microorganism. Passive immunity is resistance based on antibodies that were "preformed" in another host. Examples include the immunoglobulins passed from mother to fetus during pregnancy and the preformed antibodies given to treat a disease during the incubation period (e.g., rabies). Risks and disadvantages include possible hypersensitivity reactions to the antibodies and short life span of such antibodies. "Passive active" immunity involves giving preformed antibodies (e.g., immunoglobulins) for immediate protection and vaccinations for long-term protection against certain diseases (Levinson, 2012).

Leukocytes and the Immune System

Leukocytes, or white blood cells (WBCs), orchestrate both nonspecific immunity through the inflammatory response and adaptive immunity. A differential WBC count provides specific information related to infections and disease. Normal WBC counts range from 5000 to 10,000/mL. **Leukopenia** is defined as a reduction of the number of leukocytes in the blood to a count of less than 5000/mm³. The types and functions of the different types of leukocytes are listed in Table 2-2.

Lymphocytes and Adaptive Immunity

As mentioned earlier, the B and T lymphocytes are involved in adaptive immunity. There are two major branches of the adaptive immune response: humoral (antibody-mediated) immunity and cell-mediated immunity. Humoral immunity includes the production of antibody molecules in response to an antigen. This is mediated by the B lymphocytes (also called B cells). Mature B cells are found in bone marrow, lymph nodes, spleen, some areas of the intestine, and to a smaller extent in the bloodstream (Vizcarra, 2010). When stimulated by an antigen, they mature into plasma cells, which produce antibodies. Antibodies are also called immunoglobulins.

> Table 2-2   **TYPES AND FUNCTIONS OF WHITE BLOOD CELLS**

Type and % of Total White Blood Cells	Function
Granular	
Neutrophils: 55%–70% Segments are mature neutrophils; in presence of infection, immature neutrophils (bands) are released to engulf and destroy bacteria	Released from bone marrow or vessel surfaces and migrate to site of infection Body's first line of defense through phagocytosis Have receptors for IgG on surface that make bacteria more easily phagocytosed As neutrophils die, they form purulent drainage Note that in patients who are neutropenic, signs and symptoms such as erythema and drainage are not present
Eosinophils: 1%–3%	Reduce inflammatory response by producing enzymes that destroy histamine thus have role in allergic reactions Count is elevated in parasitic diseases and hypersensitivity diseases Weakly phagocytose bacteria
Basophils: 0.5%–1%	Release histamine, heparin, and serotonin granules as part of the inflammatory response
Agranular	
Lymphocytes: 20%–35% Found in bone marrow, thymus, spleen, and lymph nodes T cells mature in thymus	T cells: Responsible for cell-mediated immunity; recognize, attack, and destroy antigens B cells: Responsible for humoral immunity; produce immunoglobulins, and attack and destroy antigens
Monocytes: 3%–8% Similar to lymphocytes Stay in peripheral blood for 70 hours	Able to phagocytize directly as well as differentiate into macrophages, which help clean up damaged or injured tissue

Sources: Levinson, 2012; Storey & Jordan, 2008; Van Leeuwen, Poelhuis-Leth, & Bladh (2012).

Immunoglobulins circulate throughout the body, interacting with and aiding in the destruction of potentially harmful microorganisms and toxins. The main functions of these antibodies are to neutralize toxins and viruses and to make bacteria easier to phagocytize (Levinson, 2012). There are five classes of immunoglobulins:

IgG: The major immunoglobulin in the bloodstream; can enter the tissue spaces and coat microorganisms to expedite their destruction by other immune cells; the only immunoglobulin that crosses the placenta and passes immunity on to the infant (i.e., passive immunity)

IgA: Found in tears, saliva, and secretions of the respiratory and GI tracts

IgD: Remains attached to B cells and plays an important role in early B-cell response

IgE: Present in trace amounts; responsible for allergy symptoms

IgM: Present and remains in bloodstream where it effectively kills bacteria (Vizcarra, 2010)

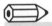 *NURSING FAST FACT!*

The absence of one or more of these substances has been linked to infection or disease processes. Regular infusion of immunoglobulin, via either the I.V. route or the subcutaneous route, may be used to treat patients with certain deficiencies in the immune system.

In contrast to humoral immunity, cell-mediated immunity does not involve antibody production. The response is mediated by the T lymphocytes, which do not produce antibodies but directly attack antigens. Cytotoxic T lymphocytes (also called T cells), activated macrophages, activated NK cells, and cytokines are produced in response to antigens. The cytotoxic T cells directly destroy antigens; they also respond to foreign tissues in the body, such as a transplanted organ. The NK cells come from the bone marrow and are involved in killing virus-infected cells; they may play a role in cancer prevention. Macrophages are large WBCs found in many organs. They remove debris and worn out cells, and they secrete monokines, which are an important chemical signal to the immune response. Cytokines include interferons, interleukins, and growth factors, which boost the immune system, repair damage, and defend against infection (Vizcarra, 2010).

Impaired Host Resistance

Many factors can result in impaired host defense. Persons who acquire an infection because of a deficiency in any of their multifaceted host defenses are referred to as compromised hosts. Persons with major defects related

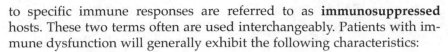

to specific immune responses are referred to as **immunosuppressed** hosts. These two terms often are used interchangeably. Patients with immune dysfunction will generally exhibit the following characteristics:

1. Infections occur frequently.
2. Infections are more severe than usual.
3. Unusual infecting agents or infections with opportunistic organisms occur.
4. Patients have incomplete response to treatment without complete elimination of the infecting agent.

Immune System Disorders

Disorders in the immune system consist of either an excessive immune response or a deficiency in response. Examples of an excessive immune response can be found with autoimmune diseases such as rheumatoid arthritis, Crohn's disease, and inflammatory skin diseases, and as a result of transplant-related rejection. In such cases, biological agents such as monoclonal antibodies may be administered to suppress the immune system.

There are two types of immune deficiencies. Primary immune deficiencies result from an inborn defect in the cells of the immune system. Deficiencies in the immune response may be due to a congenital, acquired, or inherited immune dysfunction. There are many primary immune disorders, ranging from common to rare. Examples include agammaglobulinemia and hypogammaglobulinemia.

Secondary immunodeficiencies arise from disease processes or therapies that decrease immune system organ or cell function. These deficiencies are acquired. Examples include chronic lymphocytic leukemia and human immunodeficiency virus/acquired immunodeficiency syndrome (HIV/AIDS).

 Websites:

Immune Deficiency Foundation: http://primaryimmune.org

Basic Principles of Epidemiology

Epidemiology is the study of factors determining the occurrence of diseases in human populations (Archibald, 2012). Factors and determinants leading to infection are discussed in this section.

Infection is defined as the successful **transmission** of microorganisms into a host after the microorganisms evade or overcome the host's defense mechanisms. Proliferation and invasion of organisms result in clinical signs and symptoms such as inflammation, drainage, or fever. Colonization is the presence of a microorganism on or within body sites without a detectable host immune response, cellular damage, or clinical symptoms (McGoldrick, 2010). A carrier (or colonized person) is an individual colonized with a specific microorganism and from whom the organism can be recovered but who shows no signs or symptoms of the presence of the microorganism. A carrier may have a history of previous disease. The carrier state may be transient (short term), intermediate (on occasion), or chronic (long term, permanent, or persistent).

Dissemination is the shedding of microorganisms into the immediate environment from a person carrying the microorganisms. Cultures of air samples, surfaces, and objects reveal dissemination or shedding of microorganisms. Some facilities routinely culture all or selected asymptomatic staff in an attempt to identify carriers of certain organisms; however, such surveys lack practical relevance unless they are related to a specific outbreak of disease. Usually only a fraction of colonized persons are disseminating; therefore, nondisseminators are not associated with the actual spread of infection.

The risk of dissemination is generally greater from individuals with disease caused by that organism than from individuals with subclinical infection or those who are colonized with the organism.

Chain of Infection

Infections result from interaction between infectious agents and **susceptible hosts**. This interaction is called transmission. The **chain of infection** refers to six links that make up the chain: the causative agent or microorganism; the place where the organism naturally resides (**reservoir**); a portal of exit from the reservoir; a method (mode) of transmission; a portal of entry into a host; and the susceptibility of the host. To control infection, the chain of infection must be attacked at its weakest link (Figure 2-1).

First Link: Causative Agent

The first link in the chain of infection is the microbial agent or source, which may be a bacterium, fungus, virus, or parasite. The majority of HAIs are caused by bacteria and viruses. The ability of an organism to induce disease is called its **virulence** or invasiveness. The ability of microorganisms to induce disease is referred to as **pathogenicity**, and it may be assessed via disease/colonization ratios.

Second Link: Reservoir

All organisms have a reservoir, or source of microorganisms. The source of a microorganism may be animate (e.g., humans, the patient's own

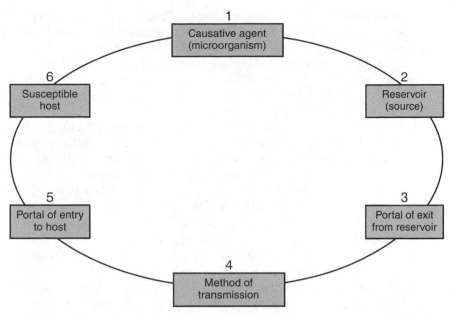

Figure 2-1 ◾ Chain of infection.

microorganisms) or inanimate (e.g., bedside tables, artificial fingernails, toys). The reservoir is where the organism maintains its presence, metabolizes, and replicates. Viruses survive better in human reservoirs, whereas the gram-negative bacteria may have human, animal, or inanimate reservoirs.

Third Link: Portal of Exit from Reservoir

The exit site is important in transmission of infection. Organisms from humans usually have a single portal of exit, but multiple portals of exit are possible. The major portals of exit are the respiratory tract, GI tract, and skin (e.g., in wounds). In addition, blood may be a portal of exit and is a concern for infusion nurses.

Fourth Link: Method (Mode) of Transmission

After a microorganism leaves its source or reservoir, it requires a means of transmission to reach another person or host through a receptive portal of entry. There are five mechanisms of transmission:

1. Contact transmission: Contact transmission can be divided into two subgroups. The first, direct transfer of organisms, involves body surface-to-body surface contact and physical transfer of microorganisms between a susceptible host and an infected or colonized person (e.g., occurs when turning a patient or performing

other patient-care activities) or through touching, biting, kissing, or sexual intercourse. The second subgroup, indirect-contact transmission, involves contact of a susceptible host with a contaminated intermediate object, usually inanimate (e.g., contaminated instruments, needles, dressing, or hands). Examples of organisms that can be transmitted via contact are *Staphylococcus* and *Enterococcus* (Siegel, Rhinehart, Jackson, & Chiarello, 2007).

2. Droplet transmission: Droplet transmission is a form of contact transmission. The mechanism of transfer of the pathogen to the host is different from that of contact transmission. Droplet transmission is considered a separate route of transmission. Transmission via large-particle droplets (>5 mm in size) requires close contact between the source and recipient, usually 3 to 6 feet. Examples of pathogens transmitted by the droplet route are *Bordetella pertussis* and *Neisseria meningitides* (Siegel, Rhinehart, Jackson, & Chiarello, 2007).

3. Airborne transmission: Airborne transmission occurs by dissemination of airborne droplet nuclei (small-particle residues, <5 μm) of evaporated droplets containing microorganisms that remain suspended in the air for long periods of time. Examples of airborne transmission are *Mycobacterium tuberculosis,* rubeola, and varicella viruses (Siegel, Rhinehart, Jackson, & Chiarello, 2007).

4. **Vehicle-borne transmission**: A vehicle is any substance that serves as an intermediate means to transport and introduces an infectious agent into a susceptible host. Examples are toys, handkerchiefs, soiled linen, and clothes.

5. Vector-borne transmission: A vector is an animal or flying or crawling insect that serves as an intermediate means for transporting an infectious agent. An example is the mosquito carrying the West Nile virus (Siegel, Rhinehart, Jackson, & Chiarello, 2007).

Fifth Link: Portal of Entry to the Susceptible Host

A person can become infected once the organism enters the body. The skin is a barrier to infectious agents; however, any break in the skin can readily serve as a portal of entry. The mucous membranes and the respiratory, GI, and urinary tracts are other portals of entry. An organism may colonize one site and cause no disease, but the same organism at another site may result in clinical disease. For example, *Escherichia coli* routinely colonizes the GI tract and under normal circumstances does not cause disease; however, *E. coli* in the urinary tract can cause infection.

Sixth Link: Host Response

A host can respond to a microorganism in one of three ways: a subclinical infection, a clinically apparent illness, or the extreme response of death. The same organism infecting different hosts can result in a clinical spectrum of disease that is the same, similar, or different in various individuals. A susceptible host is a person with inadequate defenses against the invading organism. Susceptibility is influenced by factors such as age (e.g., very young or very old), family associations, occupation, travel, access to preventive health care, vaccination status, and hospitalization (Archibald, 2012). Patients who are receiving immune suppression treatment for cancer, have a chronic illness, or have undergone a successful organ transplant are susceptible hosts.

Classification of Infections

Location

When infections can cause harm in a limited region of the body (e.g., upper respiratory tract or bladder), these infections are considered local. Systemic infections occur when the pathogens invade the bloodstream and spread through the body. A bacteremia or BSI is defined by the clinical presence of bacteria in the blood, whereas **septicemia** is symptomatic systemic infection caused by pathogenic organisms or their toxins (McGoldrick, 2010). The source of the pathogen must be identified.

Endogenous infections are caused by a person's own flora. Sources of endogenous infections include body sites inhabited by microorganisms such as the skin and the GI tract. For example, resident microorganisms on a patient's skin may lead to a BSI after venipuncture if the skin preparation and antisepsis was inadequate. **Exogenous** infections result from sources outside a person's body. It may not always be possible to determine whether a particular organism isolated from a patient with HAIs is exogenous or endogenous.

Stages

Many infections follow a fairly predictable course of events. The duration and intensity of symptoms may vary from one individual to the next.

- Incubation: The time between exposure to an infectious agent and the first appearance of symptoms
- Prodromal stage: Characterized by the first appearance of vague symptoms. Not all infections have a prodromal stage.
- Illness: The stage marked by appearance of signs and symptoms characteristic of the disease

NOTE > If the patient's immune defenses and medical treatment are ineffective, this stage can end in death of the patient.

- Decline: The stage during which the patient's immune defenses, along with any medical therapies, successfully reduce the number of pathogens. Symptoms begin to fade.
- Convalescence: Characterized by tissue repair and return to health.

Health-Care–Associated Infections

HAIs are infections that patients develop while they are receiving care in a health-care setting. In the United States, four types of HAIs account for 75% of infections. They are urinary tract infections, surgical site infections, pneumonia, and BSIs. BSI is a serious and potentially life-threatening complication of VADs. In fact, presence of a CVAD is the most common cause related to health-care–associated BSIs (O'Grady et al., 2011). The cost of care and the length of hospital stay are increased in the event of BSI. The cost of a central line–associated BSI has been estimated at $16,550 (O'Grady, 2011c).

VAD-related infections are one of the 10 hospital-acquired conditions considered a preventable adverse event; thus, their treatment is not reimbursed under CMS. Aligning payment with patient outcomes represents a significant change in government policy, and prevention of infections is a major health-care goal. Of note, greater attention to HAIs targeted by this CMS policy was reported in a national survey; at least 50% of infection preventionists reported more rapid removal of CVADs and use of antimicrobial dressings (Lee, et al., 2012). As discussed in Chapter 1, TJC (2012b) includes the prevention of CVAD infections as one of the 2013 National Patient Safety Goals for both hospitals and long-term care organizations.

Vascular Access Device-Related Infections: Scope and Terminology

Health-care institutions purchase millions of intravascular catheters each year. Estimates include over 330 million short peripheral catheters sold annually and about three million CVADs placed each year (Hadaway, 2012; TJC, 2012a). It is estimated that 80,000 catheter-related BSIs occur in intensive care units (ICUs) annually in the United States, and, if the entire hospital is included, beyond the ICUs, the estimate is 250,000 catheter-related BSIs per year (O'Grady et al., 2011). Much of the focus has been on the CVAD, particularly in the ICU setting. However, the importance and significance of BSI in hospital units beyond intensive care and those associated with peripheral I.V. catheters are just beginning to be recognized and addressed. In a systematic literature review, although the evidence indicates a low infection rate with short peripheral I.V. catheters, the large numbers of catheters used translates into potentially thousands of infections each year. A low 0.1% BSI rate would result in 165,000 BSIs per year in the United States if half of the 330 million catheters were considered to be successfully inserted (Hadaway, 2012).

There are limited current data regarding the rate of these infections in alternate sites such as nursing homes and home care settings. Indwelling devices, including VADs, were associated with higher rates of infection in the nursing home population (Montoya & Mody, 2011). In a point preva-lence study of 10,939 veterans, peripherally inserted central catheters (PICCs) were associated with increased risk for infection (Tsan et al., 2010). The rate of infections among home care patients has been histori-cally low based on studies published many years ago (Gorski, Perucca, & Hunter, 2010).

It is important to understand the terminology used to describe VAD-related infections. The terms catheter-related bloodstream infec-tion (CRBSI) and central line-associated bloodstream infection (CLABSI) are often used interchangeably, but they have different meanings. CRBSI is a more rigorous definition that requires specific laboratory testing that identifies the catheter as the source of the BSI. CLABSI is a primary BSI (i.e., no apparent infection at another site) that devel-ops in a patient with a central line in place within the 48-hour period before onset of the BSI that is not related to another site (O'Grady et al., 2011). The microorganisms most frequently implicated in CLABSIs are coagulase-negative staphylococci, *Staphylococcus aureus*, and *Candida* (O'Grady et al., 2011).

Central Line-Associated Bloodstream Infection Surveillance and Public Reporting

Historically, HAIs were perceived as being inevitable consequences of health care. That is no longer the case. Today, HAIs are considered preventable and unacceptable. This has led to public reporting of their occurrence in the United States as well as other countries. Many states require mandatory public reporting of HAIs, although there is variation in reporting requirements. In 2011, CMS expanded public reporting be-yond just the state level. Medicare-eligible hospitals are now required to track and report CLABSIs in ICUs in order to receive an annual increase in Medicare payments. The data are reported on the Hospital Compare website (www.hospitalcompare.hhs.gov). The National Healthcare Safety Network (NHSN) is the oldest and most well-developed HAI surveillance system. It is a voluntary and secure Internet-based system. Starting in 2008, all types of health-care facilities in the United States could enroll in the NHSN for data collection, reporting, and analysis (CDC, 2013).

Pathogenesis of Vascular Access Device–Related Infections

There are four potential routes for introducing microorganisms into a patient's bloodstream (O'Grady et al., 2011):

- Extraluminal: Migration of skin organisms at the insertion site into the catheter tract and along the catheter surface, thus gaining access to the external catheter surface
  - Microorganisms attach to the catheter at the tip and the external surface as the catheter enters through the epidermis. The source of the microorganisms is the patient's skin or the health-care provider's hands.
  - Microorganisms from the patient's skin can enter the catheter tract during the dwell time of the catheter.
  - Skin is considered the most common source of infection with short-term catheters in place less than 10 days (usually within the first week of catheterization).
- Intraluminal: Direct contamination of the catheter or catheter hub by contact with contaminated hands or fluids or devices. Microorganisms gain access through the internal catheter lumen of the catheter.
  - Risk is present every time the catheter is accessed. During medication or fluid administration, catheter flushing, or changing of the needleless connector or I.V. tubing, microorganisms can enter the catheter lumen. The source of the microorganisms may be the hands of the health-care provider, patient, or caregiver.
  - Risk is present if I.V. solutions are not properly handled (i.e., improper refrigeration of infusates, failure to adhere to **aseptic technique** during solution preparation, or use of multidose vials for more than one patient).
  - The intraluminal route is associated with prolonged CVAD dwell time as the number of catheter manipulations and accesses increase.
- **Hematogenous** seeding of bacteria from another type of infection present in the patient, such as a urinary tract infection. This is a less common cause.
- Infusate contamination (Figure 2-2).

Risk factors for CLABSI include both nonmodifiable and potentially modifiable factors (TJC, 2012b) (Table 2-3).

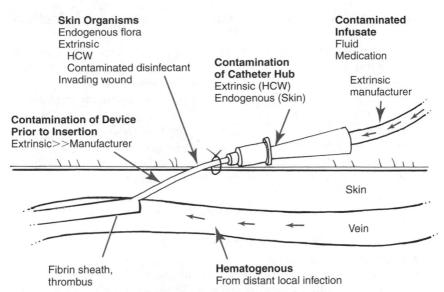

Skin Organisms
Endogenous flora
Extrinsic
   HCW
   Contaminated disinfectant
   Invading wound

**Contamination
of Catheter Hub**
Extrinsic (HCW)
Endogenous (Skin)

**Contaminated
Infusate**
Fluid
Medication

Extrinsic
manufacturer

**Contamination of Device
Prior to Insertion**
Extrinsic>>Manufacturer

Skin

Vein

Fibrin sheath,
thrombus

Hematogenous
From distant local infection

Figure 2-2 ▪ Sources of I.V. cannula-related infections. (From *Bennett &
Brachman's hospital infections* [5th ed.]. Philadelphia, PA: Lippincott Williams
& Wilkins. Used with permission.)

> Table 2-3 | **FACTORS ASSOCIATED WITH INCREASED CENTRAL LINE-ASSOCIATED BLOODSTREAM INFECTION (CLABSI) RISK**

Nonmodifiable Risk Factors

• Age: Young children, especially neonates
• Underlying diseases or conditions: Hematological deficiencies, immune system deficiencies, cardiovascular disease, gastrointestinal diseases
• Male gender

Potentially Modifiable Risk Factors

• Prolonged hospitalization prior to central vascular access device (CVAD) insertion
• Having multiple CVADs
• Receiving parenteral nutrition
• CVAD placed via the femoral or internal jugular vein (risk of infection for femoral-placed catheters may be heightened in obese patients)
• Heavy microbial colonization at CVAD insertion site
• Longer duration of CVAD placement
• Multilumen CVADs
• Failure to use maximal sterile barrier precautions (e.g., catheter inserter does not wear a sterile gown, sterile gloves, cap, and full body drape for patients) during CVAD insertion
• CVAD insertion in an intensive care unit (ICU) or emergency department

Sources: O'Grady et al., 2011; TJC, 2012a.

Intrinsic versus Extrinsic Causes of Bloodstream Infection

Potential contamination of the infusion system can occur by **extrinsic contamination,** which occurs during preparation or administration, or by **intrinsic contamination,** which occurs during manufacturing.

Extrinsic contamination of parenteral fluids can occur during administration of solutions and medications via many possible sources. Microorganisms gain access when air enters the bottles, from entry points into the administration set, from the I.V. device through the line, or at the junction between the administration set and the catheter hub. Extrinsic contamination is preventable in all settings. Examples of extrinsic contamination include:

■ During admixture procedure in the pharmacy when laminar flow hoods are not used
■ Incorrect use of admixing equipment
■ Improper refrigeration
■ Improper technique, such as failure to maintain a closed, sterile I.V. system, touch contamination of the catheter and syringe, and failure to disinfect the needleless connector

Intrinsic contamination of the infusate is considered rare but can occur during the manufacturing and sterilization processes before the containers reach the health-care organization. Damage can occur during storage and delivery. Glass containers can become cracked or damaged and plastic bags punctured. Bacteria and fungi may invade a hairline crack in an I.V. container. When intrinsic contamination occurs, it can cause epidemic device-related infections because of the large numbers of patients in multiple hospitals who may be affected (McGoldrick, 2010).

NOTE > Unopened samples of the suspect lot or lots should be quarantined and saved for analysis.

Before use, any glass container lacking a vacuum when opened should be considered contaminated. To prevent potential infection due to intrinsic causes, follow these steps prior to initiating infusions:

■ Examine containers of fluid against light and dark backgrounds for cracks, defects, turbidity, and particulate matter.
■ Squeeze plastic bags gently to check for loss of integrity.
■ Observe for droplet formation on the I.V. bag surface.
■ Inspect all protective coverings and seals.
■ Inspect the solution for clarity and check expiration dates.

Any concerns about the infusate should result in nonuse of the infusate and reporting to the U.S. Food and Drug Administration (McGoldrick, 2010).

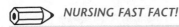 *NURSING FAST FACT!*

The most important measures to prevent BSIs from contaminated in-use (extrinsic) infusate are stringent asepsis during the preparation and compounding of admixtures in the hospital central pharmacy or in individual patient-care units. Aseptic technique should be followed at all times during infusion therapy, and the administration set should be changed at periodic intervals.

Poor technique when using and during handling of I.V. equipment can lead to contamination. Pay attention to the following:

1. *Needleless connectors:* Failure to disinfect the needleless connectors prior to flushing or medication administration is a significant problem. The Institute for Safe Medication Practices (ISMP, 2007) documented infection control problems, including failure to disinfect the needleless connector when accessing the infusion for flushing or medication administration. This increases the risk for contamination and potential BSI. TJC (2012b) states the following in the National Patient Safety Goals: "Use a standardized protocol to disinfect catheter hubs and injection ports prior to accessing the port." New products are available, including needleless connectors with built-in antimicrobial protection and disposable alcohol disinfection caps with an alcohol sponge, which are attached to the needleless connector in between intermittent infusions (Figure 2-3).

2. *Three-way stopcocks:* These adjunct devices are potential sources of transmission of bacteria because their ports, which are unprotected by sterile covering, are open to moisture and contaminants. These devices usually are connected to CVADs and arterial lines and are frequently used for drawing blood. The INS (2011, p. S31) states that use of stopcocks is *not* recommended. However, if they are used, sterile caps should be placed on the ports to provide a closed system. As with all infusion-related procedures, aseptic technique is vital when accessing the ports.

3. *Administration sets:* Intravenous administration sets must be changed based on several factors. The administration set is changed immediately when contamination is suspected or when the integrity of the system has been compromised (INS, 2011). Consider the following published account written by a mother whose young son was receiving total parenteral nutrition. Her child's I.V. tubing came unattached from his PICC and ended up on the hospital room floor. The nurse "nonchalantly picked up (the) tubing, wiped the end off with a small alcohol pad and went to reattach it to Tyler's PICC without any consideration for where that tubing had been and the

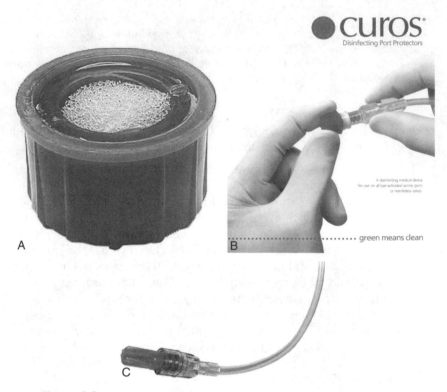

Figure 2-3 ■ Curos® alcohol disinfection cap. *A*, Cap, which is changed after each catheter access. *B*, View of cap over a needleless connector. *C*, Companion alcohol cap used to cover male end of intermittently used I.V. tubing. (Courtesy of Ivera Medical Corporation, San Diego, CA.)

contaminated (needleless connector) that had been rubbing against my son's clothing" (Bailey, 2009). This is clearly an example of compromised integrity. Any I.V.-related product should not be used when it is known to no longer be sterile. Another important aspect relates to the situation of intermittent infusions. It is also critical that a sterile, compatible covering device be aseptically attached to the end of the administration set. Failure to do so has been documented by the ISMP (2007) as another important factor contributing to increased infection risk. Administration sets used for intermittent infusions are changed at least every 24 hours (INS, 2011a, p. S55).

INS Standard Primary and secondary continuous administration sets used to administer fluids other than lipid, blood, or blood products should be changed no more frequently than every 96 hours. They shall be changed immediately when contamination is suspected or when the integrity of the product or system has been compromised. The administration set shall be changed whenever the peripheral catheter is rotated or when a new CVAD is changed (INS, 2011a, p. S55).

INS Standard To prevent the entry of microorganisms into the vascular system, the needleless connector should be consistently and thoroughly disinfected using alcohol, tincture of iodine, or chlorhexidine gluconate/alcohol combination prior to each access (INS, 2011a, p. S32).

Microorganisms most frequently encountered in catheter-related BSIs are listed in Table 2-4.

Diagnosing Infection: Culturing Techniques

When an infusion-related infection is suspected, cultures may be obtained to ascertain the source of infection. Culture specimens may include one or all of the following:

- Purulent exudate from the catheter exit site
- Catheter tip/segment
- Administration set
- Infusate
- Patient's blood

The recommended method for culturing a catheter is the semiquantitative culture technique (Procedures Display 2-1). This technique involves rolling the catheter segment across an agar plate. Colony-forming

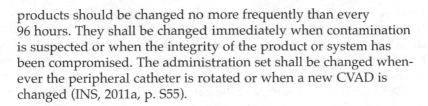

> Table 2-4	MICROORGANISMS MOST FREQUENTLY ENCOUNTERED
Source	**Pathogens**
Peripheral I.V. catheter related	Most common causative organism in bloodstream infection (BSI) is *Staphylococcus aureus*, including methicillin resistant
Central vascular access device related	Gram-positive organisms are most commonly reported causative organisms, including coagulase-negative staphylococci *S. aureus*, including methicillin resistant *Enterococcus* *Candida* species Gram-negative; most common organisms include *Escherichia coli and Klebsiella*

Sources: *Hadaway, 2012; O'Grady et al., 2011; TJC, 2012a.*

units (CFUs) are counted after overnight incubation. Disadvantages of the semiquantitative method are as follows: (1) this method may fail to detect bacteremia of the internal lumens of the catheter tip; and (2) the catheter must be removed for culturing and may not actually be the source of infection.

When culturing drainage at the catheter–skin site, do not cleanse the area to be cultured. On the other hand, when preparing to remove and culture a catheter, the skin around the insertion site must be cleansed with an antiseptic solution prior to catheter removal and allowed to air dry. If a blood culture is required, it is recommended that a phlebotomy team obtain the samples (Mermel et al., 2009).

 NURSING FAST FACT!

When obtaining blood through a catheter for culture, the first sample of blood obtained through the catheter is used to inoculate the culture bottles. This is different than the procedure followed when obtaining blood samples for laboratory studies via a catheter where the initial blood sample is discarded.

 NURSING FAST FACT!

Growth of 15 or more CFUs from a catheter tip segment represents catheter colonization (Mermel et al., 2009).

Any purulent drainage at the exit site should be collected for culture and gram staining to determine if gram-positive or gram-negative bacteria are present (INS, 2011a, p. S69). If the I.V. solution is the suspected source of infection, send the fluid container and the tubing to a laboratory for analysis.

Blood cultures are generally drawn through a peripheral vein and through the VAD. Important procedural considerations include the following: obtain the sample before any antibiotic therapy; use an antiseptic skin preparation prior to venipuncture to avoid contamination of blood specimen; use of phlebotomy teams for blood cultures is recommended; and change the needleless connector prior to drawing blood specimens through a catheter to reduce risk of obtaining a contaminated specimen (INS, 2011, p. S69).

■ Strategies for Preventing Infection

Nurses involved in maintaining VADs must have the knowledge base and competency to implement evidence-based interventions to reduce infection risk. The principles of infection prevention provide the foundation for the delivery of infusion therapy. Prevention begins with knowledge regarding the techniques used to prevent infection.

1. Standard and Transmission-Based Precautions

Standard precautions are intended to be applied to the care of all patients in all health-care settings, regardless of the suspected or confirmed presence of infectious agents, whereas transmission-based precautions are applied in the presence of known or suspected certain communicable infections. Of note, although these guidelines apply to all settings, the CDC recognizes the shift in health settings to community-based and ambulatory settings and, in 2011, released a summary guide of recommendations specifically aimed at these outpatient settings (CDC, 2011). The specific elements of standard and transmission-based precautions are as follows (Siegel, Rhinehart, Jackson, & Chiarello, 2007).

Tier One: Standard Precautions

Standard precautions incorporate the fundamentals of universal precautions (designed to reduce exposure risks to bloodborne pathogens) and body substance isolation (designed to reduce the risk of exposures to pathogens residing in moist body fluids) and require consistent use for all patients regardless of their infection status. Standard precautions are intended to protect the health-care provider as well as the patient from health-care–associated transmission of infectious agents (Siegel, Rhinehart, Jackson, & Chiarello, 2007).

Standard precautions are based on the principle that all blood, body fluids, secretions, and excretions (except sweat), nonintact skin, and mucous membranes may contain transmissible infectious agents. Standard precautions include the following infection prevention practices: **hand hygiene**; personal protective equipment (PPE) such as gloves, gowns, masks, eye protection, or face shields; and safe injection practices. The application of standard precautions is determined based on the type of interaction with the patient. For example, with peripheral venipuncture, only gloves would normally be worn. In summary, standard precautions are imposed when:

1. there is risk of exposure to blood,
2. there is risk of exposure to other body fluids, including secretions and excretions (not including sweat), whether or not evidence of blood is present,
3. nonintact skin is present, and
4. there will be contact with any mucous membranes.

There are three additional elements of standard precautions that are specifically aimed at protecting the patient. They are:

1. Respiratory hygiene/cough etiquette
2. Safe injection practices
3. Use of masks for insertion of catheters or injection of material into spinal or epidural spaces via lumbar punctures procedures (Siegel, Rhinehart, Jackson, & Chiarello, 2007)

Respiratory Hygiene/Cough Etiquette

The need for vigilance and prompt implementation of infection control measures at the first point of encounter within a health-care setting (e.g., reception and triage areas, outpatient clinics and physician offices) led to this strategy targeted at patients and accompanying family members with undiagnosed transmissible respiratory infections. The term cough etiquette is derived from recommended source control measures for *M. tuberculosis*. Respiratory hygiene/cough etiquette includes:

- Education of health-care facility staff, patients, and visitors
- Posted signs in language(s) appropriate to the population served with instructions to patients and accompanying family members or friends
- Source control measures, such as the patient covering the mouth/nose with a tissue when coughing and promptly disposing of used tissues, and the coughing patient using a face mask when tolerated and appropriate
- Hand hygiene after contact with respiratory secretions
- Spatial separation, ideally greater than 3 feet, of persons with respiratory infections in common waiting areas when possible.

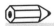 *NURSING FAST FACT!*

*Health-care personnel are advised to observe **droplet precautions** (e.g., wear a mask) and hand hygiene when examining and caring for patients with signs and symptoms of respiratory infection (Siegel, Rhinehart, Jackson, & Chiarello, 2007).*

Safe Injection Practices

Poor infection prevention practices and lack of or poor aseptic technique with injections have led to a campaign aimed at safe practices (CDC, 2011b). Areas of concern include (1) reinsertion of used needles into a multidose vial or solution container and (2) use of a single needle/syringe to administer intravenous medication to multiple patients. Whenever possible, use of single-dose vials is preferred over multidose vials, and multidose vials are only used with a single patient. Outbreaks related to unsafe injection practices indicate that some health-care personnel are unaware of, do not understand, or do not adhere to basic principles of infection control and aseptic technique. Use the CDC Injection Safety Checklist (Figure 2-4) to ensure that the health-care organization is adhering to safe injection practices.

 NURSING FAST FACT!

The use of saline extracted from I.V. bags for the purpose of catheter flushing has resulted in outbreaks of infection and is an unacceptable practice.

INJECTION SAFETY ✅ CHECKLIST

The following Injection Safety checklist items are a subset of items that can be found in the *CDC Infection Prevention Checklist for Outpatient Settings: Minimum Expectations for Safe Care.*

The checklist, which is appropriate for both inpatient and outpatient settings, should be used to systematically assess adherence of healthcare personnel to safe injection practices. (Assessment of adherence should be conducted by direct observation of healthcare personnel during the performance of their duties.)

Injection Safety	Practice Performed?	If answer is No, document plan for remediation
Injections are prepared using aseptic technique in a clean area free from contamination or contact with blood, body fluids or contaminated equipment.	Yes No	
Needles and syringes are used for only one patient (this includes manufactured prefilled syringes and cartridge devices such as insulin pens).	Yes No	
The rubber septum on a medication vial is disinfected with alcohol prior to piercing.	Yes No	
Medication vials are entered with a new needle and a new syringe, even when obtaining additional doses for the same patient.	Yes No	
Single dose (single-use) medication vials, ampules, and bags or bottles of intravenous solution are used for only one patient.	Yes No	
Medication administration tubing and connectors are used for only one patient.	Yes No	
Multi-dose vials are dated by HCP when they are first opened and discarded within 28 days unless the manufacturer specifies a different (shorter or longer) date for that opened vial. Note: This is different from the expiration date printed on the vial.	Yes No	
Multi-dose vials are dedicated to individual patients whenever possible.	Yes No	
Multi-dose vials to be used for more than one patient are kept in a centralized medication area and do not enter the immediate patient treatment area (e.g,. operating room, patient room/cubicle). Note: If multi-dose vials enter the immediate patient treatment area they should be dedicated for single-patient use and discarded immediately after use.	Yes No	

RESOURCES

Checklist: **http://www.cdc.gov/HAI/pdfs/guidelines/ambulatory-care-checklist-07-2011.pdf**

Guide to Infection Prevention for Outpatient Settings: Minimum Expectations for Safe Care:
http://www.cdc.gov/HAI/pdfs/guidelines/standatds-of-ambulatory-care-7-2011.pdf

www.oneandonlycampaign.org

Figure 2-4 ■ Centers for Disease Control and Prevention (CDC) injection safety checklist. (Courtesy of CDC. Available at http://www.cdc.gov/injectionsafety/PDF/SIPC_Checklist.pdf)

INS Standard Single-use systems include single-dose vials and prefilled syringes and are the preferred choices for flushing and locking. If multidose containers must be used, each container should be dedicated to a single patient (INS, 2011a, p. S60).

INFECTION CONTROL PRACTICES FOR SPECIAL LUMBAR PUNCTURE PROCEDURES

In October 2005, a Healthcare Infection Control Practices Advisory Committee (HICPAC) reviewed evidence related to eight cases of bacterial meningitis infection by *Streptococcus* species from oropharyngeal flora of HCWs after myelography. The conclusion warranted the additional protection of a face mask for the individual placing a catheter or injecting material into the spinal or epidural spaces (Siegel, Rhinehart, Jackson, & Chiarello, 2007).

Tier Two: Transmission-Based Precautions

Transmission-based precautions are the second tier of isolation precautions. These additional precautions are based on the known or suspected infectious state of the patient and the possible routes of transmission. It is important to recognize that there are exceptions to application of transmission-based precautions, most notably the home setting, where the risk of transmission is not well defined, an isolation room is not possible, and family members already exposed to diseases generally do not wear masks. Nurses and HCWs who care for patients with infectious diseases need to use some protection. Standard precautions should always be followed. There are three categories of transmission-based precautions:

1. *Airborne precautions,* which require special air handling and ventilation to prevent the spread of organisms. When suspended in air, infectious agents remain infectious over long distances; examples include the organisms that cause tuberculosis, varicella, and measles. The preferred patient placement is in an airborne infection isolation room (AIIR). The AIIR is a single-patient room that is equipped with special air handling and ventilation capacity that meet the American Institute of Architects/Facility Guidelines Institute standards for AIIRs (e.g., monitored negative pressure relative to the surrounding area; 12 air exchanges per hour for new construction and renovation and six air exchanges per hour for existing facilities; air exhausted directly to the outside or recirculated through high-efficiency particulate air [HEPA] filtration before return). Health-care personnel caring for the patient on airborne precautions wear a mask or respirator (HEPA or N95 respirators for patients with tuberculosis), depending on the disease-specific recommendations. The mask is donned before entering the room or, in the case of a patient at home, when entering the home setting (Siegel, Rhinehart, Jackson, & Chiarello, 2007).

2. *Droplet precautions,* which require the use of mucous membrane protection (eye protection and masks) to prevent infectious organisms from contacting the conjunctivae or mucous membranes of the nose or mouth. Examples of infections are mumps, rubella,

influenza, adenovirus, rhinovirus, and pertussis. The pathogens do not remain infectious over long distances in a health-care facility; special air handling and ventilation are not required to prevent droplet transmission. A single-patient room is preferred. Patients on droplet precautions who must be transported outside of the room should wear a mask if tolerated and follow respiratory hygiene/cough etiquette (Siegel, Rhinehart, Jackson, & Chiarello, 2007).

3. *Contact precautions*, which require the PPE use of gloves and gowns when direct skin-to-skin contact or contact with a contaminated environment is anticipated. Don PPE when entering the room and discard it before exiting the room to contain pathogens, especially those that have been implicated in transmission through environmental contamination, such as vancomycin-resistant *Enterococcus* (VRE), *Clostridium difficile*, noroviruses and other intestinal tract pathogens, and respiratory syncytial virus (RSV) (Siegel, Rhinehart, Jackson, & Chiarello, 2007).

2. Hand Hygiene

Hand hygiene has been shown to significantly decrease the risk of contamination and cross-contamination. Touch contamination is a common cause of transfer of pathogens. Although the CDC guidelines on hand hygiene published in 2002 remain current, more recent evidence-based practice guidelines were published in 2009 by the World Health Organization (WHO).

Skin Function/Barrier Protection

The stratum corneum is the most superficial layer of the top layer of the skin (the epidermis). Its function is to reduce water loss, provide protection against abrasive action and microorganisms, and act as a barrier to the environment. The barrier function results from the dying, degeneration, and compaction of underlying epidermis and from the process of synthesis of the stratum corneum occurring at the same rate as loss.

When using specific products for hand hygiene, it is important to maintain normal barrier function. The normal barrier function is biphasic: 50% to 60% of barrier recovery typically occurs within 6 hours, but complete normalization of barrier function requires 5 to 6 days (CDC, 2002).

TRANSMISSION OF PATHOGENS ON HANDS

Bacteria present on hands fall into two categories: resident and transient. **Resident flora** reside under the superficial cells of the stratum corneum and on the skin surface. *Staphylococcus epidermidis* is the most dominant resident. **Transient flora** are microorganisms acquired through patient contact and by contact with environmental surfaces; they tend to be more amenable to removal by routine hand hygiene (WHO, 2009). Transmission of health-care–associated pathogens from one patient to another via the hands of HCWs requires the following sequence of events:

1. Organisms present on the patient's skin (both normal intact skin as well as wounds) or that have been shed onto inanimate objects must be transferred to the hands of HCWs. Areas of skin that tend to be highly colonized include the perineum and inguinal area, but also the axillae, trunk, and upper extremities.
2. These organisms must be capable of surviving for at least several minutes on the hands of personnel.
3. Hand hygiene by the worker is inadequate or omitted entirely, or the agent used for hand hygiene is inappropriate.
4. The contaminated hands of the HCW must come in direct contact with another patient (WHO, 2009).

PREPARATIONS USED FOR HAND HYGIENE

Alcohol-based products are more effective for standard hand washing or hand antisepsis by HCWs than are soaps or antimicrobial soaps. Applying friction removes most microbes and should be used when placing invasive devices, when persistent antimicrobial activity is desired, and when it is important to reduce the numbers of **resident flora** in addition to transient microorganisms (CDC, 2002). Alcohols are not appropriate for use when hands are visibly dirty or contaminated and in the case of suspected or known spore-forming pathogens as discussed below.

RECOMMENDATIONS FOR HAND HYGIENE IN HEALTH-CARE SETTINGS

Recommendations are summarized as follows:
- Wash hands with either a nonantimicrobial or an antimicrobial soap and water when hands are visibly dirty or contaminated with proteinaceous material, when hands are visibly soiled with blood or body fluids, and after using the toilet. Rub hands together vigorously for at least 15 seconds (CDC, 2002).
- An alcohol-based hand rub is preferred for hand hygiene (WHO, 2009), as listed in the bullet points below, except when exposure to spore-forming pathogens is suspected or proven (e.g., presence of *C. difficile*), then soap and water should be used to wash hands.
  - Alcohol kills microbes quickly when applied on the skin. Although there is no residual activity, regrowth of bacteria occurs more slowly after use.
  - Alcohol-based hand rubs that contain humectants cause less drying and irritation than soaps.
  - When using an alcohol-based hand rub, apply a palmful and cover all surfaces of hands, rubbing until hands are completely dry (CDC, 2002); this should take 20 to 30 seconds (WHO, 2009).

- Perform hand hygiene:
  - Before and after touching a patient
  - After contact with body fluids, excretions, mucous membranes, nonintact skin, or wound dressings
  - If moving from a contaminated body site to another body site while providing care on the same patient
  - After removing gloves (sterile and nonsterile)
  - Before handling an invasive device, whether or not gloves are worn
  - After contact with inanimate object(s) in immediate vicinity of patient; this includes medical equipment such as infusion pumps

"My Five Moments for Hand Hygiene" is a model for hand hygiene that is used worldwide. It can be correlated to the indications for hand hygiene (WHO, 2009). The five moments are:

1. Before touching a patient
2. Before a clean/aseptic procedure
3. After body fluid exposure
4. After touching a patient
5. After touching a patient's surroundings

INS Standard Hand hygiene shall be a routine practice established in organizational policies, procedures, and/or practice guidelines (INS, 2011a, p. S26).

> *EBP The role of hospital surfaces (e.g., bed rails, tray tables) in transmitting certain pathogens was reported in a narrative review of the literature. It is estimated that 20% to 40% of HAIs in hospitals are attributable to cross-infection via HCW hands as a result of either directly via patient contact or indirectly through touching environmental surfaces. Pathogens that are able to survive on surfaces for prolonged periods of time include methicillin-resistant Staphylococcus aureus (MRSA), vancomycin-resistant enterococci (VRE), norovirus, Clostridium difficile, and Acinetobacter species. Critically important to reducing transmission of these pathogens are hand hygiene and attention to surface cleaning and disinfection (Weber et al., 2010).*

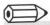 *NURSING FAST FACT!*

- *It is recommended that health-care agencies provide personnel with efficacious hand hygiene products that have a low irritancy potential, particularly when these products are used multiple times per shift.*
- *The use of gloves does not replace hand hygiene and does not provide complete protection.*
- *For insertion of peripheral catheters, good hand hygiene and wearing of gloves during catheter insertion, combined with proper aseptic technique during catheter manipulation, reduce infection risk.*

ADDITIONAL HAND HYGIENE RECOMMENDATIONS

Several studies have demonstrated that skin underneath rings is more heavily colonized than comparable areas of skin on fingers without rings. According to WHO (2009), wearing of rings or other jewelry should be discouraged during health care for several reasons: sharp surfaced rings can puncture gloves, the potential of physical danger (e.g., jewelry caught in equipment), and poorly maintained jewelry may harbor microorganisms. Additional recommendations include:

- Do not wear artificial fingernails or extenders when having direct contact with patients at high risk.
- Keep natural nail tips less than $1/4$ inch long.
- Wear gloves, as part of standard precautions, when in contact with blood or body fluids, mucous membranes, and nonintact skin, and never wear the same pair of gloves for the care of more than one patient.

3. Aseptic Technique

Aseptic technique must be followed for all clinical procedures associated with risk for infections. This includes virtually all infusion procedures. Yet, there is often confusion and misunderstanding about terminology. It is important to understand the difference between the terms sterile, aseptic, and clean technique. Although some clinicians equate aseptic with clean technique, this is not true. Take the example of peripheral I.V. site preparation. *Clean* skin is achieved with soap and water cleansing. This would be inadequate alone for I.V. insertion. Skin antisepsis also must be performed to minimize the presence of microbes on the skin prior to insertion, thus reducing risk for infection.

Once a package is opened and sterile supplies are exposed to the air, the term aseptic technique is used, in preference to sterile technique. As defined earlier in this chapter, aseptic technique is defined as a set of specific practices and procedures performed in a manner that minimizes risk of transmission of pathogenic microorganisms to patients. Aseptic no-touch technique (ANTT) is a specific type of aseptic technique in widespread use throughout the United Kingdom (Rowley, Clare, Macqueen, & Molyneux, 2010). Based on a theoretical and practice framework, hand hygiene and presence of an aseptic field promote aseptic technique, but effective "no-touch" technique ensures it. Critical to ANTT, key parts of the supplies used for an infusion must not be touched, whether with or without gloves, to ensure asepsis. Examples:

- The peripheral I.V. catheter, once taken out of the package and its protective covering removed, cannot be touched before insertion.
- The tip of the flush syringe is protected by a cap that is not to be removed until it is ready for use. The syringe tip must not be touched prior to insertion into the needleless connector.

- The male luer-end of the administration set must be protected by a cap and not touched prior to insertion into the needleless connector or the VAD.
- Needleless connectors must be appropriately disinfected prior to access.

Any I.V.-related product should not be used when it is known to no longer be sterile. Any breaks in asepsis should result in prompt disposal and replacement of the product.

4. Skin Antisepsis

Skin antisepsis prior to VAD placement and as part of site care during catheter dwell time is a critical step in reducing the risk of infection. Skin antisepsis is important because bacteria on the skin at the insertion site can travel along the external surface of the catheter during VAD catheter insertion and during catheter dwell. According to the CDC (O'Grady et al., 2011), acceptable antiseptics for skin antisepsis include 70% alcohol, tincture of iodine, or an iodophor or chlorhexidine/alcohol solution. Chlorhexidine/alcohol solution is the standard of practice and is the preferred antiseptic agent recommended by the INS (2011a); unlike the other antiseptic agents, it has a residual effect on the skin that lasts for up to 48 hours. The current exception is for children younger than 2 months; however, there is evolving evidence of chlorhexidine safety and efficacy for all age groups (Pedivan, 2010). Of note, TJC (2012b) provides guidance for prevention of catheter-associated BSIs with their National Patient Safety Goals. One of the goals addresses the requirement for use of an antiseptic cited in the scientific literature or endorsed by a professional organization for skin preparation during CVAD insertion.

For patients who are sensitive or allergic to chlorhexidine or alcohol and for children younger than 2 months, povidone-iodine is considered an acceptable disinfectant. To be most effective, povidone-iodine requires at least 2 minutes of contact time on the skin (CDC, 2002; INS, 2011; Pedivan, 2010). For patients with compromised skin integrity or infants younger than 2 months, the povidone-iodine can be removed with sterile normal saline or sterile water to prevent absorption of the product through the skin (Pedivan, 2010).

Additional important aspects of skin preparation include the following:

- Antimicrobial solutions in a single-unit use configuration should be used.
- Alcohol should not be applied after the application of povidone-iodine preparation because alcohol negates the effect of povidone-iodine.
- The antimicrobial preparation solution should be allowed to air-dry completely before proceeding with the VAD insertion procedure or as part of routine site care, prior to dressing placement.

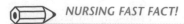 *NURSING FAST FACT!*

> ■ *It is never acceptable to speed up the drying process of skin antisepsis by "blowing" on or fanning the area!*

5. Catheter Dressings

Maintaining a clean, dry, and occlusive dressing is important in protecting the catheter insertion site and reducing the risk for infection. A dressing is placed at the time of catheter insertion and is regularly changed as part of the overall site care procedure with CVADs.

Dressing choices include transparent dressings, gauze dressings, and antimicrobial dressings. Use of a transparent versus a gauze dressing is based on the patient's preference and needs because there is no current evidence supporting one choice over the other. Most often, the transparent dressing is preferred based on the following advantages:

- Less frequent need for replacement (and associated site care)
  - Recommendations for transparent dressing changes are every 7 days (INS, 2011a; O'Grady et al., 2011)
- Ability to easily and continually visualize the insertion site for any signs of local infection without disturbing the dressing
- Less cost in supplies and in nursing time as a result of less frequent dressing changes

Gauze dressings are changed at least every 2 days (INS, 2011a; O'Grady et al., 2011). Indications for use of a gauze dressing include:

- Site drainage; for example, gauze dressings are often used on newly placed CVADs because bleeding may occur in the first 24 hours
- Patients who perspire excessively
- Patients who have a sensitivity or allergic reaction to transparent dressings

Dressings should *always* be changed earlier than the scheduled 2- or 7-day interval if they become loosened, dislodged, or wet, or if blood or drainage is present. The presence of a damp dressing or drainage around the site provides a culture medium for bacterial growth, which increases the risk of infection.

> *EBP Lack of attention to dressing care was found in an assessment of compliance with CVAD maintenance. Deficiencies were found in 31% of 420 CVAD sites observed; these included blood present under dressings, exposed insertion sites, and visible moisture under the dressings (Rupp, Cassling, & Faber, 2013). Although there was no correlation found between CVAD site maintenance and CLABSI in this single-site study, the researchers emphasize the importance of site maintenance.*

EBP Another study of CVAD dressings in ICU patients found that more than two dressing changes for disruption (e.g., undressed site or soiled dressing) was associated with a higher than threefold increase in the risk for infection (Timsit et al., 2012a). The researchers suggest that assessing the CVAD dressing and ensuring dressing integrity is an important element of post-insertion care.

Antimicrobial dressings, such as chlorhexidine-impregnated sponge dressings, are commonly used with short-term CVADs because research supports their benefits in hospitalized patients (Timsit et al., 2009). The most well-known product is a small, round sponge disc that incrementally releases chlorhexidine. It is placed around the catheter at the exit site, covered with a transparent dressing, and changed every 7 days. Note that it is not a stand alone dressing in that it is always covered with another dressing, usually a transparent one (Figure 2-5). A transparent dressing with an integrated gel pad of chlorhexidine also is available. A recently published randomized controlled trial found that chlorhexidine gel–impregnated dressings decreased the infection rate in patients with intravascular catheters in the ICU compared to a highly adhesive transparent dressing (Timsit et al., 2012b) (Figure 2-6).

Another aspect of dressing care is the importance of protecting the catheter dressing from water. The catheter and connecting device (e.g., needleless connector) should be protected with an impermeable cover during showering (O'Grady et al., 2011). There are products specifically designed for this purpose (Figure 2-7).

 NURSING FAST FACT!

Some nurses like to place a transparent dressing over the gauze dressing to secure the gauze in place. It is important to recognize that if gauze is used under the transparent dressing, it is considered a gauze dressing and must be changed at least every 48 hours (INS, 2011). A gauze dressing is often placed under the wings to stabilize the noncoring needle with implanted ports, followed by application of a transparent dressing. If the gauze does not obstruct the needle insertion site, the transparent dressing may be changed every 7 days (INS, 2011, p. S50).

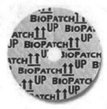

Figure 2-5 ■ Biopatch®. (Courtesy of J&J Wound Management, Division of Ethicon, Inc., Somerville, NJ.)

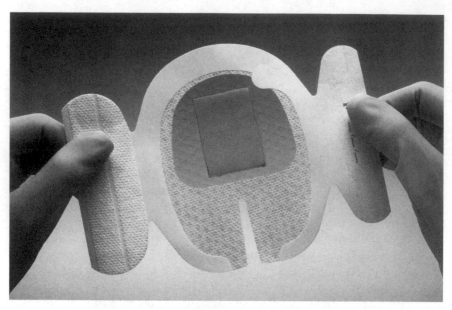

Figure 2-6 ■ Chlorhexidine (CHG) transparent semipermeable dressing. (Courtesy of 3M Medical Division, St. Paul, MN.)

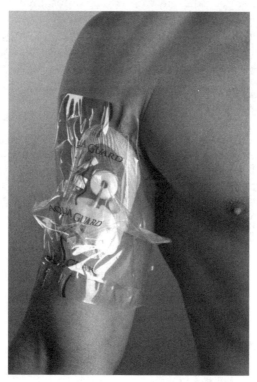

Figure 2-7 ■ Aquaguard. (Courtesy of Cenorin, LLC, Kent, WA.)

6. Catheter Stabilization

Catheter stabilization is considered an important step in the care of peripheral I.V. catheters, nontunneled CVADs, and PICCs. Catheter movement in and out of the insertion site allows pathogens on the skin to migrate into the catheter tract (McGoldrick, 2010). The concept of catheter stabilization often is confusing. Many nurses believe that the dressing itself stabilizes or secures the catheter in place or that use of surgical strips ("Steri-Strips") or sterile tape will stabilize the catheter. However, there is no evidence supporting the benefits of a dressing or tape alone in catheter hub stabilization.

Stabilization is achieved through use of an engineered stabilization device; in the case of CVADs, sutures may be used. A common type of engineered stabilization device consists of an adhesive pad and a mechanism to hold the catheter to the pad. The purpose is to control catheter movement at the catheter insertion site (Figure 2-8). Certain types of dressings in conjunction with a platform (i.e., "winged") type of peripheral I.V. catheter also may qualify as a stabilization device (Bausone-Gazsa, Lefaiver, & Walters, 2010). A newer, novel stabilization product specific for PICC stabilization is a small anchor that is placed beneath the skin in the subcutaneous tissue. Advantages to this product are no need for replacement, ease of site antisepsis, and no adhesives, which can be an issue for some patients. This product was found to be efficacious in a small study of 68 in- and outpatients in three different institutions (Egan et al., 2013) (see Chapter 5, Figure 5-21).

Because the presence of sutures may increase the risk for infection, the CDC recommends sutureless stabilization devices to reduce the risk of infection in CVADs (O'Grady et al., 2011). However, the use of sutures may be considered appropriate in special populations (e.g., pediatric patients or those with skin integrity problems), thus precluding use of tape or an engineered stabilization device (INS, 2011).

> **INS Standard** VAD stabilization shall be used to preserve the integrity of the access device, minimize catheter movement at the hub, and prevent catheter dislodgement and loss of access (INS, 2011a, p. S46).

7. Antimicrobial/Antiseptic-Impregnated Catheters

Catheters that are coated or impregnated with antimicrobial or antiseptic agents can decrease the risk for catheter-related BSIs. Several different types of materials are used to coat catheters. They include:

- Chlorhexidine/silver sulfadiazine: Newest generation available with coating over both internal and external luminal surfaces; more expensive than standard catheters

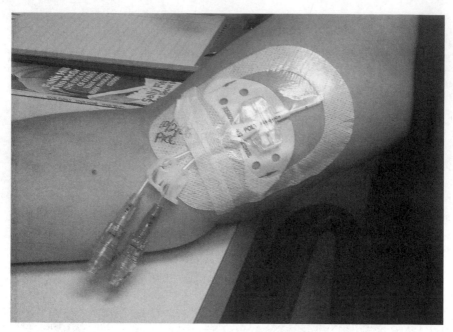

Figure 2-8 ■ Transparent dressing over a peripherally inserted central catheter with stabilization device—StatLock®. (Courtesy of Mark R Hunter CRNI, VA-BC, RN.)

- Minocycline/rifampin: Available impregnated on both external and internal surfaces. Although there is concern about development of antimicrobial resistance, this risk is low.
- Platinum/silver: Ionic metals have a broad antimicrobial activity and are being used in catheters and cuffs.

There are also new catheters with chlorhexidine chemically bound to both the internal and external catheter surfaces (see Chapter 5, Central Vascular Access Devices, for more information). Based on current data, the CDC guidelines recommend use of a chlorhexidine/silver sulfadiazine or minocycline/rifampin CVAD in patients when the expected duration of catheterization is expected to be greater than 5 days *if* the CLABSI rate has not decreased with implementation of a comprehensive strategy, which includes staff education, use of maximal sterile barrier precautions, and use of chlorhexidine/alcohol skin antisepsis prior to catheter placement (O'Grady et al., 2011).

8. Central Line Bundle

Although today many specialty nurses, in addition to physicians, are placing CVADs, nonspecialty nurses also play an important role in assisting and ensuring that CVADs are placed according to the central line bundle. Implementation of the "central line bundle" in acute care hospitals has resulted in a markedly decreased rate of central venous access device–related infections. The concept of a "bundle" was originally identified by Resar et al., 2012). A bundle is a group of evidence-based interventions that, when implemented consistently together as a "package," result in better outcomes than any component implemented individually.

The basic components of the central line bundle adopted by the IHI in its five million lives campaign include:

- Hand hygiene prior to catheter insertion
- Maximal sterile barrier precautions with insertion (catheter inserter wears a cap, mask, sterile gloves and gown, and a large sterile drape is placed over patient during insertion)
- Chlorhexidine skin antisepsis
- Avoidance of the femoral site
- Daily review of line necessity with prompt removal of unnecessary lines (Resar et al., 2012)

The origin of the bundle came from a now classic study. With implementation of the above interventions, a 66% reduction in the CLABSI rate was demonstrated across 103 ICUs in the state of Michigan (Pronovost et al., 2006). In addition to the bundle, interventions included comprehensive education, use of CVAD carts that contain all needed supplies, a checklist to ensure all procedures are followed, and the power to stop the procedure for any breaches.

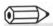 *NURSING FAST FACT!*

Bundles that include checklists to prevent central line–associated BSIs are now identified as one of the top 10 "strongly encouraged patient safety practices" (Agency for Healthcare Research and Quality [AHRQ], 2013).

EBP The employment of five evidence-based interventions, along with an improved culture for patient safety, can prevent CLABSI (Pronovost et al., 2010). In a follow-up study examining the sustainability of reduction in BSIs, it was found that the original reduction in infection rate was sustained for an additional 18 months with a mean CLABSI rate of 1.1. per 1000 central line days and a median of zero. The five evidence-based interventions included hand hygiene, use of full barrier precautions, cleansing the skin with chlorhexidine, avoiding the femoral site when possible at the time of CVAD placement, and removal of unnecessary catheters. This model led to a national effort for CLABSI reduction supported by the AHRQ (TJC, 2012a).

9. Other Aspects of Postinsertion Care

Optimal care at the time of catheter placement can prevent infections, but the risk of infection is present the entire time the catheter is in place.

Research and attention are now aimed at postinsertion care and maintenance, which is an underestimated aspect of infusion care.

Ongoing attention to the catheter site through regular skin antisepsis,
use of antimicrobial dressing products, and dressing replacement, as
discussed above, are important in preventing growth of skin microorganisms. As discussed earlier, contamination of the catheter and catheter
hub gives microbes access via the internal catheter lumen. To summarize
interventions to reduce risk, attention must be paid to the following:

- Hand hygiene
- Aseptic technique used with all access procedures
- Administration set changes as discussed earlier
- Changing needleless connectors according to manufacturer's
  recommendations
- Disinfection of needleless connectors prior to access and/or use of
  alcohol disinfection caps placed on needleless connectors between
  intermittent access for infusions

The use of antimicrobial locking solutions, such as dilute vancomycin/
heparin solution or ethanol locks, also may be considered. The CDC
recommends their use in patients with long-term CVADs who have a
history of multiple CLABSIs despite maximal adherence to aseptic technique (O'Grady et al., 2011). Although studies have demonstrated reduced
risk for infection, concerns about antimicrobial resistance limit their use as a
routine practice. There also is concern about the effect of the solution on the
catheter; for example, the use of ethanol is not recommended with certain
types of CVADs because it can break down the catheter material. Manufacturer's recommendations should always be reviewed and considered.

*EBP More comprehensive data collection submitted to and analyzed by the
NHSN is useful in designing infection prevention programs. For example, in
2010 it was found that, in the state of Pennsylvania, 71.7% of CLABSIs
occurred more than 5 days after insertion, suggesting internal lumen contamination and the need to pay more attention to catheter maintenance
procedures (Davis, 2011).*

*EBP Use of a disinfection cap impregnated with alcohol and placed on the
needleless connector significantly reduced line contamination, density of
organisms, and CLABSIs. This study was done in an acute care facility and
involved three phases: phase 1 baseline—standard scrub of needleless connector, phase 2—disinfection cap placed on all CVADs, and phase 3—back
to standard scrub. Infection rates were reduced in phase 2 and increased
back to phase 1 levels when the organization reverted back to a standard
scrub of the needleless connector (Wright et al., 2013).*

NURSING POINTS OF CARE
PREVENTION OF INFUSION-RELATED INFECTIONS

Nursing Assessments

History

- History of any exposure to pathogens in the environment, including work, recent travel, contact with people who are ill
- Past and present disease histories
- Immunization history
- Risk factors for infection (Table 2-3)

Physical Assessment
- Baseline immunologic studies: WBC count, differential (Table 2-5)
- Vital signs, especially elevated temperature and pulse rate
- Assess for signs of local infection: Erythema, inflammation, purulent drainage, tenderness, warmth at catheter site
- Assess skin turgor and mucous membranes

Key Nursing Interventions
1. Reduce exposure to pathogens through the use of aseptic technique.
2. Follow standard precautions at all times and transmission-based precautions as appropriate.
3. Maintain skin integrity and natural defenses against infection.
4. Use aseptic technique with all infusion-related procedures.
5. Pay attention to skin antisepsis at time of VAD placement and with routine site care.
6. Remove the peripheral I.V. catheter at first sign of complications or if no longer necessary.
7. Change the VAD dressing regularly (e.g., every 7 days with transparent dressing) and earlier if the dressing becomes wet, soiled, or nonocclusive.
8. Secure proximal I.V. connections with a luer-lock set.
9. Monitor for:
    a. Signs and symptoms of infection (fever, hypotension, positive blood cultures)
    b. Oxygen saturation with oximetry
10. Inspect all infusates before administering.
11. Follow central line bundle and postinsertion care interventions.

> Table 2-5 **COMMON TESTS FOR EVALUATING THE PRESENCE OR RISK OF INFUSION-RELATED INFECTIONS**

Test	Description
White blood cell (WBC) count with differential	A breakdown of the types of WBCs; normal WBC count is 5000–10,000/mm³. Constitute the body's primary defense system against foreign organisms, tissues, and other substances. Life span of a normal WBC is 13–20 days. Produced in bone marrow. Leukocytosis ((WBC), and leukopenia ((WBC). Acute leukocytosis is initially accompanied by changes in WBC count, followed by changes in individual WBCs.
Blood culture	A sample of blood is placed on culture media and evaluated for growth of pathogens. Collected whenever bacteremia or septicemia is suspected.
Panels to evaluate specific disease exposure Immunoglobulin (IgA, IgG, IgM) levels	Blood tests to evaluate exposure to specific diseases (e.g., human immunodeficiency virus [HIV], hepatitis). Identifies immunocompromised status. Blood tests to evaluate humoral immunity status. Immunoglobulins neutralize toxic substances, support phagocytosis, and destroy invading microorganisms. Evaluates humoral immunity status. IgA: Evaluates anaphylaxis associated with transfusion of blood and blood products. IgG: Chronic or recurrent infections. IgM: Viral infections.
C-reactive protein (CRP)	CRP is a glycoprotein produced by the liver in response to acute inflammation. CRP assay is a nonspecific test that determines the presence (not the cause) of inflammation; it is often ordered in conjunction with ESR.
Cold agglutinin titer	Used to diagnose atypical infections by detecting antigens in the blood. Cold agglutinins are antibodies that cause clumping or agglutination of RBCs at cold temperatures in individuals who are infected by a particular organism.
Erythrocyte (red blood cell [RBC]) sedimentation rate (ESR; or sedimentation rate)	Measures rate of sedimentation of RBCs in an anticoagulated whole blood sample over a specified period of time. The basis of the ESR test is the alteration of blood proteins by inflammatory and necrotic processes. Nonspecific indicator of widespread inflammatory reaction as a result of infection or autoimmune disorders.

Source: Van Leeuwen, A. M., Kranpitz, T. R., & Smith, L. (2006). Davis's comprehensive handbook of laboratory and diagnostic tests with nursing implications (2nd ed.). Philadelphia: F. A. Davis.

▋ Occupational Hazards

Occupational hazards specifically associated with infusion therapy include risk for exposure to bloodborne pathogens, exposure to hazardous drugs, and latex allergy. Inserting VADs, administering infusions, handling and discarding sharps, and assisting with sterile procedures and many other high-risk procedures are ordinary parts of the daily practice regimen for nurses who administer infusion therapy.

Bloodborne Pathogens

Injuries from needlesticks and other sharps are a serious concern for all HCWs. Pathogens such as hepatitis B virus (HBV), hepatitis C virus (HCV), and HIV pose grave and potentially deadly risks to HCWs. A survey sponsored by the American Nurses Association (ANA, 2008) identified three main causes of needlestick injury accounting for two thirds of the problem: while giving an injection, before activating the safety feature, and during disposal of a nonsafety device. Other less common causes include after a coworker left a sharp on a surface, in response to an action by a co-worker, and while activating a safety feature.

In 2000 Congress passed the Needlestick Safety and Prevention Act (NSPA) (http://www.gpo.gov/fdsys/pkg/PLAW-106publ430/html/PLAW-106publ430.htm), and in 2001 OSHA (2001) published an amended version of the bloodborne pathogens standard. Although these efforts have resulted in increased use of safety engineered devices in health care, there is still work to do.

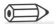 *NURSING FAST FACT!*

> The ANA performed a Health and Safety Survey in 2011 and found a significant improvement in the use of safety needles from 82% in 2001 to 96% in 2011 (Daley, 2012). Of note, only 76% of nurses said their facilities used safety needles frequently, nurses were not involved in selecting safety products 19% of the time, and 43% did not know if nurses were involved in decision making.

The International Healthcare Worker Safety Center (n.d.) at the University of Virginia drafted and circulated a consensus statement on sharps safety in 2011. Endorsed by the ANA, INS, and numerous other nursing and health-care organizations, the consensus statement focuses on the following:

- Improving sharps safety in surgical settings
- Understanding and reducing exposure risk in nonhospital settings
- Involving frontline workers in selection of safety devices
- Addressing gaps in current safety products
- Enhancing worker education and training (Daley, 2012)

There are several categories of safety devices. *Active* devices require the HCW to activate a safety mechanism. Failure to do so leaves the worker unprotected; thus, education in proper use by HCWs is critical. *Passive* safety devices remain in effect before, during, and after device use and do not require activation. The INS (2011a, p. S28) states that the nurse should advocate for passive safety engineered devices for needlestick injury prevention. An *integrated safety design* means that the safety feature is built in as an integral part of the device and cannot be removed; this is the preferred design feature. An *accessory safety device* is external to the device and must be carried to or temporarily or permanently fixed to the point of use; because this is dependent on employee compliance, it is less desirable. Types of safety devices relevant to infusion therapy are listed in Table 2-6.

Requirements of the OSHA bloodborne pathogens standard include the following:

- A written exposure control plan aimed at eliminating/minimizing exposure to bloodborne pathogens. This plan must be reviewed every year.
- Attention to adherence to standard precautions, previously addressed in this chapter
- Engineering controls and work practices to eliminate or minimize worker exposure. These are aimed at isolating or removing pathogens from the workplace and include sharps disposal containers and safety needle products.
- Input from nonmanagerial HCWs responsible for patient care in selection of engineering controls
- Prohibition from bending, recapping, or removing contaminated needles from a syringe
- Proper disposal: Use of sharps containers, not overfilling containers, no shearing or breaking of needles
- Use of PPE

> Table 2-6	SHARPS SAFETY DEVICES AND RECOMMENDATIONS
Practice	**Safety Recommendations**
Blood drawing	Shielded or self-blunting needles for vacuum tube phlebotomy Shielded, retracting, or self-blunting butterfly-type needles Automatically retracting finger/heelstick lancets Plastic (not glass) blood collection vacuum tubes Ensure that blood is never injected through the rubber stopper of a vacuum tube using an exposed needle
Infusion	Needleless infusion systems Vascular access devices with safety feature; passive safety products preferred Safety noncoring needle for implanted port access

Sources: International Healthcare Worker Safety Center (n.d.); INS, 2011.

- Free HBV vaccinations
- Postexposure evaluation and follow-up, including access to prophylaxis treatment and procedures for evaluating the circumstances surrounding exposure incidents
- Recordkeeping, including an employer sharps injury log (OSHA, 2001)

Mucocutaneous Exposure to Bloodborne Pathogens

Although most attention is paid to needlestick or sharps, mucocutaneous transmission is another route of exposure to bloodborne pathogens. This refers to blood or body fluid exposure through a break in intact skin or from mucous membrane exposure of the eyes, nose, or mouth of the HCW. Although the chance of becoming infected with HIV after mucocutaneous exposure to infected blood is 0.1% (one third the chance after a needlestick injury) and the risks of HBV and HCV infection also are lower, the risks should not be underestimated (Delisio, 2012). Exposure may occur from accidental splashing of blood into the eyes or a skin cut, when starting or removing VAD, during disposal of body fluids, or during dressing of an open wound. A 2003 study found that nurses had a higher mucocutaneous exposure rate than physicians and medical technologists. More than one third (39%) of registered nurses and one fourth (27%) of licensed practical nurses said they had experienced one or more mucocutaneous blood exposures in the previous 3 months, yet few reported their exposures (Delisio, 2012).

Prevention of Exposure to Bloodborne Pathogens

- Consider all blood, body fluids, secretions, and excretions (except sweat), nonintact skin, and mucous membranes as potentially infectious.
- Use hand hygiene.
- Follow standard precautions.
- Use appropriate PPE (gloves, gown, mask, eye protection, face shield) during care.
- Use safety products.
- Become involved in product evaluation and decision making. Nurses must realize that the right to be involved is part of the NSPA (Foley, 2012). Echoing direction from the regulations, the INS (2011a, p. S28) states that the nurse should be involved in the multidisciplinary team to develop, implement, and evaluate a plan to reduce needlestick injury.

NOTE > Safety features for needleless and needle protection systems are discussed in detail in Chapter 5.

Websites

American Nurses Association: Needlestick Injury Prevention: www.nursingworld.org/mainmenucategories/occupationalandenvironmental/occupationalhealth/safeneedles.aspx

CDC: Bloodborne infectious diseases: HIV/AIDS, Hepatitis B, Hepatitis C: www.cdc.gov/niosh/topics/bbp

Occupational Safety and Health Administration: Needlestick/Sharps Injuries: http://www.osha.gov/SLTC/etools/hospital/hazards/sharps/sharps.html#safer

International Healthcare Worker Safety Center: Safety Device List: www.healthsystem.virginia.edu/pub/epinet/new/chcklst2.pdf

 NURSING FAST FACT!

The primary barriers to protect HCWs from blood and/or body fluid exposures are gloves in conjunction with appropriate hand hygiene practices, and appropriate PPE.

Hazardous Drugs

HCWs who work with or near hazardous drugs may be exposed to these agents in the air or on work surfaces, clothing, medical equipment, or patient urine or feces. Nurses are exposed to hazardous drugs during infusion administration, such as when priming and disconnecting I.V. administration sets, changing infusion containers, and during disposal (Eisenberg, 2012). Pathways of exposure include skin contact with drugs and inhalation. Hazardous drugs have demonstrated the ability to cause chromosome breakage in circulating lymphocytes, mutagenic activity in urine, and skin necrosis after surface contact with abraded skin or damage to normal skin. Concern about exposure to hazardous drugs dates back to the 1970s, particularly in relation to antineoplastic drugs. These agents remain the main focus of concern, but other hazardous drugs include some antiviral drugs, hormones, and bioengineered drugs. OSHA published guidelines for the management of cytotoxic (antineoplastic) drugs in the workplace in 1986 and updated those guidelines in 2004 (NIOSH, 2004). NIOSH publishes periodic updated lists of hazardous drugs (NIOSH, 2012). Drugs are considered hazardous when they exhibit one or more of the following characteristics in humans or animals:

1. Carcinogenicity (e.g., leukemia, lymphoma, skin cancer)
2. Teratogenicity or other developmental toxicity (e.g., learning disabilities in offspring)

3. Reproductive toxicity (e.g., menstrual cycle changes, spontaneous abortion, infertility)
4. Organ toxicity at low doses
5. Genotoxicity (e.g., chromosomal damage)
6. Structure and toxicity of new drugs that mimic existing drugs determined hazardous by the above criteria (NIOSH, 2004)

Nurses who administer hazardous drugs require special education aimed at personal protection. Some of the guidelines from NIOSH (2004) aimed at reducing risk of exposure are accomplished by:

- Hazardous drug preparation in an area that is devoted to that purpose alone and is restricted to only authorized personnel
- Preparation of hazardous drugs inside a ventilated cabinet designed to protect workers and others from exposure and to protect all drugs that require sterile handling
- Using chemotherapy sharps disposal containers for drug-contaminated syringes and other supplies
- Cleaning and decontaminating work areas before and after each activity involving hazardous drugs and at the end of each shift.
- Cleaning up small spills of hazardous drugs immediately, using proper safety precautions and PPE. For nurses who provide chemotherapy in the home setting, a "spill kit" should be available in the homes of patients receiving such infusions.
- Wearing chemotherapy gloves and disposable, closed-front, long-sleeved gowns during drug preparation and administration.
- Using a face shield when splashes to the eyes, nose, or mouth may occur and when adequate engineering controls (e.g., sash or window on a ventilated cabinet) are not available.
- Washing hands with soap and water immediately after using personal protective clothing such as disposable gloves and gowns.

Although most organizations pay attention to the NIOSH guidelines, they are technical voluntary guidelines and have not been enforced (Eisenberg, 2012). In a published survey, a researcher found that nurses do not consistently implement safety precautions such as wearing chemotherapy gloves and gowns (Polovich & Clark, 2012). Of note, the state of Washington passed bills in 2011 requiring facilities to follow NIOSH guidelines (Eisenberg, 2012).

Latex Allergy

Natural rubber latex (NRL) allergy is a serious medical issue for HCWs. Latex allergy develops with exposure to NRL, a plant cytosol that was used extensively to manufacture medical gloves and other medical devices. The prevalence of latex allergy has been the highest in HCWs, rubber industry workers, patients with multiple injuries, and children with bladder issues (Gawchik, 2011). Allergic reactions to latex range from asthma to anaphylaxis, which can result in chronic illness, disability, career loss, and death. There is no treatment for latex allergy except complete avoidance of latex. Patients and health-care providers must be assured of safety from sensitization and allergic reaction to latex.

There are three types of reactions that occur with latex exposure:

1. Latex allergy (immediate hypersensitivity): Occurs within minutes to hours after exposure. Mild reactions include skin redness, hives, and/or itching. More severe reactions include runny nose, sneezing, itchy eyes, scratchy throat, wheezing, coughing, or difficulty breathing. Although anaphylactic shock can occur, it usually is not associated with the first exposure.
2. Irritant contact dermatitis: The most common reaction, which includes symptoms of dry, itchy, irritated skin
3. Allergic contact dermatitis (delayed hypersensitivity): Similar to a poison ivy reaction that shows up 24 to 96 hours after contact (NIOSH, 2010)

In recent years, the incidence of latex allergy in the United States has significantly decreased as a result of prevention efforts, although it remains a worldwide problem because of continued use of powdered latex gloves (Gawchik, 2011). Many other medical products may contain latex. Examples include tapes, catheters, goggles, masks, electrode pads, injection ports on I.V. administration sets, blood pressure cuffs, and stethoscopes (NIOSH, 2010). In the home setting, many objects may also contain latex, such as baby bottle nipples, balloons, erasers, carpeting, and dishwashing gloves (NIOSH, 2010). HCWs with an allergy to NRL who are providing care in the home setting should be aware of these additional objects that may place them at increased risk for an allergic response.

Nurses working in infusion therapy are at risk because of the common routes of exposure. The routes of exposure for latex reaction for infusion specialists include aerosols and glove contact. Employer recommendations to prevent latex exposure include the following:

■ Use of gloves that are latex free and resistant to bloodborne pathogens (e.g., nitrile, vinyl)
■ If latex gloves are used, the gloves should be made of reduced protein and powder free.
■ Education and training for employees
■ Medical evaluation for any employees with early symptoms
■ Frequent cleaning of areas potentially contaminated with latex dust

INS Standards Exposure to latex in the environment shall be minimized. Powdered gloves made of NRL should be eliminated from the environment. The nurse should have knowledge about evolving guidelines about preventing allergic reactions (INS, 2011a, p. S30).

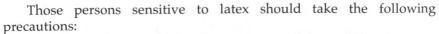

Those persons sensitive to latex should take the following precautions:

- Avoid all contact with latex.
- Avoid areas where latex is likely to be inhaled.
- Inform the employer.
- Before receiving any injections or undergoing any medical procedures, consult about any modifications in supplies used.
- Wear a medical identification bracelet (NIOSH, 2010).

To reduce the risk of an allergic response, avoid using hand lotions or lubricants that contain mineral oil, petroleum salves, and other hydrocarbon-based gels or lotions to prevent the breakdown of the glove material and maintain barrier protection. Do not reuse disposable examination gloves because disinfecting agents can damage the barrier properties of gloves. Following hand hygiene guidelines is recommended after gloves are removed and before a new pair is applied. Gloves should not be stored where they will be subjected to excessive heat, direct ultraviolet or fluorescent light, or ozone (NIOSH, 2010).

NOTE > Manufacturers of nonlatex- and nonchlorine- (nonvinyl and nonneoprene) containing gloves are listed on Davis*Plus*, along with additional website resources of latex allergy.

NURSING POINTS OF CARE:
ALLERGIC RESPONSE TO LATEX

Assessment
- Obtain a history of risk factors (persons with neural tube defects, atopic individuals including those with allergies to food products); those who possess a known or suspected NRL allergy; persons with ongoing occupational exposure to NRL (e.g., HCWs, rubber industry workers, laboratory personnel).
- Question the patient about associated symptoms of itching, swelling, and redness after contact with rubber products such as rubber gloves, balloons, and barrier contraceptives.

Key Nursing Interventions
- Treat latex-sensitive patients as if they have NRL allergy.
- Supply materials and items that are latex free.
- Collaborate with the pharmacy to have a list of latex-containing drugs available.
- Encourage wearing of MedicAlert bracelet.
- Encourage importance of carrying an emergency kit.

AGE-RELATED CONSIDERATIONS

The Pediatric Patient

The pediatric population is diverse, and the risk of infection varies with age, birthweight, underlying disease, host factors, medications, type of device, and nature of the infusion therapy. Immunity and risk for infection are of particular concern in the newborn infant. Antibodies are provided primarily through passive immunity by immunoglobulin G (IgG) transfer across the placenta during pregnancy. This maternal antibody wanes over time, with little remaining by 3 to 6 months of age (Levinson, 2012). Newborns also have less effective T-cell function.

The Older Adult

Immunity generally declines with age. There is a reduced IgG response to certain antigens, fewer T cells, and a reduced and delayed hypersensitivity response (Levinson, 2012). These conditions result in increased susceptibility to infections; also, the severity of infections is worse in older than in younger adults (Levinson, 2012; Smith & Cotter, 2012).

Home Care Issues

It is generally believed that at-home risk factors for developing a catheter-related infection are lower than are risk factors in a hospital setting. Although many home care patients are more active, and activities such as bathing, gardening, and playing with pets may pose some risk, the risk of transmission associated with multiple patients/multiple providers in the institution is eliminated in the home setting. Patients and their caregivers must take personal responsibility related to care of the vascular access device (VAD). Although available studies show that the risk for I.V.-related infections at home is low (McGoldrick, 2010), there is a need for new research to develop an understanding of which home care patients pose the greatest risk for infection and what interventions are critical for prevention.

As discussed earlier, standard precautions apply in the home setting, but transmission-based precautions must be adapted and applied as appropriate in the home setting. For example, the patient with active tuberculosis may be quarantined in the home, and home care staff providing care could be fitted for and provided N95 respirators to wear when making a home visit. In the case of multidrug-resistant organisms (MDROs), such as methicillin-resistant *Staphylococcus aureus* (MRSA), standard precautions apply unless a higher level of precautions is required. In that case, limit the use of patient care equipment utilized repeatedly (e.g., blood pressure cuff, stethoscope), leave it in the home, and transport it to an appropriate site for cleaning and disinfection (Siegel, Rhinehart, Jackson, & Chiarello, 2007). Each nurse or aide providing care in the home needs appropriate equipment and supplies related to infection control. The home health clinician typically carries a "nursing bag" from home to home. It should contain needed supplies such

Home Care Issues—cont'd

as blood pressure cuffs, stethoscope, blood glucose meter (glucometer), pulse oximeter, hand hygiene, and other medical supplies (e.g., dressings), disinfectants to clean equipment (e.g., stethoscope diaphragm) after use, and a spill kit in case a large amount of blood or body fluid spills on the floor or any other surface. Because it is recognized that microorganisms may be transferred to the nursing bag, many organizations employ "bag technique" strategies such as using a barrier under the bag, hand hygiene prior to accessing equipment, and routine bag cleaning.

> *EBP Nursing bags from four different home care agencies were cultured. It was found that approximately 84% of the outside of the bags cultured positive for human pathogens (15.9% multidrug-resistant organisms [MDROs]); 48.4% of the inside of the bags had positive cultures (6.3% MDROs), and 43.7% of patient care equipment was contaminated with human pathogens (5.6% MDROs). Although this study only described the existence of pathogens on the nursing bag, it is recognized that there is potential risk for transmission of infection from one patient to another via contaminated nursing bags (Bakunas-Kenneley & Madigan, 2009).*

The home care provider should establish policies and procedures for handling waste.
- Sharps containers must be used for all contaminated sharps generated by the nurse.
- Infusion pharmacies should deliver sharps containers to the patient's home and pick them up when therapy is completed or the containers are full.
- For "mail back" sharps container programs, the patient is provided with packaging and labeling to return the containers when they are full.
- Prepackaged kits available from a number of manufacturers include sharps disposal systems and chemotherapy spill kits.

 Patient Education

In all health-care environments, patient education is an important component in preventing infusion-related complications. Education regarding vascular access management is crucial. Information regarding catheter management should be individualized to meet the patient's needs but remain consistent with established policies and procedures for infection control.

Education should include:
■ Instructions on hand hygiene; aseptic technique; and concept of dirty, clean, and sterile

Continued

Patient Education—cont'd

- Proper methods for handling equipment
- Judicious use of antibiotics, which is a major nursing role to slow an epidemic of drug-resistant infections
- Importance of adhering to directions for prescribed antibiotics
- Dressing changes
- Assessment of the site and the key signs and symptoms to report to the home care agency, hospital health-care worker, or physician
- Information regarding emergency procedures should catheter break or rupture

Allergy
- Provide information about natural rubber latex allergy and sensitivity

Nursing Process

The nursing process is a six-step process for problem solving that guides nursing action. See Chapter 1 for details on the steps of the nursing process related to vascular access. The following table focuses on nursing diagnoses, nursing outcomes classification (NOC), and nursing interventions classification (NIC) for infection control and risk management. Nursing diagnoses should be patient specific and outcomes and interventions individualized. The NOC and NIC presented here are suggested directions for development of outcomes and interventions.

Nursing Diagnoses Related to Infection Control and Safety	Nursing Outcomes Classification (NOC)	Nursing Intervention Classification (NIC)
Allergic response: Latex, related to: Hypersensitivity to natural latex rubber protein	Allergic response: Localized or systemic, immune hypersensitivity response, symptom severity, tissue integrity, skin and mucous membranes	Allergy management, latex precautions
Skin integrity, impaired, related to: *External:* Chemical substances, mechanical factors (e.g., shearing forces, pressure, vascular access device [VAD]), medications *Internal:* Changes in turgor, immunological deficit, impaired circulation	Tissue integrity: Primary intention healing of VAD insertion site	Incision site care, skin surveillance

Continued

Nursing Diagnoses Related to Infection Control and Safety	Nursing Outcomes Classification (NOC)	Nursing Intervention Classification (NIC)
Infection, risk for, related to: Inadequate acquired immunity, inadequate primary defenses, inadequate secondary defenses, increased environmental exposure to pathogens, immunosuppression, invasive procedures (placement of intravenous catheter)	Infection control, risk control, risk detection; infection management	Infection control practices and central line bundle implementation, infection protection
Protection, ineffective, related to: Abnormal blood profile (leukopenia), drug therapy (antineoplastic), immune disorders, inadequate nutrition, drug therapies	Health-promoting behavior; immune status	Infection prevention, infection protection

Sources: Ackley & Ladwig, 2011; Bulechek, Butcher, Dochterman, & Wagner, 2013; Moorhead, Johnson, Maas, & Swanson, 2013.

Chapter Highlights

- The purpose of the immune system is to recognize and destroy invading antigens. Organs of the immune system include the thymus, bone marrow, lymph nodes, spleen, liver, Peyer's patches, appendix, tonsils and adenoids, and lungs.
- There are two types of immunity:
  - Innate or nonspecific immunity: Present before exposure to antigens
  - Adaptive or specific immunity: Develops after exposure to antigens
- The chain of infection includes six links:
  - Causative agent
  - Reservoir
  - Portal of exit
  - Method of transmission
  - Portal of entry
  - Host response
- An HAI is an infection that a patient develops while receiving care in a health-care setting.
- Infusion-related infections
  - VAD-related infection
  - Infusate-related infections: Intrinsic contamination (by manufacturer) (rare) and extrinsic contamination (during preparation and maintenance)
  - Culturing techniques: Semiquantitative method
  - Culture one or all of the following depending on symptoms and observation of catheter site.
    - Catheter–skin junction: Do not use alcohol to cleanse before culturing.
    - Catheter

　　　- Infusate with administration set
　　　- Patient's blood
- Strategies to prevent/treat infection include:
  - Following standard precautions
  - Adhering to aseptic technique
  - Performing hand hygiene
  - Using appropriate skin antisepsis
  - Regular site care including skin antisepsis and dressing replacement
  - Using catheter stabilization devices
  - Implementation of the central line bundle
  - Postinsertion care strategies
- Occupational risks associated with infusion therapy include:
  - Biological exposure to bloodborne pathogens
  - Needlestick injuries
  - Chemical exposure
  - Latex allergy

■■ Thinking Critically: Case Study

A patient is admitted with uncontrolled diabetes mellitus. She has a locked peripheral I.V. catheter in place in her left wrist area. A symptomatic drop in blood sugar level to 38 requires she receive 50 mL of 50% dextrose infused at 3 mL/min via the peripheral infusion site. She responds well, but the next day she needs another dose of dextrose via the same infusion site because of a second drop in blood sugar level. At discharge, she complains of burning and pain at the site. The nurse documents that the catheter is intact on discontinuation of the peripheral catheter, but no site assessment data or subjective patient complaints are recorded. The patient is admitted 3 days later with purulent drainage from the left wrist infusion site, temperature of 101°F, and pulse rate of 100.

Case Study Questions

1. *What is the INS standard for placement of a peripheral catheter in the wrist (cephalic vein) area?*

2. *What is the probable reason for the second admission?*

3. *What are contributing factors?*

4. *What breach of standards of practice occurred?*

5. *What are the legal ramifications of this case?*

Media Link: Answers to the case study and more critical thinking activities are provided on DavisPlus.

Post-Test

1. Which of the following constitute the first line of defense in the immune system?
   a. Phagocytosis, complement cascade
   b. Leukocytes, proteins
   c. Physical and chemical barriers
   d. Immune system and phagocytes

2. The major immunoglobulin in the bloodstream is:
   a. IgA
   b. IgE
   c. IgD
   d. IgG

3. The most common route for microorganisms to enter the bloodstream in the first 10 days is:
   a. Extraluminal
   b. Intraluminal
   c. Via hematogenous seeding
   d. Contaminated infusate

4. Transient microorganisms on the skin *(check all that apply)*:
   a. Are normally present
   b. Are acquired through patient contact
   c. Are difficult to remove with routine hand hygiene
   d. Require soap and water for removal

5. Which of the following describe the transmission of organisms from source to host? *(Select all that apply.)*
   a. Contact
   b. Airborne
   c. Vector borne
   d. Colonized person

6. A correct step in the procedure for obtaining a culture of a catheter tip is to:
   a. Always cleanse the skin at the catheter exit site with antiseptic before removal
   b. Always use clean scissors to cut the catheter from the hub
   c. Change the needleless connector after obtaining a blood culture
   d. Put the entire CVAD into the culture tube after removal

7. Which of the following is part of the central line insertion bundle?
   a. Weekly culture of catheter/skin site
   b. An ethanol catheter flush upon insertion
   c. Chlorhexidine/alcohol skin antisepsis
   d. Use of an alcohol cap on the needleless connector

8. Postinsertion care should address:
   a. Change of all administration sets every 24 hours
   b. Disinfection of the needleless connector prior to access
   c. Change of transparent dressing at least every 7 days
   d. Weekly catheter replacement

9. A passive safety device:
   a. Requires activation of a safety mechanism
   b. Does not require activation
   c. Is less desirable than an active safety device
   d. Is an external device that must be attached prior to use

10. The risks of hazardous drugs are minimized when:
   a. Drugs are prepared for administration in the patient room
   b. A standard sharps container is used for disposal of all drug-contaminated supplies
   c. Chemotherapy gloves and gown are worn during drug administration
   d. Hand hygiene is performed prior to gown removal

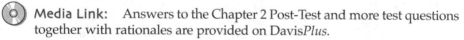 **Media Link:** Answers to the Chapter 2 Post-Test and more test questions together with rationales are provided on Davis*Plus*.

■ References

Ackley, B. J., & Ladwig, G. B. (2011). *Nursing diagnosis handbook: An evidence-based guide to planning care* (9th ed). St. Louis, MO: Mosby Elsevier.

Agency for Healthcare Policy and Research (AHRQ). (2013). *Making health care safer II: An updated critical analysis of the evidence for patient safety practices—Executive report.* Retrieved from www.ahrq.gov/research/findings/evidence-based-reports/ptsafetysum.html (Accessed March 29, 2013).

American Nurses Association (ANA). (2008). *2008 Study of nurses' views on workplace safety and needlestick injuries.* Retrieved from www.nursingworld.org/MainMenuCategories/WorkplaceSafety/Healthy-Work-Environment/SafeNeedles/2008-Study/2008InviroStudy.pdf (Accessed January 26, 2013).

Archibold, L. K. (2012). Principles of infectious diseases epidemiology. In C.G. Mayhall (ed.) Hospital epidemiology and infection control (4th ed). Philadelphia: Lippincott, Williams & Wilkins.

Bailey, R. (2009). A matter of trust. Lifeline letter. Retrieved from http://oley.org/lifeline/A_Matter_of_Trust.html (Accessed December 30, 2010).

Bakunas-Kenneley, I. & Madigan, E. A. (2009). Infection prevention and control in home health care: the nurse's bag. *American Journal of Infection Control* 37 (8), 687–688.

Bausone-Gazsa, D., Lefaiver, C. A., & Walters, S. A. (2010). A randomized controlled trial to compare the complications of 2 peripheral IV catheter stabilization systems. *Journal of Infusion Nursing, 33*(6), 371–384.

Bulechek, G. M., Butcher, H. K., Dochterman, J. M., & Wagner, C. M. (2013). Nursing interventions classification (NIC) (6th ed.). St. Louis, MO: Mosby Elsevier.

Centers for Disease Control and Prevention (CDC). (2002). Guideline for hand hygiene in health-care settings. *MMWR Morbidity Mortality Weekly Report, 51*(RR-16), 1–44.

CDC. (2011a). *Guide to infection prevention for outpatient settings: Minimum expectations for safe care.* Retrieved from www.cdc.gov/HAI/settings/outpatient/outpatient-care-gl-standard-precautions.html (Accessed January 11, 2013).

CDC. (2011b). *Injection safety checklist.* Retrieved from www.cdc.gov/injectionsafety/PDF/SIPC_Checklist.pdf (Accessed January 11, 2013).

CDC. (2011c). Vital signs: Central line-associated bloodstream infections – United States, 2001, 2008, and 2009. *MMWR 60* (8), 243–248.

CDC. (2013). *National Healthcare Safety Network: About NHSN.* Retrieved from www.cdc.gov/nhsn/about.html (Accessed May 1, 2013).

Daley, K. A. (2012). Editorial. *American Nurse Today,* (Suppl September), 1.

Davis, J. (2011). Central-line-associated bloodstream infection: Comprehensive, data-driven prevention. *Pennsylvania Patient Safety Authority, 8*(3), 100–105. Retrieved from http://patientsafetyauthority.org/ADVISORIES/AdvisoryLibrary/2011/sep8(3)/Pages/100.aspx (Accessed January 14, 2013).

Delisio, N. (2012). Bloodborne infection from sharps and mucocutaneous exposure: A continuing problem. *American Nurse Today, 7*(5).

Egan, G. M., Siskin, G. P., Weinmann, R., & Galloway, M. M. (2013). A prospective postmarket study to evaluate the safety and efficacy of a new peripherally inserted central catheter stabilization system. *Journal of Infusion Nursing, 36*(3), 181–188.

Eisenberg, S. (2012). NIOSH safe handling of hazardous drugs guidelines becomes state law. *Journal of Infusion Nursing, 35*(5), 316–319.

Foley, M. (2012). Essential elements of a comprehensive sharps injury-prevention program. *American Nurse Today,* (Suppl September), 2–4.

Gawchik, S. M. (2011). Latex allergy. *Mount Sinai Journal of Medicine, 78,* 759–772.

Gorski, L., Perucca, R., & Hunter, M. (2010). Central venous access devices: Care, maintenance, and potential complications. In M. Alexander, A. Corrigan, I. Gorski, J. Hankins, & R. Perucca (Eds.), *Infusion nursing: An evidence-based practice* (3rd ed.) (pp. 495–515). St. Louis: Saunders/Elsevier.

Hadaway, L. (2012). Short peripheral intravenous catheters and infections. *Journal of Infusion Nursing, 35*(4), 230–240.

Infusion Nurses Society (INS). (2011a). Infusion nursing standards of practice. *Journal of Intravenous Nursing, 34*(1S), S1–S110.

INS. (2011b). *Policies and procedures for infusion nursing* (4th ed.). Norwood, MA: Author.

Institute for Healthcare Improvement (IHI). (2006). *Eliminating central-line related bloodstream infections with bundle compliance.* Retrieved from www.ihi.org (Accessed June 8, 2008).

Institute for Safe Medication Practices (ISMP). (2007). *Failure to cap IV tubing and disconnect IV ports place patients at risk for infections.* Retrieved from www.ismp.org/newsletters/acutecare/articles/20070726.asp (Accessed January 26, 2013).

International Healthcare Worker Safety Center. (n.d.). *Checklist for Sharps Injury Prevention.* Retrieved from www.healthsystem.virginia.edu/pub/epinet/new/chcklst2.pdf (Accessed January 26, 2013).

Lee, G. M., Hartmann, C. W., Graham, D., Kassler, W., Dutta Linn, M. Krein, S., ... Jha, A. (2012). Perceived impact of the Medicare policy to adjust payment for health care-associated infections. *American Journal of Infection Control* 40(4), 314–319.

Levinson, W. (2012). *Review of medical microbiology & immunology* (12th ed.). New York: McGraw Hill Companies.

McGoldrick, M. (2010). Infection prevention and control. In M. Alexander, A. Corrigan, L. Gorski, J. Hankins, & R. Perucca (Eds.), *Infusion nursing: An evidence-based approach* (3rd ed.) (pp. 204–228). St. Louis, MO: Saunders Elsevier.

Mermel, L. A., Allon, M., Bouza, E., Craven, D. E., Flynn, P., O'Grady, N. P., ... Warren, D. K. (2009). Clinical practice guidelines for the diagnosis and management of intravascular catheter-related infection: 2009 update by the Infectious Disease Society of America. *Clinical Infectious Diseases, 49,* 1–45.

Montoya, A., & Mody, L. (2011). Common infections in nursing homes: A review of current issues and challenges. *Aging Health, 7*(6), 889–899.

Moorhead, S., Johnson, M., Maas, M., & Swanson E. (2013). *Nursing outcomes classification* (NOC) (5th ed.). St. Louis, MO: Mosby Elsevier.

National Institute for Occupational Safety and Health (NIOSH). (2004). *Preventing occupational exposure to antineoplastic and other hazardous drugs in health care settings.* Retrieved from www.cdc.gov/niosh/docs/2004-165/pdfs/2004-165sum.pdf (Accessed January 26, 2013).

NIOSH. (2010). *NIOSH hazard review: Occupational hazards in home healthcare.* Retrieved from www.cdc.gov/niosh/docs/2010-125/pdfs/2010-125.pdf (Accessed January 26, 2013).

NIOSH. (2012). *NIOSH list of antineoplastic and other hazardous drugs in healthcare settings 2012.* Retrieved from www.cdc.gov/niosh/docs/2012-150/pdfs/2012-150.pdf (Accessed January 26, 2013).

Occupational Safety and Health Administration (OSHA). (2001). *Bloodborne pathogens and needlestick prevention: OSHA Standards.* Washington, DC: Author. Retrieved from www.osha.gov/SLTC/bloodbornepathogens/standards.html (Accessed January 26, 2013).

O'Grady, N. P. Alexander, M., Burns, L. A., Patchen Dellinger, E., Garland, J., Heard, S. O., ... the Healthcare Infection Control Practices Advisory Committee (HICPAC). Healthcare Infection Control Practices Advisory Committee (HICPAC). (2011). Guidelines for the prevention of intravascular catheter related infections, 2011. *American Journal of Infection Control, 39*(4 Suppl):S1-S34. Retrieved from www.cdc.gov/hicpac/pdf/guidelines/bsi-guidelines-2011.pdf (Accessed September 15, 2012).

Pedivan. (2010). *Best practice guidelines in the care and maintenance of pediatric central venous catheters.* Herrrman, UT: Association for Vascular Access.

Polovich, M., & Clark, P. C. (2012). Factors influencing oncology nurses' use of hazardous drug safe-handling precautions. *Oncology Nursing Forum, 39*(3), E299–E309.

Pronovost, P., Needham, D., Berenholtz, S., Sinopoli, D., Chu, H., Cosgrove, S., … Goeschel, C. (2006). An intervention to decrease catheter-related bloodstream infections in the ICU. *New England Journal of Medicine 28*, 2725–2732.

Pronovost, P., Goeschel, C. A., & Colantuoni, E. (2010). Sustaining reductions in catheter related bloodstream infections in Michigan intensive care units: observational study. *British Medical Journal, 340*.

Resar, R., Griffin, F. A., Haraden, C., & Nolan, T. W. (2012). Using care bundles to improve health care quality. IHI Innovation Series white paper. Cambridge, MA: IHI.

Rowley, S., Clare, S., Macqueen, S., & Molyneux, R. (2010). ANTT v2: An updated practice framework for aseptic technique. *British Journal of Nursing, 19*(5 Suppl), S5–S11.

Rupp, M. E., Cassling, K., & Faber, H. (2013). Hospital-wide assessment of compliance with central venous catheter dressing recommendations. *American Journal of Infection Control, 41*, 89–91.

Siegel, J. D., Rhinehart, E., Jackson, M., & Chiarello, L. (2007). *Guideline for isolation precautions: Preventing transmission of infectious agents in healthcare settings 2007.* Retrieved from www.cdc.gov/ncidod/dhqp/hai.html (Accessed December 11, 2012).

Smith, C. M., & Cotter, V. T. (2012). *Nursing standard of practice protocol: Age-related changes in health.* Retrieved from http://consultgerirn.org/topics/normal_aging_changes/want_to_know_more (Accessed December 28, 2012).

Storey, M., & Jordan, S. (2008). An overview of the immune system. *Nursing Standard, 23*(15–17), 47–56.

The Joint Commission (TJC). (2012a). *Preventing central line–associated infections: A global challenge, a global perspective.* Retrieved from www.jointcommission.org/assets/1/18/CLABSI_Monograph.pdf (Accessed January 28, 2013).

The Joint Commission. (2012b). *National patient safety goals.* Retrieved from www.jointcommission.org/standards_information/npsgs.aspx (Accessed October 29, 2012).

Timsit, J. F., Bouadma, L., Ruckly, S., Schwebel, C., Garrouste-Orgeas, M., Bronchard, R., … Lucet, J. C. (2012a). Dressing disruption is a major risk factor for catheter-related infections. *Critical Care Medicine, 40*(6), 1704–1714.

Timsit, J. F., Mimoz, O., Mourvillier, B., Souweine, B., Garrouste-Orgeas, M., Alfandari, S., … Lucet, J. C. (2012b). Randomized controlled trial of chlorhexidine dressing and highly adhesive dressing for preventing catheter-related infections in critically ill adults. *American Journal of Respiratory Critical Care Medicine, 186*(12), 1272–1278.

Timsit, J. F., Schwebel, C., Bouadma, L., Geffroy, A., Garrouste-Orgeas, M., Pease, S., …Dressing Study Group. (2009). Chlorhexidine-impregnated sponge and less frequent dressing changes for prevention of catheter-related infections in critically ill adults. *Journal of the American Medical Association 301*(12), 1231–1241.

Tsan, L., Langberg, R., Davis, C., Phillips, Y., Pierce, J., Hojlo, C., ... Roselle, G. (2010). Nursing home infections in Department of Veterans Affairs community living centers. *American Journal of Infection Control, 38*(6), 461–466.

Van Leeuwen, A. M., Poelhuis-Leth, D. J., & Bladh, M. L. (2012). *Davis's comprehensive handbook of laboratory and diagnostic tests with nursing implications* (5th ed.). Philadelphia: F. A. Davis.

Vizcarra, C. (2010). Biologic therapy. In M. Alexander, A. Corrigan, L. Gorski, J. Hankins, & R. Perucca (Eds.), *Infusion nursing: An evidence-based approach* (3rd ed.) (pp. 299–315). St. Louis, MO: Saunders Elsevier.

Weber, D. J., Rutala, W. A., Miller, M. B., Huslage, K., & Sickbert-Bennett, E. (2010). Role of hospital surfaces in the transmission of emerging health care-associated pathogens: Norovirus, *Clostridium difficile* and *Acinetobacter* species. *American Journal of Infection Control, 38*, S25–S333.

World Health Organization (WHO). (2009). *WHO guidelines on hand hygiene in health care.* Retrieved from http://whqlibdoc.who.int/publications/2009/9789241597906_eng.pdf (Accessed December 10, 2012).

Wright, M. O., Tropp, J., & Schora, D. M. (2013). Continuous passive disinfection of catheter hubs prevents contamination and bloodstream infection. *American Journal of Infection Control, 41*, 33–38.

PROCEDURES DISPLAY 2-1

Steps in Culturing Catheter–Skin Junction, Catheter, Infusate, and Blood

Delegation
This procedure should not be delegated. It is a registered nurse's responsibility to assess and apply critical thinking skills to obtain the necessary cultures.

Procedure	Rationale
1. Verify the authorized prescriber's order.	1. A written order is a legal requirement.
2. Introduce yourself to the patient.	2. Establishes nurse–patient relationship
3. Verify the patient's identity using two patient identifiers.	3. Patient safety goal
4. Perform hand hygiene.	4. Important means of preventing the spread of infection
5. Explain procedure to patient.	5. Prepares patient for procedure

Culture: Drainage present at catheter–skin junction
Follow steps 1–5 above

6. Gather supplies: Clean gloves, culture tube, site care supplies.	6. Preparation

PROCEDURES DISPLAY 2-1

Steps in Culturing Catheter–Skin Junction, Catheter, Infusate, and Blood—*cont'd*

Procedure	Rationale
7. Don clean gloves.	7. Standard precautions
8. Remove dressing over I.V. site and discard appropriately according to organizational procedures.	8. Soiled dressings are potentially infectious and must be discarded properly.
9. Remove gloves and perform hand hygiene.	9. Standard precautions; always perform hand hygiene between glove changes.
10. Don another pair of clean gloves.	
11. Swab purulent drainage with a sterile swab and place swab into culture tube using aseptic technique according to organizational procedure.	11. To obtain culture.
12. Recap the culture tube.	
13. Perform site care per organizational procedure if catheter is to be left in place.	
14. Remove gloves, perform hand hygiene, label culture tube with patient name, date and time, and source of culture.	14. Ensures obtaining results from the correct patient.

Culture: Catheter tip
Follow steps 1–5 above.

6. Gather supplies: Sterile gloves, culture tube, antiseptic solution, gauze dressing (occlusive dressing for central vascular access device [CVAD] removal).	6. Preparation
7. Put on sterile gloves.	7. Prevents transfer of skin pathogens onto catheter.

Continued

PROCEDURES DISPLAY 2-1

Steps in Culturing Catheter–Skin Junction, Catheter, Infusate, and Blood—*cont'd*

Procedure	Rationale
8. Cleanse skin at catheter exit site with antiseptic solution and allow to dry.	8. To reduce the risk of microorganisms on the skin contaminating catheter during removal process.
9. Place sterile drape in proximity to catheter–skin junction.	9. For placement of catheter on removal; to reduce risk of contaminating catheter thus reducing risk for false-positive results.
10. Remove catheter and place on sterile drape, avoiding contact with surrounding skin according to organizational procedure, and place occlusive dressing over site. Pay special attention to reducing risk of air embolism with CVADs (see Chapter 9).	10. To reduce risk of contaminating catheter; safe catheter removal.
11. Remove gloves and perform hand hygiene.	11. Standard precautions; always perform hand hygiene between glove changes
12. Put on second pair of sterile gloves.	12. Standard precautions; maintain aseptic technique with catheter tip culture to reduce false-positive results.
13. Cut a 2-inch segment of CVAD catheter tip using sterile scissors; for short peripheral catheter, cut entire length of catheter from catheter hub.	
14. Uncap culture tube.	
15. Drop catheter segment into culture tube maintaining aseptic technique.	

PROCEDURES DISPLAY 2-1

Steps in Culturing Catheter–Skin Junction, Catheter, Infusate, and Blood—*cont'd*

Procedure	Rationale
16. Recap the culture tube and label with patient's name, date and time, and specimen type.	16. Ensures obtaining results from the correct patient.

Culture: Infusate

Follow steps 1–5.

6. Gather supplies: Gloves, syringe.	6. Preparation
7. Put on gloves.	7. Standard precautions
8. Disinfect injection port of infusate container with disinfectant (e.g., 70% alcohol, chlorhexidine/alcohol) for at least 15 seconds using a twisting motion and allow to dry.	8. Prevent cross-contamination from port site
9. Insert sterile needleless syringe into injection port of infusate bag.	9. To obtain sterile sample of infusate
10. Withdraw approximately 5 mL of infusate into syringe.	10. Amount needed for culture
11. Remove the syringe from the infusate container.	
12. Inject syringe contents into appropriate culture bottles.	
13. Label culture bottles with patient's name, date and time, and specimen type.	13. Ensures obtaining results from the correct patient.

Blood cultures

NOTE: It is recommended that dedicated staff (e.g., phlebotomy team in an inpatient setting) collect blood cultures for sample because contamination rates are lower.

Important points include the following:

■ Paired blood samples are recommended, one drawn from the catheter and one drawn via peripheral venipuncture.

■ Blood cultures are always collected before initiating any antibiotic therapy.

Continued

PROCEDURES DISPLAY 2-1

Steps in Culturing Catheter–Skin Junction, Catheter, Infusate, and Blood—*cont'd*

- Skin preparation for blood cultures drawn via peripheral venipuncture is an important aspect of care; recommended skin antiseptic agents include 70% alcohol, tincture of iodine, or chlorhexidine/alcohol; povidone-iodine should not be used; skin should be allowed to completely dry prior to venipuncture.
- The needleless connector should be changed prior to drawing a blood sample for culture through a catheter; the new needleless connector should be thoroughly scrubbed with 70% alcohol, tincture of iodine, or chlorhexidine/alcohol and allowed to dry prior to drawing blood.
- The first sample of blood obtained through the catheter is used to inoculate the culture bottles; the initial blood sample is not discarded (this is different than the procedure followed when obtaining blood samples for laboratory studies via a catheter).
- Blood cultures are collected in sets of two and special tubes or bottles are used, one aerobic (with air) and one anaerobic (without air).
- Laboratory guidelines for blood cultures must be carefully followed.

Source: INS. (2011b).

Chapter **3**

Fundamentals of Fluid and Electrolyte Balance

In the great majority of cases, the stomach of the patient is guided by other principles of selection than merely the amount of carbon or nitrogen in the diet. No doubt, in this as in other things, nature has very definite rules for her guidance, but these rules can only be ascertained by the most careful observation at the bedside.

—Florence Nightingale, 1860

Chapter Contents

■ LEARNING OBJECTIVES

On completion of this chapter, the reader will be able to:

1. Define terminology related to fluids and electrolytes.
2. Identify the three fluid compartments within the body.
3. State the functions of body fluids.
4. Differentiate between active and passive transport.
5. Define the concept of osmosis and give examples of this concept.
6. Describe the homeostatic mechanisms.
7. Compare and contrast the movement of water in hypotonic, hypertonic, and isotonic solutions.
8. Compare and contrast fluid volume deficit and fluid volume excess.
9. List the six major body systems assessed for fluid balance disturbances.
10. State the seven major electrolytes within the body fluids.
11. Differentiate between cations and anions.
12. Contrast each of the seven electrolytes and their major roles in body fluids.
13. Identify signs and symptoms of deficits of sodium, potassium, calcium, magnesium, chloride, and phosphate.
14. Identify signs and symptoms of excesses of sodium, potassium, calcium, magnesium, chloride, and phosphate.
15. Discuss patients at risk for electrolyte imbalances.
16. State the normal pH range of body fluids.
17. Identify regulatory organs of acid–base balance.
18. Compare clinical manifestations of metabolic acidosis and alkalosis.

19. Compare clinical manifestations of respiratory acidosis and alkalosis.
20. Identify nursing diagnoses and interventions related to fluid and electrolyte balance.

GLOSSARY

Acidosis   An actual or relative increase in the acidity of blood due to an accumulation of acids or an excessive loss of bicarbonate; blood pH below normal (<7.35)

Active transport   The process by which a cell membrane moves molecules against a concentration or electrochemical gradient. Metabolic work is required.

Alkalosis   An actual or relative increase in blood alkalinity due to an accumulation of alkalis or reduction of acids in the blood; blood pH above normal (>7.45)

Anion   Negatively charged electrolyte

Antidiuretic hormone (ADH)   A hormone secreted from the pituitary mechanism that causes the kidney to conserve water; sometimes referred to as the "water-conserving hormone"

Atrial natriuretic peptide (ANP)   ANP is a cardiac hormone found in the atria of the heart that is released when atria are stretched by high blood volume

Body fluid   Body water in which electrolytes are dissolved

Cation   Positively charged electrolyte

Chvostek's sign   A sign elicited by tapping the facial nerve about 2 cm anterior to the ear lobe, just below the zygomatic process; the response is a spasm of the muscles supplied by the facial nerve

Diffusion   The movement of a substance from a region of high concentration to one of lower concentration

Extracellular fluid (ECF)   Body fluid located outside the cells

Filtration   The process of passing fluid through a filter using pressure

Fingerprinting edema   A condition in which imprints are made on the hands, sternum, or forehead when the area is pressed firmly by the fingers

Fluid volume deficit (FVD)   A fluid deficiency; hypovolemia; an equal proportion of loss of water and electrolytes from the body

Fluid volume excess (FVE)   The state of exceeding normal fluid levels; hypervolemia; retention of both water and sodium in similar proportions to normal ECF

Homeostasis   The state of dynamic equilibrium of the internal environment of the body that is maintained by the ever-changing processes of feedback and regulation in response to external or internal changes

Hypertonic Having a concentration greater than the normal tonicity of plasma; solution of higher osmotic concentration than that of an isotonic solution; greater than 375 mOsm

Hypotonic Having a concentration less than the normal tonicity of plasma; solution of lower osmotic concentration than that of an isotonic solution

Insensible loss Fluid loss that is not perceptible to the individual; non-visible form of water loss that is difficult to measure (e.g., perspiration)

Interstitial fluid Body fluid between the cells

Intracellular fluid (ICF) Body fluid inside the cells

Intravascular fluid The fluid portion of blood plasma

Isotonic Having an osmotic pressure equal to that of blood; equivalent osmotic pressure; between 250 and 375 mOsm

Licensed independent practitioner (LIP) An individual permitted by law to provide care and services without direction or supervision within the scope of the individual's granted clinical privileges, license, and organizational policies

Oncotic pressure The osmotic pressure exerted by colloids (proteins), as when albumin exerts oncotic pressure within the blood vessels and helps to hold the water content of the blood in the intravascular compartment

Osmolality The number of milliosmoles per kilogram of solvent

Osmolarity The number of milliosmoles per liter of solution

Osmosis The movement of water from a lower concentration to a higher concentration across a semipermeable membrane

pH A measure of hydrogen ion (H^+) concentration; the degree of acidity or alkalinity of a substance

Sensible loss Output that is measurable (e.g., urine)

Solute The substance that is dissolved in a liquid to form a solution

Syndrome of inappropriate antidiuretic hormone secretion (SIADH) A condition in which excessive ADH is secreted, resulting in hyponatremia

Tetany Continuous tonic spasm of a muscle

Trousseau's sign A spasm of the hand elicited when the blood supply to the hand is decreased or the nerves of the hand are stimulated by pressure; elicited within several minutes by applying a blood pressure (BP) cuff inflated above systolic pressure

■ Body Fluid Composition

Body fluid is body water in which electrolytes are dissolved. Water is the largest single constituent of the body. Body water, the medium in which cellular reactions take place, constitutes approximately 60% of total body weight (TBW) in young men and 50% to 55% in women. Table 3-1 lists

> Table 3-1	PERCENTAGES OF TOTAL BODY FLUID IN RELATION TO AGE AND GENDER
Age	**Total Body Fluid (% of Body Weight)**
Full-term newborn	70–80
1 year old	64
Puberty to 39 years	Men: 60 Women: 55
40–60 years	Men: 55 Women: 47
>60 years	Men: 52 Women: 46

percentages of total body fluids in relation to age and gender. Fat tissue contains little water, and the percentage of total body water varies considerably based on the amount of body fat present. In addition, total body water progressively decreases with age, making up about 50% of body weight in elderly people (Halperin, Kamel, & Goldstein, 2010).

CULTURAL AND ETHNIC CONSIDERATIONS

A person's age, gender, ethnic origin, and weight can influence the amount and distribution of body fluid. For example, African Americans often have larger numbers of fat cells compared with other groups and therefore have less body water (Giger, 2012).

Fluid Distribution

Homeostasis is dependent on fluid and electrolyte intake, physiological factors (e.g., organ function, hormones, age, gender), disease state factors (e.g., respiratory, renal, metabolic disorders), external environmental factors (e.g., temperature, humidity), and pharmacological interventions.

Water is a neutral polar molecule in which one part is negative and one part is positive. Body water is distributed within cells and outside cells. The body water within the cells is referred to as **intracellular fluid (ICF)**. Fluid outside the cells is referred to as **extracellular fluid (ECF)** and consists of two compartments: interstitial and **intravascular fluid**. Approximately 40% of the TBW is composed of the fluid inside the cell (ICF). Another 20% is fluid outside the cell (ECF) and is divided between interstitial and intravascular spaces, with 15% in the tissue (interstitial) space and only 5% in the plasma (intravascular) space. The **interstitial fluid** lies outside of the blood vessels in the interstitial spaces between the body cells. Lymph and cerebrospinal fluids, although highly specialized, usually are regarded as interstitial fluid. Figure 3-1 shows a representation of body water distribution.

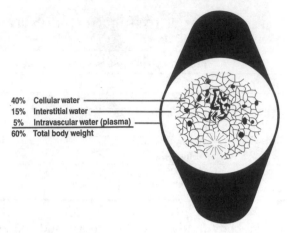

40% Cellular water
15% Interstitial water
5% Intravascular water (plasma)
60% Total body weight

Figure 3-1 ■ Percentages of body fluid.

An exchange of fluid occurs continuously among the intracellular, plasma, and interstitial compartments. Of these three spaces, the intake or elimination of fluid from the body directly influences only the plasma. Changes in the intracellular and interstitial fluid compartments occur in response to changes in the volume or concentration of the plasma.

The internal environment needs to remain in homeostasis; therefore, the intake and output (I&O) of fluid must be relatively equal, as occurs in healthy individuals. In persons who are ill, this balance is frequently upset, and intake of fluid may become diminished or even cease. Output may vary with the influences of increased temperature, increased respiration, draining wounds, or gastric suction.

Normal sources of water on a daily basis include liquids, water-containing foods, and metabolic activity. In healthy adults, the intake of fluids varies from 1000 to 3000 mL/day, and oxidation produces 200 to 300 mL.

> **NURSING FAST FACT!**
>
> Normally, I&O approximately balance only every 72 hours; thus, an appropriate target date for fluid rehydration would be 3 days (Newfield, Hinz, Tilley, et al., 2007).

The elimination of fluid is considered either **sensible** (measurable) **loss** or **insensible** (not measurable) **loss**. Water is eliminated from the body by the skin, kidneys, bowels, and lungs. Approximately 300 to 500 mL of water is eliminated through the lungs every 24 hours, and the skin eliminates about 500 mL/day of water in the form of perspiration. The amount of insensible loss in an adult is approximately 500 to 1000 mL/day. Losses through the gastrointestinal (GI) tract are only about 100 to 200 mL/day because of reabsorption of most of the fluid in the small intestines. Increased losses of GI fluids can occur from diarrhea or intestinal fistulas (Smeltzer, Bare, Hinkle, & Cheever, 2010).

The metabolic rate increases with fever; it rises approximately 12% for every 1°C (7% for every 1°F increase in body temperature). Significant sweat losses occur if a patient's body temperature exceeds 101°F (38.3°C) or if the room temperature exceeds 90°F. Fever also increases the respiratory rate, resulting in additional loss of water vapor through the lungs (Porth & Matfin, 2010). Insensible loss is also increased if respirations are increased to more than 20 per minute.

■ Fluid Function

Fluids within the body have several important functions. The ECF transports nutrients to the cells and carries waste products away from the cells via the capillary beds. Body fluids are in constant motion, maintaining living conditions for body cells. The fluid within the body also has the following functions:

1. Maintains blood volume.
2. Regulates body temperature.
3. Transports material to and from cells.
4. Serves as an aqueous medium for cellular metabolism.
5. Assists digestion of food through hydrolysis.
6. Acts as a solvent in which solutes are available for cell function.
7. Serves as a medium for excretion of waste.

Fluid Transport

Body fluids are in constant motion, maintaining healthy living conditions for body cells. The ECF interfaces with the outside world and is modified by it, but the ICF remains stable. Nutrients are transported by the ECF to the cells, and wastes are carried away from the cells via the capillary beds (Kee, Paulanka, & Polek, 2010).

Movement of particles through the cell membrane occurs through four transport mechanisms: passive transport, which consists of **diffusion, osmosis**, and **filtration**; and **active transport**. Materials are transported between the ICF and the extracellular compartment by these four mechanisms.

Passive Transport

Passive transport is also referred to as non–carrier-mediated transport. It is the movement of **solutes** through membranes without the expenditure of energy. It includes passive diffusion, osmosis, and filtration.

Passive Diffusion

Passive diffusion is the passive movement of water, ions, and lipid-soluble molecules randomly in all directions from a region of high concentration to an area of low concentration. Diffusion occurs through semipermeable membranes by the substance either passing through pores, if small enough, or dissolving in the lipid matrix of the membrane wall. If there is no force opposing diffusion, particles distribute themselves evenly. Many substances can diffuse in both directions through the cell membrane. Influencing factors in the diffusion process are concentration differences, electrical potential, and pressure differences across the pores. The greater the concentration, the greater the rate of diffusion. An increase in the pressure on one side of the membrane increases the molecular forces striking the pores, thus creating a pressure gradient. Other factors that increase diffusion include:

■ Increased temperature
■ Increased concentration of particles
■ Decreased size or molecular weight of particles
■ Increased surface area available for diffusion
■ Decreased distance across which the particle mass must diffuse

Filtration

Filtration is the transfer of water and a dissolved substance from a region of high pressure to a region of low pressure; the force behind it is hydrostatic pressure (i.e., the pressure of water at rest). The pumping heart provides hydrostatic pressure in the movement of water and electrolytes from the arterial capillary bed to the interstitial fluid. Diffusion moves in either direction across a membrane; filtration moves in one direction only because of the hydrostatic, osmotic, and interstitial fluid pressures. Filtration is likened to pouring a solution through a sieve: The size of the opening in the sieve determines the size of the particle to be filtered.

The plasma compartment contains more protein than the other compartments. Plasma protein, composed of albumin, globulin, and fibrinogen, creates an **oncotic pressure** at the capillary membrane, which prevents fluid from the plasma from leaking into the interstitial spaces. Oncotic pressure created within the plasma by the presence of protein (mainly albumin) keeps the water in the vascular system.

Starling's Law of the Capillaries maintains that, under normal circumstances, fluid filtered out of the arterial end of a capillary bed and reabsorbed at the venous end is exactly the same, creating a state of near-equilibrium (Starling, 1896). However, it is not exactly the same because of the difference in hydrostatic pressure between the arterial and venous capillary beds. The pressure that moves fluid out of the arterial end of the network totals 28.3 mm Hg. The pressure that moves fluid back into circulation at the venous capillary bed is 28 mm Hg. The small amount of excess remaining in the interstitial compartment is returned to the circulation by way of the lymphatic system (Kee, Paulanka, & Polek, 2010).

Active Transport

Active transport is similar to diffusion except that it acts against a concentration gradient. Active transport occurs when it is necessary for ions (electrolytes) to move from an area of low concentration to an area of high concentration. By definition, active transport implies that energy expenditure must take place for the movement to occur against a concentration gradient. Adenosine triphosphate (ATP) is released from the cell to enable certain substances to acquire the energy needed to pass through the cell membrane. For example, sodium concentration is greater in ECF; therefore, sodium tends to enter by diffusion into the intracellular compartment. This tendency is offset by the sodium–potassium pump, which is located on the cell membrane. In the presence of ATP, the sodium–potassium pump actively moves sodium from the cell into the ECF. Active transport is vital for maintaining the unique composition of both the extracellular and intracellular compartments (Wilkinson & Van Leuven, 2007).

Osmosis

Osmosis is the passage of water from an area of lower particle concentration toward one with a higher particle concentration across a semipermeable membrane. For a membrane to be semipermeable, it has to be more permeable to water than to solutes. This process tends to equalize the concentration of two solutions.

Osmosis governs the movement of body fluids between the intracellular and ECF compartments, therefore influencing the volumes of fluid within each. Through the process of osmosis, water flows through semipermeable membranes toward the side with the higher concentration of particles (thus from lower to higher) (Hankins, 2010).

OSMOTIC PRESSURE GRADIENTS

Osmotic pressure develops as solute particles collide against each other. Osmotic pressure is the amount of hydrostatic pressure needed to draw a solvent (water) across a membrane, and it develops as a result of a high concentration of particles colliding with one another. As the number of solutes increases, there is less space for them to move; therefore, they come in contact with one another more frequently. This results in increased osmotic pressure, which causes the movement of fluid. The osmotic pressure differs at the cell membrane and the capillary membrane. The process of osmosis depends on how much of the membrane is involved and on certain characteristics of the solution (Hankins, 2010). The colloid osmotic pressure is influenced by proteins because proteins are the only substances dissolved in the plasma and interstitial fluid that do not diffuse readily through capillary membranes. The concentration of protein in plasma is two to three times greater than that of the proteins found in the interstitial fluid. Only the substances that do not pass through the semipermeable membrane exert osmotic pressure. Therefore, proteins in the ECF spaces are responsible for the osmotic pressure at the capillary membrane. Osmotic pressure is measured in milliosmoles (mOsm).

Osmolarity Versus Osmolality

The osmotic activity of a solution may be expressed in terms of either its **osmolarity** or its **osmolality**. Osmolarity refers to the osmolar concentration in 1 L of solution. Osmolality is the osmolar concentration of 1 kg of water. Osmolarity usually refers to fluids outside the body, and osmolality refers to fluids inside the body. Because 1 L of water weighs 1 kg, the terms osmolarity and osmolality are often used interchangeably (Porth & Matfin, 2010).

Tonicity of Solutions

A change in water content causes cells to either swell or shrink. The term tonicity refers to the tension or effect that the effective osmotic pressure of a solution with impermeable solutes exerts on cell size because of water movement across a cell membrane. Tonicity is determined solely by effective solutes such as glucose, which cannot penetrate the cell membrane, thereby producing an osmotic force that pulls water into or out of the cell and causing it to change size. Solutions to which body cells are exposed can be classified as isotonic, hypotonic, or hypertonic, depending on whether they cause cells to swell or shrink. Cells placed in an isotonic solution, which has the same effective osmolality as ICFs, neither shrink nor swell (Porth & Matfin, 2010).

When cells are placed in a hypotonic solution, which has a lower effective osmolality than ICFs, they swell as water moves into the cells. When they are placed in a hypertonic solution, which has a greater effective osmolality than ICFs, they shrink as water is pushed out of the cells.

Figure 3-2 shows the movement of water by osmosis in hypotonic, isotonic, and hypertonic solutions.

Isotonic solutions, such as 0.9% sodium chloride (NaCl) and 5% dextrose in water, have the same osmolarity as normal body fluids. Solutions that have an osmolarity of 250 to 375 mOsm/L are considered isotonic solutions. They have no effect on the volume of fluid within the cell; the solution remains within the ECF space. Isotonic solutions are used to expand the ECF compartment.

Hypotonic solutions contain less salt than the intracellular space. When infused, they have an osmolarity below 250 mOsm/L and move water into the cell, causing the cell to swell and possibly burst. By lowering

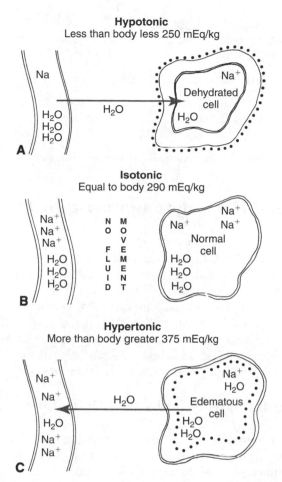

Figure 3-2 ■ Effects of fluid shifts in (A) hypotonic, (B) isotonic, and (C) hypertonic states. (From Kuhn, M. [1998]. *Pharmacotherapeutics: A nursing process approach* [4th ed., p. 128]. Philadelphia: F. A. Davis, with permission.)

the serum osmolarity, body fluids shift out of the blood vessels into the interstitial tissue and cells. Hypotonic solutions hydrate cells and can deplete the circulatory system. An example of a hypotonic solution is 2.5% dextrose in water.

Hypertonic solutions, conversely, cause the water from within a cell to move to the ECF compartment, where the concentration of salt is greater, causing the cell to shrink. Hypertonic solutions have an osmolarity of 375 mOsm/L and above. These solutions are used to replace electrolytes. When hypertonic dextrose solutions are used alone, they also are used to shift ECF from interstitial tissue to plasma. Examples of hypertonic solutions are 5% dextrose and 0.9% NaCl, or 5% dextrose and lactated Ringer's solution. Figure 3-3 illustrates tonicity (osmolarity) ranges.

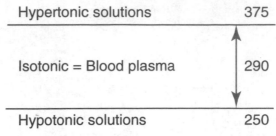

Hypertonic solutions	375
Isotonic = Blood plasma	290
Hypotonic solutions	250

Figure 3-3 ■ Tonicity osmolarity ranges of solutions.

◼ Fluid and Electrolyte Homeostatic Mechanisms

Regulation of body water is maintained through exogenous sources, such as the intake of food and fluids, and endogenous sources, which are produced within the body through a chemical oxidation process. Several homeostatic mechanisms are responsible for the balance of fluid and electrolytes within the body. When homeostasis is compromised and imbalance occurs, the nurse is responsible for managing the exogenous source of fluid replacement via the intravenous route. The endogenous sources of balancing fluid and electrolytes are various body systems such as the cardiovascular, lymphatic, renal, respiratory, nervous, and endocrine systems.

Cardiovascular System and Atrial Natriuretic Factor

The pumping action of the heart provides circulation of blood through the kidneys under pressure, which allows urine to form. Renal perfusion makes renal function possible. Blood vessels provide plasma to reach the kidneys in sufficient volume (20% of circulating blood volume) to permit regulation of water and electrolytes. Baroreceptors located in the carotid sinus and aortic arch respond to the degree of stretch of the vessel wall, which has been generated by the body's reaction to hypovolemia. The response is to stimulate fluid retention.

　　Atrial natriuretic peptide (ANP) are produced by the cardiac atria, ventricles, and other vessels in response to changes in ECF volume. When atrial pressure is increased, ANP released by the atrial and ventricular myocytes acts on the nephron to increase sodium excretion. Additionally, ANP is a direct vasodilator, lowering systemic BP (Halperin, Kamel, & Goldstein, 2010).

Lymphatic System

The lymphatic system serves as an adjunct to the cardiovascular system by removing excess interstitial fluid (in the form of lymph) and returning it to the circulatory system. Fluid overload in the interstitial compartment would result if it were not for the lymphatic system. The lymphatic system carries the excess fluid, proteins, and large particulate matter that cannot be reabsorbed by the venous capillary bed out of the interstitial compartment. This minute excess (0.3 mm Hg) accounts for 1.7 mm/min of fluid. If the lymphatic system were not continually removing this small amount of fluid, there would be a buildup of 2448 mL in the interstitial compartment over a 24-hour period of time (Porth & Matfin, 2010).

Kidneys

The kidneys are vital to the regulation of fluid and electrolyte balance. The kidney is the main regulator of sodium. The kidney monitors arterial pressure and retains sodium when arterial pressure is decreased and eliminates it when arterial pressure is increased (Porth & Matfin, 2010). The kidneys normally filter 170 L of plasma per day in the adult and excrete only 1.5 L of urine (Porth & Matfin, 2010). They act in response to bloodborne messengers such as aldosterone and **antidiuretic hormone (ADH)**. Renal failure can result in multiple fluid and electrolyte imbalances.

Functions of the kidneys in fluid balance are:
- Regulation of fluid volume and osmolarity by selective retention and excretion of body fluids
- Regulation of electrolyte levels by selective retention of needed substances and excretion of unneeded substances
- Regulation of **pH** of ECF by excretion or retention of hydrogen ions (H^+)
- Excretion of metabolic wastes (primarily acids) and toxic substances (Kee, Paulanka, & Polek, 2010).

Renin–Angiotensin–Aldosterone Mechanism

The renin–angiotensin–aldosterone system exerts its action through angiotensin II and aldosterone. Renin is a small enzyme protein that is released by the kidney in response to changes in arterial pressure, the glomerular filtration rate, and the amount of sodium in the tubular fluid. Aldosterone acts at the level of the cortical collecting tubules of the kidneys to increase sodium reabsorption while increasing potassium elimination (Porth & Matfin, 2010).

Respiratory System

The lungs are vital for maintaining homeostasis and constitute one of the main regulatory organs of fluid and acid–base balance. The lungs regulate acid–base balance by regulating the hydrogen ion (H^+) concentration. Alveolar ventilation is responsible for the daily elimination of approximately 13,000 mEq of H^+ ions. The kidneys excrete only 40 to 80 mEq of hydrogen daily. Under influence from the medulla, the lungs act promptly to correct metabolic acid–base disturbances by regulating the level of carbon dioxide (a potential acid) in the ECF. Functions of the lungs in body fluid balance are:

- Regulation of metabolic alkalosis by compensatory hypoventilation, resulting in carbon dioxide (CO_2) retention and increased acidity of the ECF
- Regulation of metabolic acidosis by causing compensatory hyperventilation, resulting in CO_2 excretion and thus decreased acidity of the ECF
- Removal of 300 to 500 mL of water daily through exhalation (i.e., insensible water loss)

Endocrine System

The glands responsible for aiding in homeostasis are the adrenal, pituitary, and parathyroid glands. The endocrine system responds selectively to the regulation and maintenance of fluid and electrolyte balance through hormonal production.

Water

Holliday and Segar (1957) established that regardless of age, all healthy persons require approximately 100 mL of water per 100 calories metabolized, for dissolving and eliminating metabolic wastes. That means a person who expends 1800 calories of energy requires approximately 1800 mL of water for metabolic purposes. Two main physiological mechanisms assist in regulating body water: thirst and ADH. Both mechanisms respond to changes in extracellular osmolality and volume.

Thirst

Thirst is controlled by the thirst center in the hypothalamus. There are two stimuli for true thirst based on water need: cellular dehydration caused by an increase in extracellular osmolality, and a decrease in blood volume, which may or may not be associated with a decrease in serum osmolality. Thirst develops when there is as little as 1% to 2% change in serum osmolality (Ayus, Achinger, & Arieff, 2008).

 NURSING FAST FACT!

Thirst is one of the earliest symptoms of hemorrhage and often is present before other signs of blood loss appear.

Antidiuretic Hormone

ADH, the pituitary hormone that influences water balance, is also called vasopressin. This hormone, which affects renal reabsorption of water, is also referred to as the "water-conserving" hormone. Functions of ADH are to maintain osmotic pressure of the cells by controlling renal water retention or excretion and controlling blood volume. Excessive secretion of ADH results in the **syndrome of inappropriate antidiuretic hormone secretion (SIADH)**.

As with thirst, ADH levels are controlled by extracellular volume and osmolality. A small increase in serum osmolality is sufficient to cause ADH release. A blood volume decrease of 5% to 10% produces a maximal increase in ADH levels. As with many other homeostatic mechanisms, acute conditions produce changes in ADH levels.

Numerous drugs (e.g., alcohol, narcotic antagonists) can block ADH activity or reduce tubular responsiveness to ADH (e.g., lithium, demeclocycline), which results in increased water loss, causing dehydration and hypernatremia. Increased ADH secretion may be the result of disease (hormone-secreting tumor, head injury) or may be related to administration of drugs such as chlorpropamide, vinca alkaloids, carbamazepine, cyclophosphamide, tricyclic antidepressants, and narcotics (Porth & Matfin, 2010).

Factors that affect ADH production include pathological changes such as head trauma and tumors of the brain or lung, anesthesia and surgery in general, and certain drugs (e.g., barbiturates, antineoplastics, and nonsteroidal antiinflammatory drugs).

Parathyroid Hormone

The parathyroid gland is embedded in the corners of the thyroid gland and regulates calcium and phosphate balance. The parathyroid gland influences fluid and electrolytes, increases serum calcium levels, and lowers serum phosphate levels. A reciprocal relationship exists between extracellular calcium and phosphate levels. When the serum calcium level is low, the parathyroid gland secretes more parathyroid hormone (PTH). PTH can increase the serum calcium level by promoting calcium release from the bone as needed. Calcitonin from the thyroid gland increases calcium return to the bone, thus decreasing the serum calcium level.

Aldosterone

The adrenal cortex is important in fluid and electrolyte homeostasis. The primary adrenocortical hormone influencing the balance of fluid is aldosterone. Aldosterone is responsible for renal reabsorption of sodium, which results in the retention of chloride and water and the excretion of potassium. Aldosterone also regulates blood volume by regulating sodium retention.

Epinephrine

Epinephrine, another adrenal hormone, increases BP, enhances pulmonary ventilation, dilates blood vessels needed for emergencies, and constricts unnecessary vessels.

Cortisol

When produced in large quantities, the adrenocortical hormone cortisol can produce sodium and fluid retention and potassium deficit. Table 3-2 summarizes the regulators of fluid and electrolyte balance.

■ Physical Assessment of Fluid and Electrolyte Needs

A body systems approach is the best method for assessing fluid and electrolyte imbalances related to infusion therapy. The nurse should begin by obtaining a history, assessing vital signs, performing a focused physical

> Table 3-2	REGULATORS OF FLUID BALANCE
Homeostatic Mechanism	**Action**
Cardiovascular	Baroreceptor in carotid sinus and aortic arch responds to hypovolemia. Atrial natriuretic peptide (ANP) is direct vasodilator, lowering blood pressure.
Lungs	Lungs excrete 400–500 mL of water daily through normal breathing.
Kidneys	Kidneys excrete 1000–1500 mL of body water daily. Water excretion may vary according to the balance between fluid intake and fluid loss.
Lymphatics	Plasma protein that shifts to the tissue spaces cannot be reabsorbed into the blood vessels. Lymphatic system promotes the return of water and protein from the interstitial spaces to the vascular spaces.
Skin	Skin excretes 300–500 mL of water daily through normal perspiration.
Electrolyte	Sodium promotes water retention. With a water deficit, less sodium is excreted via kidneys; thus, more water is retained.
Nonelectrolytes	Protein and albumin promote body fluid retention. These nondiffusible substances increase the colloid osmotic (oncotic) pressure in favor of fluid retention.
Hormones	
Antidiuretic hormone (ADH)	ADH is produced by the hypothalamus and stored in the posterior pituitary gland. ADH is secreted when there is an extracellular fluid volume deficit or an increased osmolality. ADH promotes water reabsorption from the distal tubules of the kidneys.
Aldosterone	Aldosterone is secreted from the adrenal cortex. It promotes sodium, chloride, and water reabsorption from the renal tubules.
Renin	Decreased renal blood flow increases the release of renin, an enzyme, from the juxtaglomerular cells of the kidneys. Renin promotes peripheral vasoconstriction and the release of aldosterone (sodium and water retention).

assessment, monitoring pertinent laboratory test results, and evaluating I&O. The purpose of this data gathering is to identify clients at risk for or already experiencing alterations in fluid and electrolyte balance.

Nursing history related to fluid and electrolyte balance includes questions about past medical history, current health concerns, food and fluid intake, fluid elimination, medications, and lifestyle. The physical assessment correlates data with the nursing history, validating subjective information. Focused assessment includes, but is not limited to, neurological evaluation of level of consciousness (LOC), cardiovascular system, respiratory system, skin, special senses, and weight. Laboratory data should be assessed in a comprehensive review of patient fluid and electrolyte needs.

Neurological System/Focus on Level of Consciousness

Changes in LOC occur with changes in serum osmolality or changes in serum sodium. They also can occur with acute acid–base imbalances. Fluid volume changes, along with serum sodium levels, affect the central nervous system (CNS) cells, resulting in irritability, lethargy, confusion, seizures, or coma. CNS cells shrink in sodium excess and expand when serum sodium levels decrease. Sensation of thirst depends on excitation of the cortical centers of consciousness. The use of antianxiety agents, sedatives, or hypnotic agents can lead to confusion and disorientation, causing the patient to forget to drink fluid (Heitz & Horne, 2005).

Assessment of neuromuscular irritability is particularly important when imbalances in calcium, magnesium, sodium, and potassium are suspected. Electrolyte imbalances can cause neurological system signs and symptoms. Abnormal reflexes occur with calcium and magnesium imbalances, including **Trousseau's** and **Chvostek's signs**. Hyperkalemia (increase in potassium level) can cause flaccid paralysis. Paresthesia may occur in patients with acid–base imbalances (Heitz & Horne, 2005).

There is a progressive loss of CNS cells with advancing age, along with decreases in the sense of smell and tactile sense. The thirst mechanism in elderly people may be diminished and is a poor guide for fluid needs in older patients. An ill patient may not be able to verbalize thirst or to reach for a glass of water.

Cardiovascular System

The quality and rate of the pulse are indicators of how the patient is tolerating the ECF volume. The peripheral veins in the extremities provide a way of evaluating plasma volume. Examination of hand veins can evaluate the plasma volume. Peripheral veins empty in 3 to 5 seconds when the hand is elevated and fill in the same amount of time when the hand is lowered to a dependent position. Peripheral vein filling takes longer than 3 to 5 seconds in patients with sodium depletion and extracellular dehydration (Kee, Paulanka, & Polek, 2010). Slow emptying of the peripheral veins indicates overhydration and excessive blood volume (Fig. 3-4).

A 20 mm Hg fall in systolic BP when shifting the patient from the lying to the standing position (postural hypotension) usually indicates **fluid volume deficit (FVD)**. The jugular vein provides a built-in manometer for evaluation of central venous pressure (CVP). Changes in fluid volume are reflected by changes in neck vein filling.

When a patient is supine, the external jugular veins fill to the anterior border of the sternocleidomastoid muscle. Flat neck veins in the supine position indicate a decreased plasma volume. When the patient is in a 45-degree position, the external jugular vein distends no higher than 2 cm above the sternal angle. Neck veins that distend from the top portion of the sternum to the angle of the jaw indicate elevated venous pressure (Fig. 3-5).

Edema indicates expansion of interstitial volume. Edema can be localized (usually caused by inflammation) or generalized (usually related to capillary hemodynamics). Edema should be assessed over bony surfaces of the tibia or sacrum and rated according to severity from 1+ to 4+ (Fig. 3-6). The presence of periorbital edema suggests significant fluid retention.

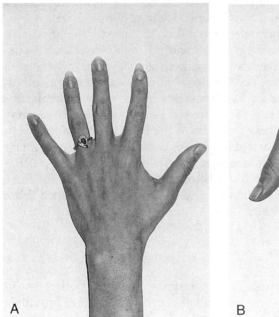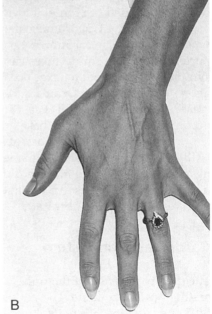

A   B

Figure 3-4 ■ Hand vein assessment. *A*, Slow emptying of the hand veins indicates overhydration and excessive blood volume. *B*, Peripheral hand vein filling can take longer than 3 to 5 seconds in patients with sodium depletion and dehydration.

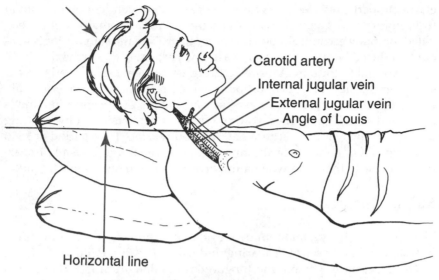

Carotid artery
Internal jugular vein
External jugular vein
Angle of Louis

Horizontal line

Figure 3-5 ▪ Jugular venous distention.

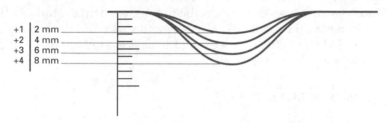

+1	2 mm
+2	4 mm
+3	6 mm
+4	8 mm

Figure 3-6 ▪ Edema.

Respiratory System

A key to the assessment of circulatory overload is an assessment of the lung fields. Changes in respiratory rate and depth may be a compensatory mechanism for acid–base imbalance. Tachypnea (>20 respirations/min) and dyspnea indicate **fluid volume excess (FVE)**. Moist crackles in the absence of cardiopulmonary disease indicate FVE. Shallow, slow breathing may indicate metabolic alkalosis or respiratory acidosis. Deep, rapid breathing may indicate respiratory alkalosis or metabolic acidosis.

Skin Appearance and Temperature

Assessments of temperature and skin surface are key in determining fluid volume changes. Pinching the area over the hand, inner thigh, sternum, or forehead can assess skin turgor. In a well-hydrated person, the pinched skin immediately falls back to its normal position when released. This elastic property, referred to as turgor, is partially dependent on interstitial fluid volume. In a person with FVD, the skin may remain slightly elevated for many seconds. In persons older than 55 years, skin turgor is generally reduced because of loss of elasticity, particularly in areas that have been exposed to the sun. A more accurate assessment can be made on the skin over the sternum. A condition in which placement of fingers firmly on the patient's skin leaves finger imprints is called fingerprinting and is associated with FVE. **Fingerprinting edema** is demonstrated by pressing a finger firmly over the sternum or other body surface for a period of 15 to 30 seconds. On removal of the finger, a positive sign is a visible fingerprint similar to that seen when a fingerprint is made on paper with ink.

Special Senses

The eyes, mouth, lips, and tongue are other key indicators of fluid volume imbalances. The absence of tearing and salivation in a child is a sign of FVD. In a healthy person, the tongue has one longitudinal furrow. In a person with FVD, the tongue has additional longitudinal furrows and is smaller because of fluid loss (Porth & Matfin, 2010).

Mucous membranes often show the first sign of dehydration. As fluid volume decreases, the mouth becomes dry and sticky and the lips dry and cracked. In FVD, the patient's eyes tend to appear sunken; in significant FVE, periorbital edema is present.

 NURSING FAST FACT!

Good oral hygiene is imperative with mouth-breathing patients. If the patient is receiving good oral care and the crusted, dry, furrowed tongue does not improve, FVD must be restored to aid in solving this problem.

Body Weight

Taking daily weights of patients with potential fluid imbalances is an important clinical tool. Accurate body weight measurement is a better indicator of gains or losses than I&O records. A loss or gain of 1 kg (2.2 lb) reflects a loss or gain of 1 L of body fluid. Generally, FVD or excess is considered severe when body weight fluctuates 15% higher or lower than the person's normal body weight.

EBP A study by Armstrong (2005) found that a systematic review demonstrated measurement of weight is a safe technique to assess hydration status, especially for dehydration that occurs over a period of 1 to 4 hours; less frequent measurement may reflect changes in respiratory water loss or gain or loss of adipose tissue. Thus, weight changes may be a less accurate indicator of hydration status.

Table 3-2 summarizes the regulators of fluid balance.

> EBP A study by Wakefield (2008) found that urine color significantly correlates with urine osmolality, serum sodium, and blood urea nitrogen (BUN)/creatinine ratios. In a hydrated person, urine should be light yellow—the color of lemonade; the color of apple juice indicates slight dehydration (Wakefield, 2008).

Laboratory Values

The review and interpretation of a patient's laboratory findings provide important objective data for analysis of alterations in fluid balance and of major electrolyte imbalances. The blood gas analysis is a key indicator, along with physical assessment, of acid–base imbalances. Tests that reflect the proper function of the heart and kidneys are of particular importance and require close scrutiny for early detection of fluid imbalances. Table 3-3 summarizes laboratory findings for monitoring fluid and electrolyte imbalances.

> Table 3-3	SUMMARY OF LABORATORY EVALUATION FOR FLUID AND ELECTROLYTE IMBALANCES
Test	**Clinical Considerations**
Kidneys	
Blood urea nitrogen (BUN)	Assess nutritional support; evaluate hydration, and renal function.
Creatinine	Evaluate for renal impairment. Assess known or suspected disorder involving muscles in the absence of renal disease.
Specific gravity	Urine concentration reflects fluid volume concentrations and hydration status.
Urine osmolarity	Monitor for fluid imbalances.
Blood Chemistry	
Calcium, ionized	Identify individuals with hypocalcemia; monitor patients with renal failure in whom secondary hyperparathyroidism may occur. Monitor patient with sepsis or magnesium deficiency.
Chloride, blood	Assist in confirming diagnosis of disorder associated with abnormal chloride values in acid–base and fluid volume imbalances. Differentiate between types of acidosis.
Magnesium, blood	Determine electrolyte balance in renal failure and chronic alcoholism. Evaluate cardiac dysrhythmias.
Potassium, blood	Assess known or suspected disorder associated with renal disease, glucose metabolism, trauma, or burns. Evaluate electrolyte imbalances (especially in the elderly). Evaluate cardiac dysrhythmias, especially during digitalis therapy. Monitor acidosis (potassium moves from red blood cells (RBCs) into extracellular fluid in acidotic states).
Sodium, blood	Determine whole body stores of sodium. Monitor effectiveness of drug therapy, especially of diuretics on serum sodium levels. Determine hydration status.

Continued

> Table 3-3   **SUMMARY OF LABORATORY EVALUATION FOR FLUID
AND ELECTROLYTE IMBALANCES—cont'd**

Test	Clinical Considerations
Complete blood count (CBC)	CBC screening for hemoglobin, hematocrit, RBC, white blood cell, and platelets prior to replacement of these components or when expanding extracellular fluid.
Blood Gases	Evaluate acid–base status.
pH, hydrogen ion	The pH, negative logarithm of the hydrogen ion concentration, determines the acidity or alkalinity of body fluids.
Bicarbonate (HCO_3^-)	Alkaline substance that is over half of the total buffer base in the blood. Role in maintaining pH of 7.35–7.45.
Partial pressure of oxygen (Pa_{CO_2})	Determines amount of oxygen available to bind with hemoglobin. Pa_{O_2} is decreased in respiratory diseases.
Partial pressure of carbon dioxide (Pa_{CO_2})	Partial pressure of carbon dioxide reflects adequacy of alveolar ventilation. The pH affects the combining power of oxygen and hemoglobin.
Miscellaneous	
Serum glucose	Monitor osmotic diuresis.

Source: Van Leeuwen, Poelhuis-Leth, & Bladh (2012).

■ Disorders of Fluid Balance

Fluid volume imbalances may reflect an increase or a decrease in total body fluid or an altered distribution of body fluids. There are two major alterations in ECF balance: FVD and FVE.

Fluid Volume Deficit (Hypovolemia)

Extracellular FVD (hypovolemia) reflects a contracted vascular compartment caused by either a significant ECF loss or an accumulation of fluid in the interstitial space. ECF deficit is also referred to as dehydration. It may be caused by an actual decrease in body water, excessive fluid loss or inadequate fluid intake, or a relative decrease in which fluid (plasma) shifts from the intravascular compartment to the interstitial space, a process called "third spacing" (Porth & Matfin, 2010). Depending on the type of fluid lost, hypovolemia may be accompanied by acid–base, osmolar, or electrolyte imbalances. Prolonged hypovolemia may lead to the development of acute renal failure (Heitz & Horne, 2005).

Etiology

FVD occurs when there is either an excessive loss of body water or an inadequate compensatory intake. The ECF consists predominantly of the electrolytes sodium and chloride, both of which tend to attract water; loss of these electrolytes also leads to loss of water. GI dysfunction is the most common cause of ECF deficit. Other common causes include overzealous use of diuretics and diaphoresis.

FVD also occurs in third spacing, which is caused by peritonitis, intestinal obstruction, postoperative conditions, thrombophlebitis, acute pancreatitis, ascites, fistula drainage, and burns. Third spaces are extracellular body spaces in which fluid is not normally present in large amounts but in which fluid can accumulate. Fluid that accumulates in third spaces is physiologically useless because it is not available for use. Common sites for collection of third space fluid include tissue spaces, abdomen, pleural spaces, and pericardial space (Porth & Matfin, 2010).

COMMON CAUSES OF ISOTONIC DEHYDRATION

- Hemorrhage resulting in loss of fluid, electrolytes, proteins, and blood cells in proportional amounts, resulting in inadequate vascular volume
- GI losses: Vomiting, diarrhea, nasogastric (NG) suction, drainage from fistulas and tubes; tend to be lost in proportional amounts
- Fever, environmental heat, and diaphoresis result in profuse sweating, causing water and sodium loss
- Burns initially damage skin and capillary membranes allow fluid, electrolytes, and proteins to escape into the burned tissue, resulting in inadequate vascular volume.
- Diuretics cause excessive loss of fluid and electrolytes in proportional amounts.
- Third space fluid shifts occur when fluid moves from the vascular space into physiologically useless extracellular spaces (Kee, Paulanka, & Polek, 2010).

COMMON CAUSES OF HYPERTONIC FLUID DEHYDRATION

- Inadequate fluid intake: Patients who are unable to respond to thirst independently (bedridden, infants, elderly who have nausea, and anorexia, those who are NPO without adequate fluid replacement)
- Decreased water intake results in ECF solute concentration and leads to cellular dehydration (Kee, Paulanka, & Polek, 2010).

Clinical Manifestations

Clinically, ECF deficit is characterized by acute weight loss, altered cardiovascular function that reflects the underlying ECF volume deficit, and complaints of nausea and vomiting. The cardiovascular assessment is the most important part of the process to determine plasma volume changes. In a patient who is hypovolemic, the heart rate increases, the BP decreases, and the peripheral pulses are weak. Symptoms reflect a dehydrated state with sunken eyeballs, poor skin turgor, and oliguria commonly seen.

Laboratory Findings

- Hemoconcentration with the serum hemoglobin, hematocrit, and proteins increased
- BUN is elevated above 20 mg/100 mL
- Urine specific gravity reflects high solute concentration greater than 1.030

NURSING POINTS OF CARE
HYPOVOLEMIA (FVD)

Nursing Assessments
1. Complete a client history identifying factors that may cause FVD, such as vomiting, diarrhea, limited fluid intake, diabetes mellitus, large draining wound, or diuretic therapy.
2. Complete a functional assessment if appropriate (especially for the elderly patient) to determine fluid and food needs and to obtain adequate intake.
3. Assess skin turgor, mucous membranes, cracked lips, and furrows on the tongue.
4. Check vital signs: Heart rate increases with blood volume decrease. Check for narrow pulse pressure.
5. Assess urine output for volume and concentration (color) and specific gravity.
6. Assess recent weight loss by percentage.
7. Assess hand or neck vein filling.
8. Review laboratory findings such as BUN, hematocrit, and hemoglobin.

Nursing Interventions
1. Monitor vital signs every 1 to 4 hours depending on severity of fluid loss.
2. Monitor I&O at least every 8 hours and sometimes hourly.
3. Provide fluid intake hourly orally or by I.V. replacement.
4. Monitor assessments frequently: Skin turgor, mucous membranes, hand filling, and urinary output. *Note*: Urine output of less than 30 mL/hr should be reported to the **licensed independent practitioner (LIP)**.
5. Monitor I.V. fluid replacement to ensure infusion rate.

 Media Link: Use Web-based interactive for case study with care plans.

Treatment

Treatment for patients with an ECF volume deficit entails fluid replacement (orally or intravenously) until the oliguria is relieved and the cardiovascular and neurological systems stabilize. Isotonic electrolyte solutions, such as 0.9% NaCl or lactated Ringer's solution, are used to treat hypotensive patients with FVD. A hypotonic electrolyte solution (0.45% NaCl) is often used to provide electrolyte and free water for renal excretion of metabolic wastes.

If the patient with severe FVD is not excreting enough urine, the LIP needs to determine whether the depressed renal function is caused by reduced renal blood flow secondary to FVD or acute tubular necrosis. A fluid challenge test is used in this situation. A typical example involves administering 100 to 200 mL of sodium chloride solution (0.9% NaCl) over 15 minutes. The goal is to provide fluids rapidly enough to attain adequate tissue perfusion without compromising the cardiovascular system (Smeltzer, Bare, Hinkle, & Cheever, 2010).

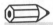 NURSING FAST FACT!

Extreme caution must be exercised in fluid replacement therapy to avoid fluid overload.

Fluid Volume Excess (Hypervolemia)

ECF volume excess causes an expansion of the ECF compartment. The primary cause of ECF excess is cardiovascular dysfunction. FVE is always secondary to an increase in total body sodium content, which causes total body water increase. Normally, the posterior pituitary decreases secretion of the ADH when excess water moves into the cells. This causes the kidney to eliminate excess fluid. However, if a patient has excessive secretion of ADH, the water will be retained, which places the patient at risk for FVE. Excessive secretion of ADH can be caused by fear, pain, and postoperative reaction 12 to 24 hours after surgery, along with acute infections.

Etiology

Conditions that cause overhydration include excessive administration of oral or I.V. fluids containing sodium, excessive irrigation of body cavities or organs, and use of hypotonic fluids to replace isotonic fluid loss. When sodium and water are retained in the same proportion, iso-osmolar FVE occurs. Edema is commonly associated with excess extracellular body fluid or excess fluid due to I.V. overhydration. Physiological factors leading to edema may be caused by various clinical conditions, such as heart failure (HF), kidney failure, cirrhosis of the liver, steroid excess, and retention of sodium (Kee, Paulanka, & Polek, 2010).

NOTE > Azotemia (increased nitrogen levels in the blood) can occur with FVE when urea and creatinine are not excreted because of decreased perfusion by the kidneys and excretion of wastes (Smeltzer, Bare, Hinkle, & Cheever, 2010).

Common Causes of Isotonic Overhydration

- Renal failure leading to decreased excretion of water and sodium
- HF leading to stasis of blood in the circulation and venous congestion
- Excess fluid intake of isotonic I.V. solutions
- High corticosteroid levels as a result of therapy, stress response, or disease causing sodium and water retention
- High aldosterone levels (stress response to adrenal dysfunction, liver damage, or metabolic problems)

Common Causes of Hypotonic Overhydration (Water Intoxication)

- More fluid is gained than solute
- Serum osmolality falls, causing cells to swell (cerebral cells most sensitive)
- Repeated plain water enemas
- Overuse of hypotonic I.V. fluids
- In young children or infants, ingestion of inappropriately prepared formula and/or excess water (use of water bottle as pacifier)
- SIADH causes kidneys to retain large amounts of water without sodium.

Clinical Manifestations

Clinically, ECF volume excess has distinct signs and symptoms, the most prominent being weight gain. A constant irritating nonproductive cough is frequently the first clinical symptom of hypervolemia. It is caused by excess fluid "backed up" into the lungs.

Edema usually is not apparent until 2 to 4 kg of fluid has been retained. Alterations in respiratory and cardiovascular function are present and include hypertension and tachycardia. Moist crackles in the lung usually indicate that the lungs are congested with fluid. Cyanosis is a late symptom of pulmonary edema resulting from hypervolemia. In addition to having the common assessment findings, some patients experience confusion, altered LOC, skeletal muscle weakness, and increased bowel sounds.

Peripheral edema present in the morning may result from inadequate cardiac, hepatic, or renal function. Peripheral edema in the evening may result from fluid stasis or dependent edema. An increase in vascular volume may be evidenced by distended neck veins, slow-emptying peripheral veins, a full and bounding pulse, and an increase in CVP.

NURSING FAST FACT!

> *Peripheral edema should be assessed in the morning before the patient gets out of bed. A weight gain of 2.2 lb is equivalent to the retention of 1 L of body water.*

Laboratory Findings

Laboratory findings are variable and usually nonspecific.

- BUN, serum protein, albumin, hemoglobin, and hematocrit may be decreased as a result of hemodilution.
- Serum osmolality will be decreased below 280 mOsm/kg.
- B-type natriuretic peptide (BNP) is increased to greater than 100 pg/mL in congestive HF.
- Serum sodium is decreased if hypervolemia occurs as a result of excessive water retention.
- Urine specific gravity is decreased if kidney is attempting to excrete excess volume.

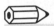 *NURSING FAST FACT!*

> *Severe or prolonged isotonic FVE in a person with a healthy heart and kidneys usually is compensated by increasing urinary output.*

NURSING POINTS OF CARE
HYPERVOLEMIA (FVE)

Nursing Assessments

- Complete a client history to identify underlying health problems that may have contributed to FVE.
- Obtain dietary history that emphasizes sodium, protein, and water intake.
- Assess vital signs; focus on the presence of a bounding pulse.
- Assess for constant irritating cough, difficulty in breathing, neck and hand vein engorgement, and lung crackles.
- Assess I&O at regular intervals to identify excessive fluid retention.
- Assess acute weight gain of 2.2 lb (1 kg) using serial daily weights.
- Assess extremities for peripheral edema (feet and ankles in ambulatory patients, and sacral region in patients confined to bed).

Continued

Key Nursing Interventions

1. Monitor vital signs; report elevated BP or bounding pulse to LIP.
2. Monitor weight daily. Check (serial) weight every morning before breakfast.
3. Observe for the presence of edema daily. Check for pitting edema in the extremities every morning.
4. Monitor diet, and teach appropriate food selections to avoid excess salt.
5. Encourage rest periods to support diuresis.

Treatment

Medical management is directed toward sodium and fluid restriction, administration of diuretics, and treatment of the underlying cause (Porth & Matfin, 2010). The treatment of FVE focuses on providing a balance between sodium and water I&O. Diuretic therapy is commonly used to increase sodium elimination. If renal function is so severely impaired that pharmacological agents cannot act efficiently, hemodialysis or peritoneal dialysis may be considered to remove nitrogenous wastes, control potassium and acid–base balance, and remove sodium and fluid (Smeltzer, Bare, Hinkle, & Cheever, 2010). Table 3-4 summarizes the fluid imbalances of hypovolemia and hypervolemia.

> Table 3-4	QUICK ASSESSMENT GUIDE FOR FLUID IMBALANCES	
Area of Clinical Assessment	Signs and Symptoms of Fluid Volume Deficit (Hypovolemia)	Signs and Symptoms of Fluid Volume Excess (Hypervolemia)
Neurological	Irritability, restlessness, lethargy, confusion (seizures and coma) Thirst	Confusion
Cardiovascular	Frank or postural hypotension Tachycardia Weak, thready pulses Decreased pulse volume Cool extremities with delayed capillary refill Flat neck veins Poor peripheral vein filling Central venous pressure (CVP) <4 cm	Galloping heart rhythm (heart S_3 sound) in adults Distended neck veins Slow emptying hand veins CVP >11 cm Bounding full pulse Peripheral edema
Respiratory	Lungs clear Respirations may be rapid and shallow	Tachypnea (>20) and dyspnea Irritated cough Hacking cough, becoming moist and productive Labored breathing Wet lung sounds (moist crackles) Decreased O_2 saturation Cyanosis

> Table 3-4	QUICK ASSESSMENT GUIDE FOR FLUID IMBALANCES—cont'd	
Area of Clinical Assessment	Signs and Symptoms of Fluid Volume Deficit (Hypovolemia)	Signs and Symptoms of Fluid Volume Excess (Hypervolemia)
Skin Appearance and Temperature	Low-grade fever Dry skin "tenting" Sunken or depressed fontanels in infants	Bulging fontanels in children <18 months Edematous skin (1+ to 4+)
Eyes	Decreased tearing and dry conjunctiva Sunken eyeballs	Periorbital edema
Lips	Dry lips, cracked	No change
Oral Cavity	Dry Increased tongue furrows, tongue coated Sticky mucous membranes	No change
Urine Volume and Concentration	Concentrated urine and low volume <30 mL/hr Specific gravity high: >1.035	Polyuria Specific gravity <1.005
Body Weight	Weight loss 5%: Mild deficit 5%–10%: Moderate deficit >15%: Severe deficit (especially important in children)	Weight gain (acute and rapid) 5%: Mild excess 5%–10%: Moderate excess >15%: Severe excess
Diagnostic Laboratory Findings	Normal or high hematocrit and blood urea nitrogen (BUN) Serum osmolarity elevated: >300 Serum sodium >150 mEq Serum glucose elevated: >120 mg/dL	Hematocrit and BUN decreased Serum osmolality low: <275 Serum sodium low: <125 mEq

Sources: Kee, Paulanka & Polek, (2010); Porth & Matfin, (2010).

■ Basic Principles of Electrolyte Balance

Chemical compounds in solution behave in one of two ways: They separate and combine with other compounds, or they remain intact. One group of compounds remains intact; these are called nonelectrolytes (e.g., urea, dextrose, creatinine). These compounds do not separate from their complex form when added to a solution. The second group of compounds, electrolytes, dissociates or separates in solution. These compounds break up into separate particles known as ions in a process called ionization. The major electrolytes in body fluids are sodium, potassium, calcium, magnesium, chloride, phosphorus, and bicarbonate.

Ions, which are the dissociated particles of an electrolyte, each carries an electrical charge, either positive or negative. Negative ions are called **anions** and positive ions are called **cations**.

Electrolytes are active chemicals that unite. The ions are expressed in terms of milliequivalents (mEq) per liter rather than milligrams. A milliequivalent measures chemical activity or combining power rather than weight. For example, when a hostess creates a guest list for a party, she does not invite 1000 lb of boys per 1000 lb of girls; rather, she invites the same number of boys and girls. In total, the milliequivalents of cations in a given compartment is equal to the milliequivalents of anions. There are 154 mEq of anions and 154 mEq of cations in the plasma. Each water compartment of the body contains electrolytes. The concentration and composition of electrolytes vary from compartment to compartment. Table 3-5 gives a diagrammatic comparison of electrolyte composition in the fluid compartments.

Most of the electrolytes have more than one physiological role; often several electrolytes work together to mediate chemical events. The physiological roles of electrolytes include:

- Maintaining electroneutrality in fluid compartments
- Mediating enzyme reactions

> Table 3-5   **COMPARISON OF ELECTROLYTE COMPOSITION IN FLUID COMPARTMENTS**

Intracellular Water (approx. mEq/L)		Extracellular Water (approx. mEq/L)			
Intracellular		*Plasma*		*Interstitial Fluid*	
Cations	Anions	Cations	Anions	Cations	Anions
205 mEq	205 mEq	154 mEq	154 mEq	154 mEq	154 mEq

Intracellular:
Na$^+$ 10
K$^+$ 160
Mg^{++} 35

Cl$^-$ 2
HCO$_3^-$ 8
HPO$_4^-$ 140
Protein$^-$ 55

Plasma Cations:
Na$^+$ 142
K$^+$ 4
Mg^{++} 3
Ca^{++} 5

Plasma Anions:
Cl$^-$ 103
HCO$_3^-$ 27
HCO$_4^-$ 2
SO$_4^-$ 1
Organic acids$^-$ 5
Protein$^-$ 16

Interstitial Fluid Cations:
Na$^+$ 145
K$^+$ 4
Mg^{++} 2
Ca^{++} 3

Interstitial Fluid Anions:
HPO$_4^-$ 2
SO$_4^-$ 1
Organic acids$^+$ 5
Protein$^+$ 1

- Altering cell membrane permeability
- Regulating muscle contraction and relaxation
- Regulating nerve impulse transmission
- Influencing blood clotting time

The electrolyte content of ICF differs from that of ECF. Usually only ECF plasma electrolytes are measured because of the special techniques required to measure the concentration of electrolytes in ICF. The serum plasma levels of electrolytes are important in the assessment and management of patients with electrolyte imbalances.

Nursing Diagnosis and Electrolyte Imbalances

Certain physiological complications that nurses monitor to detect onset or changes in status are considered collaborative problems. Nurses manage collaborative problems using physician- and nursing-prescribed interventions to minimize the complications of the events. Electrolyte imbalances are collaborative problems, and for collaborative problems nursing focuses on monitoring for onset of change in status of physiological complications.

General Diagnostic Statement

Potential complication metabolic related to electrolyte imbalance: A person with an electrolyte imbalance is experiencing or is at risk for experiencing a deficit or excess of one or more electrolytes.

Nursing goal: The nurse will manage and minimize episodes of electrolyte imbalances using laboratory values and monitor for signs and symptoms of specific electrolyte imbalance.

NOTE > For each of the following electrolytes, the Nursing Points of Care focuses on assessments and nursing interventions that support collection of data for monitoring for changes in status.

Sodium (Na$^+$)

Normal Reference Value: 135 to 145 mEq/L

Physiological Role

The physiological role of sodium includes:
- Neuromuscular: Transmission and conduction of nerve impulses (sodium pump)
- Body Fluids: Responsible for the osmolality of vascular fluids
- Cellular: Maintain water balance. Sodium shifts into cells as potassium shifts out of cells—depolarization (cell activity). When sodium shifts out of cells, potassium shifts back into cell—repolarization (enzyme activity).

■ Acid–base: Sodium combines with chloride or bicarbonate to regulate acid–base balance (Kee, Paulanka, & Polek, 2010).

 NURSING FAST FACT!

Doubling the serum sodium level gives the approximate serum osmolality.

The major function of sodium is to maintain ECF volume. Extracellular sodium level has an effect on the cellular fluid volume based on the principle of osmosis. Sodium represents about 90% of all the extracellular cations. Sodium does not easily cross the cell wall membrane and therefore is the most abundant cation of ECF.

A low serum sodium level results in dilute ECF, therefore allowing water to be drawn into the cells (lower to higher concentration). Conversely, if the serum sodium is high, water is drawn out of the cells, leading to cellular dehydration. Figure 3-7 shows the relationship between sodium and cellular fluid. The normal daily requirement for sodium in adults is approximately 100 mEq.

The kidneys are extremely important in the regulation of sodium, which is primarily accomplished through the action of the hormone aldosterone. Hyponatremia is a common complication of adrenal insufficiency because of aldosterone and cortisol deficiencies. Elderly persons have a slower rate of aldosterone secretion, which places them at risk for sodium imbalances.

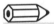 **NURSING FAST FACT!**

The cerebral cells are very sensitive to changes in serum sodium levels and exhibit adaptive changes to sodium imbalances (Ayus, Achinger, & Arieff, 2008).

Three factors can create a sodium imbalance:

1. Change in the sodium content of the ECF, such as a deficit caused by excessive vomiting
2. Change in the chloride content, which can affect both the sodium concentration and the amount of water in the ECF; when the ratio of chloride to sodium deviates from normal, it is reflected as an acid–base imbalance
3. Change in the quantity of water in the ECF

Serum Sodium Deficit: Hyponatremia

Hyponatremia is a condition in which the sodium level is below normal (<135 mEq/L). A low sodium level can be the result of an excessive loss of sodium or an excessive gain of water; in either event, hyponatremia is

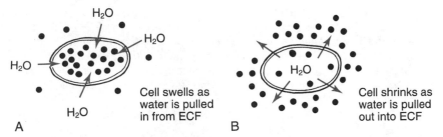

Figure 3-7 ■ Sodium and cellular fluid relationship. (*A*) Hyponatremia. The cell swells as water is pulled in from the extracellular fluid. (*B*) Hypernatremia. The cell shrinks as water is pulled out into the extracellular fluid.

caused by a relatively greater concentration of water than of sodium. Sodium deficit usually is associated with hypervolemic states.

ETIOLOGY

The pathophysiology that contributes to sodium deficit (hyponatremia) is often a sign of a serious underlying disease; there are also many causes of hyponatremia.

All GI secretions contain sodium; therefore, any abnormal loss of GI secretions can cause a sodium deficit. GI disorders such as vomiting, diarrhea, drainage from suction or fistulas, and excessive tap water enemas may also cause hyponatremia.

Other causes of hyponatremia are losses from skin as a result of excessive sweating, combined with excessive water consumption and the use of thiazide diuretics (especially dangerous with low-salt diets). In addition, excessive parenteral hypo-osmolar fluids such as dextrose in water solutions can cause hyponatremia.

Hormonal factors such as labor induction with oxytocin and SIADH reduce the amount of sodium per volume, which in turn leads to dilutional hyponatremia. Oxytocin has been shown to have an intrinsic ADH effect by increasing water reabsorption from the glomerular filtrate. Cerebral ICF excess (hyponatremic encephalopathy) is associated with the risk of seizures, coma, and death, which can occur when water shifts into the brain cells (Kee, Paulanka, & Polek, 2010). Researchers believe that physiological responses in premenopausal women place them at higher risk than men for hyponatremic encephalopathy because estrogen stimulates ADH release and antagonizes the brain's ability to adapt to swelling (Ayus, J. C., Achinger, S. G., et al., 2008). In men, androgens suppress ADH release and enhance the brain's ability to adapt to swelling. Young women account for most of the reported cases of fatalities secondary to hyponatremia. Marathon runners have been shown to develop hyponatremic encephalopathy related to dilutional hyponatremia (Rosner & Kirven, 2007).

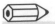 *NURSING FAST FACT!*

> *SIADH has progressed from a rare occurrence to the most common cause of hyponatremia seen in general hospitals. It occurs in patients with inflammatory disorders such as pneumonia, tuberculosis, abscess, oat cell cancer of the lung, and CNS disorders such as meningitis, trauma, stroke, and degenerative diseases (Goh, 2004).*

EBP TREATMENT OF SEVERE DILUTIONAL HYPONATREMIA. An evidence-based consensus statement concluded that both excessive fluid consumption and a decrease in urine formation contribute to dilutional effect in hyponatremia, which can lead to life-threatening and fatal cases of pulmonary and cerebral edema. Strategies for treatment include intravenous hypertonic solutions (e.g., 3% sodium chloride) to reverse the symptoms related to moderate and life-threatening hypotonic encephalopathy (Hew-Butler et al., 2005).

CLINICAL MANIFESTATIONS

Hyponatremia affects cells of the CNS. Patients with chronic hyponatremia may experience impaired sensation of taste, anorexia, muscle cramps, feelings of exhaustion, apprehension, feelings of impending doom (at Na^+ <115), and focal weaknesses (e.g., hemiparesis, ataxia). Patients with acute hyponatremia caused by water overload experience the same symptoms as well as fingerprinting edema (sign of intracellular water excess). Patients undergoing operative procedures involving irrigations (e.g., transurethral resection of prostate [TURP], endometrial ablation) may develop hyponatremia.

LABORATORY FINDINGS

- Serum sodium: Less than 135 mEq/L
- Serum osmolarity: Less than 280 mOsm/L
- Urine specific gravity: Less than 1.010 (except in SIADH)
- Urine sodium: Decreased (usually less than 20 mEq/L)
- Hematocrit: Above normal when FVD exists
- Decreased BUN

TREATMENT/COLLABORATIVE MANAGEMENT

Treatment of patients with hyponatremia aims to provide sodium by the dietary, enteral, or parenteral route. Patients able to eat and drink can easily replace sodium by ingesting a normal diet. Those unable to take sodium orally must take the electrolyte by the parenteral route. An isotonic saline or Ringer's solution (e.g., 0.9% sodium chloride (NaCl), or lactated Ringer's solution may be ordered. The immediate goal of therapy is the correction of acute symptoms, gradual return of sodium to a normal level, and, if necessary, restoration of normal ECF volume.

Acute symptomatic hyponatremia requires more aggressive treatment. Treatment must be individualized. Too rapid correction of chronic hyponatremia (lasting >24–48 hours) may cause irreversible neurological damage and death as a result of osmotic demyelination (Halperin, Kamel, & Goldstein, 2010).

General treatment guidelines for patients with hyponatremia are:

1. Replace sodium and fluid losses through diet or parenteral fluids.
2. Restore normal ECF volume.
3. Restrict water intake.
4. Increase the excretion of water without electrolytes.
5. Correct any other electrolyte losses such as potassium or bicarbonate.

Treatment of hyponatremia with fluid volume overload includes:

1. Remove or treat underlying cause such as SIADH.
2. Administer loop diuretic (thiazide diuretics should be avoided).
3. Water restriction to 1000 mL/day establishes negative water balance and increases plasma sodium levels in most adults.

 NURSING FAST FACT!

When the primary problem is water retention, it is safer to restrict water than to administer sodium. An I.V. solution that can contribute to hyponatremia is excessive administration of 5% dextrose in water.

 NURSING FAST FACT!

Permanent neurological damage may occur in patients with acute symptomatic hyponatremia as a result of failure to adequately treat hyponatremic encephalopathy. The replacement of sodium chloride solution by infusion pump should be at a rate calculated to elevate the plasma sodium level about 1 mEq/L/hr. Too rapid elevation of sodium (>25 mEq/L in the first 48 hours) can cause brain damage (Goh, 2004; Halperin, Kamel, & Goldstein, 2010).

NURSING POINTS OF CARE
HYPONATREMIA

Nursing Assessments
- Obtain a patient history of high-risk factors for hyponatremia (vomiting, diarrhea, eating disorders, low-sodium diet).
- Obtain a history of medications, with emphasis on those predisposing patients to hyponatremia (e.g., diuretics).

Continued

- Assess for signs and symptoms of hyponatremia (weight gain without peripheral edema, fingerprinting, edema, poor skin turgor, dry mucosa, headache, decreased saliva production, orthostatic fall in BP, nausea, and vomiting).
- Obtain baseline laboratory tests (e.g., serum sodium, serum osmolarity, serum potassium, serum chloride, urinary specific gravity).

Key Nursing Interventions
1. Monitor laboratory test results, with emphasis on serum sodium.
2. Monitor GI losses.
3. Monitor for signs and symptoms of hyponatremia: CNS changes (coma, headache), weakness, nausea, muscle cramps, vomiting, diarrhea, and apprehension. In severe cases status epilepticus, coma, and obtundation occur and are related to cellular swelling and cerebral edema (Smeltzer, Bare, Hinkle, & Cheever, 2010).
4. Monitor I&O, daily weight, and specific gravity.
5. Restrict water when hyponatremia is caused by hypervolemia.
6. Follow LIP orders to rate and type of I.V. fluid to administer.

Serum Sodium Excess: Hypernatremia

The serum level of sodium is elevated to above 145 mEq/L in hypernatremia. This elevation can be caused by a gain of sodium without water or a loss of water without loss of sodium. There are two primary defenses against hypernatremia: (1) thirst response and (2) excretion of maximally concentrated urine through increased production of ADH. Sodium is the major determinant of ECF osmolality; therefore, hypernatremia causes hypertonicity. Hypertonicity causes a shift of water of the cells, which leads to cellular dehydration. Dehydration of the cerebral cells results in the development of CNS symptoms (Heitz & Horne, 2005).

ETIOLOGY

Increased levels of serum sodium can occur with water loss or deprivation of water, when a person cannot respond to thirst, and during hypertonic tube feeding with inadequate water supplements. Sodium gain can occur with excessive parenteral administration of sodium-containing solutions and in near-drowning in salt water. Sodium is lost in cases of watery diarrhea (a particular problem in infants), increased insensible loss, ingestion of sodium in unusual amounts, profuse sweating, heat stroke, and diabetes insipidus when water intake is inadequate (Smeltzer, Bare, Hinkle, & Cheever, 2010).

Clinical Manifestations

Patients with hypernatremia may experience marked thirst; elevated body temperature; swollen tongue; red, dry, sticky mucous membranes; and tachycardia. In severe hypernatremia, disorientation and irritability or hyperactivity when the patient is physically stimulated can occur.

Laboratory Findings

- Serum sodium: Greater than 145 mEq/L
- Chloride may be elevated.
- Serum osmolarity: Greater than 295 mOsm/kg
- Urine specific gravity: Greater than 1.015 (except for those with diabetes insipidus)
- Dehydration test: Water is withheld for 16 to 18 hours; serum and urine osmolarity are checked 1 hour after administration of ADH; this test is used to identify the cause of polyuric syndromes (central vs. nephrogenic diabetes insipidus).

EBP Ferry (2005) found that because the aging process causes a decrease in thirst, once a geriatric client experiences thirst, he or she may have a severe water deficit and sodium excess.

Treatment/Collaborative Management

The goal of treatment of patients with hypernatremia is gradual lowering of the serum sodium level (usually over 48 hours) by infusing a hypotonic electrolyte solution such as 0.45% normal saline or 5% dextrose in water. Many clinicians consider a hypotonic sodium solution to be safer than D5W because it allows a gradual reduction in the serum sodium level, thereby decreasing the risk of cerebral edema (Porth & Matfin, 2010). The sodium level should not be lowered by more than 15 mEq/L in an 8-hour period for adults (Smeltzer, Bare, Hinkle, & Cheever, 2010).

Generally, treatment guidelines for hypernatremia are:

1. Infusion of hypotonic electrolyte solution (0.45% NaCl or 5% dextrose in water). If the sodium level is more than 160 mEq/L, 5% dextrose in water is indicated.
2. Decreasing sodium levels by use of diuretics, which induce excretion of water and sodium
3. Administration of desmopressin acetate (DDAVP) to treat central diabetes insipidus. Treating the underlying cause (e.g., fever, diarrhea) minimizes abnormal fluid loss.
4. Removal of the cause of hypernatremia, for example, discontinuing medications that cause increase sodium levels (lithium) or correcting electrolyte imbalances such as hypokalemia and hypercalcemia (Smeltzer, Bare, Hinkle, & Cheever, 2010).

NURSING POINTS OF CARE
HYPERNATREMIA

Nursing Assessments
- Obtain a patient history of high-risk factors for hypernatremia (e.g., increased sodium intake, water deprivation, increased adrenocortical hormone production, use of sodium-retaining drugs).
- Assess for signs and symptoms of hypernatremia (restlessness and weakness, disorientation, delusions, thirst), which result from dehydration of cells (Smeltzer, Bare, Hinkle, & Cheever, 2010).
- Obtain baseline values of laboratory tests, especially serum sodium.

Key Nursing Interventions
1. Monitor laboratory test results, with emphasis on serum sodium and serum osmolarity.
2. Monitor fluid I&O and daily weight.
3. Monitor for signs and symptoms of hypernatremia related to abnormal loss of water or large gains of sodium, which includes thirst, CNS effects (agitation to convulsions), weight gain and edema, elevated BP, elevated temperature, and tachycardia.
4. Monitor for signs of pulmonary edema when the patient is receiving large amounts of parenteral sodium chloride.
5. Promote increased mobility if appropriate.
6. Monitor for seizures.
7. Administer orders from LIP of hypotonic sodium monitoring rate.

Potassium (K+)

Normal Reference Value: 3.5 to 5.0 mEq/L

Physiological Role

The physiological role of potassium includes:
- Regulation of fluid volume within the cell
- Promotion of nerve impulse transmission
- Contraction of skeletal, smooth, and cardiac muscle
- Control of hydrogen ion (H^+) concentration, acid–base balance; when potassium moves out of the cell, hydrogen ions move in, and vice versa.
- Role in enzyme action for cellular energy production

Potassium is an intracellular electrolyte present as 98% in the ICF and 2% in the ECF. Potassium is a dynamic electrolyte. Cellular potassium replaces ECF potassium if it becomes depleted. Potassium is acquired through diet and must be ingested daily because the body has no effective method of potassium storage. The daily requirement is 40 mEq. Potassium influences both skeletal and cardiac muscle activity. Alterations in the concentration of plasma potassium change myocardial irritability and rhythm. Potassium moves easily into the intracellular space when the body is metabolizing glucose. It moves out of the cells during strenuous exercise, when cellular metabolism is impaired, or when the cell dies. Potassium, along with sodium, is responsible for transmission of nerve impulses. During nerve cell innervation, these ions exchange places, creating an electrical current (Kee, Paulanka, & Polek, 2010).

There is a relationship between acid–base imbalances and potassium balance. Hypokalemia can cause alkalosis, which in turn can further decrease serum potassium. Hyperkalemia can cause acidosis, which in turn can further increase serum potassium.

The regulation of potassium is related to several other processes, including:

- Sodium level: Enough sodium must be available for exchange with potassium.
- Hydrogen ion excretion: When there is an increase in hydrogen ion excretion, there is a decrease in potassium excretion.
- Aldosterone level: An increased level of aldosterone stimulates and increases excretion of potassium.
- Potassium imbalances are commonly seen in clinical practice because of their association with underlying disease, injury, or ingestion of certain medications.

Serum Potassium Deficit: Hypokalemia

Hypokalemia is a serum potassium level below 3.5 mEq/L. It usually reflects a real deficit in total potassium stores; however, it may occur in patients with normal potassium stores when alkalosis is present. Hypokalemia is a common disturbance; many factors are associated with this deficit, and many clinical conditions contribute to it.

ETIOLOGY

Many conditions can lead to potassium deficit, including GI and renal loss, increased use of diuretic, increased perspiration, shifting of extracellular potassium into the cells, and poor dietary intake. GI loss can result from diarrhea or laxative overuse, prolonged gastric suction, and protracted vomiting. Renal loss can result from potassium-wasting diuretic therapy; excessive use of glucocorticoids; ingestion of drugs such as sodium penicillin, carbenicillin, or amphotericin B; excessive ingestion of European licorice (which mimics the action of aldosterone); and excessive steroid administration.

Sweat loss can result from heavy perspiration in persons acclimated to the heat. Shifting into the cells can occur with parenteral nutrition (PN) therapy without adequate potassium supplementation, alkalosis, and excessive administration of insulin. Poor dietary intake can occur with anorexia nervosa, bulimia, and alcoholism.

CLINICAL MANIFESTATIONS

Clinical symptoms rarely develop before the serum potassium level has decreased to less than 3 mEq/L unless the rate of decline has been rapid (Smeltzer, Bare, Hinkle, & Cheever, 2010). Patients with hypokalemia may experience neuromuscular changes such as fatigue, muscle weakness, diminished deep tendon reflexes, and flaccid paralysis (late). Other symptoms include anorexia, nausea, vomiting, irritability (early), increased sensitivity to digitalis, electrocardiographic (ECG) changes, and death (in those with severe hypokalemia) caused by cardiac arrest.

LABORATORY AND ECG FINDINGS

- Serum potassium: Less than 3.5 mEq/L
- Arterial blood gas (ABG): May show metabolic alkalosis (increased pH and bicarbonate ion)
- Elevated serum glucose levels (increased insulin secretion and increased osmotic pressure)
- ECG: ST-segment depression, flattened T wave, presence of U wave, and ventricular dysrhythmias. The ECG tracing in Figure 3-8 reflects changes when potassium is below normal.

 NURSING FAST FACT!

Clinical signs and symptoms rarely occur before the serum potassium level has fallen below 3 mEq/L.

Potassium replacement must take place slowly to prevent hyperkalemia. Extreme caution should be used when potassium chloride replacement exceeds 120 mEq in 24 hours. The patient must be monitored for dysrhythmias.

TREATMENT/COLLABORATIVE MANAGEMENT

Replacement of potassium is the key concept in treating patients with potassium deficit. Replace potassium either by mouth or intravenously. The usual oral dose is 40 to 80 mEq/day in divided doses. I.V. potassium is necessary if hypokalemia is severe or if the patient is unable to tolerate oral potassium. I.V. potassium is irritating to the vessels, so the rate must be adjusted to prevent phlebitis. Potassium usually is replaced in combination with chloride or phosphate. Hypokalemia is frequently associated with ECF volume deficit and chloride loss; potassium chloride is usually

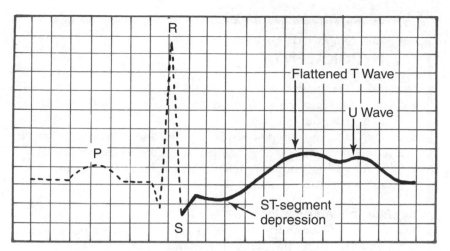

Figure 3-8 ■ Sample ECG tracing showing hypokalemia. The ECG tracing for hypokalemia has ST-segment depression, flattened T wave, and presence of a U wave.

ordered. Hypokalemia associated with metabolic acidosis may be treated with potassium bicarbonate or citrate (Heitz & Horne, 2005).

General treatment guidelines include:

1. Mild hypokalemia usually is treated with dietary increases of potassium or oral supplements.
2. Salt substitutes (e.g., Morton Salt Substitute, Co-Salt, Adolph's Salt Substitute) contain potassium and can be used to supplement potassium intake.
3. If the serum potassium is below 2 mEq/L, monitor the patient's ECG and administer potassium by a secondary piggyback set in a volume of 100 mL (Smeltzer, Bare, Hinkle, & Cheever, 2010). Table 3-6 lists guidelines for I.V. potassium.

NOTE > Never give potassium I.V. push/bolus.

 NURSING FAST FACT!

Potassium should be administered only after adequate urine flow has been established. Potassium is primarily excreted by the kidney.

Table 3-6 gives critical guidelines for nursing in I.V. administration of potassium.

NURSING POINTS OF CARE
HYPOKALEMIA

Nursing Assessments
- Obtain history of high-risk factors for hypokalemia (vomiting, renal disease, diuretic use).
- Assess for signs of hypokalemia (fatigue, anorexia, nausea, vomiting, muscle weakness, leg cramps, paresthesias, dysrhythmias).
- Obtain baseline laboratory test values (ECG reading, serum potassium, serum osmolarity).

Key Nursing Interventions
1. Monitor the laboratory test results, especially serum potassium.
2. Monitor for signs and symptoms of hypokalemia.
3. Keep accurate I&O records to assess renal function.
4. Monitor for changes in cardiac response.
5. Monitor for signs of phlebitis (potassium irritates veins) when given by I.V. route.
6. When administering potassium by I.V., always dilute and do not exceed 10 mEq/hr in adults. **Never give by I.V. push.**

> Table 3-6	CRITICAL GUIDELINES FOR ADMINISTRATION OF POTASSIUM

Never give a potassium I.V. push.

Potassium chloride (KCl) should be added to a nondextrose solution such as isotonic saline to treat severe hypokalemia because administration of KCl in a dextrose solution may cause a small reduction in the serum potassium level.

Never administer concentrated potassium solutions without first diluting them as directed.

KCl preparations >60 mEq/L **should not** be given in a peripheral vein. Concentrations >8 mEq/100 mL can cause pain and irritation of peripheral veins and lead to postinfusion phlebitis.

When adding KCl to infusion solutions, especially plastic systems, make sure the KCl is thoroughly mixed with the solution. Invert and agitate the container to ensure mixing.

Do not add KCl to a hanging container!

For patients with any degree of renal insufficiency or heart block, reduce the infusion by 50%, for example, 5–10 mEq/hr rather than 10–20 mEq/hr.

Administer potassium at a rate not to exceed 10 mEq/hr through peripheral veins.

For patients with extreme hypokalemia, rates should be no more than 40 mEq/hr while electrocardiogram is constantly monitored.

KCl administered into the subcutaneous tissue (infiltration) is extremely irritating and can cause serious tissue loss. Use extravasation protocol in this situation.

Sources: Gahart & Nazareno (2012); Smeltzer, Bare, Hinkle & Cheever (2010).

Serum Potassium Excess: Hyperkalemia

Hyperkalemia occurs less frequently than hypokalemia, but it can be more dangerous. It seldom occurs in patients who have normal renal function. Hyperkalemia is defined as a serum plasma level of potassium above 5.0 mEq/L. The main causes of hyperkalemia are (1) increased intake of potassium (oral or parenteral), (2) decreased urinary excretion of potassium, and (3) movement of potassium out of the cells and into the extracellular space.

ETIOLOGY

High levels of serum potassium can be caused by either a gain of potassium body or a shift of potassium from the ICF to the ECF. Hyperkalemia can be caused by excessive administration of potassium parentally or orally; severe renal failure resulting in reduced potassium excretion; release of potassium from altered cellular function (as occurs with burns or crush injuries); and acidosis.

Drugs that can cause a predisposition to hyperkalemias include potassium penicillin, indomethacin, amphetamines, nonsteroidal antiinflammatory drugs, alpha agonists, beta blockers, succinylcholine, cyclophosphamide, and potassium-sparing diuretics. Pseudohyperkalemia can occur with prolonged tourniquet application during blood withdrawal (Kee, Paulanka, & Polek, 2010).

CLINICAL MANIFESTATIONS

The cardiac effects of elevated serum potassium usually are not significant when the level is less than 7 mEq/L but will be present when the level is 8 mEq/L or greater (Smeltzer, Bare, Hinkle, & Cheever, 2010). Patients with hyperkalemia may experience changes that will be seen on the ECG, irregular pulse, vague muscle weakness, flaccid paralysis, anxiety, nausea, abdominal cramping, and diarrhea.

LABORATORY AND ECG FINDINGS

- Serum potassium: Greater than 5.0 mEq/L with clinical symptoms present after 7 mEq/L
- ABG values: Metabolic acidosis (decreased pH and bicarbonate ion)
- ECG: Widened QRS, prolonged PR, and ventricular dysrhythmias (Fig. 3-9)
- If dehydration is causing hyperkalemia, then hematocrit, hemoglobin, and sodium and chloride levels should be drawn.
- If associated with renal failure, creatinine and BUN levels should be drawn.

TREATMENT/COLLABORATIVE MANAGEMENT

The goal is to treat the underlying cause and return the serum potassium to a safe level. In acute hyperkalemia, administration of

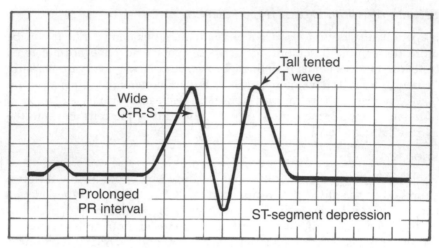

Figure 3-9 ■ Sample ECG tracing showing hyperkalemia. The ECG tracing for hyperkalemia shows progressive changes; tall, thin T waves; prolonged PR intervals; ST-segment depression; widened QRS; and loss of P wave.

I.V. calcium gluconate, glucose and insulin, beta$_2$ agonists, or sodium bicarbonate is temporary. It is usually necessary to follow these medications with a therapy that removes potassium from the body (Heitz & Horne, 2005).

The following are guidelines for the treatment of patients with hyperkalemia:

1. The goal is to treat the underlying cause and return the serum potassium level to normal.
2. Restrict dietary potassium in mild cases.
3. Discontinue potassium supplements.
4. Cation exchange resins (Kayexalate) may be given PO, NG, or via retention enema to exchange sodium for potassium in the bowel.
5. Administer I.V. calcium gluconate if necessary for cardiac symptoms. Administer I.V. sodium bicarbonate, which alkalinizes the plasma and causes a temporary shift of potassium into the cells.
6. Administer regular insulin (10–25 units) and hypertonic dextrose (10%), which causes a shift of potassium into the cells.
7. Peritoneal dialysis or hemodialysis may be ordered.
8. A beta$_2$ agonist (albuterol or salbutamol) may be ordered by nasal inhalation or I.V. to shift potassium into the cells.

Table 3-7 provides critical guidelines for nursing in the treatment of patients with potassium excess.

> Table 3-7   **CRITICAL GUIDELINES FOR REMOVAL OF POTASSIUM**

Treatment Guidelines

- **Sodium polystyrene sulfonate** is a cation exchange resin that removes potassium from the body by exchanging sodium for potassium in the intestinal tract. This method should not be the sole treatment of severe hyperkalemia because of its slow onset.
  Oral sodium polystyrene sulfonate (15–30 g); may repeat every 4–6 hours as needed. Removes potassium in 1–2 hours.
  Rectal sodium polystyrene sulfonate (50 g) as retention enema. When administered, use an inflated rectal catheter to ensure retention of the dissolved resin for 30–60 minutes. Removes potassium in 30–60 minutes. Each enema can lower the plasma potassium concentration by 0.5–1.0 mEq/L.
- **Dialysis** is used when more aggressive methods are needed. Peritoneal dialysis is not as effective as hemodialysis. Whereas peritoneal dialysis can remove approximately 10–15 mEq/hr, hemodialysis can remove 25–35 mEq/hr.
- **Glucose and insulin**
  Insulin facilitates potassium movement into the cells, reducing the plasma potassium level. Glucose administration in nondiabetic patients may cause a marked increase in insulin release from the pancreas, producing desired plasma potassium-lowering effects.
  From 250–500 mL of 10% dextrose with 10–15 units of regular insulin over 1 hour. The potassium-lowering effects are delayed about 30 minutes but are effective for 4–6 hours.
- **Emergency measures**
  Calcium gluconate: 10 mL of 10% calcium gluconate administered slowly over 2–3 minutes. Administer only to patients who need immediate myocardial protection against toxic effects of severe hyperkalemia. Protective effect begins within 1–2 minutes but lasts only 30–60 minutes.
  Sodium bicarbonate: 45 mEq (1 ampule of 7.5% sodium bicarbonate) infused slowly over 5 minutes. This temporarily shifts potassium into the cells and is helpful in patients with metabolic acidosis.

Sources: Gahart & Nazareno (2012); Heitz & Horne (2005).

NURSING POINTS OF CARE
HYPERKALEMIA

Nursing Assessments
- Obtain client history relative to high-risk factors for hyperkalemia (renal disease, potassium-sparing diuretics, excessive salt substitute use).
- Assess for signs of hyperkalemia (disturbances in cardiac conduction, skeletal muscle weakness, paralysis of respiratory and speech muscles).
- Obtain baseline ECG; assess for altered T waves.
- Obtain baseline serum potassium.

Continued

Key Nursing Interventions
1. Monitor laboratory test results, especially serum potassium.
2. Keep accurate I&O records.
3. Monitor for changes in cardiac response.
4. Monitor vital signs, with special attention to tachycardia and bradycardia.
5. Administer I.V. potassium at rate ordered by LIP following guidelines.

Calcium (Ca^{2+})

Normal Reference Value: 4.5 to 5.5 mEq/L or 9 to 11 mg/dL

Physiological Role

The physiological role of calcium includes:
- Maintaining skeletal elements; calcium is needed for strong, durable bones and teeth
- Regulating neuromuscular activity
- Influencing enzyme activity
- Converting prothrombin to thrombin, a necessary part of the material that holds cells together

Calcium ions are most abundant in the skeletal system, with 99% residing in the bones and teeth. Only 1% is available for rapid exchange in the circulating blood bound to protein. PTH is responsible for the transfer of calcium from bone to plasma. PTH also augments the intestinal absorption of calcium and enhances net renal calcium reabsorption. Calcium is acquired through dietary intake. Adults require approximately 1 g of calcium daily, along with vitamin D and protein, which are required for absorption and utilization of this electrolyte.

Calcium is instrumental in activating enzymes and stimulating essential chemical reactions. It plays an important role in maintaining the normal transmission of nerve impulses and has a sedative effect on nerve cells. Calcium plays its most important role in the conversion of prothrombin to thrombin, a necessary sequence in the formation of a clot.

Calcium and phosphate have a reciprocal relationship; that is, an increase in calcium level causes a drop in the serum phosphorus concentration, and a drop in calcium causes an increase in phosphorus level.

Calcium is present in three different forms in the plasma: (1) ionized (50% of total calcium); (2) bound (<50% of total calcium); and (3) complexed (small percentage that combines with phosphate). Only ionized calcium (iCA; i.e., calcium affected by plasma pH, phosphorus, and albumin levels) is physiologically important. A relationship between iCA and plasma pH is reciprocal; an increase in pH decreases the percentage of calcium that is ionized. The relationship between plasma phosphorus and iCA also is reciprocal. Albumin does not affect iCA, but it does affect the amount of calcium bound to proteins (Porth & Matfin, 2010).

Serum Calcium Deficit: Hypocalcemia

A reduction of total body calcium levels or a reduction of the percentage of ICA causes hypocalcemia. Total calcium levels may be decreased as a result of increased calcium loss or altered regulation (hypoparathyroidism). The most common cause of low total calcium level is hypoalbuminemia.

ETIOLOGY

Total calcium levels may be decreased because of increased calcium loss, reduced intake secondary to altered intestinal absorption, and altered regulation, as occurs in patients with hypoparathyroidism.

The most common cause of hypocalcemia is inadequate PTH secretion caused by primary hypoparathyroidism or surgically induced hypoparathyroidism. It also can result from calcium loss through diarrhea and wound exudate, acute pancreatitis, hyperphosphatemia usually associated with renal failure, inadequate intake of vitamin D or minimal sun exposure, prolonged NG tube suctioning resulting in metabolic alkalosis, and infusion of citrated blood (citrate–phosphate–dextrose).

Many drugs can lead to the development of hypocalcemia, including potent loop diuretics, Dilantin and phenobarbital, antineoplastic drugs, some radiographic contrast media, large doses of corticosteroids, heparin, and antacids (Smeltzer, Bare, Hinkle, & Cheever, 2010).

CLINICAL MANIFESTATIONS

Patients with hypocalcemia may experience neuromuscular symptoms (e.g., numbness of the fingers), cramps in the muscles (especially the extremities), hyperactive deep tendon reflexes, and a positive Trousseau's sign (Fig. 3-10) and Chvostek's sign (Fig. 3-11).

Other symptoms include irritability, memory impairment, delusions, seizures (late), prolonged QT interval, and altered cardiovascular hemodynamics that may precipitate congestive HF. In patients with hypocalcemia caused by citrated blood transfusion, the cardiac index, stroke volume, and left ventricular stroke work values have been found to be lower.

The most dangerous symptom associated with hypocalcemia is the development of laryngospasm and **tetany**-like contractions. A low magnesium level and a high potassium level potentiate the cardiac and neuromuscular irritability produced by a low calcium level. However, a low potassium level can protect patients from hypocalcemic tetany.

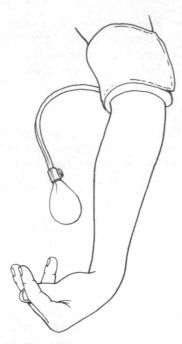

Figure 3-10 ■ Positive Trousseau's sign. Carpopedal attitude of the hand when blood pressure cuff is placed on the arm and inflated above systolic pressure for 3 minutes. A positive reaction is the development of carpal spasm.

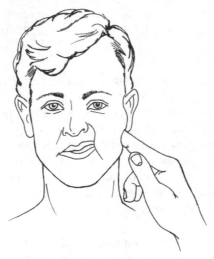

Figure 3-11 ■ Positive Chvostek's sign, which occurs after tapping the facial nerve approximately 2 cm anterior to the ear lobe. Unilateral twitching of the facial muscle occurs in some patients with hypocalcemia.

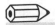 **NURSING FAST FACT!**

> *Today's blood analyzers allow measurement of the iCA level. The normal serum iCA level is 2.2 to 2.5 mEq/L or 4.25 to 5.25 mg/dL (Kee, Paulanka, & Polek, 2010).*

LABORATORY AND RADIOGRAPHIC FINDINGS

- iCA level less than 4.0 mg/dL
- Radiographic films detect bone fractures and thinning
- Bone mass density tests for signs of osteoporosis
- Potential for hypomagnesemia (1 mg/dL)
- Potential for hypokalemia (<3.5 mEq/mL)
- Hyperphosphatemia (>2.6 mEq/mL)
- Potential for elevated creatinine from renal insufficiency

TREATMENT/COLLABORATIVE MANAGEMENT

The goal of treatment is to alleviate the underlying cause. Treatment of patients with hypocalcemia consists of:

1. Administration of calcium gluconate, orally (preferred) with calcium supplements, 1000 mg/day, to raise the total serum calcium level by 1 mg/dL.
2. Patients with symptomatic hypocalcemia less than 7.5 mg/dL usually require parenteral calcium. Hypocalcemia in adults is treated with 5 to 20 mL (2.3–9.3 mEq) of a 10% solution by I.V. injection slowly *or* diluted in 1000 mL of 0.9% sodium chloride over 12 to 24 hours. Do not exceed 200 mg/min (Gahart & Nazareno, 2012).

NOTE > Follow current rate administration guidelines for safe I.V. administration of medications.

NURSING POINTS OF CARE
HYPOCALCEMIA

Nursing Assessments
- Obtain history relative to potential causes of hypocalcemia (low-calcium diet, lack of vitamin D, low-protein diet, chronic diarrhea, hormonal disorders).
- Postoperative hypoparathyroidectomy first 24 to 48 hours
- Obtain history of drugs that could predispose the patient to hypocalcemia (furosemide [Lasix], cortisone).
- Assess for signs of hypocalcemia (tetany, which is the most characteristic symptom; seizures, tingling in tips of fingers and around mouth).

Continued

■ Obtain baseline values for serum calcium, iCA serum albumin, and acid–base status.

Key Nursing Interventions
1. Observe safety precautions and prepare to adopt seizure precautions if hypocalcemia is severe.
2. Monitor laboratory test results, with emphasis on serum and ionized calcium.
3. Monitor ECGs for changes in pattern.
4. Monitor for signs of cardiac arrhythmias in patients receiving digitalis and calcium supplements.
5. Monitor for hypocalcemia in patients receiving massive transfusion of citrated blood.
6. Administer I.V. calcium slowly at prescribed rate.
7. Observe I.V. site for infiltration because of risk of extravasation and resultant cellulitis or necrosis.
8. Check LIP order to clarify which calcium salt to administer: Calcium gluconate yields 4.5 mEq of calcium and calcium chloride provides 13.6 mEq of calcium.

 NURSING FAST FACT!

> *Too rapid I.V. administration of calcium can cause cardiac arrest. Calcium should be diluted in D5W and administered as a slow I.V. bolus or a slow I.V. infusion (Smeltzer, Bare, Hinkle, & Cheever, 2010).*

Serum Calcium Excess: Hypercalcemia

Hypercalcemia is caused by excessive release of calcium from bone, almost always from malignancy, hyperparathyroidism, thiazide diuretic use, or excessive calcium intake.

ETIOLOGY

Most symptoms of hypercalcemia are present only when the serum calcium level is greater than 12 mg/dL and tend to be more severe if hypercalcemia develops quickly. Causes of hypercalcemia include hyperparathyroidism, Paget's disease, multiple fractures, and overuse of calcium-containing antacids. Patients with solid tumors that have metastasized (e.g., breast, prostate, malignant melanomas) or with hematological tumors (e.g., lymphomas, acute leukemia, and myelomas) are also at risk for developing hypercalcemia.

Drugs that predispose an individual to hypercalcemia include calcium salts, megadoses of vitamin A or D, thiazide diuretics (potentiate action of PTH), androgens or estrogen for breast cancer therapy, I.V. lipids, lithium, and tamoxifen.

CLINICAL MANIFESTATIONS

Patients with hypercalcemia may experience neuromuscular symptoms such as muscle weakness, incoordination, lethargy, deep bone pain, flank pain, and pathological fractures (caused by bone weakening). Other symptoms include constipation, anorexia, nausea, vomiting, polyuria or polydipsia leading to uremia if not treated, and renal colic caused by stone formation. Patients taking digitalis must take calcium with extreme care because it can precipitate severe dysrhythmias.

LABORATORY AND RADIOGRAPHIC FINDINGS

- Serum iCA: Greater than 5.5 mg/dL
- Serum PTH: Increased levels in primary or secondary hyper-parathyroidism
- Radiography: May reveal osteoporosis, bone cavitations, or urinary calculi

TREATMENT/COLLABORATIVE MANAGEMENT

Hypercalcemia should be treated according to the following guidelines:

1. Treat the patient's underlying disease.
2. Administer saline diuresis. Fluids should be forced to help eliminate the source of the hypercalcemia. A solution of 0.45% NaCl or 0.9% NaCl I.V. dilutes the serum calcium level. Rehydration is important to dilute Ca^{2+} ions and promote renal excretion.
3. Give inorganic phosphate salts orally (Neutra-Phos) or rectally (Fleet Enema).
4. Provide hemodialysis or peritoneal dialysis to reduce serum calcium levels in life-threatening situations.
5. Use furosemide, 20 to 40 mg every 2 hours, to prevent volume overloading during saline administration.
6. Administer calcitonin, 4 to 8 units/kg intramuscularly or subcutaneously every 6 to 12 hours. This will temporarily lower the serum calcium level by 1 to 3 mg/100 mL.
7. Give bisphosphonates to inhibit bone reabsorption. Pamidronate 60 to 90 mg in 1 L of 0.9% NaCl or 5% dextrose in water infused over 24 hours is effective (Smeltzer, Bare, Hinkle, & Cheever, 2010).

NURSING POINTS OF CARE
HYPERCALCEMIA

Nursing Assessments
- Obtain a patient history of probable cause of hypercalcemia (e.g., cancer); excessive use of calcium supplements, antacids, or thiazide diuretics; or steroid therapy.

Continued

■ Assess for signs of hypercalcemia (muscle weakness, incoordination, anorexia, nausea and vomiting, constipation; abdominal and bone pain).
■ Obtain baseline values for serum calcium and serum phosphate.
■ Obtain baseline ECG.
■ Assess client's fluid volume status and mental alertness.

Key Nursing Interventions
1. Monitor changes in vital signs and laboratory test results.
2. Encourage the patient to drink 3 to 4 L of fluid per day.
3. Encourage the patient to consume fluids (e.g., cranberry or prune juice) that promote urine acidity to help prevent formation of renal calculi.
4. Keep accurate fluid I&O records.
5. Monitor for digitalis toxicity (toxic level >2 mg/mL)
6. Handle the patient gently to prevent fractures.
7. Encourage the patient to avoid high-calcium foods.

Magnesium (Mg^{2+})

Normal Reference Value: 1.5 to 2.5 mEq/L or 1.8 to 3.0 mg/dL

Physiological Role

The physiological role of magnesium includes:
■ Enzyme action
■ Regulation of neuromuscular activity (similar to calcium)
■ Regulation of electrolyte balance, including facilitating transport of sodium and potassium across cell membranes, influencing the utilization of calcium, potassium, and protein

Magnesium is a major intracellular electrolyte. The normal diet supplies approximately 25 mEq of magnesium. Approximately one-third of serum magnesium is bound to protein; the remaining two-thirds exists as free cations. The same factors that regulate calcium balance influence magnesium balance. Magnesium balance is also affected by many of the same agents that decrease or influence potassium balance.

Magnesium acts directly on the myoneural junction and affects neuromuscular irritability and contractility, possibly exerting a sedative effect. Magnesium acts as an activator for many enzymes and plays a role in both carbohydrate and protein metabolism. Magnesium affects the cardiovascular system, acting peripherally to produce vasodilation. Imbalances in magnesium predispose the heart to ventricular dysrhythmias (Smeltzer, Bare, Hinkle, & Cheever, 2010).

Serum Magnesium Deficit: Hypomagnesemia

Hypomagnesemia is often overlooked in critically ill patients. This imbalance is considered to be one of the most underdiagnosed electrolyte deficiencies. Symptoms of hypomagnesemia tend to occur when the serum level drops below 1.0 mEq/L.

ETIOLOGY

Hypomagnesemia can result from chronic alcoholism; malabsorption syndrome, especially if the small bowel is affected; prolonged malnutrition or starvation; prolonged diarrhea; acute pancreatitis; administration of magnesium-free solutions for more than 1 week; and prolonged NG tube suctioning.

Drugs that predispose an individual to hypomagnesemia include aminoglycosides, diuretics, cortisone, amphotericin, digitalis, cisplatin, and cyclosporine. Infusion of collected blood preserved with citrate also can cause hypomagnesemia (Heitz & Horne, 2005).

CLINICAL MANIFESTATIONS

Patients with hypomagnesemia often experience neuromuscular symptoms, such as hyperactive reflexes, coarse tremors, muscle cramps, positive Chvostek's and Trousseau's signs (see Figs. 3-10 and 3-11), seizures, paresthesia of the feet and legs, and painfully cold hands and feet. Other symptoms include disorientation, dysrhythmias, tachycardia, and increased potential for digitalis toxicity.

LABORATORY AND ECG FINDINGS

- Serum magnesium: Less than 1.5 mEq/L
- Urine magnesium: Helps to identify renal causes of magnesium depletion.
- Serum albumin: A decrease may cause a decreased magnesium level resulting from the reduction in protein-bound magnesium.
- Serum potassium: Decreased because of failure of the cellular sodium–potassium pump to move potassium into the cell and because of the accompanying loss of potassium in the urine
- Serum calcium: May be reduced because of a reduction in the release and action of PTH.
- ECG: Findings of tachydysrhythmia, prolonged PR and QT intervals, widening of the QRS, ST-segment depression, and flattened T waves. A form of ventricular tachycardia (i.e., torsades de pointes) associated with all three electrolyte imbalances (magnesium, calcium, potassium) may develop.

TREATMENT/COLLABORATIVE MANAGEMENT

Treatment of patients with hypomagnesemia includes identification and removal of the cause. Magnesium sulfate is the parenteral replacement and can be administered intramuscularly or intravenously. The drug is available in strengths of 10, 12.5, and 50%. A suggested order for adults is 10 mL of a 50% solution.

1. Administering oral magnesium salts: Magnesium oxide (Mag-Ox) or magnesium chloride (Slow-Mag). Magnesium containing antacids may also be used.
2. Administering IM injection, the dosage is divided.
3. Administering IV infusion, the dosage is diluted into 1 liter of solution (Kee, Paulanka, & Polek, 2010).

NOTE > Follow current rate administration guidelines for safe I.V. administration of medications.

Table 3-8 provides critical guidelines for nurses who are administering magnesium.

 NURSING FAST FACT!

Be aware that other CNS depressants can cause further depressed sensorium when magnesium sulfate is being administered. Therefore, be prepared to deal with respiratory arrest if hypermagnesemia inadvertently occurs during administration of magnesium sulfate.

NURSING POINTS OF CARE
HYPOMAGNESEMIA

Nursing Assessments
- Obtain a patient history, being alert to factors that predispose to hypomagnesemia such as alcoholism, laxative abuse, TPN, and potassium-wasting diuretic use.
- Assess for signs and symptoms of hypomagnesemia (not all related to magnesium but resulting from secondary changes in potassium and calcium metabolism, tonic–clonic or focal seizures, laryngeal stridor, dysphagia, positive Chvostek's and Trousseau's signs, ECG changes, marked alterations in mood).
- Obtain baseline values for laboratory tests, serum magnesium, serum calcium, and serum potassium.
- Obtain baseline ECG.

Key Nursing Interventions
1. Monitor vital signs.
2. Monitor for dysphagia, nausea, and anorexia.
3. Monitor for muscle weakness and athetoid movements (slow, involuntary twisting movements).

4. Monitor closely for digitalis toxicity (toxic level >2 mg/mL).
5. Keep accurate I&O records. Monitoring urine output is essential before, during, and after magnesium administration.
6. Notify LIP if urine output drops below 100 mL over 4 hours.
7. Have calcium gluconate available to treat hypocalcemic tetany.
8. Initiate seizure precautions if necessary to protect from injury (Martin & Gonzalez et al, 2009).

Serum Magnesium Excess: Hypermagnesemia

Hypermagnesemia occurs when a person's serum level is greater than 2.5 mEq/L. The most common cause of hypermagnesemia is renal failure in patients who have an increased intake of magnesium.

ETIOLOGY

Renal factors that lead to hypermagnesemia include renal failure, Addison's disease, and inadequate excretion of magnesium by kidneys.

Other causes include hyperparathyroidism; hyperthyroidism; and iatrogenic causes such as excessive magnesium administration during treatment of patients with eclampsia, hemodialysis with excessively hard water using a dialysate inadvertently high in magnesium, or ingestion of medications high in magnesium, such as antacids and laxatives.

CLINICAL MANIFESTATIONS

The major symptoms of hypermagnesemia result from depressed peripheral and central neuromuscular transmissions. Patients with hypermagnesemia may experience neuromuscular symptoms such as flushing and sense of skin warmth, lethargy, sedation, hypoactive deep tendon reflexes, and depressed respirations, and weak or absent cry in newborns. Other symptoms include hypotension, sinus bradycardia, heart block, and cardiac arrest (serum level >15 mEq/L) and increased susceptibility to digitalis toxicity, nausea, vomiting, and seizures. The most common cause of hypermagnesemia is individuals who have renal failure with an increased intake of magnesium (Heitz & Horne, 2005).

> Table 3-8 | **CRITICAL GUIDELINES FOR ADMINISTRATION OF MAGNESIUM**

■ Double-check the order for magnesium administration to ensure that it stipulates the concentration of the solution to be used. Do not accept orders for "amps" or "vials" without further clarification.
■ Use caution in patients with impaired renal function; watch urine output.
■ Reduce other central nervous system depressants when given concurrently with magnesium preparations.
■ Therapeutic doses of magnesium can produce flushing and sweating, which occur most often if the administration rate is too fast.
■ Closely assess patients receiving magnesium.

Laboratory and ECG Findings

- Serum magnesium: Greater than 2.5 mEq/L
- ECG: Possible findings of widened QRS complex, and prolonged QT interval (at levels >2.5 mEq/L).

Treatment/Collaborative Management

The goal of treatment is to remove the cause of the hypermagnesemia, for example, by discontinuing or avoiding use of magnesium-containing medications, especially in patients with decreased renal function. Guidelines for treatment of patients with hypermagnesemia are:

1. Decrease oral magnesium intake.
2. Administer diuretics and 0.45% sodium chloride solution to enhance magnesium excretion in patients with adequate renal function.
3. Administer I.V. calcium gluconate (10 mL of 10% solution) to antagonize the neuromuscular effects of magnesium in patients with lethal hypermagnesemia.
4. Support respiratory function.
5. Administer peritoneal dialysis or hemodialysis in severe cases of hypermagnesemia.

NURSING POINTS OF CARE
HYPERMAGNESEMIA

Nursing Assessments
- Evaluate possible causes of hypermagnesemia, including renal insufficiency and chronic laxative use.
- Assess for signs of hypermagnesemia (depression of CNS and peripheral neuromuscular function, lowered BP, nausea, vomiting, weakness, facial flushing and sensations of warmth, lost deep tendon reflexes).
- Obtain baseline values for serum magnesium and serum calcium.
- Obtain baseline ECG.

Key Nursing Interventions
1. Monitor vital signs for decreased BP, pulse, and respirations.
2. Observe for flushing of the skin.
3. Monitor laboratory test results (hypochloremia).
4. Monitor for ECG changes.
5. Encourage fluid intake if not contraindicated.
6. Provide ventilatory assistance or resuscitation if necessary.
7. Follow administration guidelines by LIP for I.V. calcium gluconate.

Phosphorus (HPO$_4$–)

Normal Reference Value: 2.5 to 4.5 mg/dL

Physiological Role

The physiological role of phosphorus is:
- Essential to all cells
- Role in metabolism of proteins, carbohydrates, and fats
- Essential to energy, necessary for the formation of high-energy compounds ATP and adenosine diphosphate (ADP)
- As a cellular building block; it is the backbone of nucleic acids and is essential to cell membrane formation
- Delivery of oxygen; functions in formation of red blood cell enzyme

Approximately 80% of phosphorus in the body is contained in the bones and teeth, and 20% is abundant in the ICF. PTH plays a major role in homeostasis of phosphate because of its ability to vary phosphate reabsorption in the proximal tubule of the kidney. PTH also allows for the shift of phosphate from bone to plasma.

Phosphorus plays an important role in delivery of oxygen to tissues by regulating the level of 2,3-diphosphoglycerate (2,3-DPG), a substance in red blood cells that decreases the affinity of hemoglobin for oxygen.

 NURSING FAST FACT!

Phosphorus and calcium have a reciprocal relationship: An increase in the phosphorus level frequently causes a decrease in calcium.

Serum Phosphate Deficit: Hypophosphatemia

Phosphorus is a critical constituent of all the body's tissues. Hypophosphatemia occurs when the serum level is below the lower limit of normal (<2.5 mg/dL). This imbalance may occur in the presence of total body phosphate deficit or may merely reflect a temporary shift of phosphorus into the cells.

ETIOLOGY

Hypophosphatemia can result from overzealous refeeding, PN administered without adequate phosphorus, malabsorption syndromes, or alcohol withdrawal. GI causes of loss include vomiting and chronic diarrhea.

Hormonal influences such as hyperparathyroidism enhance renal phosphate excretion. Drugs that predispose an individual to hypophosphatemia include aluminum-containing antacids (which bind phosphorus, thereby lowering serum levels), diuretics, androgens, corticosteroids, glucagon, epinephrine, gastrin, and mannitol. Another cause is treatment of patients with diabetic ketoacidosis (dextrose with insulin causes a shift of phosphorus into cells). In hypophosphatemia, the oxygen-carrying capacity of the blood decreases due to decreased 2,3-DPG and gas exchange. With decreased 2,3-DPG levels, the oxyhemoglobin dissociation curve shifts to the right, that is, at a given oxygen tension of arterial blood (Pao_2) level, more oxygen is bound to hemoglobin and less is available to the tissues (Heitz & Horne, 2005).

CLINICAL MANIFESTATIONS

Hypophosphatemia can affect the CNS, neuromuscular, and cardiac status, and the blood. An affected patient may experience disorientation, confusion, seizures, paresthesia (early), profound muscle weakness, tremor, ataxia, incoordination, dysarthria, dysphagia, and congestive cardiomyopathy. Hypophosphatemia affects all blood cells, especially red cells. It causes a decline in 2,3-DPG levels in erythrocytes. 2,3-DPG in red cells normally interacts with hemoglobin to promote the release of oxygen. It is thought that hypophosphatemia predisposes a person to infection (Smeltzer, Bare, Hinkle, & Cheever, 2010).

LABORATORY AND RADIOGRAPHIC FINDINGS

- Serum phosphorus: Less than 2.5 mg/dL (1.7 mEq/L)
- Serum PTH: Elevated
- Serum magnesium: Decreased because of increased urinary excretion of magnesium
- Serum alkaline phosphatase: Increased with increased osteoblastic activity
- Radiography: Skeletal changes of osteomalacia or rickets

TREATMENT/COLLABORATIVE MANAGEMENT

Treatment should focus on identification and elimination of the cause, for example, by avoiding use of phosphorus-binding antacids. Treatment can also include:

1. For mild to moderate deficiency, oral phosphate supplements (e.g., Neutra-Phos, Phospho-Soda) can be administered.
2. For severe hypophosphatemia, administer I.V. sodium phosphorus or potassium phosphorus solutions.

NURSING POINTS OF CARE
HYPOPHOSPHATEMIA

Nursing Assessments
- Obtain a patient history with focus on factors that put patients at high risk for hypophosphatemia, such as alcoholism, use of TPN, and diabetic ketoacidosis.

■ Assess for signs of hypophosphatemia (irritability, fatigue, apprehension, weakness, paresthesias, dysarthria, dysphagia seizures). Obtain baseline laboratory values of serum phosphate and serum calcium.

Key Nursing Interventions
1. Monitor for cardiac, GI, and neurological abnormalities.
2. Monitor for changes in laboratory test results.
3. Keep accurate I&O records.
4. Use safety precautions when a patient is confused.
5. Monitor for refeeding syndrome once oral feeding is restarted after prolonged starvation.
6. Monitor for other electrolyte complications of phosphorus administration (hypocalcemia, hyperphosphatemia).
7. Administer I.V. sodium or potassium phosphate at prescribed rate not to exceed 10 mEq/hr.
8. Monitor for infiltration due to the potential for tissue sloughing and necrosis.

Serum Phosphate Excess: Hyperphosphatemia

ETIOLOGY

Hyperphosphatemia can result from renal insufficiency, hypoparathyroidism, or increased catabolism. It is also seen in patients with cancer states, such as myelogenous leukemia and lymphoma.

Drugs that can predispose an individual to hyperphosphatemia include oral phosphates, I.V. phosphates; phosphate laxatives; and excessive vitamin D, tetracyclines, and methicillin. Another cause is massive blood transfusions caused by phosphate leaking from the blood cells.

CLINICAL MANIFESTATIONS

Patients with hyperphosphatemia may experience many symptoms, including hypocalcemia; tetany (short-term); soft tissue calcification (long-term); mental changes, such as apprehension, confusion, and coma; and increased 2,3-DPG levels in red blood cells.

LABORATORY AND RADIOGRAPHIC FINDINGS

■ Serum phosphorus: Greater than 4.5 mg/dL (2.6 mEq/L)
■ Serum calcium: Useful in assessing potential consequences of treatment
■ Serum PTH: Decreased in those with hypoparathyroidism
■ BUN: To assess renal function
■ Radiography: Skeletal changes of osteodystrophy

Treatment/Collaborative Management

Treatment should include the following regimen:

1. Identify the underlying cause of hyperphosphatemia.
2. Restrict dietary intake.
3. Administer the intake of phosphate-binding gels (e.g., Amphojel, Basaljel, Dialume).
4. Administer vitamin D preparations such as calcitriol, which is available in oral (Rocaltrol) and parenteral (Calcijex) forms.

NURSING POINTS OF CARE
HYPERPHOSPHATEMIA

Nursing Assessments
- Obtain a patient history for factors that place patients at high risk for hyperphosphatemia (e.g., renal insufficiency, laxative use).
- Assess for signs and symptoms of hyperphosphatemia (tetany with tingling sensation in the fingertips and around the mouth; anorexia, nausea, vomiting, bone and joint pain, muscle weakness, tachycardia).
- Obtain baseline laboratory values for serum phosphate.
- Assess 24-hour urinary output; less than 600 mL/day increases serum phosphate levels.

Key Nursing Interventions
1. Monitor for cardiac, GI, and neuromuscular abnormalities.
2. Monitor changes in laboratory test results.
3. Keep accurate I&O records.
4. Observe the patient for signs and symptoms of hypocalcemia; when phosphate levels increase, calcium levels decrease.

Table 3-9 summarizes clinical problems associated with electrolyte imbalances.

Chloride (Cl⁻)

Normal Reference Value: 95 to 108 mEq/L

Physiological Role

The physiological role of chloride is:
- Regulation of serum osmolarity
- Regulation of fluid balance; when sodium is retained chloride is also retained, causing water retention and increased fluid volume.

> Table 3-9   **CLINICAL PROBLEMS ASSOCIATED WITH ELECTROLYTE IMBALANCES**

Clinical Problem	Sodium (Na⁺)	Potassium (K⁺)	Calcium (Ca²⁺)	Magnesium (Mg²⁺)
Cardiovascular				
Myocardial infarction	Na⁺↓ (hypervolemia)	K⁺↓	—	Mg²⁺↓
Heart failure (HF)	Na⁺↑	K⁺ Normal	—	Mg²⁺↓/N
Gastrointestinal				
Vomiting and diarrhea	Na⁺↓	K⁺↓	Ca²⁺↓	Mg²⁺↓
Malnutrition	Na⁺↓	K⁺↓	Ca²⁺↓	Mg²⁺↓
Anorexia	Na⁺↓	K⁺↓	Ca²⁺↓	Mg²⁺↓
Intestinal fistula	Na⁺↓	K⁺↓		Mg²⁺↓
GI surgery	Na⁺↓	K⁺↓		Mg²⁺↓
Chronic alcoholism	Na⁺↓	K⁺↓	Ca²⁺↓	Mg²⁺↓
Hyperphosphatemia			Ca²⁺↓	
Transfused citrated blood			Ca²⁺↓	
Endocrine				
Cushing's syndrome	Na⁺↑	K⁺↓		Mg²⁺↓
Addison's disease	Na⁺↓	K⁺↑		Mg²⁺↓
Diabetic ketoacidosis	Na⁺↑	K⁺↑ Diuresis K⁺↓	Ca²⁺↓ Ionized	Mg²⁺↓
Hypoparathyroidism			Ca²⁺↓	
Hyperparathyroidism			Ca²⁺↓	Diuresis Mg²⁺↓
Renal				
Acute renal failure	Na⁺↑	Oliguria K⁺↑ Diuresis K⁺↓		Mg²⁺↑
Chronic renal failure	Na⁺↑		Ca²⁺↑/↓	Mg²⁺↑
Miscellaneous				
Cancer	Na⁺↓	K⁺↓/↑	Ca²⁺↑	Mg²⁺↓
Burns	Na⁺↓	K⁺↓/↑	Ca²⁺↓	Mg²⁺↓
Acute pancreatitis			Ca²⁺↓	
Syndrome of inappropriate antidiuretic hormone secretion (SIADH)	Na⁺↓			
Metabolic acidosis		K⁺↓	Ca²⁺↓	
Metabolic alkalosis		K⁺↓		

■ Control of acidity of gastric juice
■ Regulation of acid–base balance
■ Role in oxygen–carbon dioxide exchange (chloride shift)

Chloride is the major anion in the ECF. Changes in serum chloride concentration usually are secondary to changes in one or more of the other electrolytes. Chloride has a reciprocal relationship with bicarbonate (HCO_3^-). For example, a decrease in HCO_3^- concentrations results in a reciprocal rise in chloride level; when chloride level decreases, HCO_3^- level increases in compensation. Chloride exists primarily combined as sodium chloride or hydrochloric acid. Serum chloride is most frequently measured for its inferential value.

Reabsorption of chloride by the renal tubules is one of the major regulatory functions of the kidneys. As sodium chloride is reabsorbed, water follows through osmosis. It is through this function that vascular blood volume is maintained.

Chloride plays its most important role in acid–base balance. Its role in the pH balance of the ECF is referred to as the "chloride shift." The chloride shift is an ionic exchange that occurs within red blood cells. This shift preserves the electrical neutrality of the red blood cells and maintains the 1:20 ratio of carbonic acid and HCO_3^- that is essential for pH balance of the plasma.

NOTE > Chloride is discussed further under acid–base balance. Imbalances in chloride are reflected in metabolic alkalosis and metabolic acidosis.

■ Acid–Base Balance

Regulation of the hydrogen ion concentration of body fluids is actually the key component of acid–base balance. The pH of a fluid reflects the hydrogen ion concentration of that fluid. The normal pH of arterial blood ranges from 7.35 to 7.45. A solution is either basic or acidic depending on the concentration of hydrogen ions in the solution, and the pH scale is used to describe the hydrogen ion concentration. The pH scale is a logarithmic scale with values from 0.00 to 14.00. A neutral solution (i.e., neither acidic nor basic) has a pH of 7.00 (Porth & Matfin, 2010).

The inverse proportion of the pH to the concentration of hydrogen ions is reflected in the concept that the higher the pH value, the lower the hydrogen ion concentration. Conversely, the lower the pH value, the higher the hydrogen ion concentration. Therefore, a pH below 7.35 reflects an acidic state, whereas a pH greater than 7.45 indicates alkalosis and a lower hydrogen ion concentration. A variation from 7.35 to 7.45 of 0.4 in either direction can be fatal. Figure 3-12 shows the pH scale.

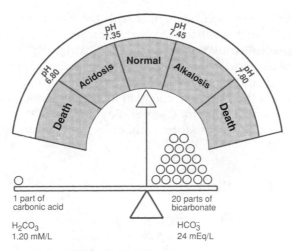

Figure 3-12 ■ Acid–base scale.

Three mechanisms operate to maintain the appropriate pH of the blood:

1. Chemical buffer systems in the ECF and within the cells
2. Removal of carbon dioxide by the lungs
3. Renal regulation of the hydrogen ion concentration

Chemical Buffer Systems

The buffer systems are fast-acting defenses that provide immediate protection against changes in the hydrogen ion concentration of the ECF. The buffers also serve as transport mechanisms that carry excess hydrogen ions to the lungs.

A buffer is a substance that reacts to minimize pH changes when either acid or base is released into the system. There are three primary buffer systems in the ECF: the hemoglobin system, the plasma protein system, and the bicarbonate system. The capacity of a buffer is limited; therefore, after the components of a buffer system have reacted, they must be replenished before the body can respond to further stress.

The hemoglobin and deoxyhemoglobin found in red blood cells, together with their potassium salts, act as buffer pairs. The electrolyte chloride shifts in and out of the red blood cells according to the level of oxygen in the blood plasma. For each chloride ion that leaves a red blood cell, a bicarbonate ion enters the cell; for each chloride ion that enters a red blood cell, a bicarbonate ion is released.

Plasma proteins are large molecules that contain the acid (or base) and salt form of a buffer. Proteins then have the ability to bind or release hydrogen ions.

The bicarbonate buffer system maintains the blood's pH in the range from 7.35 to 7.45, with a ratio of 20 parts bicarbonate to 1 part carbonic acid by a process called hydration of carbon dioxide, which is a means of buffering the excess acid in the blood. If a strong acid is added to the body, the ratio is upset. In this acid imbalance, the largest amount of carbon dioxide diffuses in the plasma to the red blood cells; carbon dioxide then combines with plasma protein. Carbon dioxide that is dissolved in the blood combines with water to form carbonic acid (Smeltzer, Bare, Hinkle, & Cheever, 2010).

Respiratory Regulation

In healthy individuals, the lungs form a second line of defense in maintaining the acid–base balance. When carbon dioxide combines with water, H_2CO_3 is formed. Therefore, an increase in the acid carbon dioxide lowers the pH of blood, creating an acidotic state; a decrease in the carbon dioxide level increases the pH, causing the blood to become more alkaline. After H_2CO_3 is formed, it dissociates into carbon dioxide and water. The carbon dioxide is transferred to the lungs, where it diffuses into the alveoli and is eliminated through exhalation. Therefore, the rate of respiration affects the hydrogen ion concentration. An increase in respiratory rate causes carbon dioxide to be blown off by the lungs, resulting in an increase in pH. Conversely, a decrease in respiratory rate causes retention of carbon dioxide and thus a decrease in pH. This means that the lungs can either hold the hydrogen ions until the deficit is corrected or inactivate the hydrogen ions into water molecules to be exhaled with the carbon dioxide as vapor, thereby correcting the excess. It takes from 10 to 30 minutes for the lungs to inactivate the hydrogen molecules by converting them to water molecules (Smeltzer, Bare, Hinkle, & Cheever, 2010).

Renal Regulation

The kidneys regulate the hydrogen ion concentration by increasing or decreasing the HCO_3^- ion concentration in the body fluid by a series of complex chemical reactions that occur in the renal tubules. The regulation of acid–base balance by the kidneys occurs chiefly by increasing or decreasing the HCO_3^- ion concentration in body fluids. Hydrogen is secreted into the tubules of the kidney, where it is eliminated in the urine. At the same time, sodium is reabsorbed from the tubular fluid into the ECF in exchange for hydrogen and combines with HCO_3^- ions to form the buffer $NaHCO_3$.

The kidneys help to regulate the extracellular concentration of HCO_3^-. Two buffer systems help the kidney to eliminate excess hydrogen in the urine: the phosphate buffer system and the ammonia buffer system.

With each of these systems, an excess of hydrogen is secreted and HCO_3^- ions are formed; sodium is reabsorbed, thus forming $NaHCO_3$. The time it takes for a change to occur in the acid–base balance can range from a fraction of a second to more than 24 hours. Although the kidneys are the most powerful regulating mechanism, they are slow to make major changes in the acid–base balance (Halperin, Kamel, & Goldstein, 2010; Smeltzer, Bare, Hinkle, & Cheever, 2010).

◼ Major Acid–Base Imbalances

There are two types of acid–base imbalances: (1) metabolic (base bicarbonate deficit and excess) **acidosis** and **alkalosis**, and (2) respiratory (carbonic acid deficit and excess) acidosis and alkalosis. The balanced pH of the arterial blood is 7.4, and only small variations of up to 0.05 can exist without causing ill effects. Deviations of more than five times the normal concentration of H+ in the ECF are potentially fatal (Porth & Matfin, 2010).

Metabolic Acid–Base Imbalances

Bicarbonate: Normal Reference Value: 22 to 26 mEq/L

Metabolic Acidosis: Base Bicarbonate Deficit

Metabolic acidosis (HCO_3^- deficit) is a clinical disturbance characterized by a low pH and a low plasma HCO_3^- level. This condition can occur by a gain of hydrogen ion (H^+) or a loss of HCO_3^-. Metabolic acidosis can be divided clinically into two forms, according to the values of the serum anion gap: high anion gap acidosis and normal anion gap acidosis. The anion gap reflects normally unmeasured anions (phosphates, sulfates, and proteins) in the plasma (Smeltzer, Bare, Hinkle, & Cheever, 2010).

ETIOLOGY

Metabolic acidosis occurs with loss of HCO_3^- from diarrhea, draining fistulas, and administration of TPN. Diabetes mellitus, alcoholism, and starvation cause ketoacidosis. Respiratory or circulatory failure, ingestion of certain drugs or toxins (e.g., salicylates, ethylene glycol, methyl alcohol), some hereditary disorders, and septic shock cause lactic acidosis. It also can result when renal failure leads to excessive retention of hydrogen ions.

 NURSING FAST FACT!

Hyperkalemia usually is present in clinical cases of acidosis due to shift of potassium out of the cells. Later as the acidosis is corrected, potassium moves back into the cells (Smeltzer, Bare, Hinkle, & Cheever, 2010).

CLINICAL MANIFESTATIONS

Patients with metabolic acidosis may experience CNS-related symptoms such as headache, confusion, drowsiness, increased respiratory rate, and Kussmaul respirations. Other symptoms include nausea, vomiting, decreased cardiac output, and bradycardia (when serum pH is <7.0).

LABORATORY AND ECG FINDINGS

- ABG values: pH less than 7.35, HCO_3^- less than 22 mEq/L
- $PaCO_2$: Less than 38 mm Hg
- Serum HCO_3^-: Less than 22 mEq/L
- Serum electrolytes: Elevated potassium possible because of exchange of intracellular potassium for hydrogen ions in the body's attempt to normalize the acid–base environment
- ECG: Dysrhythmias caused by hyperkalemia

COMMON CAUSES OF METABOLIC ACIDOSIS

- GI abnormalities: Starvation, severe malnutrition, chronic diarrhea
- Renal abnormalities: Kidney failure
- Hormonal influences: Diabetic ketoacidosis, hyperthyroidism, thyrotoxicosis
- Other: Trauma, shock, excess exercise, severe infection, fever

TREATMENT/COLLABORATIVE MANAGEMENT

Patients with metabolic acidosis are treated by

1. Reversing the underlying cause (e.g., diabetic ketoacidosis, alcoholism related to ketoacidosis, diarrhea, acute renal failure, renal tubular acidosis, poisoning, lactic acidosis)
2. Eliminating the source (if the cause is excessive administration of sodium chloride)
3. Administering $NaHCO_3$ (7.5% 44.4 mEq/50 mL or 8.4% 50 mEq/50 mL I.V. when pH is ≤7.2). Concentration depends on severity of acidosis and presence of any serum sodium disorders.
4. Potassium replacement: Hyperkalemia usually is present, but potassium deficit can occur. If a deficit of less than 3.5 mEq/L is present, the potassium deficit must be corrected before $NaHCO_3$ is administered because the potassium shifts back into the ICF when the acidosis is correct.

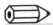 *NURSING FAST FACT!*

Give $NaHCO_3$ cautiously to avoid having patients develop metabolic alkalosis and pulmonary edema secondary to sodium overload.

NURSING POINTS OF CARE
METABOLIC ACIDOSIS

Nursing Assessments
- Obtain a patient history of health problems that relate to metabolic acidosis, such as diabetes or renal disease.
- Obtain baseline vital signs with focus on the respiration and cardiac functioning.
- Assess for symptoms of metabolic acidosis (headache, confusion, drowsiness, increased respiratory rate and depth, decreased BP, cold and clammy skin, dysrhythmias, and shock. Cardiac output decreased when pH drops to <7).
- Obtain baseline values for ABGs and laboratory tests. Note serum electrolytes, serum CO_2 content, HCO_3^-, and blood sugar level.

Key Nursing Interventions
1. Provide safety precautions when a patient is confused.
2. Monitor for signs and symptoms of metabolic acidosis.
3. Monitor the patient's dietary and fluid I&O record.
4. Monitor laboratory test results for changes.
5. Monitor the patient for changes in vital signs, especially changes in respiration, cardiac function, and CNS signs.
6. Monitor serum potassium level.
7. Administer sodium bicarbonate at prescribed rate.

Metabolic Alkalosis: Base Bicarbonate Excess

Metabolic alkalosis (i.e., HCO_3^- excess) is a clinical disturbance characterized by a high pH and a high plasma HCO_3^- concentration. It can be produced by a gain of HCO_3^- or a loss of hydrogen ion.

ETIOLOGY

Metabolic alkalosis occurs with GI loss of hydrogen ions from gastric suctioning and vomiting. Renal loss of hydrogen ions occurs from potassium-losing diuretics, excess of mineralocorticoid, hypercalcemia, and hypoparathyroidism. In patients with hypokalemia and carbohydrate refeeding after starvation, hydrogen ions shift from ECF into the cells, depleting serum levels. This also occurs when excessive ingestion of alkalis (e.g., antacids such as Alka-Seltzer), parenteral administration of $NaHCO_3$ during cardiopulmonary resuscitation, and massive blood transfusions increase serum levels of HCO_3^- (Porth & Matfin, 2010).

Clinical Manifestations

Patients with metabolic alkalosis may experience dizziness and depressed respirations in addition to impaired mentation, tingling of fingers and toes, circumoral paresthesia, and hypertonic reflexes. Other symptoms include hypotension, cardiac dysrhythmias, hyperventilation, hypokalemia, and decreased iCA (i.e., carpopedal spasm).

Laboratory and ECG Findings

- ABG values: pH greater than 7.45; HCO_3^- greater than 26 mEq/L
- $PaCO_2$: Greater than 42 mm Hg
- Serum HCO_3^-: Greater than 26 mEq/L
- Serum electrolytes: Low serum potassium (<4 mEq/L) and low serum chloride
- ECG: Assess for dysrhythmias (Smeltzer, Bare, Hinkle, & Cheever, 2010).

Common Causes of Metabolic Alkalosis

- Chloride depletion: Loss of gastric secretions, vomiting, NG tube drainage, diarrhea
- Potassium depletion: Primary aldosteronism, mineral corticoid excess, laxative abuse
- Hypercalcemic states: Hypercalcemia of malignancy, acute milk alkali syndrome
- Miscellaneous: Medication (bicarbonate ingestion, carbenicillin, ampicillin), refeeding syndrome, hypoproteinemia

 NURSING FAST FACT!

> *Hypokalemia is often present in patients with alkalosis.*

Treatment/Collaborative Management

Patients with metabolic alkalosis are treated by

1. Reversing the underlying cause
2. Administering sufficient chloride for the kidney to excrete the excess HCO_3^-. Usually isotonic sodium chloride infusion corrects the deficit.
3. Replacing potassium if K^+ is low. Usually potassium chloride is preferred because chloride losses can be replaced simultaneously. Carbonic anhydrase inhibitors such as acetazolamide (Diamox) are useful for correcting metabolic alkalosis in patients who cannot tolerate rapid volume expansion. Acetazolamide causes a large increase in renal secretion of HCO_3^- and K^+, so it may be necessary to supplement potassium prior to administration of medication.

4. Administering acidifying agents such as diluted HCl and ammonium chloride (NH_4Cl). There are serious side effects, so this solution is not commonly used (Smeltzer, Bare, Hinkle, & Cheever, 2010).

NURSING POINTS OF CARE
METABOLIC ALKALOSIS

Nursing Assessments
- Obtain history of health problems related to metabolic alkalosis (e.g., peptic ulcer, vomiting, **adrenocortical hormone** abnormalities).
- Obtain baseline vital signs.
- Assess for signs and symptoms of metabolic alkalosis related to decreased calcium ionization (tingling of fingers and toes, dizziness, hypertonic muscles; respirations depressed as a compensatory action, atrial tachycardia).
- Obtain baseline values for ABGs and serum electrolyte, serum CO_2 content, and HCO_3^-.

Key Nursing Interventions
1. Use safety precautions for hyperexcitability states.
2. Monitor the patient's fluid I&O.
3. Monitor renal and hepatic function.
4. Monitor laboratory test results for changes (ABGs, potassium, chloride).
5. Monitor the patient for changes in vital signs, with particular attention to respirations and CNS.
6. Monitor for changes in cardiac rhythm, especially in patients taking cardiac glycosides.
7. Administer sodium chloride at prescribed rate. KCl may be used to replace both the Cl and K ions.

Respiratory Acid–Base Imbalances

Normal Reference Value: Partial pressure of carbon dioxide ($Paco_2$): 38 to 42 mm Hg

Respiratory Acidosis: Carbonic Acid Excess

Respiratory acidosis is caused by inadequate excretion of carbon dioxide and inadequate ventilation resulting in increased serum levels of carbon dioxide and H_2CO_3. Acute respiratory acidosis usually is associated with emergency situations.

Etiology

Acute respiratory acidosis can result from pulmonary, neurological, and cardiac causes, such as pulmonary edema; aspiration of a foreign body; pneumothorax; severe pneumonia; severe, prolonged exacerbation of acute asthma; overdose of sedatives; cardiac arrest; and massive pulmonary embolism.

Chronic respiratory acidosis results from emphysema, bronchial asthma, bronchiectasis, postoperative pain, obesity, and tight abdominal binders (Kee, Paulanka, & Polek, 2010).

Clinical Manifestations

Acute signs and symptoms include tachypnea; dyspnea; dizziness; seizures; warm, flushed skin; and ventricular fibrillation. Chronic signs and symptoms occur if $Paco_2$ exceeds the body's ability to compensate and include respiratory symptoms.

Laboratory and Radiographic Findings

- ABG values: *Acute:* pH less than 7.35, $Paco_2$ greater than 42 mm Hg, HCO_3^- greater than 26 mEq/L. *Chronic:* pH less than 7.35, $Paco_2$ greater than 42 mm Hg, HCO_3^- normal or slight increase
- Serum HCO_3^-: Reflects acid–base balance; initial values normal unless mixed disorder is present
- Serum electrolytes: Usually not altered
- Chest radiography: Determines the presence of underlying pulmonary disease
- Drug screen: Determines the quantity of drug if patient is suspected of taking an overdose

Common Causes of Respiratory Acidosis

Acute:
- Pulmonary/thoracic disorders: Severe pneumonia, acute respiratory distress syndrome (ARDS), flail chest, pneumothorax, smoke inhalation
- Increased resistance to air flow: Upper airway obstruction, aspiration, laryngospasm, severe bronchospasm
- CNS depression: Sedative overdose, anesthesia

Chronic:
- Obstructive diseases: Emphysema, chronic bronchitis, cystic fibrosis, obstructive sleep apnea
- Restriction of ventilation: Kyphoscoliosis, hydrothorax, severe chronic pneumonitis, obesity–hypoventilation (pickwickian syndrome)
- Neuromuscular abnormalities: Spinal cord injuries, poliomyelitis, muscular dystrophy, multiple sclerosis

■ Depression of respiratory center: Brain tumor, chronic sedative overdose

TREATMENT/COLLABORATIVE MANAGEMENT

The goal is to treat the underlying cause. Respiratory acidosis is treated by carrying out the following:

■ Restore normal acid–base balance: Support respiratory function.
■ Administer bronchodilators or antibiotics for respiratory infections as indicated.
■ Administer oxygen as indicated.
■ Administer adequate fluids (2–3 L/day) to keep mucous membranes moist and help remove secretions.

NURSING POINTS OF CARE
RESPIRATORY ACIDOSIS

Nursing Assessments
■ Obtain history of pneumonia, chronic obstructive pulmonary disease (COPD), narcotic use, or emphysema.
■ Obtain baseline vital signs.
■ Assess for signs and symptoms of respiratory acidosis (dyspnea, tachycardia, disorientation, weakness, skin flushed and warm, increased pulse and respiratory rate, increased BP, mental cloudiness).
■ Obtain baseline values for laboratory tests, especially $Paco_2$.

Key Nursing Interventions
1. Provide safety precautions when a patient is confused.
2. Monitor laboratory test results for changes, especially pH and $Paco_2$.
3. Monitor for changes in vital signs.
4. Monitor oxygen and mechanical ventilator when in use.
5. Elevate the head of the patient's bed.
6. Perform pulmonary hygiene measures when necessary to clear the respiratory tract of mucus and problem purulent drainage
7. Encourage adequate hydration to keep the mucous membranes moist.

Respiratory Alkalosis: Carbonic Acid Deficit

Respiratory alkalosis usually is caused by hyperventilation, which causes "blowing off" of carbon dioxide and a decrease in H_2CO_3 content. Respiratory alkalosis can be acute or chronic.

Etiology

Acute respiratory alkalosis results from pulmonary disorders that produce hypoxemia or stimulation of the respiratory centers. Underlying causes of hypoxemia include high fever, pneumonia, congestive HF, pulmonary emboli, hypotension, asthma, and inhalation of irritants. Causes of stimulation of respiratory centers include anxiety (most common), excessive mechanical ventilation, CNS lesions involving the respiratory center, and salicylate overdose (an early sign).

Clinical Manifestations

Respiratory alkalosis causes light-headedness, the inability to concentrate, numbness and tingling of the extremities (circumoral paresthesia), tinnitus, palpitations, epigastric pain, blurred vision, precordial pain (tightness), sweating, dry mouth, tremulousness, seizures, and loss of consciousness.

Laboratory and ECG Findings

- ABG values: pH greater than 7.45, $Paco_2$ less than 38 mm Hg, HCO_3^- less than 22 mEq/L
- Serum electrolytes: Presence of metabolic acid–base disorders
- Serum phosphate: May fall to less than 0.5 mg/dL
- ECG: Determines cardiac dysrhythmias

Common Causes of Respiratory Alkalosis

- Caused by hyperventilation "blowing off of CO_2"
- Hypoxemia: Pneumonia, hypotension, severe anemia, congestive HF
- Stimulation of pulmonary or pleural receptors: Pulmonary emboli, pulmonary edema, asthma, inhalation of irritants
- Central stimulation of respiratory center: Anxiety, pain, intracerebral trauma
- Hyperventilation, mechanical: Fever, sepsis (gram negative), hepatic disease (Kee, Paulanka, & Polek, 2010).

Treatment/Collaborative Management

In respiratory alkalosis, the underlying disorder must be treated. Treatment of patients with respiratory alkalosis consists of the following:

1. Treat underlying cause of respiratory alkalosis.
2. Treat the source of anxiety (instruct patient to breathe slowly into a paper bag).
3. Administer a sedative as indicated.
4. Administer oxygen therapy if hypoxemia is causative factor.
5. Adjust mechanical ventilators: Check settings and make adjustments to ventilatory parameters in response to ABG results (Smeltzer, Bare, Hinkle, & Cheever, 2010).

Table 3-10 provides a summary of acute acid–base imbalances.

> Table 3-10 | **SUMMARY OF ACUTE ACID–BASE IMBALANCES**

Body's Reaction to Acid–Base Imbalance

Condition	pH	$Paco_2$	HCO_3^-	How the Body Compensates
Respiratory acidosis	↓	↑	Normal	
With compensation	↓	↑	↑	Kidneys conserve HCO_3^- and eliminate H^+ to increase pH
Respiratory alkalosis	↑	↓	Normal	
With compensation	Slightly or normal	↓	↓	Kidneys eliminate HCO_3^- and conserve H^+ to decrease pH
Metabolic acidosis	↓	Normal	↓	
With compensation	↓	↓	↓	Hyperventilation to blow off excess CO_2 and conserve HCO_3^-
Metabolic alkalosis	↑	Normal	↑	
With compensation	Slightly ↓ or normal	↑	↑	Hypoventilation to CO_2, or normal kidneys keep H^+ and excrete HCO_3^-

Common Causes of Acid–Base Imbalance

Respiratory acidosis	Asphyxia, respiratory depression, central nervous system depression
Respiratory alkalosis	Hyperventilation, anxiety, PE (causing hyperventilation)
Metabolic acidosis	Diarrhea, renal failure, salicylate overdose such as acetylsalicylic acid (ASA; aspirin)
Metabolic alkalosis	Hypercalcemia, overdose on an alkaline substance such as antacid

NURSING POINTS OF CARE
RESPIRATORY ALKALOSIS

Nursing Assessments
- Obtain a patient history of hysteria, fever, or severe infection.
- Check for signs and symptoms of respiratory alkalosis (light-headedness, numbness and tingling, tinnitus, occasional loss of consciousness) (Heitz & Horne, 2005).
- Obtain baseline vital signs.
- Obtain ABG and electrolyte values.

Key Nursing Interventions
1. Encourage the patient who is hyperventilating to breathe slowly.

Continued

2. Have the patient rebreathe expired air by breathing into a paper bag.
3. Administer a sedative as directed.
4. Listen to the patient who is in emotional distress.
5. Monitor for respiratory alkalosis.
6. Determine the cause of hyperventilation.
7. Monitor ABG values and electrolyte levels (potassium, calcium).

AGE-RELATED CONSIDERATIONS
The Pediatric Client

Physiological differences in pediatric clients, which include body surface area, immaturity of renal structures, high rate of metabolism, and immaturity of the endocrine system in promoting homeostatic control, predispose this age group to various fluid and electrolyte imbalances. Pediatric clients are additionally at risk for acid–base imbalances because the transport system for ions and bicarbonate is weaker than in older children and adults (Kee, Paulanka, & Polek, 2010).

Infants have proportionately more body fluid (70%–80% of body weight) than any other age group. Infants are at higher risk for FVD during times of increased external temperatures. In infants (children younger than 18 months), sunken or depressed fontanels can indicate FVD and bulging fontanels can indicate FVE. In addition, in children, skin turgor begins to diminish after 3% to 5% of body weight is lost. Factors that increase insensible fluid loss are hyperthermia, increased activity, hyperventilation, radiant warmers, and phototherapy (Kee, Paulanka, & Polek, 2010).

> *EBP Recommendations by Aker (2002) for pediatric NPO times have been revised to allow clear liquids up to 2 hours preoperatively for pediatric clients younger than 6 months and up to 3 hours preoperatively for pediatric clients 6 months and older.*

Assessment begins with observations of the infant's/child's general appearance and behavioral changes. The following assessments should be performed and documented in the medical records:
• Monitor vital signs according to the severity of the illness. Vital signs of seriously ill infants and children must be monitored every 15 minutes. With each temperature increase of 1°, the metabolic need for oxygen increases by 7% and respiratory rate increases by four breaths per minute (Kee, Paulanka, & Polek, 2010).

- Assess skin and mucous membranes. The extremities often become cold and mottled with the presence of fever and severe FVD.
- Skin elasticity can be assessed by pinching the skin on the abdomen or inner thigh (dent test). Common areas for assessing edema include the extremities, face, perineum, and torso.
- Tears and salivation are decreased or absent with dehydration. Dehydration causes the fontanels and eyeballs to appear soft and sunken. With FVE the fontanels bulge and feel taut.
- Tingling fingers and toes, abdominal cramps, muscle cramps, light-headedness, nausea, and thirst are important symptoms of electrolyte imbalances in infants and children.
- Monitor weight daily. Small weight changes are crucial in fluid balance problems.
- Monitor I&O. The immature development of the renal structures in the infant limits the kidney's ability to concentrate urine and increases the infant's risk for dehydration. Establish a baseline for normal output; normal output ranges for infants are 2 to 3 mL/kg/hr. Specific gravity should be evaluated (Kee, Paulanka, & Polek, 2010).

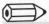 *NURSING FAST FACT!*

> *Knowledge of variations in serum electrolyte ranges for infants and children can help prevent complications.*

> *EBP A study of children with gastroenteritis demonstrated the treatment with oral rehydration fluids for children was generally as effective as intravenous fluids, and I.V. fluids did not shorten the duration of gastroenteritis and are more likely to cause adverse effects than oral rehydration therapy (Banks & Meadows, 2005).*

The Older Adult
During the normal aging process the pulmonary, renal, cardiac, GI, and integumentary systems undergo structural changes that decrease their functional efficiency; therefore, their ability to compensate for fluid and electrolyte imbalances may be decreased (Kee, Paulanka, & Polek, 2010).

Fluid balance in elderly persons is affected by physiological changes associated with aging. Older people do not possess the fluid reserves of younger individuals or the ability to adapt readily to rapid changes. Alterations in fluid and electrolyte balance frequently accompany illness. The total body water in the elderly is reduced by 6%, which creates a potential for FVD. In an elderly person, the thirst mechanism is less effective than it is in a younger person. Older persons are more prone to dehydration. Cardiovascular and respiratory

Continued

changes in the elderly combine to contribute to a slower response to the stress of blood loss, fluid depletion, shock, and acid–base imbalances (Kee, Paulanka, & Polek, 2010).

 NURSING FAST FACT!

> *The thirst mechanisms may be diminished in the aging person, so the attempt to reach homeostasis based on thirst is compromised (Hankins, 2010).*

The elderly client has a decreased ability to adapt to rapid increases in intravascular volume and can quickly develop fluid overload. Sodium and fluid overload is common in hospitalized elderly clients and can result in increased morbidity and mortality in surgical clients (Zarowitz & Lefkovitz, 2008). Dehydration and chronic hyponatremia can lead to confusional states that interfere with fluid intake in elderly people, who are very susceptible to dehydration.

 NURSING FAST FACT!

> *Clinical practice guidelines on HF suggest that daily weight monitoring leads to early recognition of excess fluid retention, which when reported can be offset with additional medication to avoid hospitalization from HF decompensation (Jessup et al., 2009).*

> *EBP Dehydrated older adults have significantly lower systolic and diastolic BPs and significantly higher BUN levels but similar creatinine levels compared with nondehydrated adults (Bennett, Thomas, & Riegel, 2004).*

Hypokalemia is a common deficit experienced by older adults. Potassium is not conserved well at any age; however, older adults often receive diuretics and steroids, which tend to decrease serum potassium levels.

 Home Care Issues
- Consider home health care for patients with diabetes mellitus, cardiovascular disorders, and severe GI disorders.
- Consider home health care for patients taking drug therapy (diuretics) for edema.
- Consider home health care for dietary follow-up.
- Provide instructions on use of pressure stockings.
- Assess patient taking oral electrolyte supplements for adherence.

Patient Education

- Teach patient risk factors for development of FVD or FVE.
- Explain to client and family the reasons for I&O records.
- Teach the client to keep track of oral liquids consumed.
- Assess the patient's understanding of the type of fluid loss being experienced.
- Give verbal and written instructions for fluid replacement (drink at least 3 quarts of liquid).
- Teach the patient to increase fluid intake during hot days and in the presence of fever or infection, and to decrease activity during extreme weather.
- Teach how to observe for dehydration (especially in infants).
- Instruct the patient to seek medical consultation for continued dehydration.
- Teach appropriate use of laxatives, enemas, and diuretics.
- Inform the patient to notify the physician if he or she has excessive edema or weight gain (more than 2 lb) or increased shortness of breath.
- Provide literature on low-salt diets; consult with dietitian if necessary.
- Provide dietary education on sodium and potassium and teach to avoid adding salt while cooking; provide information on salt substitutes.
- Teach to avoid caffeine because it acts as a mild diuretic.
- Provide written material and verbal instructions regarding any medications.
- Provide information on predisposing factors associated with specific electrolyte imbalances.
- Review indicators of digitalis toxicity, if appropriate.
- Provide information on dietary sources of electrolytes in deficit situations when appropriate.
- Provide information on over-the-counter medications (e.g., magnesium and aluminum hydroxide, antacids and phosphorus-binding antacids, laxatives, multivitamin and mineral supplements) when appropriate.
- Educate the patient with cancer about symptoms of hypercalcemia.
- Educate the patient on the high phosphorus content of processed foods, carbonated beverages, and over-the-counter medications when appropriate.

Nursing Process

The nursing process is a five- or six-step process for problem-solving to guide nursing action. Refer to Chapter 1 for details on the steps of the nursing process related to vascular access. The following tables focus on nursing diagnoses and nursing outcomes for patients with fluid, electrolyte, and acid–base imbalances. Nursing diagnoses should be patient specific and outcomes and interventions individualized. The Nursing Outcomes Classification (NOC) and Nursing Interventions Classification (NIC) presented here are suggested directions for development of outcomes and interventions.

Nursing diagnoses and interventions are specific to the underlying pathophysiological process. In addition, the following may be considered.

Nursing Diagnoses to Fluid and Related Imbalance Electrolyte	Nursing Outcomes Classification (NOC)	Nursing Interventions Classification (NIC)
Activity intolerance risk for: Muscle weakness or neuromuscular irritability secondary to electrolyte imbalance	Activity tolerance, energy conservation	Energy management
Cardiac output decreased related to: Altered heart rate; altered heart rhythm, altered contractility associated with reduced myocardial functioning from severe phosphorus depletion Electrical alterations associated with tachydysrhythmias or digitalis toxicity; possible dysrhythmia from electrolyte imbalance	Cardiac pump effectiveness, circulation status, tissue perfusion, vital signs	Cardiac care
Fluid volume deficit or excess related to: Failure of regulatory mechanisms; active fluid volume loss or gain	Electrolyte and acid–base balance, fluid balance, hydration	Fluid management, hypovolemia management, shock management: volume, fluid monitoring
Note: This nursing diagnosis overlaps with risk for falls, risk for trauma, and ineffective protection (Ackley & Ladwig [2011]). *Injury risk for related to:* **External: human:** *cognitive and psychomotor factors and physical* **Internal:** *neurosensory alterations:* Altered mental functioning, drowsiness, and weakness; sensory or neuromuscular dysfunction from hypophosphatemia-induced central nervous system disturbances	Personal safety; risk control; safe home environment Knowledge to remain free of injury	Health education; environmental modification

Nursing Diagnoses to Fluid and Related Imbalance Electrolyte	Nursing Outcomes Classification (NOC)	Nursing Interventions Classification (NIC)
Altered sensorium from primary hypernatremia or cerebral edema occurring with too rapid correction of hypernatremia Tetany—precipitation of calcium phosphate in the soft tissue and periarticular region of the large joints sensory or neuromuscular dysfunction as a result of hypomagnesemia Tetany and seizures related to neurosensory alterations from severe hypocalcemia		
Knowledge deficit related to cognitive limitations, information misinterpretation, unfamiliarity with information resources	Knowledge of diet, disease process, health behavior, health resources, medication, treatment regimen	Teaching: disease process, learning facilitation
Nutrition altered: more than body requirements, related to: Excessive intake in relation to metabolic needs: excess intake of phosphate containing compounds; oral and I.V. magnesium supplements and chronic use of drugs containing magnesium	Nutritional status, nutrient intake	Nutrition management
Nutrition altered: less than body requirements, related to: Inadequate nutritional intake, chronic alcoholism, intravenous fluid (including total parenteral nutrition) with lack of phosphate additive, magnesium related to history of poor intake, anorexia, or alcoholism Effects of vitamin D deficiency, renal failure, malabsorption, laxative use	Nutritional status; food and fluid intake, nutrient intake	Feeding, nutrition management
Perfusion, tissue ineffective (peripheral) related to: Aggravating factors	Circulation status, fluid balance, hydration, tissue perfusion: peripheral	Circulatory care and monitoring
Gas exchange, impaired related to: Alveolar–capillary membrane changes; ventilation–perfusion imbalance secondary to hypercapnia; hypercarbia; hypoxemia; hypoxia	Respiratory status: gas exchange	Acid–base management, airway management
Injury risk for, related to: *Internal:* abnormal blood profile; tissue hypoxia	Personal safety behavior; risk control	Education to prevent iatrogenic harm

Continued

Nursing Diagnoses to Fluid and Related Imbalance Electrolyte	Nursing Outcomes Classification (NOC)	Nursing Interventions Classification (NIC)
Perfusion, tissue, cardiac, decreased risk for related to: Decreased hemoglobin concentration in blood; hypoventilation; impaired transport of oxygen; mismatch ventilation with blood flow	Cardiac pump effectiveness, circulation status, tissue perfusion cardiac, tissue perfusion: cellular, vital signs	Circulatory care: arterial insufficiency Dysrhythmia management, vitals signs monitoring, shock management: cardiac

Sources: Ackley & Ladwig (2011); Bulechek, Butcher, Dochterman, & Wagner (2013); Moorhead, Johnson, Maas, & Swanson (2013).

Chapter Highlights

■ Fluid is distributed in three compartments: intracellular (40%), intravascular (5%), and interstitial (15%). TBW in water is 60% for an average adult.

■ Fluid is transported passively by filtration, diffusion, and osmosis.

■ Electrolytes are actively transported by ATP on cell membranes and by the sodium–potassium pump.

■ Osmosis is the movement of water from a lower concentration to a higher concentration across a semipermeable membrane.

■ The osmolarity of I.V. solutions has the following ranges:
  ■ Isotonic solutions: 250 to 375 mOsm/L
  ■ Hypotonic solutions: Less than 250 mOsm/L
  ■ Hypertonic solutions: Greater than 375 mOsm/L

■ The homeostatic organs that regulate fluid and electrolyte balance include the kidneys; heart and blood vessels; lungs; and adrenal, parathyroid, and pituitary glands.

■ There are six areas to assess for fluid balance: neurological status, cardiovascular, respiratory, and integumentary systems, special senses, and body weight.

■ Fluid imbalances fall into two categories:
  ■ FVD caused primarily by disorders of the GI system. Signs and symptoms reflect a dehydrated individual. Treatment is aimed at rehydration with isotonic sodium chloride.
  ■ FVE caused primarily by cardiovascular dysfunction, renal or endocrine dysfunction, and too rapid administration of I.V. fluids. Signs and symptoms reflect fluid overload. Treatment is aimed at decreasing the sodium level, using diuretics to increase the excretion of fluids, and treating the underlying cause.

■ The seven major electrolytes and their symbols are:
  ■ *Cations:* Sodium: Na^+, potassium: K^+, calcium: Ca^{2+}, magnesium: Mg^{2+}
  ■ *Anions:* Chloride: Cl^-, phosphate: HPO_4^-, bicarbonate: HCO_3^-

■ The prefix *hypo-*: Deficit in an electrolyte

■ The prefix *hyper-*: Excess in an electrolyte

- Key nursing interventions for electrolyte imbalances reflect collaborative practice and are specific to the imbalance.
- Key laboratory values that the nurse must recognize:
  - Sodium (N^+): 135 to 145 mEq/L
  - Potassium (K^+): 3.5 to 5.0 mEq/L
  - Calcium (Ca^+): 4.5 to 5.5 mEq/L or 9 to 11 mg/dL
  - Magnesium (Mg^{2+}): 1.5 to 2.5 mEq/L or 1.8 to 3.0 mg/dL
  - Phosphorus (HPO_4^-): 2.5 to 4.5 mg/dL
  - Chloride (Cl^-): 95 to 108 mEq/L
- Critical guidelines for infusion potassium include:
  - Never give potassium I.V. push.
  - Concentrations of potassium greater than 60 mEq should not be given in a peripheral vein.
  - Concentrations greater than 8 mEq/100 mL can cause pain and irritation of peripheral veins, leading to phlebitis.
  - Do not add potassium to a hanging container.
  - Administer potassium at a rate not exceeding 10 mEq/hr through peripheral veins.
- Calcium and phosphate have a reciprocal relationship: When one is elevated, the other is decreased.
- Patients with calcium imbalances may need seizure precautions. The most dangerous symptom of hypocalcemia is laryngospasm.
- The four major acid–base imbalances in the body are respiratory acidosis (carbonic acid excess), respiratory alkalosis (carbonic acid deficit), metabolic acidosis (base bicarbonate deficit), and metabolic alkalosis (bicarbonate excess).
- Acid–base balance is maintained through three major reaction-specific buffer systems that regulate hydrogen ion concentration: the carbonic acid–bicarbonate system, the phosphate buffer system, and the protein buffer system.

■■ Thinking Critically: Case Study

A 28-year-old woman who became ill on a cruise to the Bahamas was admitted to the hospital after 6 days of severe diarrhea and poor intake. She weighed 120 lb on admission (132 lb before illness). Her BUN was 40 mg/dL, and serum creatinine was 1.3 mg/dL. Her potassium level was 3.2 mEq/mL, and sodium was 133 mEq/mL. Her skin turgor was poor, and urine output was 15 mL/hr (specific gravity 1.030). Blood gases were pH 7.47 and $HCO3^-$ 30 mEq/L; BE +4; BP was 120/80 mm Hg recumbent and fell to 98/60 mm Hg when the patient was upright. Her pulse was 110, weak, and regular, with respiratory rate of 14. Her reflexes were hyperactive, and she complained of "tingling of fingers."

Case Study Questions

1. *What percentage of body weight did she lose?*
2. *What concerns would the nurse have regarding the patient's laboratory test results?*

3. *What nursing diagnoses would apply to this woman?*
4. *What nursing interventions would be implemented?*
5. *What collaborative orders would you anticipate?*

 Media Link: Answers to the case study questions are provided on DavisPlus.

Post-Test

1. The nurse administering 0.45% sodium chloride in 5% dextrose in water understands that this solution will hydrate the intravascular and intracellular spaces based on which of the following transport mechanisms?

   a. Diffusion
   b. Osmosis
   c. Filtration
   d. Sodium–potassium pump

2. You have just completed a physical assessment of a 68-year-old man. He knows who he is but is unsure of where he is (previous orientation normal). His eyes are sunken, his mouth is coated with an extra longitudinal furrow, and his lips are cracked. Hand vein filling takes more than 5 seconds, and tenting of the skin appears over the sternum. His vital signs are BP 128/60 mm Hg, pulse 78, and respiratory rate 16 (previously 150/78, 76, 16, respectively). Your assessment would lead you to suspect:

   a. Fluid volume deficit
   b. Hyponatremia
   c. Fluid volume excess
   d. Hypernatremia

3. If the external temperature is 101°F (38.4°C), which of the following age groups is at highest risk for fluid volume deficit?

   a. Infants
   b. School-aged children
   c. Adolescents
   d. Middle-aged adults

4. Which of the following could be the etiology for a nursing diagnosis of fluid volume excess? (*Select all that apply.*)

   a. Excessive infusion of 0.9% sodium chloride solution
   b. Use of diuretics
   c. SIADH
   d. Congestive heart failure

5. Which of the following laboratory values is consistent with fluid volume deficit?

   a. Urine specific gravity 1.005
   b. BUN 6 mg/100 mL
   c. Hematocrit 52%
   d. Serum osmolarity 305 mOsm/kg

6. The three most important buffer systems in body fluids are the bicarbonate buffer system, the plasma protein buffer system, and which of the following?

   a. Calcium buffer system
   b. Sodium chloride buffer system
   c. Hemoglobin buffer system
   d. Phosphate buffer system

7. Treatment for a patient with metabolic alkalosis includes which of the following? (*Select all that apply.*)

   a. Removal of underlying cause
   b. I.V. fluid administration with NaCl
   c. Replacement of potassium deficit
   d. Administration of I.V. solution with sodium bicarbonate

8. To correct metabolic acidosis, the parenteral fluid of choice is:

   a. $NaHCO_3$
   b. NaCl
   c. Albumin
   d. 5% Dextrose in water

9. A nursing diagnosis that would be appropriate for a patient with calcium deficit would be:

   a. Ineffective breathing pattern related to biochemical imbalances
   b. Altered comfort related to injuring agent
   c. Risk for protection ineffective: risk of tetany and seizures related to neurosensory alterations from severe hypocalcemia
   d. Altered urinary elimination pattern related to changes in renal function.

10. A frail 80-year-old man has experienced nausea, vomiting, and diarrhea for several days. When he became weak and confused he was admitted to the hospital. As the best indicator of the client's rehydration status, the nurse should assess the client's:

    a. Mucous membranes
    b. Weight gain of 2.2 lb
    c. Urinary output
    d. Skin turgor

Media Link:　Answers to the Chapter 3 Post-Test and more test questions together with rationales are provided on Davis*Plus*.

■ References

Ackley, B. J., & Ladwig, G. B. (2011). *Nursing diagnosis handbook: An evidence-based guide to planning care* (9th ed.). St. Louis: Mosby Elsevier.

Aker, J. (2002). Pediatric fluid management. *Current Review of Pain, 24*(7), 73-84.

Armstrong, L. E. (2005). Hydration assessment techniques. *Nutrition Reviews, 63*(6 Pt 2), S40-S54.

Ayus, J. C., Achinger, S. G., & Arieff, A. (2008). Brain cell volume regulation in hyponatremia: Role of sex, age, vasopressin and hypoxia. *American Journal of Physiology. 295*(3), 619-624.

Banks, J. B., & Meadows, S. (2005). Intravenous fluids for children with gastroenteritis. *American Family Physician, 71*(1), 121.

Bennett, J. A., Thomas V., & Riegel, B. (2004). Unrecognized chronic dehydration in older adults: Examining prevalence rate and risk factors. *Journal of Gerontology Nursing, 30*(11), 22-28.

Bulechek, G., Butcher, H., Dochterman, J., & Wagner, C. (2013). *Nursing interventions classification (NIC)* (6th ed.). St. Louis: MO: Mosby Elsevier.

Ferry, M. (2005). Strategies for ensuring good hydration in the elderly, *Nutr Rev, 63*(6 Part 2); S22-S29.

Gahart, L., & Nazareno, A. R. (2012). *Intravenous medications* (29th ed.). Philadelphia, PA: Elsevier Mosby Saunders.

Giger, J. N. (2012). *Transcultural nursing: Assessment and intervention* (6th ed.). Philadelphia, PA: Elsevier Mosby Saunders.

Goh, K. P. (2004). Management of hyponatremia. *American Family Physician, 69*(10), 2387-2394.

Halperin, M. L., Kamel S., & Goldstein, M. B. (2010). *Fluid, electrolyte, and acid-base physiology: A problem-based approach* (4th ed.). Philadelphia, PA: Saunders Elsevier.

Hankins, J. (2010). Fluids and electrolytes. In M. Alexander, A. Corrigan, L. Gorski, J. Hankins, & R. Perucca (Eds.), *Infusion Nurses Society infusion nursing: An evidence-based approach* (3rd ed.) (pp. 178-203). St. Louis, MO: Saunders Elsevier.

Heitz, Y., & Horne, M. M. (2005). *Pocket guide to fluid, electrolyte and acid-base balance* (5th ed.). St. Louis, MO: C. V. Mosby.

Hew-Butler, T., Almond C., Ayus, J. C., et al. (2005). Consensus statement of the 1st International Exercise-Associated Hyponatremia Development Conference, Cape Town, South Africa. *Clinical Journal of Sports Medicine, 15*, 208-213.

Holliday, M. A., & Segar, W. E. (1957). The maintenance need for water in parenteral fluid therapy. *Pediatrics, 19*, 823-832.

Jessup, M., Abraham, W. T., Casety, D. E., et al. (2009). 2009 focused update: ACCF/AHA guidelines for the diagnosis and management of heart failure in adults. Online www.jacc.org. (Accessed August 29, 2012).

Kee, J. L., Paulanka, B. J., & Polek, C. (2010). *Fluids and electrolytes with clinical applications: A programmed approach* (8th ed.). Clifton Park, NY: Delmar Cengage Learning.

Martin, K. G., Gonzalez, E. A., & Slatopolsy, E. (2009). Clinical consequences and management of hypomagnesemia. *Journal American Society of Nephrology, 20,* 2291-2965.

Moorhead, S., Johnson, M., Maas, M., & Swanson, E. (2013). *Nursing outcomes classification (NOC)* (5th ed.). Philadelphia, PA: Mosby Elsevier.

Newfield, S. A., Hinz, M. D., Tilley., D. S., Sridaromont, K. L., & Maramba, P. J. (2007). *Cox's clinical applications of nursing diagnosis,* Philadelphia: F.A. Davis.

Porth, C. M,. & Matfin, G. (2010). *Pathophysiology: Concept of altered health states* (8th ed.). Philadelphia, PA: Lippincott, Williams & Wilkins.

Rosner, M. H., & Kirven, J. (2007). Exercise-associated hyponatremia. *American Society of Nephrology, 2,* 151-161.

Smeltzer, S. C., Bare, B. G., Hinkle, J. L., & Cheever, K. H. (2010). *Brunner & Suddarth's textbook of medical-surgical nursing* (12th ed.). Philadelphia: Lippincott, Williams & Wilkins.

Starling, E. H. (1896). On the absorption of fluids from connective tissues spaces. *Journal of Physiology, 19*(3), 12-26.

Van Leeuwen, A. M., Poelhuis-Leth, D. J., & Bladh, M. L. (2012). *Davis's comprehensive handbook of laboratory and diagnostic tests with nursing implications* (5th ed.). Philadelphia, PA: F. A. Davis.

Wakefield, B. (2008). Fluid management guideline. In B. Ackley, G. Ladwig, & B. Swan (Eds.), *Evidence based nursing care guidelines: Medical–surgical interventions.* Philadelphia, PA: Mosby Elsevier.

Wilkinson, J. M., & Van Leuven, K. (2007). *Fundamentals of nursing: Theory, concepts, and applications.* Philadelphia, PA: F. A. Davis.

Zarowitz, B., & Lefkovitz, A. (2008). Recognition and treatment of hyperkalemia. *Geriatric Nursing, 29*(5), 333-339.

Chapter 4

Parenteral Solutions

Let the patient's taste decide. You will say that, in cases of great thirst, the patient's craving decides that it will drink a great deal of tea, and that you cannot help it. But in these cases be sure that the patient requires diluents for quite other purposes than quenching the thirst; he wants a great deal of some drink, not only of tea, and the doctor will order what he is to have, barley water or lemonade, or soda water and milk, as the case may be.
—*Florence Nightingale, 1859*

Chapter Contents

▧ GLOSSARY

Balanced solution   Parenteral solution that contains electrolytes in proportions similar to those in plasma; also contains bicarbonate or acetate ion

Body surface area   The surface area of the body expressed in square meters; used in calculating pediatric dosages, managing burn patients, and determining radiation and chemotherapy doses

Caloric method   Calculation of metabolic expenditure of energy, used in pediatric fluid maintenance and replacement

Catabolism   The breakdown of chemical compounds by the body; an energy-producing metabolic process

Colloid   A substance (e.g., blood, plasma, albumin, dextran) that does not dissolve into a true solution and is not capable of passing through a semipermeable membrane

Crystalloid A substance that forms a true solution and is capable of passing through a semipermeable membrane (e.g., lactated Ringer's solution, isotonic saline)

Dehydration A deficit of body water; can involve one fluid compartment or all three

Hydrating solution A solution of water, carbohydrate, sodium, and chloride used to determine adequacy of renal function

Hypertonic solution A solution with an osmolarity higher than that of plasma, above 375 mOsm

Hypotonic solution A solution with an osmolarity lower than that of plasma, usually below 250 mOsm

Isotonic solution A solution with the same osmolarity as plasma, usually 250 to 375 mOsm

Maintenance therapy Fluids that provide all nutrients necessary to meet daily patient requirements; usually water, glucose, sodium, and potassium

Meter square method Formula using a nomogram to determine surface areas of a pediatric client for maintenance of fluid needs

Normal saline Solution of salt (0.9% sodium chloride)

Osmolality The number of milliosmoles per kilogram of water and measures the *activity* of all solutes present in a sample of plasma or urine.

Osmolarity The number of milliosmoles per liter of solutions; measures the concentration of the most significant ions.

Parenteral therapy Introduction of substances other than through the gastrointestinal tract; particularly to the introduction of substances into an organism by intravenous route, or subcutaneous, intramuscular, or intramedullary injection

Plasma volume expander A high molecular weight compound in a solution suitable for intravenous use

Replacement therapy Replenishment of losses when maintenance cannot be met and when patient is in a deficit state

Restoration therapy Reconstruction of fluid and electrolyte needs on a continuing basis until homeostasis returns

Weight method Formula based on weight in kilograms to estimate the fluid needs of the pediatric client

■ Rationales and Objectives of Parenteral Therapy

Objectives of Delivery of Infusion Therapy

The nurse has the main responsibility of delivery of **parenteral fluid therapy**. The nurse initiates the written parenteral therapy order, monitors for patient response, and must be knowledgeable about the contents of parenteral fluids, their purposes, their action on the body, and the complications that may occur once they are delivered to the patient. The complex subject of fluids and electrolytes is covered in Chapter 3, which provides the requisite background knowledge for this chapter on parenteral therapy. To understand the use of parenteral solutions, the nurse must understand two important concepts: (1) the reason or objective for the licensed independent practitioner (LIP) order of infusion therapy and (2) the type of solution ordered, together with the composition and clinical use of that solution (Phillips, 2010). The goals for administration of parenteral therapy fall into three broad categories:

1. **Maintenance therapy** for daily body fluid requirements
2. **Replacement therapy** for present losses
3. Providing fluids and electrolytes necessary to replace ongoing losses (restoring homeostasis)

These three objectives differ with regard to the time necessary to complete the therapy, the purpose of the I.V. fluid, and the type of patient who is to receive the I.V. solution. Factors affecting the choice of objective in prescribing parenteral fluid and the rate of administration by the physician are the patient's renal function, daily maintenance requirements, existing fluid and electrolyte imbalance, clinical status, and disturbances in homeostasis as a result of parenteral therapy.

Maintenance Therapy

Maintenance therapy provides nutrients that meet the daily needs of a patient for water, electrolytes, and dextrose. Water has priority. Water is also an important dilutor for waste products excreted by the kidneys. Approximately 30 mL of fluid is needed per kilogram of body weight (i.e., 15 mL/kg) for maintenance needs. The typical patient profile for maintenance therapy is an individual who is allowed nothing by mouth (NPO) or whose oral intake is restricted for any reason. Remember that insensible loss is approximately 500 to 1000 mL every 24 hours. Maintenance therapy should be 1500 mL per square meter (m^2) of body surface over 24 hours. For example, a man weighing 85 kg (187 lb) has a **body surface area** (BSA) of 2 m^2, so 1500 times 2 equals 3000; therefore, he needs 3000 mL of fluids for maintenance therapy.

Solutions for maintenance therapy include water, daily needs of sodium and potassium, and glucose. Glucose, a necessary component in maintenance therapy, is converted to glycogen by the liver. It has four main uses in maintenance parenteral therapy:

1. Improves hepatic function
2. Supplies necessary calories for energy
3. Spares body protein
4. Minimizes ketosis

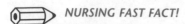 *NURSING FAST FACT!*

> *The basic caloric requirement for an adult varies with age. On average, a 70-kg adult under the age of 60 years needs approximately 1600 calories/day at rest. He needs approximately 100 to 150 g of carbohydrates daily to minimize pro-tein **catabolism** and prevent starvation. One liter of 5% dextrose in water contains 50 g of dextrose (Porth & Matfin, 2010).*

Replacement Therapy

Replacement therapy is necessary to take care of the fluid, electrolyte, or blood product deficits of patients in acute distress. This type of therapy is supplied over a 48-hour period. Examples of conditions of patients needing replacement infusion therapy (and their replacement requirements) are:

- Hemorrhage (for replacement of cells and plasma)
- Low platelet count (for replacement of clotting factors)
- Vomiting and diarrhea (for replacement of losses of electrolytes and water)
- Starvation (for replacement of losses of water and electrolytes)

When the maintenance requirements of the body cannot be met, the physician should institute replacement therapy. The physician must figure the losses and calculate replacement over a 48-hour period. Renal function is the first thing that should be checked before replacement therapy is begun. Patients requiring replacement therapy, except those in shock, require potassium. Patients under stress from tissue injury, wound infection, or gastric or bowel surgery also require potassium.

Most hospitalized patients receiving additional saline or glucose infusions are prone to developing potassium deficiency. In addition, hospitalized patients usually are under physiological stress. Excretion of potassium in their urine can increase to 60 to 120 mEq/day even with limited intake. Tissue injury significantly increases the loss of potassium. Normal dietary intake of potassium is 80 to 200 mEq/day. Potassium is often included as part of replacement therapy (Porth & Matfin, 2010).

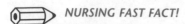 *NURSING FAST FACT!*

> *Never give more than 120 mEq of potassium in a 24-hour period unless cardiac status is monitored continuously, because it can create a life-threatening situation. Key nursing assessment: Check renal function before administering potassium in replacement therapy.*

Carefully monitor replacement solutions with potassium for the following patients:

1. Those with dysfunction of the:
   - Renal system
   - Cardiovascular system

- Adrenal glands
- Pituitary gland
- Parathyroid gland
2. Those with deficits of:
   - Sodium
   - Calcium
   - Base bicarbonate
   - Blood volume (hypovolemic)
3. Those with excess of:
   - Base bicarbonate
   - Extracellular potassium
   - Extracellular calcium

Vitamins are necessary for utilization of the nutrients and are often added to postoperative replacement therapy. Vitamin C and vitamin B complex are used frequently in postoperative parenteral therapy to assist in replacement and to promote wound healing. Vitamin B complex has a role in metabolism of carbohydrates and maintenance of gastrointestinal (GI) function.

Restoration: Providing Fluids and Electrolytes to Restore Ongoing Losses

When maintenance and replacement therapy do not meet the needs of the patient, fluid and electrolyte management is accomplished with **restoration therapy**. When restoring ongoing losses (e.g., nasogastric tubes to suction, bleeding) critical evaluation of the source of the loss is done at least every 24 hours. Accurate documentation of intake and output (I&O) is extremely important in this type of management of fluid and electrolyte therapy. Restoration of homeostasis depends on the nursing assessment of intake of I.V. fluids as well as on the documentation of all body fluid losses. The types of clinical patients who require 24-hour evaluation are those with draining fistulas, abscesses, nasogastric tubes, burns, and abdominal wounds. With these types of patients, you will see frequent changes in the types of solutions ordered, in the amounts of electrolytes ordered based on laboratory test results, and in the rate of infusion.

Third-space shifts, as occurs in peritonitis, bowel obstruction, burns, ascites, some cancers, major surgery involving extensive tissue trauma, and sepsis, are considered ongoing losses that require special consideration when determining fluid needs (Heitz & Horne, 2005). Third spacing refers to a shift of fluid from the vascular space into a portion of the body from which it is not easily exchanged with the rest of the extracellular fluid (ECF). The trapped fluid is sequestered and not available for functional use. Fluid can be sequestered from the intravascular space into body spaces (pleural or peritoneal), or it can become trapped in the bowel by obstruction or in the interstitial space as edema after burns (Porth & Matfin, 2010).

A major consideration in differentiating the fluid volume deficit associated with third spacing from that associated with fluid lost through vomiting or diarrhea is that measurable fluid can be replaced using replacement therapy whereas third-space fluid cannot; in addition, decreased body weight does not occur in third spacing. Accurate dosing of fluid therapy requires monitoring, and treatment is directed at correcting the cause of the third-space shift of body fluids and is tailored to the patient's response.

Parkland Formula: Burn Resuscitation

Fluid resuscitation is complicated. The Parkland formula is often used to calculate fluid resuscitation. This formula states that one-half of the amount is given over the first 8 hours, one-fourth is administered in the second 8 hours, and one-fourth of the total is given in the third 8-hour period after the burn. Lactated Ringer's solution is administered at 4 mL/kg per percent total body surface area (TBSA) burned. In the second 24 hours, the solution of choice is 25% albumin plus 5% dextrose in water with volume to maintain desired urine output.

> **Example:** A child who weighs 10 kg sustains an estimated TBSA burn of 50% from a house fire. The Parkland formula of fluid resuscitation is used to determine the amount of fluid that this child requires. According to this formula, a nurse should intravenously administer ____ mL of fluid to the child in the first 8 hours from the time of the injury. Fill in the blank.
>
> **Answer:** 1000
>
> **Rationale:** The Parkland formula is:
> 4 mL of lactate solution × kg of body weight × % of TBSA (total body surface area) burned
> 4 mL × 10 kg × 50% TBSA = 2000 mL

▪ Key Elements in Parenteral Solutions

The key elements that make up **crystalloid** parenteral fluids include water, carbohydrates (glucose), protein, vitamins, and electrolytes. The pH of crystalloid solutions can affect the initial response to crystalloid administration and must be considered by nurses providing the infusion.

Water

Two main physiological mechanisms assist in regulating body water: thirst and antidiuretic hormone (ADH). Thirst is primarily a regulator of water intake, and ADH is a regulator of water output. Both mechanisms respond to changes in extracellular **osmolality** and volume (Porth &

Matfin, 2010). The human body is a contained fluid environment of water and electrolytes. Holliday and Segar (1957) established that, regardless of age, all healthy persons require approximately 100 mL of water per 100 calories metabolized, for dissolving and eliminating metabolic wastes. This means that a person who expends 1800 calories of energy requires approximately 1800 mL of water for metabolic purposes. These water needs are increased in patients with sensible water losses (e.g., respiratory rate >20 breaths/min, fever, diaphoresis, located in a low-humidity environment); in patients with decreased renal concentration ability; and in elderly people. The average adult loses 500 to 1000 mL in the form of insensible water every 24 hours. Water must be provided for adequate renal function.

Carbohydrates (Glucose)

Glucose, a nutrient included in maintenance, restoration, and replacement therapies, is converted into glycogen by the liver, which improves hepatic function. By supplying calories for energy, it spares body protein. Sources of carbohydrates include dextrose (glucose) and fructose. When glucose is supplied by infusion, all the parenteral glucose is bioavailable. The addition of 100 g of glucose per day minimizes starvation. Every 2 L of 5% dextrose in water contains 100 g of glucose.

Amino Acids

Amino acids (protein) are the body-building nutrients whose major functions are contributing to tissue growth and repair, replacing body cells, healing wounds, and synthesizing vitamins and enzymes. Amino acids are the basic units of protein. The parenteral proteins currently used are elemental, provided as synthetic crystalline amino acids. These proteins are available in concentrations of 3.5% to 15% and are used in parenteral nutrition (PN) centrally or peripherally. When administered by infusion, protein bypasses the GI and portal circulation (Porth & Matfin, 2010). The usual daily requirement is 1 g of protein per kilogram of body weight. For example, a 54-kg woman needs 54 g of protein per day.

Vitamins

Vitamins are added to restorative and replacement therapies. Certain vitamins (i.e., the fat-soluble A, D, E, and K and the water-soluble B and C vitamins) are necessary for growth and act as catalysts for metabolic processes. Some disease conditions alter vitamin requirements. Vitamins B and C are the most frequently used in parenteral therapy. Vitamin B complex is important in the metabolism of carbohydrates and the maintenance of GI function, which is especially important in postoperative patients. Vitamin C promotes wound healing.

Electrolytes

Electrolytes are the major additives to replacement and restorative therapies. Correction of electrolyte imbalances is important in preventing the serious complications associated with excess or deficit of electrolytes. There are seven major electrolytes in normal body fluids, and the same seven major elements are supplied in manufactured I.V. solutions. (Chapter 3 reviews these electrolyte functions.) The electrolytes of major importance in parenteral therapy are potassium, sodium, chloride, magnesium, phosphorus, calcium, and bicarbonate or acetate ion (important for acid–base balance).

pH

The pH reflects the degree of acidity or alkalinity of a solution. Blood pH is not a significant problem for routine parenteral therapy. Normal kidneys can achieve an acid–base balance as long as enough water is supplied. The USP (U.S. Pharmacopeial Convention) standards require that solution pH must be slightly acidic (pH between 3.5 and 6.2). Many solutions have a pH of 5. The acidity of solutions allows them to have a longer shelf life.

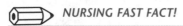 *NURSING FAST FACT!*

> *As the acidity of a solution increases, the solution's ability to irritate vein walls increases.*

■ Osmolality and Osmolarity of Parenteral Solutions

The osmotic activity of a solution may be expressed in terms of either its **osmolarity** or its osmolality. Osmolarity refers to the osmolar concentration in 1 L of solution expressed in units of measurement called the osmole (osm). Osmolality is the osmolar concentration and is expressed in 1 kg of water (mOsm/kg of H_2O) or mOsm/L. Osmolality assesses the activity of all solutes present in a sample of plasma or urine. Osmolality is a better measure of the true physiological condition than is osmolarity because it takes into account a wider range of solutes and the movement of fluid between physiological compartments (Cockerill & Reed, 2012).

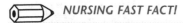 *NURSING FAST FACT!*

> *Osmolarity usually is used when referring to fluids outside the body (I.V. solutions). Osmolality is used for describing fluids inside the body, such as laboratory test values from urine or plasma.*

Extracellular osmolality is primarily determined by the sodium level because it is the main solute found in ECF. A rough estimation of extracellular osmolality can be made by multiplying the plasma sodium concentration by 2 (Porth & Matfin, 2010).

The term *tonicity* refers to the tension or effect that the effective osmotic pressure of a solution with impermeable solutes exerts on cell size because of water movement across the cell membrane. Tonicity is determined solely by effective solutes such as glucose that cannot penetrate the cell membrane, thereby producing an osmotic force that pulls water into or out of the cell and causing it to change size.

Solutions to which body cells are exposed can be classified as isotonic, hypotonic, or hypertonic depending on whether they cause cells to swell or shrink. Cells placed in an **isotonic solution**, which has the same effective osmolality as intracellular fluids (ICFs; 280–295 mOsm/L) neither shrink nor swell. When cells are placed in **hypotonic solution**, which has a lower effective osmolality than ICFs, they swell as water moves into the cell. When cells are placed in a **hypertonic solution**, which has a greater effective osmolality than ICF, they shrink as water is pulled out of the cell. Administration of intravenous fluids is guided by the tonicity of the solution and falls into three categories: isotonic or iso-osmolar, hypotonic, and hypertonic. The effect of I.V. fluid on the body fluid compartments depends on how the osmolarity of the I.V. solution compares with the patient's serum osmolality. Intravenous fluids can change the fluid compartment in one of three ways:

1. Expand the intravascular compartment
2. Expand the intravascular compartment and deplete the intracellular and interstitial compartments
3. Expand the intracellular compartment and deplete the intravascular compartment

---

NOTE > Review Chapter 3 for further information on osmolarity and diagrams of fluid shifts.

Isotonic or Iso-osmolar Fluids

Isotonic solutions have an osmolarity of 250 to 375 mOsm/L. Blood and normal body fluids have an osmolarity of 285 to 295 mOsm/kg. These fluids are used to expand the ECF compartment. No net fluid shifts occur between isotonic solutions because the osmotic pressure gradient is the same inside and outside the cells. Many isotonic solutions are available. Examples include 0.9% sodium chloride, 5% dextrose in water, and lactated Ringer's solution.

Isotonic solutions are commonly used to treat fluid loss, **dehydration**, and hypernatremia (sodium excess). Five percent dextrose solution is used for dehydration because it replaces fluid volume without disrupting the interstitial and intracellular environment. However, this solution becomes hypotonic when dextrose is metabolized; the solution should be used cautiously in patients with renal and cardiac disease because of the increased risk of fluid overload. This solution also does not provide enough daily calories and can lead to protein breakdown if used for extended periods of time (Crawford & Harris, 2011; Smeltzer, Bare, Hinkle, & Cheever, 2010).

Caution: The danger with the use of isotonic solutions is circulatory overload. These solutions do not cause fluid shifts into other compartments. The problem with overexpanding the vascular compartment is that the fluid dilutes the concentration of hemoglobin and lowers hematocrit levels.

Hypotonic Fluids

Hypotonic fluids have an osmolarity lower than 250 mOsm/L. By lowering serum osmolarity, the body fluids shift out of blood vessels into cells and interstitial spaces. The resulting osmotic pressure gradient draws water into the cells from the ECF, causing the cells to swell. Hypotonic solutions are used for patients who have hypertonic dehydration, water replacement, and diabetic ketoacidosis after initial sodium chloride replacement. Examples of hypotonic solutions include 0.45% sodium chloride (half-strength saline), 0.33% sodium chloride, and 2.5% dextrose in water.

Hypotonic solutions hydrate cells and can deplete the circulatory system. Water moves from the vascular space to the intracellular space when hypotonic fluids are infused (Crawford & Harris, 2011; Smeltzer, Bare, Hinkle, & Cheever, 2010).

Caution: Do not give hypotonic solutions to patients with low blood pressure because it will further a hypotensive state.

Hypertonic Fluids

Hypertonic fluids have an osmolarity of 375 mOsm/L or higher. The resulting osmotic pressure gradient draws water from the intracellular space, increasing extracellular volume and causing cells to shrink. Examples of hypertonic fluids include 5% dextrose in 0.45% sodium chloride, 5% dextrose in 0.9% sodium chloride, 5% dextrose in lactated Ringer's, 10% dextrose in water, and **colloids** (albumin 25%, plasma protein fraction, dextran, and hetastarch).

These fluids are used to replace electrolytes, to treat hypotonic dehydration, and for temporary treatment of circulatory insufficiency and shock. When hypertonic dextrose solutions are used alone, they also are used to shift ECF from the interstitial fluid to the plasma (Crawford & Harris, 2011; Smeltzer, Bare, Hinkle, & Cheever, 2010).

Caution: Hypertonic solutions are irritating to vein walls and may cause hypertonic circulatory overload. Some hypertonic solutions are contraindicated in patients with cardiac or renal disease because of the increased risk for congestive heart failure and pulmonary edema. Give hypertonic solutions slowly to prevent circulatory overload.

▪ Types of Parenteral Solutions

Crystalloid Solutions

Crystalloids are materials capable of crystallization (i.e., have the ability to form crystals). Crystalloids are solutes that, when placed in a solution, mix with and dissolve into a solution and cannot be distinguished from the resultant solution. Because of this, crystalloid solutions are considered true solutions that are capable of diffusing through membranes. The vascular fluid is 25% of the ECF, and 25% of any crystalloid administered remains in the vascular space. Crystalloids must be given in three to four times the volume to expand the vascular space to a degree equal to that brought about by a colloid solution. Types of crystalloid solutions include dextrose solutions, sodium chloride solutions, balanced electrolyte solutions, and alkalizing and acidifying solutions (Crawford & Harris, 2011).

Crystalloid Physiological Initial and Therapeutic Responses

INITIAL RESPONSE EFFECT ON THE VEIN INTIMA AND RED BLOOD CELLS

Crystalloid administration can be divided into two phases: the initial response and the therapeutic response. The initial response is the immediate reaction that occurs when the I.V. solution is introduced into the circulation (Cook, 2003). As the solution enters the bloodstream, it comes into immediate contact with red blood cells (RBCs) and the cells of the vein intima. The initial response of crystalloid therapy to the vein intima may be dramatic but is not life threatening. The intima, at the point of fluid injection, will be repeatedly subjected to the fluid. Hypotonic and hypertonic solutions change the immediate surroundings of the cell. Isotonic solutions do not alter the tonicity of the ECF; therefore, the RBCs are not initially affected (Cook, 2003).

Hypotonic fluids will cause the endothelial cells to swell as they absorb water; hypertonic solutions will draw fluid from the endothelial cells. The rate of swelling and the risk of lysis increase as the tonicity of the fluid decreases. The cells will return to their normal shape as they move into a more isotonic environment (Hill & Petrucci, 2004).

Hypertonic solutions draw fluid from the endothelial cells, causing shrinkage of the RBCs. The risk of cellular dehydration increases as the tonicity of fluid increases. As red cells move toward a more isotonic environment, they regain their original shape (Hill & Petrucci, 2004). The administration of hypertonic saline or dextrose preparations greater than 10% through small veins is associated with phlebitis as a result of this cellular dehydration (Cook, 2003).

THERAPEUTIC RESPONSE/SYSTEMIC EFFECTS

The therapeutic response of crystalloid administration occurs as the fluid disperses through the ECF and ICF. The therapeutic response is predictable and is the reason for the choice of one fluid over another. The therapeutic response to isotonic solutions administered by the intravenous route is the tonicity of the plasma remains unchanged. The 0.9% sodium chloride and lactated Ringer's solutions remain isotonic even after they disperse into the interstitial spaces; therefore, the tonicity of the interstitial space is unchanged. The interstitial space is three times as large as the intravascular space; 75% of the fluid will be dispersed interstitially and 25% will remain in the plasma.

The solution of 5% dextrose in water is considered isotonic in the initial response, but the mechanics are different than with isotonic electrolyte solutions. Dextrose in water is an electrolyte-free solution. As the fluid disperses throughout the ECF, the dextrose is absorbed into the cells to be used for energy. What is left is free water that dilutes the osmolality of the ECF (Porth & Matfin, 2010). The cells are suddenly suspended in a hypotonic environment and osmosis will occur, with the cells absorbing the fluid until the two compartments are isotonic. The intracellular compartment is two-thirds the size of the ECF; 67% of the water will enter the cells and 33% will remain in the ECF. The dispersion of 1 L (1000 mL) of 5% dextrose in water will be 667 mL intracellularly, approximately 250 mL into the interstitial space, and 83 mL into plasma.

Many crystalloid solutions are made up of a combination of dextrose and electrolyte solutions, most of which are hypertonic initially. The therapeutic response to these fluids can be predicted based on the tonicity of the solution. Once the cells use the dextrose, the remaining sodium chloride and electrolytes will be dispersed as isotonic electrolyte solution, hydrating only the ECF. The dispersion of the solution to ECF and ICF will be dependent on the osmolarity of the solution. Remember that 5% dextrose when added to other solutions rapidly is absorbed into the cells to be used for energy. The remaining electrolyte solution is dispersed between the ECF and ICF. The only true hypertonic crystalloid solutions are 3% and 5% sodium chloride. These remain consistently hypertonic and can cause severe cellular dehydration.

Dextrose Solutions

Carbohydrates can be administered by the parenteral route as dextrose, fructose, or invert sugar. Dextrose is the most commonly administered carbohydrate. The percentage solutions express the number of grams of solute per 100 g of solvent. Thus, a 5% dextrose in water (D5W) infusion contains 5 g of dextrose in 100 mL of water.

 NURSING FAST FACT!

One mL of water weighs 1 g, and 1 mL is 1% of 100 mL. Milliliters, grams, and percentages can be used interchangeably when calculating solution strength. Thus, 5% dextrose in water equals 5 g of dextrose in 100 mL, and 1 L of 5% dextrose in water contains 50 g of dextrose. (Example: 250 mL of 20% dextrose in water solution contains 50 g of dextrose.)

When carbohydrate needs are inadequate, the body will use its own fat to supply calories. Dextrose fluids are used to provide calories for energy, reduce catabolism of protein, and reduce protein breakdown of glucose to help prevent a negative nitrogen balance.

The monohydrate form of dextrose used in parenteral solutions provides 3.4 kcal/g. It is difficult to administer enough calories by I.V. infusion, especially with 5% dextrose in water, which provides only 170 calories per liter. One would have to administer 9 L to meet calorie requirements, and most patients cannot tolerate 9000 mL of fluid in 24 hours. Concentrated solutions of carbohydrates in 20% to 70% dextrose are useful for supplying calories. These solutions, which contain high percentages of dextrose, must be administered slowly for adequate absorption and utilization by the cells.

Dextrose is a nonelectrolyte, and the total number of particles in a dextrose solution does not depend on ionization. Dextrose is thought to be the closest to the ideal carbohydrate available because it is well metabolized by all tissues. The tonicity of dextrose solutions depends on the particles of sugar in the solution. Dextrose 5% is rapidly metabolized and has no osmotically active particles after it is in the plasma. The osmolarity of a dextrose solution is determined differently from that of an electrolyte solution. Dextrose is distributed inside and outside the cells, with 8% remaining in the circulation to increase blood volume. The USP pH requirements for dextrose is 3.5 to 6.5 (Gahart & Nazareno, 2012).

Dextrose in water is available in various concentrations, including 2.5% (25 g/L), 5% (50 g/L), 10% (100 g/L), 20% (200 g/L) 30% (300 g/L), 38.5% (385 g/L), 40% (400 g/L), 50% (500 g/L), 60% (600 g/L), and 70% (700 g/L). Dextrose is also available in combination with other types of solutions. The 5% and 10% concentrations can be given peripherally. Concentrations higher than 10% are given through central veins. A general exception is the administration of limited amounts of 50% dextrose given slowly through a peripheral vein for emergency treatment of hypoglycemia (usually 3 mL/min) (Gahart & Nazareno, 2012).

Advantages

- Acts as a vehicle for administration of medications
- Provides nutrition
- Can be used for treatment of hyperkalemia (using high concentrations of dextrose)
- Can be used for treatment of patients with dehydration
- Provides free water

Disadvantages

- The main disadvantage of dextrose solutions intravenously is vein irritation, which is caused by the slightly acidic pH of the solution. Vein irritation, vein damage, and thrombosis may result when hypertonic dextrose solutions are administered in a peripheral vein.
- Hyponatremic encephalopathy can develop rapidly in postoperative patients who receive excessive infusion of 5% dextrose in water. Postoperative hyponatremia can affect any patient but is much more serious in women of childbearing age. Premenopausal women who develop hyponatremic encephalopathy are 25 times more likely to have permanent brain damage or to die compared to men (Ayus, Achinger, & Arieff, 2008).

EBP Siegel (2007) discusses research presented on the treatment of acute onset of hyponatremia with a sodium concentration <135 mEq/L with 3% sodium chloride for emergency treatment of moderate and life-threatening symptoms.

- Solutions of 20% to 70% dextrose, when infused rapidly, act as an osmotic diuretic and can pull interstitial fluid into plasma, causing severe cellular dehydration. Any solution of dextrose infused rapidly can place the patient at risk for dehydration. To prevent this adverse reaction, infuse the dextrose solution at the prescribed rate.
- Rapid infusion of 20% to 70% dextrose can also lead to transient hyperinsulinism reaction, in which the pancreas secretes extra insulin to metabolize the infused dextrose. Sudden discontinuation of any hypertonic dextrose solution may leave a temporary excess of insulin. To prevent hyperinsulinism, infuse an isotonic dextrose solution (5%–10%) to wean the patient off hypertonic dextrose. The infusion rate should be gradually decreased over 48 hours. When administering dextrose solutions, remember that they do not provide any electrolytes.
- Dextrose solutions cannot replace or correct electrolyte deficits, and continuous infusion of 5% dextrose in water places patients at risk for deficits in sodium, potassium, and chloride.

■ Dextrose cannot be mixed with blood components because it causes hemolysis (pseudoagglutination; i.e., agglomeration) of the cells.

NOTE > Before adding any medication to a dextrose solution, check the compatibility information. Dextrose may also affect the stability of admixtures.

EBP: Use of 3% Sodium Chloride to Treat Hypotonic Encephalopathy: An evidence-based consensus statement concluded that both excessive fluid consumption and decreased urine formation contribute to a dilutional effect in hyponatremia that can lead to life-threatening and fatal cases of pulmonary and cerebral edema. Strategies for prevention and treatment include intravenous hypertonic solutions, such as 3% sodium chloride, to reverse the symptoms related to moderate and life-threatening hypotonic encephalopathy. Further studies are needed to investigate dilutional hyponatremia (Hew-Butler et al., 2005).

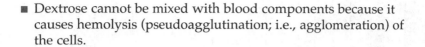 *NURSING FAST FACTS!*

• *Do not play "catch up" if the solution infusion is behind schedule. Make sure the I.V. solution does not "run away" and that it does not infuse rapidly into the patient.*
• *All dextrose solutions are acidic (pH 3.5–5.0) and may cause thrombophlebitis. Assess the I.V. site frequently.*

EBP A study by van Wissen and Breton (2004) concluded that intraoperative fluid replacement should not contain glucose because plasma cortisol increases during surgery, which in turn causes hyperglycemia.

Table 4-1 provides a summary of dextrose solution osmolarity, pH, and electrolyte content. Table 4-2 lists indications and precautions.

Sodium Chloride Solutions

Sodium chloride solutions are available as hypotonic—0.25% (1/4 NS) and 0.45% (1/2 NS); isotonic—0.9% (NS) and bacteriostatic isotonic NS, which contains benzyl alcohol as a preservative; and hypertonic—3% and 5% concentrations. Sodium chloride 0.9% solution, often referred to as **normal saline**, has 154 mEq of both sodium and chloride, which is about 9% higher than normal plasma levels of sodium and chloride ions

Text continued on page 218

> Table 4-1   CONTENTS OF AVAILABLE INTRAVENOUS FLUIDS

Solution	Osmolarity	Dextrose, g/100 mL	pH	Cal/100 mL	Na	Cl	K	Ca	Mg	Acetate	Lactate
Dextrose in Water (D/W)											
5% D/W	Isotonic—252	5	4.8	17							
10% D/W	Hypertonic—505	10	4.7	34							
20% D/W	Hypertonic—1010	20	4.8	68							
50% D/W	Hypertonic—2526	50	4.6	170							
70% D/W	Hypertonic—3532	70	4.6	237							
Sodium Chloride (NaCl)											
0.225% NaCl (1/4 strength)	Hypotonic—77		4.5		34	34					
0.33% NaCl	Hypotonic—115		4.5		51	51					
0.45% NaCl (1/2 strength)	Hypotonic—154		5.6		77	77					
0.9% NaCl (full strength)	Isotonic—308		6.0		154	154					
3% NaCl	Hypertonic—1027		6.0		513	513					
5% NaCl	Hypertonic—1711		6.0		855	855					
0.25% D and 0.9% NaCl	Isotonic—321	2.5	4.5	8	154	154					
Dextrose and Sodium Chloride (D/NaCl)											
5% D and 0.225% NaCl	Isotonic—321	5	4.6	17	34	34					
5% D and 0.45% NaCl	Hypertonic—406	5	4.6	17	77	77					
5% D and 0.9% NaCl	Hypertonic—560	5	4.4	17	154	154					

Balanced Electrolyte Solutions

Solution	pH	Tonicity—mOsm/L	Na	Cl	K	Ca	Mg	Cal	Anion
Lactated Ringer's solution	6.5	Isotonic—273	130	109	4	3			28
Ringer's injection	5.5	Isotonic—309	147	156	4	4			
Normosol-R*	7.4	Isotonic—295	140	98	5		3		27
D5 and Normosol-M*	5.0	Isotonic—363	40	98	40		3	17	16
Specialty Solutions									
1/6 M Sodium	6.5	Isotonic—335 lactate	167						167
10% Mannitol	5.7	Hypertonic—549							
20% Mannitol	5.7	Hypertonic—1098							
NaHCO$_3$	8.0	Isotonic—333	595						595

Ca = calcium; Cal = calories; Cl = chloride; K = potassium; Mg = magnesium; Na = sodium; NaCl = sodium chloride.
*Hospira Pharmaceuticals.

> Table 4-2   **QUICK-GLANCE CHART OF COMMON I.V. FLUIDS**

Solutions	Indications	Precautions
Dextrose Solutions		
5% Dextrose 10% Dextrose 20% Dextrose 50% Dextrose 70% Dextrose	Spares body protein. Provides nutrition. Provides calories. Provides free water. Acts as a diluent for I.V. drugs. Treats dehydration. Treats hyperkalemia.	Possible compromise of glucose tolerance by stress, sepsis, hepatic and renal failure, corticosteroids, and diuretics. **Does not provide any electrolytes.** **May cause vein irritation.** Possible agglomeration of red blood cells. **Use cautiously in the early postoperative period to prevent water intoxication** Antidiuretic hormone (ADH) secretions as a stress response to surgery. Use with caution in patients with known subclinical or overt diabetes mellitus. Hypertonic fluids may cause hyperglycemia, osmotic diuresis, hyperosmolar coma, or hyperinsulinism.
Sodium Chloride (NaCl) Solutions		
0.225% NaCl 0.45% NaCl 0.9% NaCl 3% NaCl 5% NaCl	Replaces extracellular fluid (ECF) and electrolytes. Replaces sodium and chloride. Treats hyperosmolar diabetes. Acts as diluent for I.V. drug administration. Used for initiation and discontinuation of blood products. Replaces severe sodium and chloride deficit. Helps to correct water overload. Acts as an irrigant for intravascular devices.	**Fluid and/or solute overload, with potential congested states or pulmonary edema** Calorie depletion Hypernatremia or hyperchloremia Deficit of other electrolytes Can induce hyperchloremic acidosis because of a loss of bicarbonate ions. Does not provide free water or calories. **Use with caution in older adults.**
Combination Dextrose and Sodium Chloride Solutions		
5D/0.225% NaCl (hydration solution) 5D/0.45% NaCl (hydration solution) 5D/0.9% NaCl	Assesses renal function. Hydrates cells. Promotes diuresis. For temporary treatment of circulatory insufficiency hydrating fluids. Replaces nutrients and electrolytes. Supplies some calories. Reduces nitrogen depletion. Used in place of plasma expanders.	**Use with caution in patients with edema and those with cardiac, renal, or liver disease.** Do not use in patients in diabetic coma. Do not use in patients who are allergic to corn.

> Table 4-2 | QUICK-GLANCE CHART OF COMMON I.V. FLUIDS—cont'd

Solutions	Indications	Precautions
Balanced Electrolyte Solutions		
Normosol-M and dextrose 5% Balanced maintenance solution	Parenteral maintenance of routine fluid and electrolyte requirements with minimal carbohydrate calories. Magnesium helps prevent iatrogenic Mg^{2+} deficiency. Provides free water, calories, and electrolytes. Provides routine maintenance. Relieves physiological stress leading to inappropriate release or ADH.	**Fluid or solute overload, overhydration with congested states, or pulmonary edema** Dilution of serum electrolyte concentrations Use with care in patients with congestive heart failure and severe renal insufficiency. Solutions with dextrose should be used with caution in patient with known subclinical or overt diabetes mellitus.
Normosol-R Balanced solution for replacement of acute losses of ECF in surgery, trauma, burns, or shock	Provides calories and electrolytes. Provides fluid and electrolyte replacement. Provides calories. Spares protein. Replaces ECF losses and electrolytes. Sodium acetate provides an alternate source of bicarbonate by metabolic conversion in the liver.	Use with care in patients with congestive heart failure, with severe renal insufficiency, or in clinical states of sodium retention. Hyperkalemia Use with caution in patients with metabolic or respiratory alkalosis. **Fluid or solute overloading, overhydration, and congested states or pulmonary edema** *Elderly have increased risk of developing fluid overload and dilutional hyponatremia.*
5% D in Ringer's injection	Provides calories Spares body protein Replaces ECF losses and electrolytes Composition similar to plasma	Contraindicated in patients with renal failure Use with caution in patients with congestive heart failure Tolerated well by patients with hepatic disease.
5% Dextrose and lactated Ringer's solutions (ionic composition similar to plasma)	Treats mild metabolic acidosis Replaces fluid losses from burns and trauma Contains bicarbonate precursor Replaces fluid losses from alimentary tract Rehydrates in all types of dehydration Ionic composition similar to plasma	Contraindicated in patients with lactic acidosis Circulatory overload May cause metabolic acidosis Hypernatremia Fluid overload Contraindicated in patients with renal failure Use with caution in patients with congestive heart failure Composition similar to plasma Tolerated well by patients with hepatic disease Contraindicated in patients with lactic acidosis Circulatory overload May cause metabolic acidosis Ionic composition similar to plasma Contains bicarbonate precursor

Bold type indicates the most common precaution or risk.

without other plasma electrolytes. Sodium chloride has a pH of 4.5 to 7 (Gahart & Nazareno, 2012).

There are many clinical uses of sodium chloride solutions, including treatment of shock and of hyponatremia, use with blood transfusions, resuscitation in trauma situations, fluid challenges, metabolic alkalosis hypercalcemia, and fluid replacement in diabetic ketoacidosis. Sodium chloride solutions should be used cautiously in patients with congestive heart failure, edema, or hypernatremia because it replaces ECF and can lead to fluid overload.

ADVANTAGES

- Provides ECF replacement when chloride loss is greater than or equal to sodium losses (e.g., a patient undergoing nasogastric suctioning)
- Treats patients with metabolic alkalosis in the presence of fluid loss (the 154 mEq of chloride helps compensate for the increase in bicarbonate ions)
- Treats patients with sodium depletion
- Initiates or terminates a blood transfusion (the saline solutions are the only solutions to be used with any blood product [Gahart & Nazareno, 2012])

DISADVANTAGES

- Provides more sodium and chloride than patients need, causing hypernatremia. The adult dietary sodium requirements are 90 to 250 mEq daily. Three liters of sodium chloride (0.9%) provides a patient with 462 mEq of sodium, a level that exceeds normal tolerance. To prevent this overload of electrolytes, assess for signs and symptoms of sodium retention.
- Can cause acidosis in patients receiving continuous infusions of 0.9% sodium chloride because sodium chloride provides one-third more chloride than is present in ECF. The excess chloride leads to loss of bicarbonate ions, leading to an imbalance of acid.
- May cause low potassium levels (i.e., hypokalemia) because of the lack of other important electrolytes over a period of time.
- Can lead to circulatory overload. Isotonic fluids expand the ECF compartment, which can lead to overload of the cardiovascular compartments.

 NURSING FAST FACT!

> *During stress, the body retains sodium, adding to hypernatremia.*

Hypotonic saline (0.45%) can be used to supply normal daily salt and water requirements safely. Hypertonic saline solution (3%–5%) is used only to correct severe sodium depletion and water overload.

Hyperosmolar saline (3% or 5% NaCl) can be dangerous when administered incorrectly. Nurses should follow these steps to ensure safe administration of hyperosmolar sodium chloride (3% and 5%).
- Check serum sodium level before and during administration.
- Administer only in intensive care settings.
- Monitor aggressively for signs of pulmonary edema.
- Administer only small volumes of hyperosmolar fluids.
- Use a volume-controlled device or electronic infusion pump.

Table 4-1 provides a summary of sodium chloride solution osmolarity, pH, and electrolyte content. Table 4-2 lists indications and precautions.

Dextrose Combined with Sodium Chloride

When sodium chloride is infused, the addition of 100 g of dextrose prevents the formation of ketone bodies. Dextrose prevents catabolism, which is the breakdown of chemical compounds by the body. Consequently, there is a loss of potassium and intracellular water.

Carbohydrates and sodium chloride fluid combinations are best used in cases of excessive loss of fluid through sweating, vomiting, or gastric suctioning. Table 4-1 provides a summary of available dextrose and sodium chloride solution osmolarity, pH, and electrolyte content. Table 4-2 lists indications and precautions.

ADVANTAGES

- Temporarily treats patients with circulatory insufficiency and shock caused by hypovolemia in the immediate absence of a plasma expander
- Provides early treatment of burns, along with plasma or albumin
- Replaces nutrients and electrolytes
- Acts as a **hydrating solution** to assist in checking renal function before replacement of potassium

DISADVANTAGE

- Same as for sodium chloride solutions (see previous section): hypernatremia, acidosis, and circulatory overload

Hydrating Solutions (Combinations of Dextrose and Hypotonic Sodium Chloride)

Solutions that contain dextrose and hypotonic saline provide more water than is required for excretion of salt and are useful as hydrating fluids. Hydrating fluids are used to assess the status of the kidneys. The administration of a hydrating solution at a rate of 8 mL/m^2 of body surface per minute for 45 minutes is called a fluid challenge. When urinary flow is established, it indicates that the kidneys have begun to function; the hydrating solution may then be replaced with a specific electrolyte solution. If urinary flow is not restored after 45 minutes, the rate of infusion should be reduced and monitoring of the patient should continue without administration of electrolyte additives, especially potassium. Carbohydrates in hydrating solutions reduce the depletion of nitrogen and liver glycogen and are also useful in rehydrating cells.

Hydrating solutions are potassium free. Potassium is essential to the body but can be toxic if the kidneys are not functioning effectively and therefore are unable to excrete the extra potassium. Table 4-1 provides a summary of the types of hydrating fluids.

Combination solutions can be used by hypodermoclysis or subcutaneous route for hydration in clients with poor venous access. The use of 5% dextrose in 0.45% sodium chloride for rehydration using hypodermoclysis or subcutaneous infusion was found in two randomized controlled studies to be comparably safe and effective as intravenous delivery of the solutions for rehydration in this client population.

ADVANTAGES

- Help assess the status of the kidneys before replacement therapy is started
- Hydrate patients in dehydrated states
- Promote diuresis in dehydrated patients

DISADVANTAGE

- Require cautious administration in edematous patients (e.g., patients with cardiac, renal, or hepatic disease).

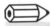 *NURSING FAST FACT!*

> *Do not give potassium to any patient unless renal function has been established. Use hydrating fluid to check renal function.*

Balanced Electrolyte Solutions

A variety of balanced electrolyte fluids are available commercially. Balanced fluids are available as hypotonic or isotonic maintenance and replacement solutions. Maintenance fluids approximate normal body electrolyte needs; replacement fluids contain one or more electrolytes in amounts higher than those found in normal body fluids. Balanced fluids also may contain lactate or acetate (yielding bicarbonate), which helps to combat acidosis and provides a truly "**balanced solution.**"

Table 4-1 provides a summary of balanced electrolyte solution osmolarity, pH, and electrolyte content. Table 4-2 lists indications and precautions.

NURSING FAST FACTS!

- *Multiple electrolyte fluids are recommended for use in patients with trauma, alimentary tract fluid losses, dehydration, sodium depletion, acidosis, and burns.*
- *Do not use gastric replacement fluid in patients with hepatic insufficiency or renal failure.*

Many types of balanced electrolyte replacement fluids are available. Special fluids available from manufacturers for gastric replacement provide the typical electrolytes lost by vomiting or gastric suction. These isotonic fluids usually contain ammonium ions, which are metabolized in the liver to hydrogen ions and urea, replacing hydrogen ions lost in gastric juices. Lactated Ringer's injection is considered an isotonic multiple electrolyte solution.

Hypertonic multiple electrolyte solutions are also used as replacement fluids. Usually 5% dextrose has been added, which raises the osmolarity of the solution.

Ringer's Solution and Lactated Ringer's

The Ringer's solutions (i.e., Ringer's injection and lactated Ringer's injection) are classified as balanced or isotonic solutions because their fluid and electrolyte contents are similar to those of plasma. They are used to replace electrolytes at physiological levels in the ECF compartment.

RINGER'S SOLUTION (INJECTION)

Ringer's injection is a fluid and electrolyte replenisher, which is used rather than 0.9% sodium chloride for treating patients with dehydration after reduced water intake or water loss. Ringer's solution (injection) is similar to normal saline (i.e., 0.9% sodium chloride) with the substitution of potassium and calcium for some of the sodium ions in concentrations equal to those in the plasma. However, Ringer's injection is superior to 0.9% sodium chloride as a fluid and electrolyte replenisher, and it is preferred to normal saline for treating patients with dehydration after drastically reduced water intake or water loss (e.g., with vomiting, diarrhea, or fistula drainage). This solution has some incompatibilities with medications, so it is necessary to check drug compatibility literature for guidelines.

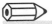 *NURSING FAST FACT!*

Ringer's injection does not contain enough potassium or calcium to be used as a maintenance fluid or to correct a deficit of these electrolytes.

Ringer's injection is used for the following:
■ Treatment of any type of dehydration
■ Restoration of fluid balance before and after surgery
■ Replacement of fluids resulting from dehydration, GI losses, and fistula drainage

Use this solution instead of lactated Ringer's when the patient has hepatic disease and is unable to metabolize lactate.

ADVANTAGES

■ Tolerated well in patients who have hepatic disease
■ May be used as blood replacement for a short period of time

DISADVANTAGES

■ Provides no calories
■ May exacerbate sodium retention, congestive heart failure, and renal insufficiency
■ Contraindicated in renal failure

LACTATED RINGER'S SOLUTION

This solution is also called Hartmann's solution. Lactated Ringer's is the most commonly prescribed solution, with an electrolyte concentration closely resembling that of the ECF compartment. This solution is commonly used to replace fluid loss resulting from burns, bile, and diarrhea.

Lactated Ringer's is used for the following:
■ Rehydration in all types of dehydration
■ Restoration of fluid volume deficits
■ Replacement of fluid lost as a result of burns
■ Treatment of mild metabolic acidosis
■ Treatment of salicylate overdose

 NURSING FAST FACT!

Lactated Ringer's solution has some incompatibilities with medications, so it is necessary to check drug compatibility literature for guidelines.

ADVANTAGES

■ Contains the bicarbonate precursor to assist in acidosis
■ Most similar to body's extracellular electrolyte content

DISADVANTAGES

■ Three liters of lactated Ringer's solution contains about 390 mEq of sodium, which can quickly elevate the sodium level in a patient who does not have a sodium deficit.
■ Lactated Ringer's solution should not be used in patients with impaired lactate metabolism, such as those with hepatic disease,

Addison's disease, severe metabolic acidosis or alkalosis, profound hypovolemia, or profound shock or cardiac failure.
■ In the above conditions, serum lactate levels may already be elevated.

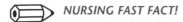 *NURSING FAST FACT!*

At present, isotonic sodium chloride is recommended as the first-line fluid in resuscitation of hypovolemic trauma patients (Bulger & Maier, 2007).

Alkalizing and Acidifying Infusion Fluids

ALKALIZING FLUIDS

Metabolic acidosis can occur in clinical situations in which dehydration, shock, hepatic disease, starvation, or diabetes causes retention of chlorides, ketone bodies, or organic salts or when too large an amount of bicarbonate is lost. Treatment consists of infusion of an alkalizing fluid. Two I.V. fluids are available when excessive bicarbonate losses and metabolic acidosis occur: 1/6 molar isotonic sodium lactate and 5% sodium bicarbonate injection. The lactate ion must be oxidized to carbon dioxide in the body before it can affect the acid–base balance. Sodium lactate to bicarbonate requires 1 to 2 hours. Oxygen is needed to increase bicarbonate concentrations. The isotonic solution sodium bicarbonate injection provides bicarbonate ions in clinical situations of excessive bicarbonate losses.

Alkalizing fluids are used in treating vomiting, starvation, uncontrolled diabetes mellitus, acute infections, renal failure, and severe acidosis with severe hyperpnea (sodium bicarbonate injection).

The 1/6 molar sodium lactate solution is useful whenever acidosis has resulted from sodium deficiency; however, it is contraindicated in patients suffering from lack of oxygen and in those with hepatic disease. Patients receiving this fluid should be watched for signs of hypocalcemic tetany.

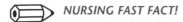 *NURSING FAST FACT!*

Sodium bicarbonate injection is used to relieve dyspnea and hyperpnea. The bicarbonate ion is released in the form of carbon dioxide through the lungs, leaving behind an excess of sodium.

ACIDIFYING FLUIDS

Metabolic alkalosis is a condition associated with an excess of bicarbonate and deficit of chloride. Isotonic sodium chloride (0.9%) provides conservative treatment of metabolic alkalosis. Ammonium chloride is the solution used to treat metabolic alkalosis. Acidifying fluids are used for severe metabolic alkalosis caused by a loss of gastric secretions or pyloric stenosis.

An advantage is that the ammonium ion is converted by the liver to hydrogen ion and to ammonia, which is excreted as urea. However, a disadvantage is that ammonium chloride must be infused at a slow rate to enable the liver to metabolize the ammonium ion. In fact, rapid infusion can result in toxicity, causing irregular breathing and bradycardia.

 NURSING FAST FACT!

> *Ammonium chloride must be used with caution in patients with severe hepatic disease or renal failure and is contraindicated in any condition in which a high ammonium level is present.*

NURSING POINTS OF CARE
CRYSTALLOID ADMINISTRATION

Nursing Assessments
- Obtain history of present illness of fluid loss.
- Observe ability to ingest and retain fluids.
- Obtain vital signs.
- Obtain weight.
- Perform initial physical assessment for signs and symptoms of fluid imbalance.
- Review licensed independent practitioner (LIP) order for accuracy and match the solution to the order.

Nursing Management
1. Administer I.V. fluids at room temperature.
2. Administer I.V. medications at prescribed rate and monitor for results.
3. Use open containers immediately.
4. Monitor I.V. site during infusion.
5. Monitor for
   a. signs and symptoms of fluid overload
   b. urine output and specific gravity
   c. trending of pertinent laboratory test results (electrolytes, prothrombin time [PT], partial thromboplastin time [PTT], serum amylase)
   d. complications associated with infusion therapy (phlebitis, erratic flow rates, infiltration)
6. Monitor for I.V. patency before administering I.V. medications.
7. Follow Infusion Nurses Society standards of practice for vascular access device removal (INS, 2011, p. 44).

8. Replace fluid containers according to established organizational policies, procedures, and/or current practice guidelines.
9. Flush vascular access devices prior to each infusion as part of the steps to assess catheter function and after each infusion to clear the infused medication from the catheter lumen to prevent contact between incompatible medications. Follow flushing and locking guidelines (INS, 2011, p. 45). Record I&O.
10. Provide information outlining current I.V. therapy.
11. Maintain standard precautions.

Colloid Solutions

Patients with fluid and electrolyte disturbances occasionally require treatment with colloids. Colloid solutions contain protein or starch molecules that remain distributed in the extracellular space and do not form a "true" solution. Colloid solutions are referred to as **plasma volume expanders**. When colloid molecules are administered, they remain in the vascular space for several days in patients with normal capillary endothelia. These fluids increase the osmotic pressure within the plasma space, drawing fluid to increase intravascular volume. Colloid solutions do not dissolve and do not flow freely between fluid compartments. Infusion of a colloid solution increases intravascular colloid osmotic pressure (pressure of plasma proteins). The most common colloid volume expanders are dextran, albumin, hetastarch, mannitol, and gelatin.

Ideal colloid solutions have the following advantages:

■ Distributed to intravascular compartment only
■ Readily available
■ Long shelf life
■ Inexpensive
■ No special storage or infusion requirements
■ No special limitations on volume that can be infused
■ No interference with blood grouping or crossmatching
■ Acceptable to all patients and no religious objections

Albumin

Albumin is a natural plasma protein prepared from donor plasma. Albumin is the predominant plasma protein and remains the standard against which other colloids are compared. Colloid osmotic pressure is influenced by proteins. The concentration of protein in plasma is two to three times greater than that of proteins found in the interstitial fluid (i.e., plasma 7.3 g/dL; interstitial fluid 2–3 g/dL) (Hankins, 2006). This colloid is available as a 5%, 20%, or 25% solution. The 5% percent albumin solution is osmotically and oncotically equivalent to plasma. The 5% solution usually is indicated in hypovolemic patients and cardiopulmonary bypass. The initial dose is

5%, which is available in 50-mL, 250-mL, 500-mL, and 1000-mL containers, 12.5 to 25 g. The 5% solution is isotonic.

The 25% solution is equivalent to 500 mL of plasma or two units of whole blood. It is indicated for patients whose fluid and sodium intake should be minimized. The 25% solution (25 g/100 mL) is available in 20-mL, 50-mL, and 100-mL vials. The 20% solution is available in 100-mL vials from one manufacturer. The 25% solution is used in hypoproteinemia, hypovolemia and burns, acute nephrosis, hemodialysis, RBC resuspension, and cardiopulmonary bypass (Gahart & Nazareno, 2012). The 20% and 25% solutions are hypertonic. In well-hydrated patients, each volume of the 25% solution draws about 300 to 500 mL in intravascular volume for every 100 mL infused (Hankins, 2006).

NOTE > These products are subject to an extended heating period during preparation and therefore do not transmit viral disease.

ADVANTAGES

- Free of danger of serum hepatitis
- Expands blood volume proportionately to amount of circulating blood
- Improves cardiac output
- Prevents marked hemoconcentration
- Aids in reduction of edema; raises serum protein levels
- Maintains electrolyte balance and promote diuresis in presence of edema
- Acts as a transport protein that binds both endogenous and exogenous substances, including bilirubin and certain drugs

DISADVANTAGES

- May precipitate allergic reactions (e.g., urticaria, flushing, chills, fever, headache)
- May cause circulatory overload (greatest risk with 25% albumin)
- May cause pulmonary edema
- May alter laboratory findings

EBP In 2004, a prospective, multicenter, double-blind controlled trial published in the New England Journal of Medicine looked at albumin versus saline in critically ill patients (Finfer, Bellomo & Boyce, et al., 2004). One of the largest prospective clinical studies to date, the SAFE (Saline versus Albumin Fluid Evaluation) trial randomized a heterogeneous group of 7000 critically ill patients requiring fluid resuscitation to receive iso-oncotic albumin or isotonic crystalloid. Overall, 28-day mortality was 21% and did not differ according to treatment assignment.

Table 4-3 provides a summary of albumin osmolarity, expansion, and side effects.

Dextran

Dextran fluids are polysaccharides that behave as colloids, which are plasma volume expanders. They are available as low molecular weight dextran (dextran 40) and high molecular weight dextran (dextran 70). Low molecular weight dextran (Dextran 40) is a rapid but short-acting plasma volume expander. It increases plasma volume by once or twice its own volume. It improves microcirculatory flow and prevents sludging in venous channels. It mobilizes water from body tissues and increases urinary output. The initial 500 mL may be given rapidly. The remainder of any desired daily dose should be evenly distributed over 8 to 24 hours (Gahart & Nazareno, 2012).

High molecular weight dextran 70 approximates colloidal properties of human albumin. It dilutes total serum proteins and hematocrit values. It is used as adjunct treatment of impending shock or shock states related to burns, hemorrhage, surgery, or trauma (AHFS, 2013). The rate of administration is variable depending on indication, present blood volume, and patient response. The initial 500 mL may be given at a rate of 20 to 40 mL/min if the

> Table 4-3   **COMMON COLLOID VOLUME EXPANDERS**

Solution	Molecular Wt.	Osmolality	Max Volume* Expansion (%)	Duration of Expansion	Side Effects
Albumin 4%, 5%	69	290	70–100	12–24 hours	Allergic reactions
Albumin 20%, 25%	69	310	300–500	12–24 hours	Allergic reactions
Starches Hetastarch 3%, 6%, 10%	450	300–310	100–200	8–36 hours	Renal dysfunction
Starches Pentastarch 10%	280	326	100–200	12–24 hours	Renal dysfunction
Dextrans % 10% Dextran-40	40	280–324	100–200	1–2 hours	Anaphylactoid reactions
3% Dextran–60 6% Dextran–70	70	280–324	80–140	<8–24 hours	Anaphylactoid reactions
Gelatins Succinylated and cross-linked: 2.5%, 3%, 4% Urea-linked: 3.5%	30–35	300–350	70–80	<4–6 hours	High calcium content (urea-linked forms)

Max volume expansion % is expressed as a percentage of administered volume.
Adapted from Martin & Matthay, 2004.

patient is hypovolemic. If additional high molecular weight dextran is required, the flow rate should be reduced to the lowest possible (Gahart & Nazareno, 2012).

It is important to monitor the patient's pulse, blood pressure, and urine output every 5 to 15 minutes for the first hour of administration of dextran and then every hour after that.

These products are used when blood or blood products are not available. They are not a substitute for whole blood or plasma proteins. Hydration status is important.

ADVANTAGE

■ Intravascular space is expanded in excess of the volume infused.

DISADVANTAGES

■ Possibility of hypersensitivity reactions (i.e., anaphylaxis)
■ Increased risk of bleeding
■ Circulatory overload
■ For I.V. use only

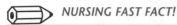 NURSING FAST FACT!

> Dextran is contraindicated in patients with severe bleeding disorders, congestive heart failure, and renal failure. It is important to draw blood for typing and crossmatching before administering dextran.

Table 4-3 provides a summary of dextran osmolarity, expansion, and side effects.

Hydroxyethyl Starches: Hetastarch and Pentastarch

Hetastarch (hydroxyethyl glucose) is a synthetic colloid made from starch and is similar to human albumin. It is available under the name Hespan® as a 6% or 10% solution, diluted in isotonic sodium chloride in a 500-mL container. These starches are not derived from donor plasma and therefore are less toxic and less expensive. Hetastarch is equal in plasma volume expansion properties to 5% human albumin.

Pentastarch is another polydisperse formulation of hydroxyethyl starch with a lower molecular weight. Pentastarch has a greater colloid osmotic pressure than hetastarch. In 2007 the FDA approved Voluven®, a 6% hydroxyethyl starch injection, for the prevention and treatment of dangerously low blood volume (AHFS, 2013).

> EBP In clinical trials of 10% pentastarch with 5% albumin, it was found that pentastarch over 5% albumin may provide greater plasma volume expansion for the volume infused, with faster onset and more rapid elimination than albumin or hetastarch (Brutocao, Bratton, Thomas, et al., 1996).

ADVANTAGES

- Hetastarch and pentastarch do not interfere with blood typing and crossmatching, as do other colloidal solutions.
- Provides hemodynamically significant plasma volume expansion in excess of the amount infused for about 24 hours (Gahart & Nazareno, 2012).
- Permits retention of intravascular fluid until hetastarch is replaced by blood proteins.

DISADVANTAGES

- Possibility of allergic reaction including anaphylaxis
- Anemia and/or bleeding as a result of hemodilution and/or factor VIII deficiency, and other coagulopathies, including disseminated intravascular coagulopathy (DIC).
- Increased intracranial bleeding

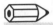 *NURSING FAST FACT!*

Use hetastarch cautiously in patients whose conditions predispose them to fluid retention.

Table 4-3 provides a summary of hydroxyethyl starches, osmolarity expansion, and side effects.

Mannitol

Mannitol is a hexahydroxy alcohol substance that is available in concentrations of 5%, 10%, 15%, 20%, and 25%. It is classified as an osmotic diuretic. This solution is limited to the extracellular space, where it draws fluid from the cells because of its hypertonicity (275–1375 mOsm). Mannitol increases the osmotic pressure of the glomerular filtrate, thereby inhibiting reabsorption of water and electrolytes.

Administration of this solution causes excretion of water, sodium, potassium chloride, calcium, phosphorus, magnesium, urea, and uric acid.

No further dilution of this product is necessary; however, any crystals present in the solution must be completely dissolved before administration (Gahart & Nazareno, 2012).

ADVANTAGES

- Used to promote diuresis in patients with oliguric acute renal failure
- Promote excretion of toxic substances in the body
- Reduce excess cerebrospinal fluid (CSF)
- Reduce intraocular pressure; treats intracranial pressure and cerebral edema
- Can reduce excess CSF within 15 minutes

DISADVANTAGES

- Fluid and electrolyte imbalances are the most common and may be severe.
- May induce dehydration with hyperkalemia, hypokalemia, or hyponatremia.
- The solution is irritating to the vein intima and may cause phlebitis. Extravasation of mannitol may lead to skin irritation and tissue necrosis (Gahart & Nazareno, 2012).
- May interfere with laboratory tests.

NOTE ＞ Mannitol solution requires cautious use in patients with an impaired cardiac or renal system. It is contraindicated in the presence of anuria, severe pulmonary and cardiac congestion, and intracranial bleeding. A test dose may be required for these patients (Gahart & Nazareno, 2012).

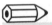 *NURSING FAST FACT!*

The nurse needs to monitor the administration of mannitol for crystal formation. It is recommended that an inline filter be used during administration of 15%, 20%, and 25% solutions.

Gelatins

Gelatin is the name given to the proteins formed when the connective tissue of animals is boiled. It has the property of dissolving in hot water and forming a jelly when cooled. Thus, gelatin is a large molecular weight protein formed from hydrolysis of collagen. Several modified gelatin products are available, and they have been collectively called the new-generation gelatins. Three types of gelatin solutions are currently in use: succinylated or modified fluid gelatins (e.g., Gelofusine®, Plasmagel®, Plasmion®); urea-cross-linked gelatins (e.g., Polygeline®); and oxypolygelatins (e.g., Gelifundol®) (Van der Linden & Hert, 2005). They have no preservatives, and all gelatins have a recommended shelf-life of 3 years when stored at temperatures less than 30°C. Gelatin is rapidly excreted by the kidney following infusion. Gelatins (GEL) have the advantage of their unlimited daily dose recommendation and minimal effect on hemostasis (Grocott, Mythen, & Gan, 2005; van der Linden et al., 2005).

ADVANTAGES

- Used to replace intravascular volume as a result of acute blood loss
- Priming heart–lung machines
- Least effect on hemostasis (Grocott, Mythen, & Gan, 2005)

DISADVANTAGES

- Are associated with anaphylactic reactions; also may cause depression of serum fibronectin
- Urea-linked gelatin has much higher calcium and potassium levels than succinylated gelatin (Kelley, 2005).
- Risks are associated with bovine-derived gelatin because of the association between new-variant Creutzfeldt–Jakob disease and bovine spongiform encephalitis. There are no known cases of transmission involving pharmaceutical gelatin preparations, but awareness of this issue is important (Grocott, Mythen, & Gan, 2005).

Table 4-3 provides a summary of gelatins osmolarity, expansion, and side effects.

NURSING POINTS OF CARE
COLLOID ADMINISTRATION

Nursing Assessments
- Carefully assess for history of allergic responses.
- Assess and record vital signs.
- Assess urinary output for renal function prior to administration.

Key Nursing Interventions
1. Monitor for signs and symptoms of localized allergic reaction.
2. Monitor laboratory test result values (serum protein levels, sodium, serum hemoglobin, and hematocrit).
3. Monitor central venous pressure (CVP) or jugular venous distention when appropriate.
4. Monitor infusion rate frequently.
5. Monitor and record input and output (I&O).
6. Monitor for the need for additional fluid in dehydrated patients.
7. Monitor for signs of fluid overload.
8. Monitor/assess bleeding postinfusion.
9. Auscultate breath sounds for development of crackles.

AGE-RELATED CONSIDERATIONS
The Pediatric Client

Factors Affecting Fluid Needs in Pediatric Clients
The most common cause of increased fluid and calorie needs in children is temperature elevation. A 1-degree increase in temperature increases a child's calorie needs by 12%. Fluid requirements of a child who is hypothermic decrease by 12% (Frey & Pettit, 2010). In children, loss of GI fluids,

Continued

ongoing diarrhea, and small intestinal drainage can seriously affect fluid balance.

 NURSING FAST FACT!

To ensure accuracy in determining fluid needs, most pediatric patients should be on strict I&O monitoring, including diaper weighing. When weighing an infant's diaper, consider the weight of the diaper before it was wet. The weight difference between a dry and a wet piece of linen represents the amount of liquid that it has absorbed. The weight of the fluid measured in grams is the same as the volume measured in milliliters (Hockenberry & Wilson, 2006).

There are three general methods for assessment of 24-hour maintenance of fluids in the pediatric client: meter square, weight, and caloric. (*Note:* These are general formulas, and each specific age group has different fluid/electrolyte/replacement needs.)

1. Meter Square Method

For calculation of maintenance of fluid requirements, use the following formula:

$$1500 \text{ mL/m}^2 \text{ per 24 hours}$$

Example: If a child's surface area is 0.5 m², then the formula would be: $1500 \text{ mL} \times 0.5 \text{ m}^2 = 750 \text{ mL/24 hr}$

A nomogram used to determine the BSA of the patient is the **meter square method**. To use a nomogram in this method, draw a straight line between the point representing the patient's height on the left vertical scale to the point representing the patient's weight on the right vertical scale. The point at which the line intersects indicates the BSA in square meters.

The following are advantages of the meter square method:
• Provides calculation of BSA to help determine the amount of fluid and electrolytes to be infused and assists with computing rate of infusion
• Helps to calculate adult and pediatric dosages of I.V. medications
• Is simple to calculate

The following is a disadvantage of the meter square method:
• Difficulty in accessibility to visual nomogram

2. Weight Method

The **weight method** uses the child's weight in kilograms to estimate fluid needs. This method uses 100 to 150 mL/kg for estimating maintenance fluid requirements and is most useful for children weighing less than 10 kg (use of the meter square method is recommended for children weighing more than 10 kg).

The following is an advantage of the weight method:
• Simple to use

The following is a disadvantage of the weight method:
• Inaccurate in children who weigh more than 10 kg

3. Caloric Method

The formula for calculating fluid requirement is:

100 to 150 mL per 100 calories metabolized

Example: If the weight of the child is 30 kg and the child expends 1700 cal/day, fluid requirement is 1700 to 2550 mL/24 hours.

The **caloric method** calculates the usual metabolic expenditure of fluid. It is based on the following metabolic expenditure:

Children weighing 0 to 10 kg expend approximately 100 cal/kg per day.

Children weighing 10 to 20 kg expend approximately 1000 cal/kg per day plus 50 cal/kg for each kilogram over 10 kg.

Children weighing 20 kg or more expend approximately 1500 calories plus 20 cal/kg for each kilogram over 20 kg.

The following is an advantage of the caloric method:
• Easy to calculate

The following is a disadvantage of the caloric method:
• Not totally accurate unless actual calorie requirements and energy intake are continuously assessed (Broyles, Reiss, & Evans, 2007; London, Ladewig, 2007).

The Older Adult

Physiological changes related to older adults and their effect on drug dosage and volume limitations, pharmacological actions, interactions, side effects, monitoring, parameters, and response to infusion therapy must be taken into account with administration of parenteral solutions (Fabian, 2010). Be aware of the increased dangers of administering sodium chloride solutions to elderly patients, patients with severe dehydration, and patients with chronic glomerulonephritis.

Geriatric clients have a higher risk of developing dehydration than do younger clients. Dehydrated geriatric clients who are to undergo surgery should receive I.V. fluids preoperatively in an effort to prevent complications from dehydration.

Dextrose administered without a pump to elderly patients can lead to cerebral edema more rapidly than in younger patients (Fabian, 2010; Phillips, 2010).

 Home Care Issues

Many infusion medications or fluids can be administered in the home setting, including antimicrobials, chemotherapy, TPN, opioid analgesics, blood products, and hydration fluids.

Intravenous fluids may be administered for patients who are dehydrated as a result of:
• Hyperemesis gravidarum
• Intractable diarrhea

Continued

- Drug-related side effects (e.g., chemotherapy [before and after])
- Short bowel syndrome

    Short-term therapy lasts from 1 to 7 days and usually is administered via a peripheral lock or long-term access device, if there is one already in place.

    Educate patients about the need for therapy, aseptic technique, setup and administration of specific solution, and possible complications.

Patient Education

- Instruct the patient on the reason for therapy (e.g., replacement fluid, vitamins, nutrition, volume replacement).
- Instruct the patient to report signs and symptoms of complications (e.g., burning at infusion site, redness, any discomfort).
- Explain the need for increased oral intake if appropriate.
- Teach the patient how to follow sodium and fluid restriction if appropriate.
- Teach the patient to weigh self daily.
- Review signs and symptoms of dehydration and overhydration with patient.
- Teach the patient to change positions slowly if any dizziness or light-headedness occurs.
- Teach the patient to report to the nurse any pain, swelling, leaking, redness, or hardness at the I.V. site.

■ Nursing Process

The nursing process is a five- or six-step process for problem-solving to guide nursing action. Refer to Chapter 1 for details on the steps of the nursing process related to vascular access. The following table focuses on nursing diagnoses, nursing outcomes classification (NOC), and nursing interventions classification (NIC) for patients with parenteral fluid needs. Nursing diagnoses should be patient specific, and outcomes and interventions individualized. The NOC and NIC presented here are suggested directions for development of outcomes and interventions.

Nursing Diagnoses Related to Parenteral Solution Administration	Nursing Outcomes Classification (NOC)	Nursing Interventions Classification (NIC)
Fluid volume deficit related to: Active loss of body fluids or failure of regulatory mechanisms	Fluid and electrolyte balance, hydration	Fluid management, hypovolemia management
Fluid volume excess related to: Compromised regulatory mechanism; excess fluid intake; excess sodium intake	Electrolyte and acid–base balance, fluid balance, hydration	Fluid monitoring, fluid management
Knowledge deficit related to: Inadequate information: new procedure and maintaining infusion therapy	Knowledge of disease process; infusion therapy treatment regimen	Teaching: Disease process, treatment
Tissue integrity, impaired related to: Mechanical factors; damaged tissue (irritating solutions on intima of vein)	Tissue integrity: Skin	Skin care, skin surveillance, wound care
Perfusion ineffective, risk for: Cerebral–renal related to fluid volume imbalance	Acute confusion level, tissue perfusion: Cerebral, agitation level, neurological status, cognition	Neurological monitoring, cerebral perfusion promotion, fall prevention, cognitive stimulation, environmental management: safety
Collaborative problem Allergic reaction related to: hypersensitivity and release of mediators to specific substances (antigens) secondary to colloid administration	Allergic response: Systemic	Allergy management

Sources: Ackley & Ladwig (2011); Bulechek, Butcher, Dochterman, & Wagner (2013); Moorhead, Johnson, Maas, & Swanson (2013).

Chapter Highlights

- The three main objectives of I.V. therapy are to:
  - Maintain daily requirements
  - Replace previous losses
  - Provide fluids and electrolytes to restore ongoing losses
- Solutions have an osmolarity that is hypotonic, isotonic, or hypertonic:
  - Hypotonic is 250 mOsm/L or below.
  - Isotonic ranges from 250 to 375 mOsm/L.
  - Hypertonic is above 375 mOsm/L.
- Give hypertonic solutions slowly to prevent circulatory overload.
- As the acidity of the solution increases, irritation to the vein wall increases.

- Do not play "catch up" with I.V. solutions that are behind schedule; recalculate the infusion.
- Always check compatibility before adding medication to dextrose solutions.
- Do not give potassium solutions to any patient unless renal function has been established.
- Infusates are categorized as:
  - *Crystalloids:* Solutions that are considered true solutions and whose solutes, when placed in a solvent, mix, dissolve, and cannot be distinguished from the resultant solutions. Crystalloids are able to move through membranes. Examples are dextrose and sodium chloride solutions and lactated Ringer's solution.
  - *Colloids:* Substances whose particles, when submerged in a solvent, cannot form a true solution because their molecules cannot dissolve but remain suspended and distributed in the fluid. Examples are dextran, albumin, mannitol, hetastarch, and gelatins.

◼◼ Thinking Critically: Case Study

Over a 16-hour period of time a 6-year-old child was inadvertently given 800 mL of 3% sodium chloride solution instead of the prescribed 0.33% sodium chloride. She developed lethargy, convulsions, and coma before the error was discovered. Despite resuscitative efforts the child died.

Case Study Questions
1. *Identify the mEq of each electrolyte in the I.V. solutions.*
2. *Identify the osmolality/tonicity of each of the electrolyte solutions.*
3. *Refer to Chapter 1 on legal aspects for factors involved in malpractice. Who was liable?*
4. *What types of safeguards should be in place for the pediatric patient receiving I.V. fluids? (Refer to Chapter 6 for pediatric peripheral infusions.)*

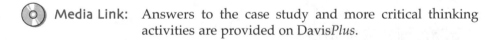 Media Link: Answers to the case study and more critical thinking activities are provided on Davis*Plus*.

Post-Test

1. A patient admitted to the emergency department with intractable vomiting was started on 5% dextrose and 0.9% sodium chloride to support which of the following objectives of infusion therapy?
   a. Maintenance of daily requirements
   b. Replacement of current losses
   c. Restore ongoing losses

2. The functions of glucose in parenteral therapy include which of the following? (*Select all that apply.*)
   a. Provides calories for energy
   b. Helps to prevent negative nitrogen balance
   c. Reduces catabolism of protein
   d. Serves as vehicle for blood transfusions

3. Maintenance solutions are used for patients who are:
   a. Ingesting nothing by mouth for a short period of time
   b. Experiencing hemorrhage
   c. Dehydrated from GI losses
   d. Experiencing draining fistulas

4. What is the most commonly used balanced electrolyte solution?
   a. 5% Dextrose in water
   b. 0.9% Sodium chloride
   c. Lactated Ringer's solution
   d. 5% Dextrose and sodium chloride

5. Which of the following is the *most* common complication of the colloid dextran?
   a. Fluid overload
   b. Hypersensitivity reactions
   c. Hyponatremia
   d. Hyperkalemia

6. What is the purpose of a colloid solution?
   a. To expand the interstitial compartment
   b. To replace electrolytes
   c. To expand the intravascular compartment
   d. To correct acidosis

7. Dextrose and hypotonic sodium chloride solutions are considered hydrating fluids because they:
   a. Provide more water than is required for excretion of sodium
   b. Provide fluid to determine renal filtration
   c. Maximize retention of potassium in the cell
   d. Maximize the retention of sodium

8. The expected outcome of administering a hypertonic solution is to:
   a. Shift ECF from the intracellular space to plasma
   b. Hydrate cells
   c. Supply free water to the vascular space

9. Which of the following solutions is used to prime the administration set when blood is to be administered?

   a. 5% Dextrose in water
   b. Lactated Ringer's
   c. 0.9% Sodium chloride
   d. 5% Dextrose and 0.45% sodium chloride

10. Before administering a prescribed intravenous solution that contains potassium chloride, the nurse should assess for:

    a. Poor skin turgor with "tenting"
    b. Behaviors indicating irritability and confusion
    c. Urinary output of 200 mL during the previous shift
    d. Minimum urinary output of 30 mL per hour.

Media Link: Answers to the Chapter 4 Post-Test and more test questions together with rationales are provided on Davis*Plus*.

⬛ References

Ackley, B. J., & Ladwig, G. B. (2011). *Nursing diagnosis handbook: An evidence-based guide to planning care.* St. Louis, MO: Mosby Elsevier.

American Society Health-System Pharmacists (ASHP). *AHFS drug information 2013.* Bethesda, MD: American Society of Health System Pharmacists. Author.

Ayus, J., Achinger, S. C., & Arieff, A. (2008). Brain cell regulation in hyponatremia: Role of sex, age, vasopressin and hypoxia. *Renal Physiology, 295*(3). 1619-1624.

Broyles, B. E., Reiss, B. S., & Evans, M. E. (2007). *Pharmacological aspects of nursing care* (7th ed.). Clifton Park, NY: Thomson Delmar Learning.

Brutocao, D., Bratton, S. L., Thomas, J. R., Schrader, P. F., Coles, P. G., & Lynn, A. M. (1996). Comparison of hetastarch with albumin for postoperative volume expansion in children after cardiopulmonary bypass. *Journal of Cardiothoracic and Vascular Anesthesia, 10* (3), 348-351.

Bulechek, G., Butcher, H., Dochterman, J., & Wagner, C. (2013). *Nursing interventions classification (NIC)* (6th ed.). St. Louis: MO: Mosby Elsevier.

Bulger, E. M., & Maier, R. V. (2007). Prehospital care of the injured: What's new. *Surgical Clinics of North America, 87*(1), 37.

Cockerill, G., & Reed, S. (2012). *Essential fluid, electrolyte and pH homeostasis.* Madden, MA: Wiley Blackwell.

Cook, L. S. (2003). IV fluid resuscitation. *Journal of Infusion Nursing, 26*(5), 2003.

Crawford, A., & Harris, H. (2011). I.V. fluid: What nurses need to know. *Nursing, 41*(5):30-38.

Fabian, B. (2010). Infusion therapy in the older adult. In M. Alexander, A. Corrigan, L. Gorski, J. Hankins, & R. Perucca (Eds.), *Infusion Nurses Society infusion nursing: An evidence-based approach* (3rd ed.) (pp. 571-582). St. Louis, MO: Saunders Elsevier.

Finfer, S., Bellomo, R., Boyce, N., French, J., Myburgh, J., Norton, R.; & SAFE Study Investigators. (2004). A comparison of albumin and saline for fluid resuscitation in the intensive care unit. *New England Journal of Medicine, 350*(22):2247-2256.

Frey, A. M., & Pettit, J. (2010). Infusion therapy in children. In M. Alexander, A. Corrigan, L. Gorski, J. Hankins, & R. Perucca (Eds.), *Infusion Nurses Society infusion nursing: An evidence-based approach* (3rd ed.) (pp. 550-569). St. Louis, MO: Saunders Elsevier.

Gahart, L., & Nazareno, A. R. (2012). *2013 Intravenous medications* (29th ed.). Philadelphia, PA: Elsevier, Mosby, Saunders.

Grocott, M., Mythen, M. G., & Gan, T. J. (2005). Perioperative fluid management and clinical outcomes in adults. *International Anesthesia Research Society, 100,* 1093-1096.

Hankins, J. (2006). The role of albumin in fluid and electrolyte balance. *Journal of Infusion Nursing, 29*(5), 260-265.

Heitz, U., & Horne, M. M. (2005). *Pocket guide to fluid, electrolyte, and acid-base balance* (5th ed.). St. Louis, MO: C. V. Mosby.

Hew-Butler, T. Almond, C., Ayus, J. C., et al. (2005). Consensus statement of the 1st International Exercise-Associated Hyponatremia Consensus Development Conference, Cape Town, South Africa. *Clinical Journal of Sports Medicine, 15,* 208-213.

Hill, J. W., & Petrucci, R. H. (2004). *General chemistry: An integrated approach* (3rd ed.). Upper Saddle River, NJ: Prentice Hall.

Hockenberry, M. J., & Wilson, D.(2006). *Wong's nursing care of infants and children* (8th ed). St. Louis: MO: Mosby Elsevier.

Holliday, M. A., & Segar, W. E. (1957). The maintenance need for water in parenteral fluid therapy. *Pediatrics, 19,* 823-832.

Infusion Nurses Society (INS). (2011). *Infusion nursing standards of practice.* Philadelphia, PA: Lippincott Williams & Wilkins.

Kelley, D. M. (2005). Hypovolemic shock: An overview. *Critical Care Nurse, 28*(1), 2-19.

London, M. L., Ladewig, P. W., Ball, J., & Bindler, R. C. (2007). *Maternal and child nursing care* (2nd ed). Upper Saddle River, NJ: Pearson Prentice Hall.

Martin, G. S., & Matthay, M. A. (2004). Evidence based colloid use in the critically ill. Consensus conference statement subcommittee of the American Thoracic Society critical care assembly. *American Journal of Respiratory and Critical Care Medicine, 170*(11), 1247-1259.

Moorhead, S., Johnson, M., Maas, M., & Swanson. (2013). *Nursing outcomes classification (NOC)* (5th ed.). St. Louis, MO: Mosby Elsevier.

Phillips, L. D. (2010). Parenteral solutions. In M. Alexander, A. Corrigan, L. Gorski, J. Hankins, & R. Perucca. (2010). *Infusion Nurses Society infusion nursing: An evidence-based approach* (3rd ed.) (pp. 229-241). St. Louis, MO: Saunders Elsevier.

Porth, C. M., & Matfin, G. (2010). *Pathophysiology: Concept of altered health states* (8th ed.). Philadelphia, PA: Lippincott Williams & Wilkins.

Siegel, A. J. (2007). Hypertonic (3%) sodium chloride for emergent treatment of exercise-associated hypotonic encephalopathy. Conference paper. *Sports Medicine, 37*(94-95), 459-462.

Smeltzer, S. C. Bare, B. G., Hinkle, J. L., & Cheever, K. H. (2010). *Brunner & Suddarth's textbook of medical-surgical nursing* (12th ed.). Philadelphia, PA: Lippincott Williams & Wilkins.

van der Linden, P. J., De Hert, S. G., Deraedt, D., Cromheecke, S., De Decker, K., De Paep, R., ... Trenchant, A. (2005). Hydroxyethyl starch 130/0.4 versus modified fluid gelatin for volume expansion in cardiac surgery patients: The effects on perioperative bleeding and transfusion needs. *International Anesthesia Research Society, 101,* 629-634.

van Wissen, K., & Breton, C. (2004). Perioperative influences on fluid distribution. *MEDSURG Nursing, 13*(5), 304-311.

Chapter **5**

Infusion Equipment

In the future, which I shall not see, for I am old, may a better way be opened! May the methods by which every infant, every human being will have the best chance of health, the methods by which every sick person will have the best chance of recovery, be learned and practiced! Hospitals are only an intermediate state of civilization never intended, at all events, to take in the whole sick population.
—*Florence Nightingale, 1860*

Chapter Contents

■ **LEARNING OBJECTIVES** *On completion of this chapter, the reader will be able to:*

1. Define the terminology related to I.V. equipment.
2. Identify the types and characteristics of solution containers.
3. Identify proper use of vented versus nonvented administration sets.
4. Identify the types and characteristics of peripheral I.V. catheters and central vascular access devices.
5. Identify the characteristics and uses of electronic infusion devices (EIDs).
6. Describe the use of filters in the infusion of solutions and blood products.
7. Describe the appropriate use of add-on devices to aid in the administration of safe infusions.
8. Describe interventions aimed at reducing risk of infection related to needleless connectors.
9. Identify the Infusion Nurses Society (INS) and the Centers for Disease Control and Prevention (CDC) recommendations for standards of practice related to equipment safety and use.

GLOSSARY

Backcheck valve   A device that functions to prevent retrograde solution flow

Cannula   A flexible tube that may be inserted into a duct, cavity, or blood vessel to deliver medication or drain fluid. It may be guided by a sharp, pointed instrument (stylet); also called a catheter.

Catheter (intravenous)   A cannula inserted into a vein to administer fluids or medications or to measure pressure

Coring   Visible, as well as microscopic, particles of rubber bung displaced by the spike during piercing of the glass container or needle during access of implanted vascular access devices

Drip chamber   Area of the intravenous administration set usually found under the spike where the solution drips and collects before running through the I.V. tubing

Drop factor   The number of drops needed to deliver 1 mL of fluid

Elastomeric pump   A portable infusion device with a balloon (elastomeric reservoir) made of soft rubberized material that is inflated with medication to a predetermined volume; when the tubing is unclamped, positive pressure is exerted to deliver the infusion

Electronic infusion device   An infusion pump powered by electricity or battery; programmed to regulate the I.V. flow rate either in drops per minute or milliliters per hour

Filter   A special porous device used for eliminating certain elements, as in particles of a certain size in a solution

Gauge   Size of cannula opening; a standard of measurement

Hub   Female connection point of an I.V. cannula where the I.V. administration set or syringe is attached

Implanted vascular access port   A catheter surgically placed into a vessel or body cavity and attached to a reservoir

Infusate   Refers to medications or solutions administered via an infusion

Lumen   The space within a tubular structure, such as an artery, vein, or catheter

Luer-lock   A design that incorporates a threaded sleeve on a male Luer

Macrodrip   In I.V. therapy, an administration set that is used to deliver measured amounts of I.V. solutions at a specific flow rate based on the size of the drops of the solution

Microaggregate   Microscopic collection of particles, such as platelets, leukocytes, and fibrin, that can exist in stored blood

Microdrip   In I.V. therapy, an administration set that delivers small amounts of I.V. solutions; drop factor of 60 drops/mL

Midline catheter   Longer peripheral I.V. catheter placed in a peripheral vein, generally inserted at about the antecubital fossa, with the catheter tip residing below the axillary line. In infants, a midline catheter may be placed in a scalp vein with the tip terminating in the external jugular vein.

Multichannel pump   Electronic infusion device that delivers multiple drug or solutions simultaneously or intermittently from bags, bottles, or syringes

Needleless connector   A device attached to the hub of the peripheral I.V. catheter or central vascular access device that allows the tip of a syringe or male Luer end of the I.V. administration set to be attached

Over-the-needle catheter   A device that consists of needle with a catheter sheath; the needle is removed leaving a plastic catheter in place; the most common type of peripheral I.V. catheter

Patient-controlled analgesia (PCA)   A drug delivery system that dispenses a preset intravascular dose of a narcotic analgesic when the patient pushes a switch on an electric cord

Peripherally inserted central catheter (PICC)   A central vascular access device placed via the peripheral veins and advanced to the superior vena cava

Port   Point of entry

Primary administration set   Device used for delivery of parenteral solutions

psi   Pounds per square inch; a measurement of pressure: 1 psi equals 50 mm Hg or 68 cm H_2O

Radiopaque   Material used in I.V. catheter that can be identified by radiographic examination

Secondary administration set   Administration set that has short tubing used for delivery of 50 to 150 mL (or sometimes greater volumes of up to 500 mL) of infusion attached to primary administration set for intermittent delivery of medication or solutions

Stylet   Needle or guide that is found inside a catheter used for vein penetration and removed after catheter insertion

Syringe pump   Piston-driven pumps that provide precise infusion by controlling the rate of drive speed and syringe size

Subcutaneously tunneled catheter   A long-term type of central vascular access device; the proximal end of the catheter is tunneled subcutaneously from the insertion site and brought out through the skin at an exit site

🖥 Infusion Therapy Equipment

Infusion therapy involves the use of many types of equipment and, often complex technology. Equipment includes single-use devices, such as disposable solution containers, tubing, and **catheters**, and durable medical equipment such as infusion pumps, I.V. poles, and visualization technologies such as ultrasound units. It is important that nurses are well educated and competent in clinical application and proper use of equipment.

Furthermore, the nurse should participate in the decision-making process of equipment acquisition. Referring back to Chapter 2, remember that the U.S. Occupational Safety and Health Administration (OSHA) Bloodborne Pathogen Standard actually requires that staff have input into safe controls to reduce exposure. There is a relationship between the industry that manufacturers the equipment, the health-care providers, and the patient that is collaborative and mutually dependent.

The public holds industry, medical institutions, and professionals accountable for the safe and effective delivery of health care. Medical products and equipment are the collective responsibility of industry and medical professionals.

■ Solution Containers

Solution containers, for use with general hydration/electrolyte solutions, medications, blood products, and nutritional products, are made of either plastic or glass. Although today the use of glass containers is relatively rare, glass is still used for medications or solutions that are not compatible with the chemicals or properties of plastic (Fig. 5-1). The history of

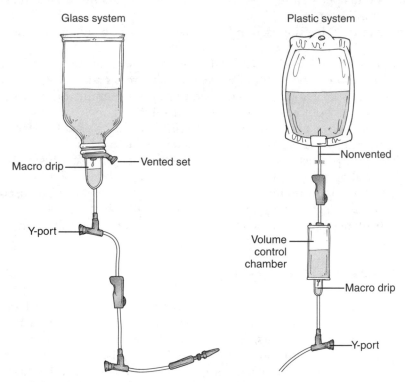

Figure 5-1 ■ Comparison of glass and plastic infusion delivery systems.

sterile evacuated glass containers dates back to 1929. In 1950, plastic containers became accessible for the storage and delivery of blood products. Today, plastic containers are used 90% to 95% of the time for administering solutions and blood products.

Glass Containers

Glass containers available in the United States are made not just of glass but of a combination of glass, plastic, rubber, and metal. Because glass does not collapse, venting is required to allow air to enter the bottle during infusion. A vented administration set must be used with glass bottles.

The closed glass system has a stopper, also called the rubber bung, which is covered with a removable seal. This seal must be removed, and the bottle should be used immediately to ensure sterility (Hadaway, 2010). During insertion of the spike of the administration set, **coring** can occur, which results in the introduction of fragments of the rubber core into the solution. Pushing the spike through the rubber bung can potentially displace visible and microscopic particles from the rubber. Because of the combination of materials in the glass system, some disadvantages have been experienced when using this system during heat sterilization procedures.

Checking the Glass Solution Containers for Clarity

To ensure safety in the administration of solutions, the nurse must check the clarity of the solution and the expiration date before connecting it to the administration set. To check a glass container, hold the glass bottle up to the light and check for flashes of light, floating particles, or discoloration. The solution should be crystal clear; if it is not, mark the container as contaminated and return it to the pharmacy. An unusual occurrence report should be completed per the organizational policy (see Chapter 1).

ADVANTAGES

- Crystal clear; allows good visualization of contents
- Graduations on glass easy to read
- Inert; has no plasticizers

DISADVANTAGES

- More easily broken during transport
- Storage problems
- Particulate matter due to coring
- Cumbersome disposal
- Rigidity
- Container constructed of mixed materials

NOTE > Once the glass system is opened by a pharmacist during introduction of an admixture, it is sealed with a tamper-proof closure to prevent alteration of the **infusate**. The nurse must check the closure for integrity; if the closure is torn, the nurse must not use it and should consult the pharmacy.

Plastic Containers

Most commonly, infusate solutions are packaged in flexible or semirigid plastic containers (Fig. 5-2). Flexible plastic containers have several unique features. The entire structure that comes in contact with the fluid, including the closure, is made of the same material. The most common plastic used in solution containers is polyvinylchloride (PVC). However, some drugs adsorb, or adhere, to the surface of the plastic container, which has led to the development of new plastics such as polyolefin and ethyl vinyl acetate (Hadaway, 2010).

NOTE > Di(2-ethylhexyl) phthalate (DEHP), a plasticizer, is added to PVC to make solution containers soft and pliable. However, DEHP is a known toxin and can seep from the plastic into the bloodstream, particularly with certain types of solutions. DEHP is lipophilic and leaches into lipid based-solutions. The greatest risk of exposure to DEHP occurs with neonatal patients. Some procedures identified with the highest risk include parenteral nutrition, exchange transfusions, and multiple procedures in sick neonates (Shaz, Grima, & Hillyer, 2011). Exposure is associated with disorders of reproductive development.

EBP DEHP concentrations significantly increased in 17 of 22 children after a 12-hour infusion of parenteral nutrition. There were no traces of DEHP in a control group of 20 children (Kambia et al., 2013).

Premixed plastic solution containers are provided in 1000-mL and 500-mL bags for primary infusions and in 50- to 150-mL bags for secondary infusions. Larger plastic bags, up to 4000 mL, are available for mixing large-volume infusions, such as parenteral nutrition solutions. Plastic containers are flexible and collapsible and do not need air to replace fluid flowing from the container. A nonvented administration set is used with plastic containers because they collapse as they empty. Depending on the manufacturer, there may be one or two extensions or entry **ports**

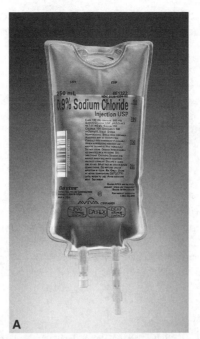

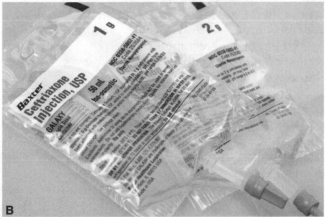

Figure 5-2 ■ Plastic infusion system. Large-volume flexible plastic container (A) and secondary solution container of 50 mL (B). (Courtesy of Baxter Healthcare Corp., Round Lake, IL.)

protruding from the bottom of the bag. If two ports protrude, one is the administration set port, encased in a protective and easily removable plastic pigtail that maintains the port's sterility before spiking with the administration set. The second extension is an injection port for adding medication. A membrane seals both the medication and the administration ports of the container, and entry of air into this system is prevented. Spiking the plastic container is accomplished by a simple twisting motion.

Because the plastic can be easily perforated during use, careful attention should be paid to the integrity of this container during preparation and infusion delivery.

NOTE > As with glass, tamper-proof additive caps are available for use with plastic solution containers. The cap fits over the medication port and indicates that a pharmacist has added medication to the infusate.

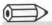 *NURSING FAST FACT!*

Never write directly on a flexible plastic bag with a ballpoint or indelible marker; the pen may puncture the bag, and the marker ink may adsorb into the plastic (INS, 2011, p. S24).

The outer wrap must remain on until use with PVC bags because of I.V. fluid loss through the bag. Non-PVC bags do not contain an outer wrap; rather, they have a multilayer film.

Semirigid, hard plastic containers made of polyolefin contain no plasticizers, the fluid level marks are easier to read, and the containers are impermeable to moisture. However, semirigid containers crack more easily and are not as tolerant to temperature extremes. Semirigid containers must be vented to add air to the infusion system because they do not collapse.

ADVANTAGES

- Closed system
- Flexible
- Lightweight
- Container composed of one substance
- Easier storage

DISADVANTAGES

- Punctures easily
- Fluid level difficult to determine
- Composed of plasticizers
- Not completely inert (potential for leaching)

Checking the Plastic System for Clarity

The plastic container should be held up to the light and checked for clarity. If there is any discoloration or floating particles in the solution, the solution should not be used and should be considered potentially contaminated. Squeeze the plastic container to check for pinholes and thus leakage and loss of integrity. Check the expiration date on the label to ensure patient safety, and be sure the outer wrap of the plastic system is free of pooled solution. Any abnormalities should result in return of the container and unusual occurrence reporting to the pharmacy per the organizational policy.

 NURSING FAST FACT!

It is important that the nurse providing infusion therapy read the information provided on the solution bag.

Use-Activated Containers

Use-activated containers (Fig. 5-3) consist of a solution (e.g., dextrose 5% in water) and a separate compartment with a premeasured drug and diluent that are mixed just prior to administration. Although more expensive, these containers are useful for infusions that have a short shelf life after admixture. They are commonly used in all nursing departments including outpatient and home care settings.

To activate the container, the nurse deliberately ruptures the container seal or diaphragm by compressing opposing parts or applying pressure to

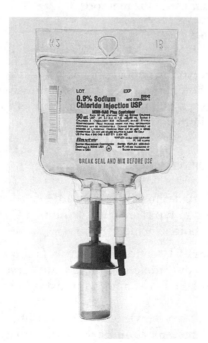

Figure 5-3 ■ Medication Additive System®. (Courtesy of Baxter Healthcare Corp., Round Lake, IL.)

rupture the internal reservoir. The primary disadvantage of the system occurs when this step is not completed appropriately and the medication is not added to the solution (Hadaway, 2010).

 NURSING FAST FACT!

Another concern with use-activated containers is belated rupture of the medication reservoir such that a potentially harmful concentration of drug is administered (Hadaway, 2010).

The Syringe as a Solution Container

Syringes are also solution containers. Prefilled flush syringes of heparin and saline are used in all settings. Of note, the syringes used most often are packaged in "clean" wrap, also known as a sterile fluid pathway, which means that the inside of the syringe and the flush solution are sterile. If the flush syringe needs to be dropped onto a sterile field, it is important to ensure that the flush syringe is packaged in sterile wrap versus a sterile fluid pathway.

Medications may also be provided in syringes, such as medications used with **syringe pumps**, discussed later in this chapter, and medications delivered via an I.V. bolus method.

Infusion Pump Specific

Some containers are specific and applicable for use with only a single, unique type of infusion pump. These types of infusion pumps often have certain limitations, such as the type of infusion therapy that can be delivered (e.g., only chemotherapy).

■ Administration Sets

The tubing choices or administration sets are manufactured with varying materials. The common types are PVC or non-PVC (usually polyolefin). Administration set choices include:

1. PVC with DEHP: Used for a majority of administration sets; however, not compatible with lipids and some drugs.
2. PVC without DEHP: Used for administration of lipids and some drugs.
3. Non-PVC lined (polyethylene lined): Inner **lumen** is lined with non-PVC material; used for administration of nitroglycerin or paclitaxel.
4. Non-PVC: Is more rigid plastic than PVC; may not be compatible with some I.V. infusion pumps.

Basic Components of Administration Sets

The most frequently used administration sets (**primary, secondary,** Y-set) among manufacturers have the same basic components but may vary in **drop factor** (Fig. 5-4). The basic components include:

1. *Spike:* The spike is a sharply tipped plastic tube designed to be inserted into the solution container. It is connected to the flange, drop orifice, and **drip chamber** (Fig. 5-5).
2. *Flange:* The flange is a plastic guard that helps prevent touch contamination during insertion of the spike.
3. *Drop orifice:* The drop orifice is an opening that determines the size and shape of the fluid drop. The size of this drop orifice determines the drop factor.

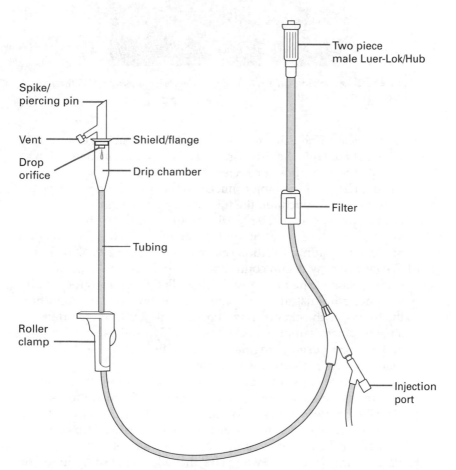

Figure 5-4 ▪ Basic administration set components.

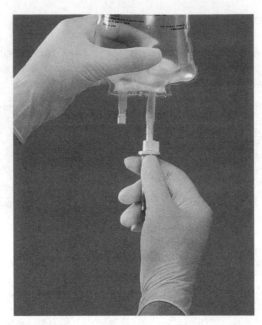

Figure 5-5 ■ Spiking an I.V. container. (Courtesy of Baxter Healthcare Corp., Round Lake, IL.)

4. *Drip chamber:* The drip chamber is a pliable, enlarged clear plastic tube that contains the drop orifice and allows for visualization of the falling drops. It is connected to the tubing.
5. *Tubing:* The plastic tubing connects to the drip chamber. Depending on the manufacturer, the tubing may have a variety of clamps, ports, connectors, or **filters** built into the system. The average length of primary tubing is 66 to 100 inches. The length of secondary administration sets averages from 32 to 42 inches.
6. *Clamp:* The flow clamp control device operates on the principle of compression of the tubing wall. The roller clamp is found on all standard administration sets and controls flow rate by occluding the tubing as the clamp is tightened. Some sets also include a slide or pinch clamp; such clamps are only used as on-off controls and are never used to regulate the flow. Be sure to check the manufacturer's instructions for use.
7. *Injection ports:* Injection ports serve as an access into the tubing and are located at various points along the administration set. Usually the ports are used for medication administration. They are accessed with a blunt plastic **cannula**, the plastic tip of a syringe, or the male end of the administration set.
8. *Backcheck valve:* A one-way valve that allows the solution to flow in one direction; most often used with secondary administration

set, thus allowing the primary solution to resume after the piggyback is completed.

9. *Hub:* The adaptor to connect the administration set to the I.V. catheter or a needleless system is also called the male **luer-lock** or Luer slip.

10. *Final filter:* The final filter removes foreign particles from the infusate. It may be an integral part of the administration set, or it may be added on separately.

Primary Continuous

Primary continuous administration sets are defined as the main administration sets used to deliver solutions and medications (INS, 2011, p. S107). These administration sets are available as vented or nonvented. Vented sets have an air filter attached to the spike pin that allows air to enter the container, and they are used with glass containers. Nonvented sets have a straight spike pin without an air vent device. The tubing of the set distal to the drip chamber terminates in a male Luer Lok end that connects to the vascular access device (VAD) hub or a **needleless connector** attached to the VAD (Fig. 5-6). Primary sets are available in **macrodrip** form (10–20 drops/mL) or in **microdrip** form (60 drops/mL).

Primary sets may have one, two, or three injection ports, backcheck valves, and often inline filters. The drop factor is clearly specified on the packaging of each administration set as well as in the accompanying

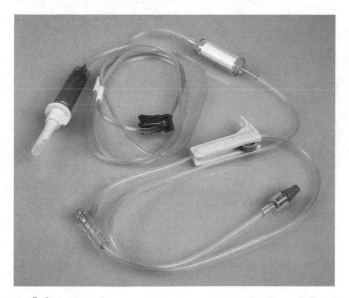

Figure 5-6 ▪ Primary administration set. (Courtesy of Baxter Healthcare Corp., Round Lake, IL.)

literature (Fig. 5-7). The microdrip set, also called a minidrip or pediatric set, is used when small amounts of fluid are required.

The backcheck valve is a device that functions to prevent retrograde flow of the fluid. When the fluid is flowing in the proper direction, from the bag to the patient, the valve is open. If the fluid is flowing in the wrong direction, from the patient toward the solution container, the valve closes. Backcheck valves are required with secondary medication administration. The secondary administration set ("piggyback") is attached to the injection port on the upper third of the primary administration set. The backcheck valve is located between the primary fluid container and the upper injection port; this prevents the secondary medication from flowing into the primary infusion container. The primary container must hang lower than the secondary container. Backcheck valves are inline components of many primary administration sets (Fig. 5-8).

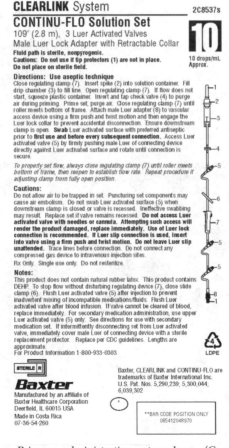

Figure 5-7 ■ Primary administration set package. (Courtesy of Baxter Healthcare Corp., Round Lake, IL.)

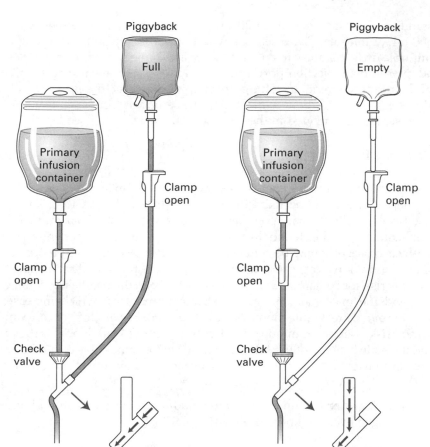

Figure 5-8 ◼ Secondary administration set. Note check valve (also called backcheck valve), which acts to prevent retrograde solution flow.

INS Standard Primary and secondary *continuous* administration sets used to administer fluids other than lipid, blood, or blood products should be changed no more frequently than every 96 hours. The administration set shall be changed immediately upon suspected contamination or when the integrity of the product or system has been compromised. All administration sets shall be of luer-lock design (INS, 2011, p. S55).

Secondary

A secondary administration set is defined as an administration set attached to the primary administration set for a specific purpose, usually to administer medications; it is commonly called the piggyback set (INS, 2011, p. S107). The piggyback set has short tubing (30–36 inches) with a standard drop factor of 10 to 20 drops/mL. It is used to deliver up to 500 mL of infusate. These sets are widely used for the administration of multiple drug therapies to patients. They are connected with a needleless adapter into an injection port immediately distal to the backcheck valve of the primary tubing. In setting up the piggyback set, the primary infusion container is positioned lower than the secondary container, using the extension hook provided in the secondary line packaging (see Fig. 5-8).

Primary Intermittent

The primary intermittent set is defined as an administration set that is connected and disconnected with each use (INS, 2011, p. S107). The set itself is generally the same one used for a continuous primary infusion. The set may be connected to the needleless connector of the patient's VAD with each use, or it may be connected to another primary continuous set. It is important to recognize that with every connection and disconnection, there is risk for contamination at the catheter hub, the needleless connector, and the male luer end of the administration set, which increases risk for bloodstream infection (INS, 2011, p. S55). Because of the contamination risk, aseptic technique with access and careful attention to protecting the male luer end of the set with a new, sterile compatible covering device after each use are critical. An example of an antimicrobial product used for this purpose is shown in Figure 5-9.

INS Standard Primary *intermittent* administration sets should be changed every 24 hours (INS, 2011, p. S55).

Metered Volume Chamber

Used less often today because of the preference for infusion pumps and syringe pumps, the metered volume chamber set is used for intermittent administration of measured volumes of fluid with a calibrated chamber (Hadaway, 2010). These sets are calibrated in much smaller increments than other infusion devices, which limits the amount of solution available to the patient (usually for safety reasons). Most chambers hold 100 to 150 mL of solution, but neonatal chambers may hold only 10 to 50 mL.

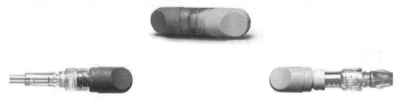

Figure 5-9 ■ Dual Cap System™. Antimicrobial protection for end of intermittently used I.V. administration sets and for the needleless connector. (Courtesy of Catheter Connections, Salt Lake City, UT.)

The volume-controlled set is most frequently used for pediatric patients and critically ill patients when small, well-controlled delivery of medication or solution is required (Fig. 5-10).

Primary Y

The primary Y administration set is used for rapid infusion or for administration of more than one solution at a time. Each leg of the Y set is capable of being the primary set. The Y set has two separate spikes with a separate drip chamber and short length of tubing with individual clamps. Primary Y sets are made up of large-bore tubing; the purpose of this tubing is to infuse large amounts of fluid in acute situations. Use of the primary Y set is associated with the risk for air embolism because air can be drawn into the administration set if one container is allowed to empty.

Blood Component

Blood is only administered with administration sets specifically designed for this use. These sets are designed for the viscous properties of blood, allow for rapid flow as needed, and can provide a dual line (Y tubing) for infusion of 0.9% sodium chloride after the transfusion. Blood transfusions are administered via a gravity infusion and also via an **electronic infusion device** (EID), if it is listed as an indication for use. Most blood

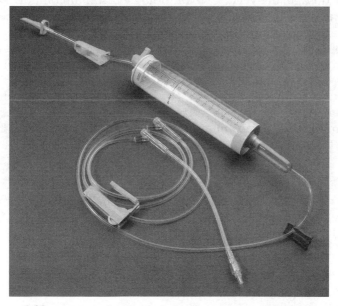

Figure 5-10 ▪ Volume chamber control set for intermittent infusion. (Courtesy of Baxter Healthcare Corp., Round Lake, IL.)

administration Y sets contain inline filters with a pore size of 170 to 260 microns and have a drop factor of 10 to allow for the safe infusion of blood cells (Fig. 5-11) (Sink, 2011).

> **INS Standard** Administration sets used for blood and blood product components should be specific to blood transfusion and include a filter; the administration sets should be replaced every 4 hours (INS, 2011, p. S56).

Lipid

Lipids or fat emulsions are supplied in glass or non-DEHP plastic containers. Lipid-containing solutions are known to leach DEHP from bags and tubing made of PVC; therefore, they must be administered through DEHP-free administration sets (INS, 2011, p. S56).

Specialty Sets: Pump/Medication Specific

The pump-specific administration set is made specifically for use with the EID for which it is designed. These sets may or may not allow priming of the set outside of the EID. For specifics on each pump administration set, see the literature that accompanies each EID.

Some drugs (e.g., nitroglycerin, insulin) are readily adsorbed into many plastics, including PVC plastics, which affects the accuracy of drug dosage delivery. Use of non-PVC administration sets and glass containers is recommended. Paclitaxel leaches DEHP from both plastic infusion containers and PVC-containing plastic containers, so it should be administered in glass containers or in polypropylene or polyolefin containers and polyethylene-lined administration sets (Gahart & Nazareno, 2012). Special administration non-DEHP sets are used for propofol infusions. The administration set should be replaced every 12 hours, when the vial is changed, and according to the manufacturer's recommendations (INS, 2011, p. S56; O'Grady et al., 2011).

> **INS Standard** When units of intravenous fat emulsion (IVFE) are administered consecutively, the administration set shall be changed every 24 hours. IVFE administration sets shall be changed immediately upon suspected contamination or when the integrity of the product or system has been compromised (INS, 2011, p. S56).

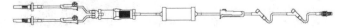

Figure 5-11 ■ Diagram of Y administration set used for blood administration. (Courtesy of Baxter Healthcare Corp., Round Lake, IL.)

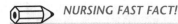

NURSING FAST FACT!

It is important that all administration sets be changed using aseptic technique, that they be of luer-lock design, and that they be anti-free flow.

Add-On Devices

A variety of "add-on devices" are used with infusion therapy. They are defined as additional components added to the administration set or VAD (INS, 2011, S101). Add-on devices include the following:
- Extension sets
- Catheter connection devices
- Stopcocks
- Needleless connectors
- Filters

In general, use of add-on devices should be limited because of the risk for contamination, accidental disconnections, or misconnections (INS, 2011, p. S31). However, there are circumstances when it makes sense to use an add-on device. It is important to have a well-defined purpose for their use (Hadaway, 2010). It is also important for any add-on device to have a luer-lock configuration to ensure a secure junction and reduce the risk of disconnection.

Extension Sets

Extension tubing may be added to the administration set or VAD. Extension sets may be straight, may be in a Y configuration, or may have multiple entries. Straight extension sets may be connected to the VAD with a needleless connector added to the end of the set to increase the length. This is common with home care patients, in whom the extra length allows easier access to scrub the needleless connector and self-infuse a medication (Fig. 5-12). Y-configured extension sets usually have a clamp on both segments and can be added to allow simultaneous or separate administration of solutions. Multientry extension sets may have three or more "pigtails" allowing entry into the infusion system. Both Y-configured and multientry sets may have clamps, additional injection ports, or backcheck valves (Alexander et al., 2013). When used with power injectable catheters, an extension set with such capability must be used (Fig. 5-13).

Catheter Connection Devices (or Catheter Extension Sets)

A catheter connection device such as a J loop or T connector added to the peripheral I.V. catheter makes it easier to convert from a continuous to an intermittent infusion with less manipulation at the catheter insertion site.

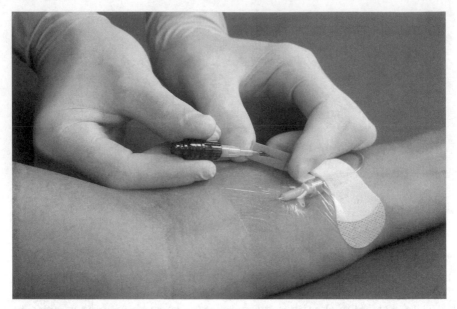

Figure 5-12 ■ Extension tubing connected to access device and hub of catheter, with slide clamp. (Courtesy of Baxter Healthcare Corp., Round Lake, IL.)

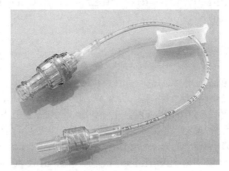

Figure 5-13 ■ Power injectable extension set. (Courtesy of Baxter Healthcare Corp., Round Lake, IL.)

These devices come in many configurations (with one, two, or three lumens), and some have power injectable capability.

Stopcocks

A stopcock is a device that controls the direction of flow of an infusate through manual manipulation of a direction-regulating valve. A stopcock is usually a three- or four-way device. A three-way stopcock connects two lines of fluid to a patient and provides a mechanism for either one to run to the patient (similar to a faucet). With a four-way stopcock, the valve can be manipulated so that one or both lines can run to the patient, either alone or in combination.

The general use of stopcocks for administration of medications or I.V. infusions and for collection of blood samples creates a potential portal of entry for microorganisms and is strongly discouraged because of the issue of contamination (INS, 2011, p. S31; O'Grady et al., 2011). When the stopcock portals are uncapped, they are vulnerable to touch contamination. The stopcock itself is small and requires handling in such a way that sterility can easily be compromised. Syringes are frequently attached to I.V. push administration, and the portal is poorly protected after use. The use of stopcocks is not recommended; however, if used, each port of the stopcock should be covered with a sterile cap between uses (INS, 2011, p. S31). Aseptic technique is followed for all add-on device changes.

> **INS Standard**   When add-on devices are used, they should be changed with each catheter or administration set replacement, or whenever the integrity of either product is compromised (INS, 2011, p. S31).

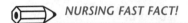 *NURSING FAST FACT!*

    Caution should be exercised when using a stopcock because of the risk of contamination of the I.V. system. The risks for inadvertent infusion interruptions and incorrect drug administration are present with stopcock use.

Needleless Connectors

A needleless connector is attached to the hub of the peripheral I.V. catheter or central vascular access device (CVAD), allowing the tip of a syringe or male luer end of the I.V. administration set to be attached. Although "needleless connector" is the current term recommended by INS, other commonly used terms are injection caps, or injection ports or valves. The development and use of needleless connectors have reduced the risk of needlestick injuries to health-care workers (O'Grady et al., 2011). Needleless connectors allow for venous access without removal of the connector, thus maintaining a closed infusion system. Many types of needleless connectors are available, and it is important to understand how they work and the implications related to flushing technique. Needleless connectors are classified into two broad categories:

- Simple: A simple device has no internal mechanisms so that fluid flows straight through the internal lumen. Simple devices include those with a split septum, which opens when a blunt plastic cannula attached to the syringe or administration set is passed through the septum (Fig. 5-14).

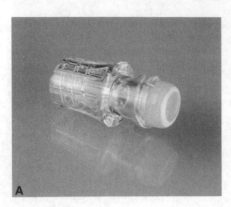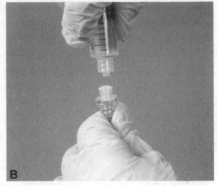

Figure 5-14 ■ Split septum needleless connectors. *A*, INTERLINK. (Courtesy of Baxter Healthcare Corp., Round Lake, IL.) *B*, BD Q-Syte™ Luer Access Split Septum. (Courtesy of BD Medical, Sandy, UT.)

■ Complex: These include mechanical valves with an internal mechanism that controls the flow of fluid through the device, allowing both infusion and aspiration of blood (Hadaway & Richardson, 2010).

Needleless connectors can be further classified based on function as follows:

■ Negative fluid displacement: Blood is pulled back into the catheter lumen (reflux) when I.V. tubing or a syringe is disconnected and the tubing is not clamped first before disconnection or when an infusion container runs dry. A positive fluid displacement technique is required to overcome blood reflux with negative fluid displacement connectors. This is accomplished when pressure is maintained on the flush syringe while the catheter clamp is being closed. Negative fluid displacement connectors are less commonly used today.

■ Positive fluid displacement: With these devices, an internal reservoir within the needleless connector holds a small amount of fluid. When the syringe or I.V. tubing is disconnected, fluid is pushed out to overcome blood reflux. Important to the use of positive needleless connectors is clamping the catheter after syringe/tubing disconnection to allow positive fluid displacement.

■ Neutral displacement: Blood reflux is prevented during connection and disconnection of I.V. tubing or syringes. Function of a neutral displacement device is not dependent on clamping technique. The catheter can be clamped either before or after disconnection (Hadaway & Richardson, 2010).

An example of a "complex" needleless connector is shown in Figure 5-15. Some needleless connectors contain an antimicrobial barrier.

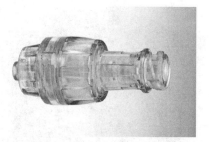

Figure 5-15 ▪ Example of a complex needleless connector (NC). ONE-LINK neutral displacement NC. (Courtesy of Baxter Healthcare Corp., Round Lake, IL.)

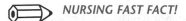 *NURSING FAST FACT!*

Blood reflux, and thus the risk for catheter occlusion, is dependent on proper flushing technique based on whether the connector is a positive or negative fluid displacement device. Refer to Chapter 6 for steps in flushing. It is important that all nurses understand which type of device is being used.

NURSING FAST FACT!

For all catheters that are supplied with a clamp, the clamp should be closed when it is not in use to prevent the risk of air embolism or exsanguination with accidental dislodgement of the needleless connector.

Infection Prevention Concerns

Important aspects of infection prevention related to needleless connectors include the frequency of changing the device and attention to aseptic technique when accessing the connector. Failure to disinfect the needleless connector before accessing has been an important problem and area of concern. The catheter hub and needleless connector are known sources of microbial contamination and present a source for development of a bloodstream infection. Although traditional practice is to scrub the needleless connector prior to any access (e.g., flushing), emerging research also supports the use of alcohol disinfection caps (Sweet, Cumpston, Briggs, Craig, & Hamadani, 2012; Wright, Tropp, & Schora, 2013). These plastic caps, which contain a sponge saturated with 70% alcohol, are placed on the end of the needleless connector in between intermittent infusions, thus protecting the end. If they are left in place for a certain length of time, based on manufacturer guidelines, the needleless connector does not require scrubbing prior to access (Fig. 5-16). Products specifically designed for site disinfection that require less scrubbing time also

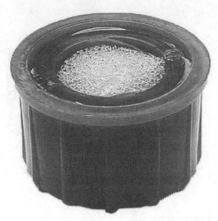

Figure 5-16 ■ Curos® alcohol disinfection cap, which is changed after each catheter access. (Courtesy of Ivera Medical Corporation, San Diego, CA.)

are available. For longer-term VADs, the needleless connector must also be changed as follows:

- The CDC recommends changing the needleless connector at the same interval as the I.V. administration set—no more often than every 72 hours and according to manufacturer's recommendations (O'Grady et al., 2011).
- INS (2011, p. S32) states that the optimal frequency for changing the needleless connector has not been determined and recommends changing the needleless connector in the following circumstances:
  - When it is removed for any reason
  - If visible blood or debris is present
  - Prior to drawing a blood sample for culture
  - On contamination
  - According to organizational policies and procedures
- In home care, needleless connectors are routinely changed at least every 7 days with intermittent infusions and more often based on INS criteria (Gorski, Perucca, & Hunter, 2010).

EBP The ports of four types of needleless connectors were inoculated with bacteria (Staphylococcus epidermidis, Staphylococcus aureus, Pseudomonas aeruginosa, and Candida albicans). After inoculation, the membranous septa were allowed to air dry for 18 hours. The ports were then disinfected for 15 seconds with 70% alcohol alone or 3.15% chlorhexidine/70% alcohol. Saline flush solutions were collected and cultured. Disinfection either with 70% alcohol alone or with 3.15% chlorhexidine/70% alcohol for 15 seconds was found to be effective. All models of needleless access ports were effectively disinfected using these two methods. The researchers recommend a 15-second scrub using friction (twisting motion) based on their in vitro research (Kaler & Chinn, 2007).

Filters

Filters are used during the infusion of intravenous solutions to prevent the administration of any particulate matter, air, microorganisms, or endotoxins that may be in the infusion system. Unwanted matter is present in all types of solutions, and the United States Pharmacopeia (USP) has set standards regarding the amount of particulate matter allowable. The addition of medications and administration sets potentially increases the amount of particulate matter (Hadaway, 2010). The ultimate location of particulates is the pulmonary capillaries, where the average diameter is about 5 microns. It is likely that even 1 L of I.V. fluid could introduce enough particles to occlude significant areas of pulmonary circulation (Hadaway, 2010).

Current recommendations for filtration include blood transfusions, parenteral nutrition solutions (i.e., lipid-containing), intraspinal infusions, and specific medications/solutions as recommended by the manufacturer (e.g., certain biologicals) (INS, 2011, p. S34; O'Grady et al., 2011). However, filter use in critically ill patients is an important area of current research.

> EBP In a randomized trial involving critically ill children, subjects were randomly assigned to a control group (n = 406) or a filter group (n = 401). Inline filtration was used with 1.2-micron filters for lipid-containing solutions and 0.2-micron filters for aqueous solutions. There was a significant reduction in the overall rate of complications (systemic inflammatory response syndrome [SIRS], sepsis, organ failure, and thrombosis) in the filtration group. In particular, the rate of SIRS was significantly lower (22.4% versus 30.3%) with filtration. The researchers concluded that filtration is efficacious and safe in preventing major complications in critically ill pediatric patients (Jack et al., 2012).

Filters are available as add-on devices or as inline components as an integral part of the administration set. Advantages to the inline filter include reduced risk for contamination and no risk of filter-tubing separation. Disadvantages include the need for an entire administration set change should the filter clog. The location of the filter may also be a disadvantage. If the filter is located at the upper portion of the tubing, it retains only substances that enter the tubing above the filter. Add-on filters are easily changed if they become clogged and can be placed at the distal end of the tubing.

Inline filters are available in a variety of forms, sizes, and materials. Common filter sizes used with common I.V. solutions and medications are:
- 0.2 micron: Most common, air eliminating, bacterial retentive
- 0.45 micron: Remove fungi or bacteria, may be air eliminating
- 1.2 micron: Used with three-in-one parenteral nutrition solutions, usually air eliminating

Examples of filters are shown in Figures 5-17, 5-18, and 5-19.

INS Standard Add-on bacteria and particulate-retentive and air-eliminating membrane filters should be located as close as possible to the catheter insertion site (INS, 2011, p. S34).

Membrane Filters

Membrane filters are screen filters with uniformly sized pores. Filters range in size from 170 microns (largest) to 0.2 micron (smallest). They allow liquids but not particles to pass through them. The finer the membrane, the more fully it will filter the liquid. A 5-micron screen will retain on the flat portion of the membrane all particles larger than 5 microns. A 0.2-micron filter is used to retain bacteria and fungi and for air retention. A 0.2-micron air-venting filter automatically vents air through a nonwettable (hydrophobic) membrane and permits uniform high-gravity flow through a large wettable (hydrophilic) membrane.

To be effective, an infusion membrane filter must have the ability to:

- Maintain high flow rates.
- Automatically vent air.
- Retain bacteria, fungi, particulate matter, and endotoxins.
- Tolerate pressures generated by infusion pumps.
- Act in a nonbinding fashion to drugs.

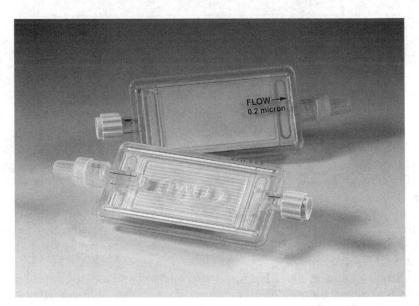

Figure 5-17 ■ Posidyne® ELD 0.2-micron filter with 96-hour bacterial and endotoxin retention. (Provided compliments of Pall Corporation, Port Washington, NY. Copyright Pall Corporation, 2013.)

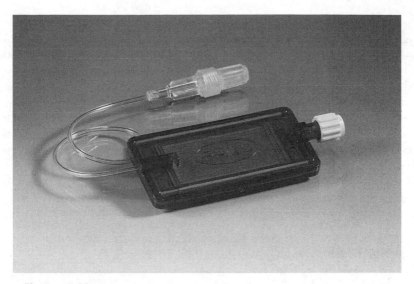

Figure 5-18 ■ Lipopor™ TNA filter set for total nutrient admixture administration with 1.2-micron air- and particle-eliminating filter. (Provided compliments of Pall Corporation, Port Washington, NY. Copyright Pall Corporation, 2013.)

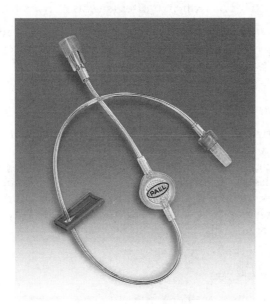

Figure 5-19 ■ Neonatal filter. Posidyne® NEO 0.2-micron filter with 96-hour bacterial and endotoxin retention. (Provided compliments of Pall Corporation, Port Washington, NY. Copyright Pall Corporation, 2013.)

A 0.2-micron filter is *contraindicated* with administration of blood or blood components and lipid emulsions. Other contraindications include the administration of low-volume medications (total amount <5 mL over 24 hours), I.V. push medications, medications with pharmacological properties that are altered by the filter membrane, and medications that adhere to the filter membrane.

All filters have a certain pressure value at which they will allow the passage of air from one side of a wetted hydrophilic membrane to the other. Filters are also rated according to the pounds per square inch (**psi**) of pressure they can withstand. The filter should withstand the psi exerted by the infusion pump or rupture may occur. If the psi rating of the housing is less than that of the membrane, excess force will break the housing.

INS Standard When an EID is used, consideration should be given to the psi rating of a filter (INS, 2011, p. S34).

Blood Filters

The American Association of Blood Banks states that blood components must be transfused through special tubing with a filter designed to remove blood clots and potentially harmful particles (Sink, 2011). Commercially available filters include the standard clot filter, the **microaggregate** filter, and the leukocyte reduction filter (see also Chapter 11).

INS Standard Blood and blood component filters appropriate to the therapy shall be used to reduce particulate matter, microaggregates, or leukocytes in infusions of blood and blood products (INS, 2011, p. S34).

Standard Clot Filter

Blood administration sets have a standard clot filter of 170 to 260 microns. These filters are intended to remove coagulated products, microclots, and debris resulting from collection and storage. They allow passage of smaller particles called microaggregates, which are composed of nonviable leukocytes, primarily granulocytes, platelets, and fibrin strands. The microaggregates can cause pulmonary dysfunction (e.g. acute respiratory distress syndrome [ARDS]) when large quantities of stored bank blood are infused.

Microaggregate Filters

Microaggregate filters are not routinely used products. They are most often used for reinfusion of shed autologous blood collected during and after surgery (Sink, 2011). The 20- to 40-micron microaggregate blood filters remove fibrin strands and clumps of dead cells.

LEUKOCYTE REDUCTION FILTERS

Leukocyte reduction filters are used to remove leukocytes (including leukocyte-mediated viruses) from red blood cells and platelets. Use of these filters decreases the risk for febrile transfusion reactions, human leukocyte antigen (HLA) alloimmunization, and cytomegalovirus transmission. Additional information on leukocyte depletion filters is provided in Chapter 11.

 Website

American Association of Blood Banks; www.aabb.org

Catheter Stabilization Devices

Catheter stabilization devices are defined as devices/systems specifically designed and engineered to control movement at the catheter hub, thereby decreasing catheter movement within the vessel and risk of catheter malposition (INS, 2011, p. S102). Attention to catheter stabilization is important because limiting movement of the catheter in and out of the insertion site (called pistoning) reduces the risk of accidental dislodgement and other complications such as infiltration, phlebitis, and infection (Alekseyev et al., 2012). Catheter stabilization is pertinent to both central and peripheral VADs. Historically, nonsterile tape was used to secure peripheral I.V. catheters, and sutures were used most often to secure central lines. Because the use of sutures is associated with increased risk for infection and health-care provider needlestick injury, their use is not recommended (INS, 2011; O'Grady et al., 2011). Because tape is not as effective as a defined stabilization device, its use is not recommended by INS (2011, p. S46).

There are a variety of catheter stabilization products on the market as well as claims of several types of catheter securement dressings. A common type of product consists of an adhesive pad and a mechanism for holding the catheter to the pad (Fig. 5-20). A newer, novel stabilization product used with **peripherally inserted central catheter** (PICC) stabilization is a small metal anchor that is placed beneath the skin in the subcutaneous tissue. Advantages to this product are no need for replacement, ease of site antisepsis, and no adhesives, which can be an issue for some patients. This product was found to be efficacious in a small study of 68 inpatients and outpatients in three different institutions (Fig. 5-21) (Egan, Siskin, Weinmann, & Galloway, 2013).

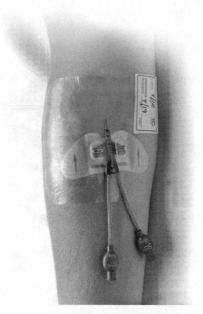

Figure 5-20 ■ StatLock® PICC Plus Catheter stabilization device. (© 2013 C.R. Bard, Inc. Used with permission.)

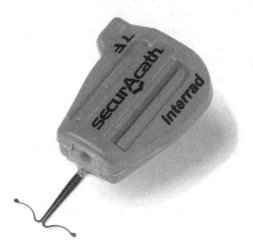

Figure 5-21 ■ Catheter stabilization device, securAcath®. Metal anchor of device sits in subcutaneous tissue. (Courtesy of Interrad Medical, Plymouth, MN.)

EBP In an integrative review of the literature, a group of nurses reviewed research studies or outcomes-based studies addressing catheter stabilization. A total of 13 studies met the study inclusion criteria and were classified, summarized, and analyzed. Although a major limitation was the fact that most of the published studies were descriptive in nature and few were randomized, the authors concluded that a significant decrease in complication rates was associated with use of specific I.V. stabilization devices as compared to tape and surgical strips. However, the authors also identified the need for further research in this area, including randomized clinical trials (Alekseyev et al., 2012).

INS Standard VAD stabilization shall be used to preserve the integrity of the access device, minimize catheter movement at the hub, and prevent catheter dislodgement and loss of access (INS, 2011, p. S46).

■ Site Protection and Joint Stabilization Devices

Site protection refers to the use of methods or products that protect the catheter site. Examples include clear plastic site protectors placed over the site, used most often with children, and mittens. Such strategies may be necessary with patients who exhibit confusion or other cognitive deficits. Hiding or camouflaging the site may reduce inadvertent manipulation at the I.V. site (Fig. 5-22).

Although areas of joint flexion should be avoided with peripheral I.V. placement (see Chapter 6), at times this is not possible. An arm board should be used and applied in a manner that allows ongoing visual assessment of the catheter and vein path. Arm boards may be flat or contoured to fit the extremity, should be padded for comfort, and should support the area of flexion to assist in maintaining a functional position (INS, 2011).

INS Standard Joint stabilization and site protection devices should be used in such a manner that preserves circulation, prevents skin impairment and nerve pressure, and provides the ability to visually inspect and assess the VAD site (INS, 2011, p. S48).

■ Peripheral Intravenous Catheters

A peripheral I.V. (PIV) catheter has a tip that terminates in the peripheral vasculature. There are three categories of PIVs:

1. The stainless steel winged needle, often called a "scalp vein needle" or a "butterfly." Flexible plastic wings extend from either

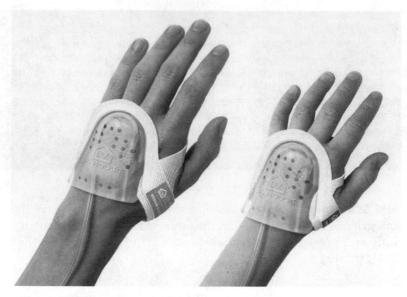

Figure 5-22 ■ I.V. House UltraDressing®, which consists of flexible fabric with thumb holes and a polyethylene dome that wraps around the patient's hand after an I.V. is started. This provides site protection and accidental snagging of the loop or catheter hub. (Courtesy of I.V. House, Inc., Chesterfield, MO.)

side of the needle hub, and a short length of tubing is attached to the needle. This type of device is indicated for obtaining blood. It may be used for single-dose I.V. medication administration and then promptly removed. It is never left in place because the risk of infiltration is high. Stainless steel needles are available in the following **gauges** (odd-numbered)—17, 19, 21, 23, 25, and 27—and in lengths from 0.5 to 1.0 inch. The wings attached to the shaft are made of rubber or plastic, and the flexible tubing extending behind the wings varies from 3 to 12 inches in length (Fig. 5-23).

2. The **over-the-needle catheter** leaves a plastic-type catheter in place and is the most common type of PIV catheter used. It can remain in place for days.
3. The **midline catheter** is a longer PIV catheter that is placed in a peripheral vein, generally inserted about the antecubital fossa, with the catheter tip residing below the axillary line. In infants, a midline catheter may be placed in a scalp vein with the tip terminating in the external jugular vein.

Catheters have **radiopaque** material or stripping added to ensure radiographic visibility. Radiopacity aids in the identification of a catheter embolus, which is a rare complication. The hub of a cannula is plastic and

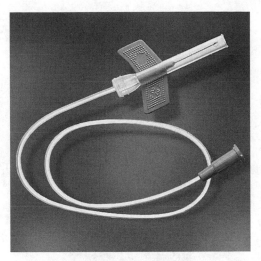

Figure 5-23 ■ Butterfly-winged scalp vein needle. (Courtesy of BD Medical, Sandy, UT.)

color coded to indicate the length and gauge. A short peripheral catheter is often defined as one that is shorter than 3 inches in length.

Catheters are made of various biocompatible materials such as steel polytetrafluoroethylene (Teflon), polyurethane, silicone, and Vialon. Teflon is considered the most thrombogenic and silicone the least thrombogenic (Alexander et al., 2013).

INS Standard The catheter selected shall be of the smallest gauge and length possible with the fewest number of lumens and shall be the least invasive device to accommodate and manage the prescribed therapy (INS, 2011, p. S37).

Over-the-Needle Catheters

The most widely used infusion device is the over-the-needle catheter, which consists of a flexible catheter in tandem with a rigid needle or **stylet** that is used as a guide to puncture and insert the catheter into the vein. The stylet connects with a clear chamber that allows for visualization of blood return indicating successful venipuncture. The hub of the catheter is plastic and color coded to indicate length and gauge. Figure 5-24 shows examples of over-the-needle catheters. The point of the stylet extends beyond the tip of the catheter. After venipuncture, the needle (stylet) is withdrawn and discarded, leaving a flexible catheter within the vein. The peripheral short catheter consists of a catheter with a length of 0.5 to 3.0 inches and gauges of even numbers ranging from 12 to 24. Recommendations related to catheter size are addressed in Chapter 6.

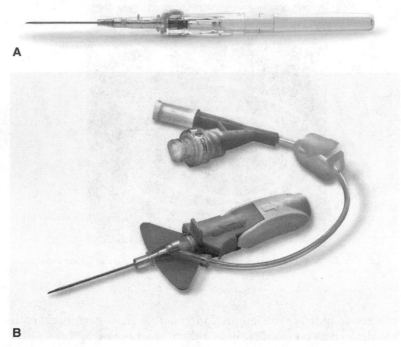

A

B

Figure 5-24 ■ Over-the-needle catheters. *A,* BD Insyte™ Autoguard™ BC Shielded IV Catheter. *B,* Nexiva™ closed I.V. catheter system. (Courtesy of BD Medical, Sandy, UT.)

 NURSING FAST FACT!

> With any catheter, use the shortest length and the smallest gauge to deliver the ordered therapy. Also, use a vein large enough to sustain sufficient blood flow because this will decrease irritation to the vein wall.

Catheter Features

Thin Walled

The thin-walled over-the-needle catheter is constructed of plastic. Its thinner wall provides higher flow rates because of its larger internal lumen. Thin-walled catheters are smoother on insertion because they have a more tapered fit to the inner stylet. Because of its thin-walled construction, the catheter becomes less able to hold its shape once it is inserted and warmed to body temperature. This soft, "flimsy" catheter is easier on the intima of the vein but collapses with negative pressure.

Flashback Chambers

The flashback chamber is a small space at the hub of the stylet. When the stylet punctures the vein during catheter insertion, the increased pressure in the vein is immediately relieved into the catheter stylet with a flow of blood in the flashback chamber. This allows the nurse to see that blood return is continuing as the catheter is advanced and secured. The safest catheters use a flashback chamber that allows the rapid return of blood but prohibits any blood spillage.

Blood Control

Exposure to blood from the hub of the catheter after stylet removal has been a risk for the nurse. New technology within the hub of the catheters stops the flow of blood out of the catheter on removal of the stylet, allowing the nurse to place a needleless connector on the hub of the catheter without being exposed to blood. The risks of mucocutaneous transmission of blood and body fluids are addressed in Chapter 2.

Addition of Wings

Adding wings to the design of I.V. catheters and scalp vein needles is intended to improve insertion technique and catheter stabilization. The wings are usually flexible plastic protrusions from the hub of the device. Winged catheters provide more control when the catheter is manipulated, thereby preventing contamination.

Color Coding

Short PIV catheters are color coded based on international color-coding standards. Universal color-coding standards allow visual recognition of the catheter gauge size. This standard has not been applied to gauge sizes of midline catheters or CVADs.
- Violet: 26-gauge
- Blue: 24-gauge
- Yellow: 22-gauge
- Pink: 20-gauge
- Green: 18-gauge
- Gray: 16-gauge

 NURSING FAST FACT!

Color coding should never substitute for reading the package label (INS, 2011).

Needle Protection: Active and Passive Sharps Safety

Two categories of safer needle devices incorporate prevention techniques for I.V. catheters: active design and passive design.

Active design safety needles require health-care workers to activate a safety mechanism after use to protect against accidental needlesticks. The user can bypass these safety mechanisms, leaving him or her at risk for injury. If a nurse forgets to activate the safety mechanism or if the safety mechanism fails to activate once the needle is removed from the patient, the nurse is at risk. The passive design deploys automatically during use.

> **INS Standard** Nurses should be trained in the use of engineered sharps safety mechanisms and how to engage the safety mechanism (INS, 2011, p. S28).

Dual-Lumen Peripheral Catheters

The dual-lumen peripheral catheter is available in a range of catheter gauges with corresponding lumen sizes. Two totally separate infusion channels exist, making it possible to infuse two solutions simultaneously. They are available as 16-gauge catheters with 18- and 20-gauge lumens or as 18-gauge catheters with 20- and 22-gauge lumens. Dual-lumen catheters are also available as midline catheters.

 NURSING FAST FACT!

Controversy still exists regarding simultaneous infusions of known incompatible solutions or medications through a dual-lumen peripheral catheter because of the limited hemodilution achievable in any peripheral vein.

Midline Catheters

Midline catheters are peripheral I.V. catheters designed for intermediate-term therapies of up to 4 weeks of isotonic or near-isotonic therapy. The catheters are generally between 3 and 8 inches long and are made of polyurethane or silicone. The catheter is placed midline in the antecubital region in the basilic, cephalic, or median antecubital site and is then advanced into the larger vessels of the upper arm for greater hemodilution. The catheter is placed using sterile technique and a traditional breakaway peripheral introducer or via a modified Seldinger technique. Midline catheters are often placed using ultrasound guidance.

ADVANTAGES

The major advantages over the conventional peripheral short catheter have been:
- Drug hemodilution
- Dwell time 1 to 4 weeks

DISADVANTAGE
- Potential for phlebitis

INS Standard The nurse should consider selection of a midline catheter for therapies anticipated to last from 1 to 4 weeks (INS, 2011, p. S37).

Vein Illumination Devices

The use of illumination devices has affected the practice of intravenous access and infusion therapy for patients who are in need of I.V.s but have veins that can neither be seen nor palpated. The transilluminator works by directing a high-intensity cool light down into the subcutaneous tissue and creating a uniform area of orange-like reflection from the fatty tissue. The light is flush with the skin; by moving the light around the extremity, a dark line can be seen. The vein's deoxygenated blood absorbs the light, whereas the fatty tissue reflects the light (Fig. 5-25).

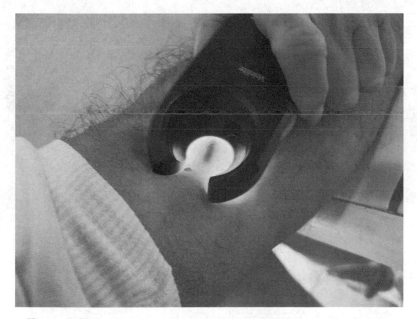

Figure 5-25 ■ Transillumination device Veinlite®. (Courtesy of Translite LLC, Sugar Land, TX.)

Near-infrared imaging devices are also used to visualize veins. One device offers a headset, hands-free device. In a study investigating the use of such technology, volunteer subjects in a large urban hospital consented to an evaluation study involving 768 observations of 384 subjects. The researchers found that use of near-infrared technology increased the visibility of veins in subpopulations of African American and Asian ethnicity and those with obesity compared to normal, unassisted eyesight (Chiao et al., 2013). Such technology also offers the advantage of being able to visualize venous flow (Figs. 5-26 and 5-27).

Ultrasound

Ultrasound allows for real-time imaging of selected blood vessels and nearby anatomic structures before and during placement of midline catheters and PICCs. Ultrasound-guided catheter insertion requires training. A thorough understanding of the vascular system and the veins accessed (basilic, brachial, and cephalic) is required.

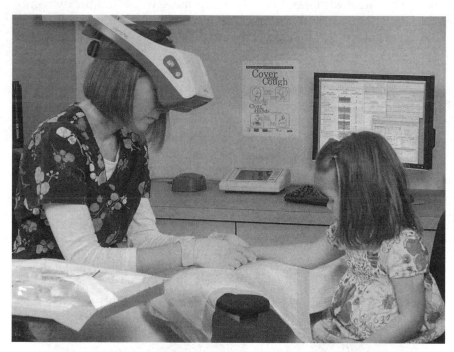

Figure 5-26 ■ Near-infrared imaging to visualize vein using VueTekVein-site™. (Courtesy of VueTek Scientific, Gray, ME.)

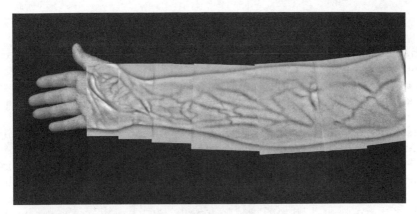

Figure 5-27 ■ View of upper-extremity veins seen with the VueTek Veinsite. (Courtesy of VueTek Scientific, Gray, ME.)

■ Central Vascular Access Devices

A CVAD is defined by the location of the catheter tip in a central vein. The CVAD catheter tip should reside in the lower one-third of the superior vena cava, above the right atrium.

CVADs are made of soft, radiopaque medical-grade silicone elastomers or thermoplastic polyurethane. They are commercially available in many designs. Polyurethane catheters are the most commonly used catheters because of the material's versatility, malleability (tensile strength and elongation characteristics), and biocompatibility. CVADs are available with single or multiple lumens. New technologies such as power injectable central catheters, catheter coatings, and addition of impregnated cuffs are addressed in Chapter 8. There are four main categories of CVADs.

NOTE > Additional information on catheter materials and designs is given in Chapter 8.

Nontunneled CVADs

The nontunneled CVAD is a percutaneously placed catheter that is usually placed via the subclavian or internal jugular vein. The nontunneled catheter is considered a short-term catheter and is used primarily in the acute care setting. These catheters may be single lumen, or they may have two, three, or four separate lumens. Physicians, radiologists, and some advanced practice specialist nurses place nontunneled catheters.

Peripherally Inserted Central Catheters

The PICC is the most common type of CVAD used in all settings, including acute care, long-term care, outpatient care, and home care. The PICC may be placed for short-term needs in the acute care setting and may be used on a longer-term basis for patients who require longer-term infusion therapy beyond the hospital. The PICC is usually placed in an insertion site above the antecubital fossa, via the cephalic, basilic, or median veins and threaded to its central location in the superior vena cava.

The PICC is composed of silicone elastomers or polyurethane. Silicone elastomer is soft, flexible, nonthrombogenic, and biocompatible. Single-, double-, and triple lumen catheters are available. PICCs range in size from 16 to 23 gauge and 50 to 60 cm in length. PICCs may be placed by the infusion nurse who has completed education, training, and competency requirements, or they may be placed in the radiology suite by interventional radiologists. Many organizations have successful nurse-led PICC teams. PICCs may also be placed via the internal or external jugular vein (EJ PICC). Although not common, EJ PICCs can be used for nonemergent access when other veins cannot be accessed (INS, 2008).

INS Standard Veins that should be considered for PICC cannulation are the basilic, median cubital, cephalic, and brachial veins. For neonatal and pediatric patients, additional site selections include the temporal vein and posterior auricular vein in the head and the saphenous vein in the lower extremities (INS, 2011, p. S41).

Figures 5-28 and 5-29 show examples of PICCs.

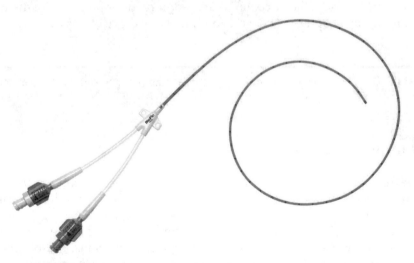

Figure 5-28 ■ BioFlo PICC made of a thromboresistant material. (Courtesy of Angiodynamics, Marlborough, MA.)

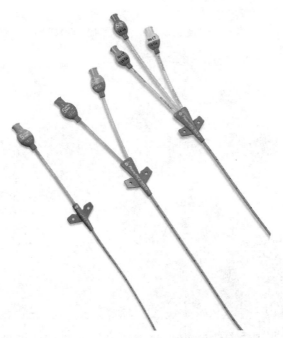

Figure 5-29 ■ Power PICC Solo®2 catheters, single, double, and triple lumen. Valve located in catheter hub. (© 2013 C.R. Bard, Inc. Used with permission.)

Subcutaneously Tunneled CVADs

The **subcutaneously tunneled catheter** is a surgically placed CVAD. It is placed in the operating room or in the interventional radiology suite. The tunneled catheter is considered a long-term catheter for patients who require lifelong or long-term infusion therapy such as total parenteral nutrition or chemotherapy. The catheter is "tunneled" in the subcutaneous tissue between an "entrance" and an "exit" site. The exit site is where the catheter extrudes, usually in the lower area of the chest. The entrance site is where the catheter enters the venous circulation, generally in the area of the clavicle, and will appear as an incision. A synthetic "cuff" is attached to the catheter and located in the tunnel. Over time, tissue attaches to the cuff, stabilizing and holding the catheter in place. The tunneling/cuff also serves to seal the path from the exit site to the vein, thus reducing the risk of bloodstream infection.

Subcutaneously tunneled catheters are made of soft, medical-grade silicone elastomers. Commonly called Broviac and Hickman catheters (Bard Access Systems), named after the physicians who developed them, these catheters are 20 to 30 inches long and have a 17- to 22-gauge internal lumen diameter. The thickness of the silicone wall varies by manufacturer. Silicone catheters can be single, dual, triple, or quadruple lumen (Fig. 5-30).

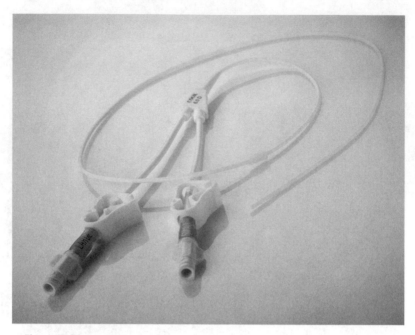

Figure 5-30 ■ Subcutaneously tunneled catheter. (Permission for use granted by Cook Medical Inc., Bloomington, IN.)

Implanted Vascular Access Ports

The **implanted vascular access port** is a completely closed system consisting of an implanted device with a reservoir, or port, with a self-sealing system connected to an outlet catheter. The device is surgically implanted into a convenient body site in a subcutaneous pocket. The self-sealing septum can withstand approximately 2000 needle punctures, as defined by the manufacturer. This device provides venous access for blood withdrawal and for intravenous infusions of hypertonic solutions, blood components, and chemotherapy (Fig. 5-31). The **implanted vascular access port** must be accessed with a noncoring (Huber) needle for safe and proper penetration of the septum of the port. The needles are sized from 19 to 24 gauge and range from 0.5 to 1.5 inches in length. The needles are available in 90-degree or straight-needle designs. Removal of the noncoring needle is associated with risk for needlestick injury. A safety noncoring needle system should be used (Figs. 5-32 and 5-33).

Catheter Features

Other distinctions with CVADs can be made in terms of catheter features. As noted earlier, there are choices in the number of lumens. Multiple lumens allow concurrent administration of medications and solutions, which is an

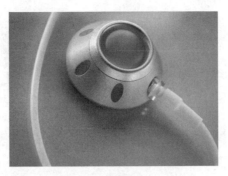

Figure 5-31 ■ Example of an implanted venous access port. (Permission for use granted by Cook Medical Inc., Bloomington, IN.)

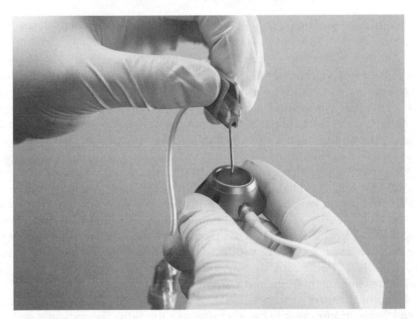

Figure 5-32 ■ View of an implanted port model showing noncoring needle access. (Permission for use granted by Cook Medical Inc., Bloomington, IN.)

advantage in the hospitalized patient who is likely to require more than one type of medication and/or I.V. solution. In addition to multilumen external catheters, two-lumen implanted ports are available. With these devices, the interior port body has two separate reservoirs to accommodate the dual-lumen catheter. With skill and knowledge, the nurse is able to palpate the two port lumens through the skin.

The device with the least number of lumens needed for the patient's infusion therapy should be selected. With multiple lumens there is more access and manipulation of the CVAD, creating the potential for microbial

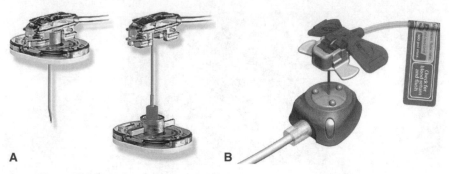

A

B

Figure 5-33 ■ *A*, SafeStep® Huber needle set. Needle locks into plastic base upon removal. *B*, PowerLoc® Safety infusion set used with power implanted port for power injection. (© 2013 C.R. Bard, Inc. Used with permission.)

contamination and increasing the risk for catheter-associated bloodstream infection.

Another characteristic of catheters is "power injectability." A power injectable catheter can tolerate the high pressures required for rapid injection of contrast material used in computed tomographic (CT) scans. However, potential confusion and risk may result if a nonpower injectable catheter is used for that purpose, increasing the risk of catheter rupture. When planning to use a CVAD for power injection, power injection capability should be identified at the time of access and immediately prior to power injection. This is particularly important with implanted ports because there is no reliable external method for determining the type of port. Some power injection-capable ports have unique characteristics that can be identified by palpation, but palpation should not be the only identification method used. It is recommended that at least two identification methods be used, including product labeling; identification cards, wristbands, or key chains provided by the manufacturer; review of operative procedure documentation; and palpation of the port.

Another feature of some CVADs is the presence of a valve built into the catheter, either into the catheter tip or in the hub. Theoretically, with a valved catheter there is less blood reflux back into the catheter and reduced risk of catheter occlusion. The first valved catheter was designed with a closed internal catheter tip with a valve near the tip (Groshong, Bard Access, Salt Lake City, UT). This valve appears as a "slit" in the catheter that only opens when infusing or withdrawing blood. With the hub-based valve, a disk opens inward on infusion and outward when withdrawing blood (PASV, Boston Scientific, Natick, MA). The manufacturers' instructions for both of these valved catheters state that the catheters do not require heparin to maintain patency and that 0.9% sodium chloride (i.e., normal saline) should be used.

Lastly, some CVADs are impregnated or coated with antiseptic or antimicrobial agents such as chlorhexidine and silver sulfadiazine (CHSS), minocycline and rifampin (MR), or silver. These catheters are not recommended for routine use but should be used in hospitals that have higher rates of infection, in patients with limited venous access and a history of recurrent catheter-associated infections, in facilities where bloodstream infection rates remain high even after implementation of standard evidence-based practices (e.g., central line bundle; see Chapter 9), or in patients who are at heightened risk for severe consequences from an infection, such as those with prosthetic heart valves (O'Grady et al., 2011).

Flow-Control Devices

Historically, control of the I.V. rate was regulated with a roller clamp, which the nurse adjusted manually with the roller or screw clamp on the administration set. Although roller clamp rate control is still useful in certain circumstances, numerous mechanical infusion devices and EIDs are available to assist nurses in maintaining an accurate infusion rate. The term flow-control device refers to any manual, mechanical, or electronic infusion device used to regulate the I.V. flow rate (INS, 2011, p. S104). Infusion flow control may rely on gravity or positive pressure to facilitate the flow of the infusion. Stationary pumps that are mounted on an I.V. pole and ambulatory pumps are available. The type of flow-control device used is guided by factors such as patient age, condition, type of infusion therapy, type of VAD, and care setting (INS, 2011).

Mechanical Infusion Devices

Mechanical flow-control devices use nonelectric methods to regulate the infusion rate. Manual flow regulators are devices that are built into the administration set or are separate add-on devices. They are used as an alternative to roller clamps, which are standard on administration sets. They are manually set to deliver specified volumes of fluid per hour. They are available as dials, with clocklike faces, or barrel-shaped devices with cylindrical controls. Flow markings on the dials help to approximate the drops per minute based on the set drop factor. Because these devices are gravity based, it is important to recognize that a number of factors affect the accuracy of the flow, such as patient position change or decreased volume in the solution container (Hadaway, 2010). Flow rate should be verified by counting the drops (Fig. 5-34). These devices are not a replacement for an EID but are useful in certain situations where some variation in flow rate is not critical. Examples include home infusions of subcutaneous fluids or certain antibiotics.

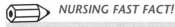 **NURSING FAST FACT!**

1psi and 50 mm Hg exert the same amount of pressure.

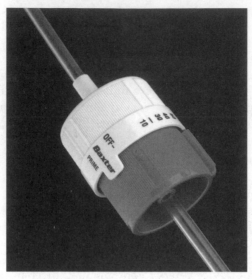

Figure 5-34 ■ Mechanical controller: Rate flow regulator. (Courtesy of Baxter Healthcare Corp., Round Lake, IL.)

Nonelectric Disposable Pumps

Nonelectric disposable infusion pumps have been in clinical use for more than 20 years. Disposable infusion pumps are used extensively in home care settings. A wide range of disposable pumps is available. Applications of disposable pumps include:

1. Continuous analgesia for postoperative pain management
2. **Patient-controlled analgesia (PCA)**
3. Delivery of chemotherapy drugs and opioids for cancer treatment
4. Delivery of antimicrobials in the home
5. Pediatric applications

All nonelectric disposable pumps exploit the same physical principles: mechanical restriction within the flow path determines the speed of pressurized fluid. The pressure on the fluid is generated by a variety of mechanisms using nonelectric power, including a stretched elastomer or compressed spring. The restriction of flow in all disposable pumps is caused by narrow-bore tubing. Tubing diameter has a determining influence on the device's flow rate.

Elastomeric Infusion Pumps

The **elastomeric pump** system is a portable device with an elastomeric reservoir, or balloon. The balloon, which is made of a soft rubberized material capable of being inflated to a predetermined volume, is safely encapsulated inside a rigid, transparent container. When the reservoir is filled, the balloon exerts positive pressure to administer the medication with an integrated flow restrictor that controls the flow rate. This system requires no batteries or electronic programming and is not reusable (Fig. 5-35).

Elastomeric balloon devices are used most often in home or outpatient settings. They may be used to deliver a variety of infusion therapies including I.V. antibiotics, chemotherapy, and analgesics. Volumes for these devices range from 50 to 250 mL. Elastomeric pumps infuse at rates of 0.5 to 500 mL/hr.

ADVANTAGES

- Portability
- Simplicity
- Disposable

DISADVANTAGES

- Cold infusates slow infusion rate; infusion solutions should be at room temperature.
- Viscosity of fluid will have an inverse effect on flow rate.
- Atmospheric pressure can affect flow accuracy.
- Changing the pump's position relative to the infusion site might affect accuracy.

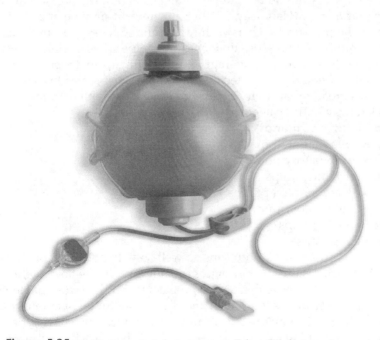

Figure 5-35 ■ Elastomeric infusion pump. Eclipse™ elastomeric pump. (Courtesy of Kimberly-Clark, Neenah, WI.)

■ Partial filling of a disposable pump can affect the internal pressure of an elastomeric balloon.

Additional nonelectric disposable pumps include spring-powered infusion pumps, negative-pressure infusion pumps, and disposable PCA pumps.

> **NURSING FAST FACT!**
>
> *Allow nonelectric infusion pumps to warm after storage and before infusion for accurate flow rate.*

Electronic Infusion Devices

Electronic infusion devices (EIDs) are powered by electricity or battery and are programmed to regulate the I.V. flow rate in either drops per minute or milliliters per hour. EIDs use positive pressure to deliver the infusion. The normal pumping pressure is slightly lower than the occlusion pressure. Some pumps have a preset or fixed occlusion pressure, whereas others allow the nurse to change the occlusion pressure.

It is important to recognize that occlusion pressures are a safety feature, and nurses should be cautious when changing the pressure to avoid setting off alarms (Hadaway, 2010). Sometimes it may be appropriate to increase the pressure, such as with high-volume high-pressure infusions, arterial infusions, and those delivered in a hyperbaric chamber. Positive-pressure infusion pumps average 10 psi, with up to 15 psi considered to be safe, although newer technology has the psi set as low as 0.1 psi. Pressures greater than 15 to 20 psi should be used with extreme caution.

Hadaway (2010) categorizes EIDs as follows:
■ Volumetric pumps
  ■ Pole-mounted pumps
  ■ Ambulatory pumps
■ Peristaltic pumps
  ■ Pole-mounted pumps
  ■ Ambulatory pumps
■ Syringe pumps
■ PCA pumps

EIDs are used in I.V. infusions as well as with subcutaneous, arterial, and epidural infusions. These devices provide an accurate flow rate, are easy to use, and have alarms that signal problems with the infusion. However, regular assessment, responsibility, and accountability for safe infusion still lie with the professional nurse. To use these devices effectively, the nurse should know (1) indications for their use, (2) their mechanical operation, (3) how to troubleshoot, (4) their psi rating, and (5) safe usage guidelines.

Volumetric Pumps

Volumetric pumps calculate the volume delivered by measuring the volume displaced in a reservoir that is part of the disposable administration set. The pump calculates every fill and empty cycle of the reservoir. The reservoir is manipulated internally by a specific action of the pump. The industry standard for the accuracy of electronic volumetric infusion pumps is ±5%, although some have even better accuracy of ±2% (Hadaway, 2010). All volumetric pumps require special tubing.

 NURSING FAST FACT!

To ensure safe, efficient operation, review the literature that accompanies the pump to become familiar with the operation of the pump. Observe all precautions.

 NURSING FAST FACT!

All positive-pressure pumps should have an "anti–free-flow" alarm to prevent inadvertent free-flowing solution.

Peristaltic Pumps

Peristaltic refers to the controlling mechanisms: a peristaltic device moves fluid by intermittently squeezing the I.V. tubing. The device may be rotary or linear. In a rotary peristaltic pump, a rotating disk or series of rollers compresses the tubing along a curved or semicircular chamber, propelling the fluid when pressure is released. In a linear device, one or more projections intermittently press the I.V. tubing. Peristaltic pumps are used primarily for infusion of enteral feedings.

Ambulatory Pumps

Ambulatory pumps are lightweight, compact infusion pumps. They have made a significant breakthrough in long-term care. These devices allow the patient freedom to resume a normal life. Ambulatory pumps range in size and weight; most weigh less than 6 pounds and are capable of delivering most infusion therapies. Features include medication delivery, delivery of several different dose sizes at different intervals, memory of programs, and safety alarms. The main disadvantage of ambulatory pumps is limited power supply; they function on a battery system that requires recharging or replacement of disposable batteries (Fig. 5-36).

Syringe Pumps

Syringe pumps are pumps that use a traditional syringe as the solution container, which is filled with prescribed medication and positioned in a

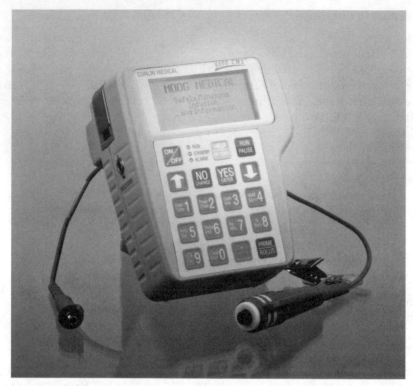

Figure 5-36 ■ Ambulatory pump: 6000CMS Ambulatory electronic infusion device. Capable of infusion modes including continuous infusion, patient-controlled analgesia, patient-controlled epidural analgesia, subcutaneous infusion, total parenteral nutrition, and intermittent infusions. (Courtesy of Moog Medical Devices Group, Salt Lake City, UT.)

special pump designed to hold it. Syringe pumps are piston-driven infusion pumps that provide precise infusion by controlling the rate by drive speed and syringe size, thus eliminating the variables of the drop rate. Syringe pumps are valuable for critical infusions of small doses of high-potency drugs. They are precisely accurate delivery systems that can be used to administer very small volumes. Some models have program modes capable of administration in milligrams per kilogram per minute, micrograms per minute, and milliliters per hour. The syringe is filled in the pharmacy and stored until used.

These pumps are used most frequently for delivery of antibiotics and small-volume parenteral therapy. Syringe pump technology is available for PCA infusion devices. Syringe pumps are used frequently in the areas of anesthesia, oncology, pediatrics, home care, and obstetrics.

The volume of the syringe pump is limited to the size of the syringe; a 60-mL syringe is usually used. However, the syringe can be as small as 5 mL. The tubing usually is a single, uninterrupted length of kink-resistant tubing with a notable lack of Y injection ports. Syringe pumps can use primary or secondary sets, depending on the intended use (Fig. 5-37).

Patient-Controlled Analgesia Pumps

PCA pumps are used for pain management in the acute care setting, long-term care, hospice, and home. PCA pumps can be used to deliver medication via the I.V., subcutaneous, and intraspinal routes. These pumps are unique from other EIDs in that a remote bolus control allows the patient to deliver a bolus of medication at set intervals by pressing a button on a cord. PCA pumps are available in ambulatory or pole-mounted models and, as mentioned earlier, PCA technology is available with syringe pumps as well.

The PCA pump can be programmed to deliver a continuous infusion, a demand infusion, or both. All three afford pain control with varying degrees of patient interaction. Some pumps offer oxygen saturation monitoring, which sets off alarms and potentially stops the infusion in the event of hypoxemia (Fig. 5-38).

- The continuous infusion is designed for patients who need maximum pain relief without the need for on-demand dosing. It usually does not fluctuate from hour to hour and should relieve pain with a constant effect.
- The demand mode infusion dose is delivered by intermittent infusion when a button attached to the pump is pushed. The demand dose can be used alone or with a continuous basal type of infusion.
- The basal mode refers to the continuous delivery of pain medicine in conjunction with the demand mode. Should the patient require additional pain medication, for example, as associated with increased activity or a painful procedure, the demand dose is delivered in conjunction with the basal rate.

 NURSING FAST FACT!

PCA pumps must be programmed with parameters to prevent overmedication. These pumps are designed with a special key or locking device for security of the medications.

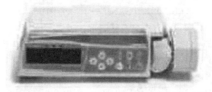

Figure 5-37 ■ Perfusor® Space Syringe Pump. (Courtesy of B. Braun, Bethlehem, PA.)

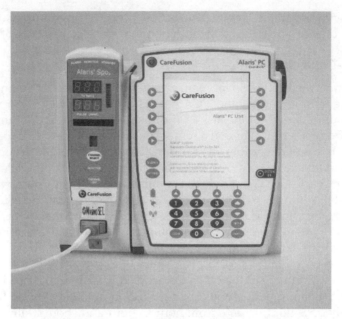

Figure 5-38 ■ Alaris® PCA pump with SpO_2 monitoring. (Courtesy of Care-Fusion, San Diego, CA.)

INS Standard The nurse should assess the patient for appropriateness of PCA therapy and the patient's comprehension of, and ability to participate in, the intended therapy.

The RN should have knowledge of appropriate drugs that can be used with PCA, including their pharmacokinetics and equianalgesic dosing, contraindications, side effects and their management, appropriate administration modalities, and anticipated outcomes (INS, 2011, pp. S89-S90).

Multichannel Pumps

Multiple-drug delivery systems are computer generated, and many use computer-generated technology. **Multichannel pumps** can deliver several medications and fluids simultaneously at multiple rates from bags, bottles, or syringes. Multichannel pumps (usually with two to four channels) require manifold-type sets to set up all channels, whether or not they are in use; each channel must be programmed independently. Programming a multichannel pump can be challenging (Fig. 5-39).

Dual-channel pumps offer a two-pump mechanism assembly, with a common control and programming panel. This type of pump uses one administration set for each channel.

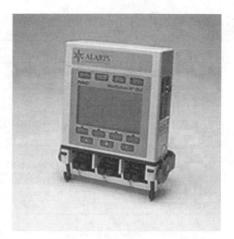

Figure 5-39 ■ Alaris® multichannel pump. (Courtesy of CareFusion, San Diego, CA.)

Smart Pumps

Smart pumps are EIDs with an imbedded computer system. The computer software is aimed at reducing drug dosing errors through the presence and use of a drug library. The drug library must be individualized to the organization's medications and dosing limits. The organization must also make decisions related to whether the programmer (e.g., nurse) can override the dosing limits. Major issues related to the effectiveness of smart pumps include lack of compliance with proper pump use, which prevents the ability to determine how effective they are in medication error prevention (Hertzel & Souza, 2009). Features of smart pumps are listed in Table 5-1.

Smart pumps are not without limitations. The accuracy of information entered into the smart pump (e.g., patient weight) is dependent on correct data. If the nurse bypasses the drug library and manually enters the infusion rate and volume, the dose error reduction software will not be able to identify potential errors (ISMP, 2009). The implementation of independent double checking of drug prescription and data entry remains important for certain high-risk medications. If there are many drug concentrations to choose from, for example, the risk for selecting the wrong concentration is increased (ISMP, 2009).

Smart pump technology is incorporated into the pumps shown in Figures 5-38 and 5-39.

INS Standard Dose-error reduction systems shall be considered in the selection and use of EIDs. Only EIDs with administration set-based anti–free-flow mechanisms shall be used (INS, 2011, p. S34).

> Table 5-1   SMART PUMP FEATURES

Feature	Description
Drug library	Includes drug names, concentrations, dosing units, hard and soft dose limits Maximum rates, volumes
Soft limit	An alert that can be overridden by the user Medication can still be infused without changing the smart pump settings
Hard limit	An alert that cannot be overridden by the user Indicates that the dose is out of the organization's safe range
Clinical advisory	An alert that prompts the nurse to consider actions that are relevant to the medication, such as prompting the use of a certain type of tubing or the use of a filter
Pump logs	Data are continuously collected, including alerts, medications, programmed doses, actions taken Useful in quality improvement efforts
Continuous display	Drug name and dosage displayed on screen at all times

 NURSING FAST FACT!

Because of the many pumps on the market, it is important to refer to the manufacturer's recommendations for setup and troubleshooting guidelines of each EID.

Electronic Infusion Devices: Pump Programming

EIDs must be programmed based on the parameters of the specific infusion therapy. The nurse typically programs the pump at the bedside. In some settings, such as home care, the pharmacist often enters the program prior to dispensing the EID to the home. Parameters include:

- *Rate:* Amount of time over which a specific volume of fluid is delivered. Infusion pumps deliver in increments of milliliters per hour. The most common rate parameters for regular infusion pumps are 1 to 999 mL/hr. Many newer pumps are capable of setting rates that offer parameters of 0.1 mL in increments of 0.1 to 99.9 mL, then in 1-mL increments up to 999 mL. Many newer pumps are capable of setting rates that satisfy both regular infusion and microinfusion needs. Some pumps offer combination rates that do not allow the rate to be set above 99.9 without a deliberate act to enter the adult values.
- *Volume infused:* Measurement that tells how much of a given solution has been infused. This measurement is used to monitor the amount of fluid infused in a shift. It can also be used in home

health to monitor the infusion periodically during the day or over several days. The "counter" is generally returned to 0 at the beginning of each shift.

■ *Volume to be infused:* Usually the amount of solution hanging in the solution container. A pump is designed to sound an alarm when the volume to be infused is reached.

■ *Tapering or ramping:* These terms are used to describe the progressive increase or decrease of the infusion rate. Tapered infusion rates are often used with parenteral nutrition infusions that are administered over part of each day (e.g., 14 hours per day). Tapering at the beginning or end of the infusion allows a more gradual infusion, allowing the body to adjust to high glucose and electrolyte concentrations. The pump mathematically calculates the ramping rate once the duration of infusion and total volume to be infused are entered into the program.

■ *Timed infusion:* This refers to an infusion governed by a 24-hour clock within the device. With timed infusion, the device must have a sufficient internal backup battery to maintain the clock accurately at all times. Timed infusions are used for ramping and tapering, automatic piggybacking, and intermittent dosing.

Alarm Terminology

■ *Air-in-line:* Designed to detect air in the line and may include air detection and air removal.

■ *Occlusion:* Detects absence of fluid flowing upstream (between pump and the infusion container) or downstream (between the patient and the pump).

■ *Infusion complete:* Alarm triggered by a preset volume limit ("infusion complete"). These alarms are helpful in preventing the fluid container from running dry because they can be set to sound before the entire solution container is infused.

■ *Low battery or low power:* Gives the user ample warning of the pump's impending inability to function. A low-battery alarm means that the batteries need to be replaced or an external power source needs to be connected. As a protective measure, when low-battery and low-power alarms are continued over a preset number of minutes, the pumps usually convert to a keep-vein-open (KVO) rate. The preset KVO rate is usually between 0.1 and 5 mL.

■ *Nonfunctional or malfunctional:* Alarm that means the pump is operating outside parameters and the problem cannot be resolved. When this alarm sounds, the pump should be disconnected from the patient and returned to biomedical engineering or to the manufacturer for evaluation. The alert signifying a nonfunctional alarm may be worded in many ways, depending on the manufacturer.

■ *Not infusing:* Indicates that all of the pump infusion parameters are not set. This feature prevents tampering or accidental setting changes. The pump must be programmed or changed and then told to "start."

■ *Tubing:* Ensures that the correct tubing has been loaded into the pump. If tubing is incorrectly loaded, this alarm will sound.

■ *Door:* Indicates that the door that secures the tubing is not closed. Cassette pumps may give a "cassette" alarm if the cassette is unable to infuse within device operating parameters.

 NURSING FAST FACT!

In a number of EIDs, the pressure is "user" selectable from 0.10 to 10 psi. Occlusion alarms at low psi settings are common because the pumps are sensitive to even slight changes in pressure and very small I.V. catheter or patient movement. Many of the current EIDs infuse fluids using very low infusion pressures, often lower than the pressure of a gravity delivery. These devices are not, however, designed to detect infiltrations. When an infiltration occurs, the inline pressure may actually drop; therefore, the EID will not detect the infiltration. Visual monitoring of the I.V. site by the nurse is mandatory for patients with EIDs.

Many other functions have been added to newer pumps. These include:

■ Preprogrammed drug compatibility
■ Retrievable patient history data
■ Central venous pressure monitor
■ Positive-pressure fill stroke
■ Modular self-diagnosing capability
■ Printer readout
■ Nurse call system
■ Remote site programming
■ Syringe use for secondary infusion
■ Adjustable occlusion pressures
■ Secondary rate settings
■ Lock level for security
■ Barcoding

Infusion Pump Safety

Because better infusion pump design and engineering can reduce infusion pump problems, the U.S. Food and Drug Administration (FDA) launched an initiative in 2010 to address safety issues related to infusion pumps. From 2005 through 2009, the FDA received approximately 56,000 reports of adverse events associated with the use of infusion pumps, including numerous injuries and deaths (FDA, 2010). These adverse event reports and associated device recalls have not been isolated to a specific manufacturer, type of infusion pump, or use environment; rather, they have occurred across the board. Causes of these adverse events include user errors and deficiencies in design and engineering, such as software defects and mechanical and electrical failures. The FDA provides guidance to the nurse to reduce infusion pump risks (Table 5-2).

> Table 5-2	INFUSION PUMP RISK REDUCTION STRATEGIES FOR CLINICIANS
Plan ahead	Have a backup plan in case of an infusion pump failure that details: ■ How to obtain a working infusion pump and infusion tubing quickly when caring for high-acuity patients. ■ How to handle high-risk infusions when the infusion pump fails. This may include staying with and closely monitoring the patient while another staff member obtains a working infusion pump if one is not readily available. ■ How to handle infusions when the infusion pump fails in vulnerable patient populations (e.g., individuals sensitive to fluid overload). This may include clamping and disconnecting the infusion tubing from the patient to prevent overinfusion prior to obtaining a new infusion pump. Participate in educational activities designed to promote the safe use of infusion pumps. Consider a secondary method of checking the expected volume infused, such as a time strip indicator or a buretrol.
Label	Label the infusion pump channels with the name of the medication or fluid if your infusion pump does not display the name. Label the infusion pump tubing at the port of entry with the medication or fluid name.
Check	Verify that the infusion pump is programmed for the right dosage, at the right rate and volume to be infused. This is especially important at a change of shift, when any change is made to the infusion pump settings, when a new bag of medication/fluid is hung, or when new infusion tubing is primed. Obtain an independent double-check of infusion pump settings by a second clinician per your hospital/facility policy when infusing high-risk medications (e.g., insulin, heparin, vasopressors, Diprivan, total parenteral nutrition, morphine, etc.). An independent double-check involves two clinicians separately checking (alone and apart from each other, then comparing results) the infusion settings in accordance with the physician's order. Monitor for signs of overinfusion or underinfusion of high-risk medications by using other patient monitoring systems, such as cardiac monitoring, pulse oximetry, end-tidal CO_2 measurement, and glucose meters, when applicable. Monitor the patient and infusion per your facility's protocol.

Continued

> Table 5-2	INFUSION PUMP RISK REDUCTION STRATEGIES FOR CLINICIANS—cont'd
Use	Use available resources, such as your Clinical/Biomedical Engineering Department, your area's "super-users," and infusion pump instructions or troubleshooting guides, when experiencing problems with an infusion pump. Use the drug library when applicable. Promptly respond and pay close attention to displayed alerts and cautions. Use the "five rights" for safe medication administration: the right patient, the right drug, the right dose, the right route, and the right time.
Report problems	Remove from use, tag with the specific problem and clinician contact information, and sequester any infusion pump that shows signs of breakage or damage, including small chips or cracks, if an unexplained alarm occurs or if the pump does not function as expected. Follow your hospital/facility protocol for reporting events where the infusion pump may have caused or contributed to a death or serious injury. You are also encouraged to report any other infusion pump safety concerns through your hospital/facility protocol. You are encouraged to file a voluntary report with the U.S. Food and Drug Administration (FDA) for any pump problem that you may encounter. Health Insurance Portability and Accountability Act of 1996 (HIPAA) restrictions do not apply to reports submitted to the FDA.

Source: www.fda.gov/MedicalDevices/ProductsandMedicalProcedures/GeneralHospitalDevicesandSupplies/ InfusionPumps/ucm205406.htm

NURSING POINTS OF CARE

MANAGEMENT OF INFUSION EQUIPMENT

Focus Assessment
- Appropriate supplies and equipment used in administration of infusion therapy
- Appropriate VAD for length and type of therapy
- Safety issues related to infusion pumps

Key Nursing Interventions
1. Monitor the patient and the infusion system for:
   a. Breaks in the integrity of the infusion equipment.
   b. Patient's knowledge of equipment.
2. Help the patient and/or family identify potential areas of conflict; for example, cultural mores or cost.
3. Select and prepare the appropriate administration set and appropriate add-on devices.
4. Use filters when appropriate.

5. Inspect fluid containers, administration sets, and cannulas for integrity before use.
6. Select and prepare infusion pumps as indicated.
7. Follow the manufacturer's guidelines on the setup and maintenance of specific EIDs.
8. Set alarm limits on equipment as appropriate.
9. Respond to equipment alarms appropriately.
10. Consult with other health-care team members and recommend equipment and devices for patient use.
11. Compare machine-derived data with nurse's perception of the patient's condition.
12. Follow INS Standards of Practice in solution container, administration set, and add-on device changes.
13. Maintain the integrity of the infusion site and equipment at all times.

Developing and Participating in Product Evaluation

Product Problem Reporting

The FDA regulates products in the United States, including over-the-counter and prescription drugs and pharmaceuticals, food, cosmetics, veterinary products, biological devices, and medical devices. A medical device is defined as any instrument, apparatus, or other article that is used to prevent, diagnose, mitigate, or treat a disease or to affect the structure or function of the body, with the exception of drugs.

Nurses use many medical devices and are usually the primary reporters of device problems. The Safe Medical Device Act of 1990 imposed significant reporting requirements on the medical device industry and users of medical devices. Medical device reporting is the mechanism for the FDA to receive information about adverse events from manufacturers and user facilities (e.g., hospitals and nursing homes). As discussed earlier, the reporting of adverse events associated with infusion pumps led to the FDA's 2010 initiative to improve infusion pump safety. Any deaths related to the medical device must be reported to both the FDA and the device manufacturer, whereas serious injury (life-threatening, permanent functional impairment/body structure damage, intervention required to prevent damage) must be reported to the device manufacturer (FDA, 1996).

Nurses play a critical role in reporting adverse events. When a device failure is noted, it is important to follow the following steps:

1. Identify previously recorded lot numbers and expiration dates of products.

2. If possible, retain sample and return to manufacturer to aid in investigation of failure.
3. Complete an unusual occurrence report.
4. Inform the supervisor.
5. Notify the Risk Management Department.

It is the responsibility of the organization's risk management department to notify the manufacturer and the FDA. Completion of these steps satisfies the legal requirement of identifying and reporting products that may have caused a patient harm.

Product Selection and Evaluation

The infusion nurse plays an important role in product selection and evaluation. Ongoing evaluation of new products and those products in current use is important in the delivery of high-quality patient care. The infusion nurse specialist's participation with his or her colleagues from other departments enhances commitment to the specialty and to the facility. Participation in product evaluation is an ongoing responsibility of professional practitioners.

Inappropriate use of medical devices may contribute to pain and suffering. The act of "jerry-rigging" or otherwise manipulating a device to overcome a small problem results in liability for problems arising from use of that piece of equipment in the institution. For example, as discussed earlier in relation to smart infusion pumps, the problem of bypassing the drug library is a concern because the computer software will not be able to identify potential errors. The law states that the responsibility shifts to the institution when a practitioner interferes with the design of a piece of equipment.

Certainly, not all medical device problems are serious as defined by the FDA, but many are significant to clinical practice. The following are examples of medical device problems related to infusion therapy practice:

- Loose or leaking catheter hubs
- Defective infusion pumps
- Misleading labeling
- Inadequate packaging
- Cracked or leaking I.V. solution bag

INS Standard All infusion equipment and supplies shall be inspected for product integrity before, during, and after use. Product integrity shall be determined by verification of the expiration date, if applicable, and visual inspection of the product. If the integrity is compromised, or expiration date passed, it shall not be used (INS, 2011, p. S23).

Websites

http://www.fda.gov/MedicalDevices/Safety/ReportaProblem/
default.htm#1
www.ecri.org/PatientSafety

> **INS Standard** The nurse shall be involved in the evaluation of infusion-related technologies, including attention to clinical application, expected outcomes, performance, infection prevention, safety, efficacy, reliability, and cost (INS, 2011, p. S23).

 ## Home Care Issues

Equipment and supplies used in home care management may include:

- Vascular access devices (VADs): Required for home infusion therapy; the most common VAD used in home care is the peripherally inserted central catheter (PICC).
- Infusion administration supplies: I.V. administration sets, needleless connectors, alcohol wipes, site care kits including antiseptic agent, sterile gloves, mask, dressings, and tape
- Infusion delivery systems: Syringe pumps, elastomeric infusion pumps, ambulatory pumps
- Premixed medications including prefilled saline/heparin syringes for flushing

Ambulatory infusion pumps are designed to allow the patient maximum portability and freedom of movement. The aim is small, quiet, lightweight infusion pumps with pouches that enclose both the pump and the infusion container. Equipment and supplies used at home must offer safety features, because the patient or a caregiver are expected to participate in the patient's care.

It is important to assess factors that affect the patient's ability to learn how to use and safely manage life with an infusion pump. Various factors may affect the ability to learn, including physical status (e.g., pain, weakness, fatigue), mental status (e.g., stress, diagnosis), manual dexterity and coordination, cognition (e.g., forgetfulness), willingness to learn, and literacy. Problematic issues should be addressed in the plan of care; involvement of a willing caregiver may be appropriate. Environmental factors may affect learning and success of home infusion therapy. Some examples include the following:

- Poor lighting affects ability to see pump display.
- Noise and/or hearing impairment affects ability to hear alarms.
- Clutter may affect ability to maneuver within home and protect pump from food and drink.

The home care nurse must address such challenges and consider ways to mitigate home/patient limitations.

NOTE > Reimbursement is an important issue to be addressed while planning for home care. The home care agency and the home infusion pharmacy are resources for reimbursement questions and will assess and verify reimbursement sources, and potential patient co-payments, before providing home care. There may be limits on the number of home visits that the insurance company will cover.

Patient Education

Patient education in the hospital and home care settings is necessary for patient safety and to decrease anxiety related to highly technical equipment. The following is important in equipment education:

■ Instruct the patient by demonstrating the preparation and administration of therapy.
■ Teach the patient and family how to operate equipment, as appropriate.
■ Have patient demonstrate how to use equipment safely.
■ Teach the patient about pump alarms and actions to take.
■ Make sure home care patients have 24-hour telephone number (home care agency, home infusion pharmacy) to call about any problems or issues related to the infusion or access device.
■ Instruct the patient on how to use the demand dose function with PCA pumps for pain control.
■ Teach the patient and family the expected patient outcomes and any potential problems associated with using the equipment.
■ Document the patient's and family's understanding of the education provided to them.

■ Nursing Process

The nursing process is a six-step process for problem-solving to guide nursing action. Refer to Chapter 1 for details on the steps of the nursing process. The following table focuses on nursing diagnoses, nursing outcomes classification (NOC), and nursing intervention classification (NIC) for patients using infusion equipment. Nursing diagnoses should be patient specific and outcomes and interventions individualized. The NOC and NIC presented here are suggested directions for development of outcomes and interventions.

Nursing Diagnoses Related to Management of Infusion Equipment	NOC: Nursing Outcomes Classification	NIC: Nursing Intervention Classification
Anxiety (mild, moderate, or severe) related to: Situational crises (new equipment technology); role function; environment	Anxiety level, anxiety self-control, coping	Anxiety reduction techniques
Knowledge deficit related to: Equipment: Unfamiliarity with information resources, cognitive limitation, and information misinterpretation	Knowledge: Procedure (equipment use), health resources	Teaching: Use written educational materials, demonstrate equipment with return demonstration, observe ability and readiness to learn
Injury, risk for (external) related to: Physical environmental conditions: Equipment	Patient safety behavior Safe home environment	Accuracy of patient identification Effectiveness of communication Medication safety Education on equipment

Source: Ackley & Ladwig (2011); Bulechek, Butcher, Dochterman, & Wagner (2013); Moorhead, Johnson, Maas, & Swanson (2013).

Chapter Highlights

- Types of solution containers include glass containers, plastic containers, and syringes.
- Check all solutions for clarity and expiration date. Squeeze to check for leaks, floating particles, and clarity.
- Concerns over DEHP: The plasticizer phthalate (DEHP) is added to some PVC plastics for flexibility. DEHP is a toxin and can leach into particularly lipid-based I.V. solutions. Non-DEHP products are available.
- Administration sets
  - Single-line sets: Most frequently used; follow INS standards for frequency of set changes. Available in vented and nonvented sets.
  - Primary (standard) sets, volume-controlled sets
  - Primary Y sets
  - Pump-specific sets: Used with EIDs.
  - Lipid administration sets: Used with fat emulsion, which are supplied in glass containers with special vented tubing.
  - Specialty sets: e.g., nitroglycerin administration sets
  - Blood administration sets
- Filters
  - Inline I.V. solution filters
  - Depth: Filters in which pore size is not uniform
  - Membrane (screen): Air-venting, bacteria-retentive, 0.22-micron filter

- Blood filters include standard clot: 170 to 220 microns; used on blood administration sets to remove coagulated products, microclots, and debris, microaggregates, and leukocyte depletion.
- Stopcocks
  - Control the direction of flow of an infusate through manual manipulation of a direction regulation valve. Are sources of contamination and potential bloodstream infection; their use should be avoided.
- Needleless connectors
  - Attach to the hub of the catheter and convert the catheter into an intermittent device
- Peripheral I.V. catheters
  - Stainless steel winged needles: For single dose infusions; odd-numbered gauges
  - Over-the-needle catheters: Most common type of device used; even-numbered gauges
  - Midline catheters: Placed in area of antecubital fossa; for infusion therapy duration 1 to 4 weeks
- Central vascular access devices (CVADs):
  - Nontunneled catheters: Short-term CVAD used primarily in acute care settings.
  - Peripherally inserted central catheters (PICCs): Inserted peripherally and threaded to the SVC; can be placed by physicians or nurses.
  - Subcutaneously tunneled catheters: Long-term catheters
  - Implanted vascular access ports: Closed system composed of implanted device with reservoir, port, and self-sealing system; requires use of a noncoring needle to access port.
- Flow-control devices
  - Mechanical infusion devices: Nonelectric methods such as mechanical flow devices and elastomeric infusion pumps.
  - Electronic infusion devices (EIDs): Powered by electricity/battery; includes volumetric pumps, syringe pumps, patient-controlled analgesia (PCA) pumps.
  - PCA: Can be used at home or in hospital to deliver pain medication.
  - Multichannel pumps: EIDs that can deliver several medications and fluids simultaneously.
  - Ambulatory infusion pumps: EIDs that can be carried in a pouch; used primarily in home infusion therapy.
  - Smart pumps: EIDs with an embedded computer system including a drug library.
  - Syringe: Piston-driven pump that controls rate of infusion by drive speed and syringe size.
  - Peristaltic: Calibrated in milliliters per hour; used primarily for delivery of enteral feedings; have a rotary disk or rollers to compress tubing.

- Product evaluation: When a device failure is noted, it is important to follow the following steps.
    - Identify previously recorded lot numbers and expiration dates of products.
    - Complete a designated internal report.
    - Inform the supervisor.
    - Notify the Risk Management Department.
    - Note problem.
    - Identity name, title, and practice specialty of the device's user.

■■ Thinking Critically: Case Study

A 45-year-old postoperative hysterectomy patient has an order to convert her continuous I.V. to a Luer-activated needleless connector.

Case Study Questions
1. *What are the steps in flushing this device? Note: Refer to Chapter 6 for procedure.*
2. *What infection prevention technique should be used prior to accessing the needleless connector with each catheter access?*

 Media Link: Answers to the case study and more critical thinking activities are provided on Davis*Plus*.

Post-Test

1. Match the term in Column I with the definition in Column II.

Column I	Column II
A. Cannula	a. A female connection point of an I.V. cannula where the tubing or other equipment attaches
B. Drip chamber	b. Point of entry
C. Lumen	c. Area of the I.V. tubing usually found under the spike where the solution drips and collects
D. Hub	d. Space within an artery, vein, or catheter
E. Port	e. A tube used for infusing fluids; also called a catheter

2. When using a flexible plastic system, what type of administration set could you choose?
   a. Vented
   b. Nonvented
   c. Vented or nonvented; both work with this system

3. A disadvantage of the glass solution containers is that it:
   a. Is breakable and difficult to store.
   b. Reacts with some solutions and medications.
   c. May be difficult to read fluid levels.
   d. May develop leaks.

4. Which of the following situations would be appropriate for a 0.22-micron filter? (*Select all that apply.*)
   a. Low-volume medication
   b. Red blood cell transfusion
   c. Infusion of 10% dextrose and amino acids via central line
   d. Total parenteral nutrition with lipids

5. The standard blood administration set has a clot filter of how many microns?
   a. 170
   b. 40
   c. 20
   d. 10

6. Microaggregate filters are used to:
   a. Administer protein solutions
   b. Reinfuse shed autologous blood
   c. Remove bacteria for infusion
   d. Filter air from the set

7. New research supports which of the following techniques to prevent infections with needleless connectors?
   a. Scrubbing needleless connectors prior to access
   b. Use of alcohol disinfection caps
   c. Leaving needleless connectors in place until the I.V. catheter is disconnected
   d. Use of negative displacement systems

8. Which of the following reduce the risk for needlestick injuries?
   a. Elastomeric pumps
   b. Luer-locks
   c. Needleless systems
   d. Three-way stopcocks

9. The limit to operating pressure at which an alarm is triggered on an electronic infusion device is known as:
   a. Air-in-line alarm
   b. Parameters or timed out
   c. Occlusion alarm
   d. Not infusing alarm

10. The nurse identifies errors in programming an infusion pump. What should the nurse do? (*Select all that apply.*)

  a. Report the device malfunction to the supervisor.
  b. Fill out appropriate hospital form.
  c. Notify Emergency Care Research Institute (ECRI) on appropriate form.
  d. Notify the Risk Manager.

Media Link: Answers to the Chapter 5 Post-Test and more test questions together with rationales are provided on Davis*Plus*.

■ References

Ackley, B. J., & Ladwig, G. B. (2011). *Nursing diagnosis handbook: An evidence-based guide to planning care* (9th ed). St. Louis, MO: Mosby Elsevier.

Alekseyev, S., Byrne, M., Carpenter, A., Franker, C., Kidd, C., & Hulton, L. (2012). Prolonging the life of a patient's IV: An integrative review of intravenous securement devices. *MedSurg Nursing, 21*(5), 285-292.

Alexander, M., Gorski, L. A., Corrigan, A., & Phillips, L. (2013). Technical and clinical application. In M. Alexander, A. Corrigan, L. Gorski, & L. Phillips (Eds.). *Core curriculum for infusion nursing,* 4th ed. Lippincott Williams & Wilkins, Philadelphia. (pp. i-xx).

Bulechek, G. M., Butcher, H. K., Dochterman, J. M., & Wagner, C. M. (2013). *Nursing interventions classification (NIC)* (6th ed.). St. Louis, MO: Elsevier Mosby.

Chiao, F. B., Resta-Flarer, F., Lesser, J., Ng, J., Ganz, A., Pino-Luey, D., ... Witek, B. (2013). Vein visualization: Patient characteristic factors and efficacy of a new infrared vein finder technology. *British Journal of Anaesthesia, 110* (6), 966-971.

Egan, G. M., Siskin, G.P., Weinmann, R. & Galloway, M. M. (2013). A prospective post-market study to evaluate the safety and efficacy of a new peripherally inserted central catheter stabilization system. *Journal of Infusion Nursing, 36* (3), 181-188.

Food and Drug Administration (FDA). (1996). *Medical device reporting for user facilities.* Retrieved from http://www.fda.gov/downloads/MedicalDevices/DeviceRegulationandGuidance/GuidanceDocuments/UCM095266.pdf (Accessed February 21, 2013).

FDA. (2010). *White paper: Infusion pump improvement initiative.* Retrieved from http://www.fda.gov/MedicalDevices/ProductsandMedicalProcedures/GeneralHospitalDevicesandSupplies/InfusionPumps/ucm205424.htm (Accessed February 21, 2013).

Gahart, B. L., & Nazareno, A. R. (2012). *Intravenous medications* (28th ed.). St. Louis, MO: Elsevier Mosby.

Gorski, L., Perucca, R., Hunter, M. (2010). Central venous access devices: care, maintenance, and potential complications. In M. Alexander, A. Corrigan, L. Gorski, J. Hankins, & R. Perucca (Eds.), *Infusion Nursing: An evidence-based practice* (3rd ed.) (pp. 495-515). St. Louis: Saunders/Elsevier.

Hadaway, L. (2010). Infusion therapy equipment. In M. Alexander, A. Corrigan, L. Gorski, J. Hankins, & R. Perucca (Eds.), *Infusion nursing: An evidence-based practice* (3rd ed.) (pp. 391-436). St. Louis: Saunders/Elsevier.

Hadaway, L. & Richardson, D. (2010). Needleless connectors: A primer on terminology. *Journal of Infusion Nursing, 33*(1), 22-31.

Hertzel, C. & Sousa, V. D. (2009). The use of smart pumps for preventing medication errors. *Journal of Infusion Nursing, 32*(5), 257-267.

Infusion Nurses Society (INS). (2008). *The role of the registered nurse in the insertion of external jugular peripherally inserted central catheters (EJ PICC) and external jugular peripheral intravenous catheters (EJ PIV).* Position Paper. Norwood MA: Author.

INS. (2011). Infusion nursing standards of practice. *Journal of Intravenous Nursing, 34*(1S), S1-S110.

ISMP. (2009). Proceedings from the ISMP summit on the use of smart infusion pumps: guidelines for safe implementation and use. Retrieved from http://www.ismp.org/tools/guidelines/smartpumps/comments/printerVersion.pdf. Accessed August 19, 2013.

Jack, T., Boehne, M., Brent, B. E., Hoy, L., Köditz, H., Wessel, A., & Sasse, M. (2012). In-line filtration reduces severe complications and length of stay on pediatric intensive care unit: a prospective, randomized, controlled trial. *Intensive Care Medicine, 38*(6), 1008-1016.

Kaler, W., & Chinn, R. (2007). Successful disinfection of needleless access ports: A matter of time and friction. *Journal of the American Medical Association, 12*(3), 140-142.

Kambia, N., Dine, T., Gressier, B., Lucykx, M., Brunet, C., Guimber, D., ... Michaud, L. (2013). Strong variability of di(2-ethylhexyl)phthalate (DEHP) plasmatic rate in infants and children undergoing 12-hour cyclic parenteral nutrition. *Journal of Parenteral and Enteral Nutrition, 37*(2), 229-335.

Moorhead, S., Johnson, M., Maas, M., & Swanson, E. (2013). *Nursing outcomes classification (NOC)* (5th ed.). St. Louis, MO: Elsevier Mosby.

O'Grady, N. P., Alexander, M., Burns, L. A., Dellinger, E. P., Garland, J., Heard, S. O., ... Healthcare Infection Control Practices Advisory Committee (HICPAC). (2011). Guidelines for the prevention of intravascular catheter related infections, 2011. *Am J Infect Control.* 2011; 39 (4 supp): S1-S34. Also available at: http://www.cdc.gov/hicpac/pdf/guidelines/bsi-guidelines-2011.pdf. Accessed September 15, 2012.

Shaz, B. H., Grima, K., & Hillyer, C. D. (2011). 2-(diethylhexyl)phthalate in blood bags: Is this a public health issue? *Transfusion, 51*, 2510-2517.

Sink, B. L. S. (2011). Administration of blood components. In J. D. Roback, B. J. Grossman, T. Harris, & C. D. Hillyer (Eds.), *Technical manual* (17th ed.) (pp. 617-629). Bethesda, MD: American Association of Blood Banks.

Sweet, M. A., Cumpston, A. C., Briggs, F., Craig, M., & Hamadani, M. (2012). Impact of alcohol-impregnated port protectors and needleless neutral pressure connectors on central-line associated bloodstream infections and contamination of blood cultures in an inpatient oncology unit. *American Journal of Infection Control, 40*, 931-934.

Wright, M. O., Tropp, J., & Schora, D. M. (2013). Continuous passive disinfection of catheter hubs prevents contamination and bloodstream infection. *American Journal of Infection Control, 41*, 33-38.

Chapter **6**

Techniques for Initiation and Maintenance of Peripheral Infusion Therapy

It may seem a strange principle to enunciate as the very first requirement in a hospital that it should do the sick no harm. It is quite necessary to lay down such a principle.
—Florence Nightingale, 1859

Procedures Displays

LEARNING OBJECTIVES

On completion of this chapter, the reader will be able to:

1. Define the terminology related to peripheral venous access.
2. Recall the anatomy and physiology related to the venous system.
3. Describe characteristics of the two main layers of the skin.
4. Identify peripheral veins appropriate for venipuncture.
5. List the factors affecting site selection.
6. Demonstrate Phillips' 16-step approach for initiating peripheral-short infusion therapy.
7. List the three sites that require labeling.
8. Identify the key areas for documentation related to peripheral infusion therapy.
9. Recall the steps in performing a saline lock.
10. Describe strategies to reduce pain during peripheral I.V. catheter insertion.
11. Describe techniques to assist with venipuncture visualization and dilation in patients with sclerotic veins, altered skin integrity, obesity, and edema.
12. Identify physiological characteristics that differentiate infusion therapy for neonates, infants, children, and older adults.
13. Locate the most appropriate sites for venipuncture in pediatric and older adult patients.
14. Identify the types of needles and catheters available for pediatric patients.
15. Describe special considerations for successful venipuncture of neonates, infants, and older adults.

GLOSSARY

Bevel   Slanted edge on opening of a needle or cannula device

Cannulation   Introduction of a tube (e.g., I.V. catheter) through a passage (e.g., vein)

Dermis   The layer of the skin immediately below the epidermis; composed of connective tissue, blood vessels, nerves, muscles, lymphatics, hair follicles, and sebaceous/sweat glands

Distal   Farther from the heart; farthest from the point of attachment (below the previous site of cannulation)

Drop factor   The number of drops needed to deliver 1 mL of fluid

Endothelium   The single layer of cells lining the blood vessels and heart

Epidermis   The outermost layer of skin covering the body, which is composed of squamous cells and is devoid of blood vessels

Gauge   Size of a cannula (catheter) opening; gradual measurements of the outside diameter of a catheter

Macrodrop   I.V. tubing with a drop factor of 10 to 20 drops/mL

Microabrasion   Superficial break in skin integrity that may predispose the patient to infection

Microdrop   I.V. tubing with a drop factor of 60 drops/mL

Midline Catheter   A longer peripheral catheter placed in the peripheral veins, generally inserted above the antecubital fossa, with the catheter tip inserted via the basilic, cephalic, or brachial vein and the tip located below the axillary line. In infants, a midline may be placed in a scalp vein with the tip terminating in the external jugular vein.

Palpation   Examination by touch

Peripheral intravenous (PIV) catheter   Catheter inserted into the peripheral veins for delivery of short-term infusion therapies; often called a "short" PIV to differentiate from a midline

Prime   To flush the air from the administration set or any add-on devices (e.g., needleless connector) with a solution before use

Proximal   Nearest to the heart; closest point to attachment (above the previous site of cannulation)

Purpura   Discolorations on skin that do not blanch; may be caused by bleeding underneath skin

Spike   A sharp object (piercing pin) used to puncture an object (e.g., a bag of intravenous fluid) permitting fluids within the object (bag) to flow out

Transillumination   Passage of light through a solid or liquid substance for diagnostic examination

Anatomy and Physiology Related to I.V. Practice

In order to place **peripheral intravenous (PIV) catheters** with the goal of providing positive vascular access outcomes, the nurse must understand the anatomy and physiology of the skin and venous system and be familiar with the physiological responses of veins to heat, cold, and stress. It is also important for the nurse to become familiar with skin thickness and consistency at various sites to perform venous access proficiently.

Skin

The skin is an important organ of the body with major functions including protection, temperature regulation, metabolism, sensation, synthesis (e.g., synthesize vitamin D), and communication (Baranoski et al., 2012). The skin consists of two main layers, the **epidermis** and the **dermis**, which overlie the subcutaneous tissue, which is also called the hypodermis. The epidermis, composed of squamous cells that are less sensitive than underlying structures, is the first line of defense against infections. It is thin, varying between 0.05 to 1.0 mm, and is an avascular layer (Thayer, 2012). The epidermis repairs and regenerates itself every 28 days (Baranoski et al., 2012). Two types of cells are common to the epidermis: Merkel and Langerhans. Merkel cells are receptors that transmit stimuli to axons through a chemical synapse. Langerhans cells are believed to play a significant role in cutaneous immune system reactions. The epidermis is thickest on the palms of the hands and soles of the feet and is thinnest on the inner surfaces of the extremities. Thickness varies with age and exposure to the elements, such as wind and sun.

It is also important to recognize that there are many microbes that live on the epidermis including *Staphylococcus, Corynebacterium, Propionibacterium,* and many others. These normal flora are protective through competitively inhibiting less desirable organisms (Thayer, 2012).

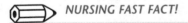 NURSING FAST FACT!

> *Prior to placing any vascular access device, skin antisepsis and hand hygiene are critical steps in minimizing any microbes on the skin (of both patient and health-care provider) to prevent device-associated infection.*

The dermis, a much thicker layer, is located directly below the epidermis. The dermis consists of blood vessels, hair follicles, sweat glands, sebaceous glands, small muscles, and nerve endings. As with the epidermis, the thickness of the dermis varies with age and physical condition. The skin is a special-sense touch organ, and the dermis reacts quickly to painful stimuli, temperature changes, and pressure sensation. As a result of the extensive network of nerves in the dermal layer, the patient feels pain during the venipuncture procedure.

The hypodermis, or subcutaneous tissue, attaches the dermis to underlying structures. Its function is to promote an ongoing blood supply to the dermis (Baranoski et al., 2012). The hypodermis consists primarily of adipose tissue, which provides a cushion between the layers of the skin, bones, and muscles (Fig. 6-1).

Sensory Receptors

There are five types of sensory receptors, four of which are important in relation to infusion therapy. The sensory receptors transmit along afferent fibers. Many types of stimulation, such as heat, light, cold, pain, pressure, and sound, are processed along the sensory receptors. Sensory receptors related to infusion therapy include:

1. Mechanoreceptors, which process skin tactile sensations and deep tissue sensation (e.g., **palpation** of veins, placement of dressings, tape placement and removal)
2. Thermoreceptors, which process cold, warmth, and pain (e.g., warm compresses)
3. Nociceptors, which process pain (venipuncture)
4. Chemoreceptors, which process osmotic changes in blood and decreased arterial pressure (decreased circulating blood volume) (Hadaway, 2010a).

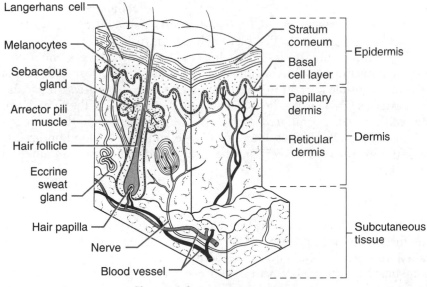

Figure 6-1 ▪ Anatomy of skin.

> **NURSING FAST FACT!**
>
> *To decrease pain during venipuncture, keep the skin taut by applying traction to it and move quickly through the skin layers.*

Nerves

When planning to place a PIV, it is important to recognize that certain sites should be avoided and/or used with caution because of nerve proximity. The radial nerve in the base of the wrist above the thumb is particularly vulnerable to injury. The radial artery, radial nerve, and cephalic vein are very superficial in this area. An anatomic study of the wrists/forearms of cadavers demonstrated that the radial nerve can be found in variable locations along the cephalic vein and that the nerve crosses over the vein up to three times in the first 4 to 5 inches above the thumb (Vialle et al., 2001).

The median nerve is the largest nerve in the arm; it is located in the center of the antecubital fossa. The median nerve advances down the central inner aspect of the forearm into the inner aspect of the wrist, branching into the palm of the hand. Injury in this area can result in scar tissue and carpal tunnel syndrome. Placement of a PIV into the antecubital area, along with phlebotomy procedures, can result in nerve damage. Although the radial and median nerves are also present on the dorsum of the hand, reported nerve injuries in that area are rare (Masoorli, 2007).

Venous System

Two series of blood vessels distribute blood to the capillaries (via the arteries) and return blood to the heart (via the veins): pulmonary and systemic. The systemic circulation, particularly the veins of the systemic circulation, is the focus of PIV placement and infusion.

The walls of all arteries and veins consist of three layers: the tunica intima (innermost layer), the tunica media (middle layer), and the tunica adventitia (outer layer) (Fig. 6-2). Veins are thinner and less muscular than arteries (Table 6-1). The wall of a vein is only 10% of the total diameter of the vessel, compared with 25% in the artery. Thus the vein can distend easily, allowing for storage of large volumes of blood under low pressure. Approximately 75% of the total blood volume is contained in the veins.

Tunica Adventitia

The outermost layer, called the tunica adventitia, consists of connective tissue that surrounds and supports a vessel. The blood supply of this layer, called the vasa vasorum, nourishes both the adventitia and media layers. Sometimes during venipuncture, you can feel a "pop" as you enter the tunica adventitia.

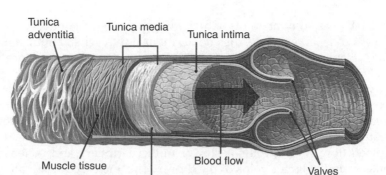

Figure 6-2 ■ Anatomy of a vein. (Courtesy of Medical Economics Publishing, Montvale, NJ, with permission.)

> Table 6-1 | COMPARISON OF ARTERY AND VEIN

Artery*	Vein*
Thick-walled	Thin-walled
Wall is 25% of total diameter	Wall is 10% of total diameter
Pulsates	Greater distensibility
Lacks valves	Valves present

*Has three tissue layers: tunica intima, tunica media, and tunica adventitia.

Tunica Media

The middle layer, called the tunica media, is composed of muscular and elastic tissue with nerve fibers for vasoconstriction and vasodilation. The tunica media in a vein is not as strong and rigid as it is in an artery, so it tends to collapse or distend as pressure decreases or increases. Stimulation by change in temperature or mechanical or chemical irritation can produce a response in this layer. For instance, cold blood or solutions can produce spasms that impede blood flow and cause pain. Application of heat promotes dilation of the vein, which can relieve a spasm or improve blood flow.

Tunica Intima

The innermost layer, called the tunica intima, has one thin layer of cells, the **endothelium**. The surface is smooth, allowing blood to flow through vessels easily. The endothelial cells of the tunica intima can be easily damaged by various I.V. insertion- and care-related factors, such as too rapid catheter advancement, insertion of a catheter too large for the vein, catheter motion caused by inadequate catheter stabilization, microorganisms entering the vein during **cannulation** because of inadequate site antisepsis, and infusion of irritating solutions (see Chapter 9 for complications).

Valves can be found in most veins, except very small and very large ones. Valves, made up of endothelial leaflets, help prevent the **distal** reflux of blood. Valves occur at points of branching, producing a noticeable bulge in the vessel when veins are distended, for example, when a tourniquet is applied (Hadaway, 2010a). There are no diagrams listing specific locations for valves within superficial veins used for venipuncture because there is great variation among individual patients (Hadaway, 2010a). The significance of valves may be recognized when blood withdrawal is attempted. The valves may compress and close the vein lumen during the process of aspiration, thus not allowing a blood return.

Blood flow via the veins is slower in the periphery and increases in turbulence in the larger veins of the thorax. This increased flow rate is an important aspect in administering hypertonic fluids because they should be administered in larger veins. The following is the amount of blood flow in milliliters per minute through each of the major veins used to deliver intravenous solutions:

- Cephalic and basilic veins: 45 to 95 mL/min
- Subclavian vein: 150 to 300 mL/min
- Superior vena cava: 2000 mL/min

Veins of the Hands and Arms

The venous system of the hands and arms is abundant, with acceptable veins for PIV catheter placement (Figs. 6-3 and 6-4). When selecting the best site, many factors must be considered, such as ease of insertion and access, type of needle or catheter that is to be used, and comfort and safety

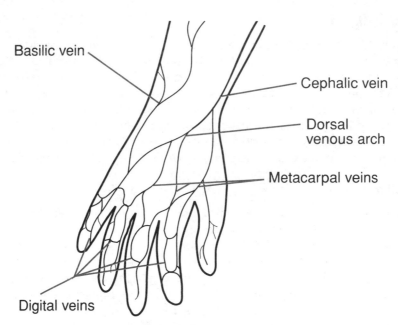

Figure 6-3 ■ Superficial veins of the dorsum of the hand. (Courtesy of BD Medical, Sandy, UT.)

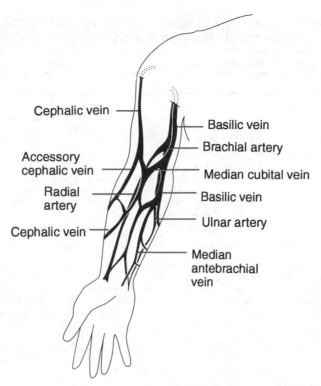

Figure 6-4 ■ Superficial veins of the forearm. (Courtesy of BD Medical, Sandy, UT.)

for the patient. The main veins used for insertion of PIV catheters are the superficial veins in the hand and forearm.

- The *metacarpal* veins located on the dorsum of the hand are easily visualized, palpated, and accessible. Their use may be limited because of excessive fat in infants and loss of subcutaneous tissue and skin turgor in older adults.
- The *cephalic* vein follows along the radius side of the forearm; it is a larger vein and relatively easy to access. The *accessory cephalic* vein branches off of the cephalic vein along the radius.
- The *basilic* vein follows along the ulnar side of the forearm to the upper arm; it is easily palpated but moves more easily, so it is important to stabilize the vein with traction during access.
- The antecubital veins, including the *median cephalic* (radius side), *median basilic* (ulnar side), and *median cubital* (in front of elbow), are located in the bend of the elbow. These large veins should be reserved for blood sampling and emergency, rather than routine, placement of a PIV.

Table 6-2 summarizes information on identifying and selecting the most effective I.V. site for clinical situations.

> Table 6-2   **SELECTING AN INSERTION SITE FOR SUPERFICIAL VEINS OF DORSUM OF HAND AND ARM**

Vein and Location	Insertion Device	Considerations
Digital		
Lateral and dorsal portions of the fingers		*Avoid* use because of small size and in areas of flexion because of increased risk for infiltration.
Metacarpal		
Dorsum of the hand formed by union of digital veins between the knuckles	20- to 24-gauge to ¾–1 inch in length over the needle catheter 21- to 25-gauge steel needle (one-time use for short infusion only)	Often, good site to begin therapy Usually easily visualized Small veins that should be avoided if infusing irritating antibiotics, potassium chloride, or chemotherapeutic agents or using high rates of infusion
Cephalic		
Radial portion of the lower arm along the radial bone of the forearm	18- to 24-gauge cannulas, usually over-the-needle catheter	Large vein, easy to access *Avoid* area of cephalic vein for about 4–5 inches above the thumb due to risk for nerve damage First use most distal section and work upward for long-term therapy Useful for infusing blood and chemically irritating medications
Basilic		
Ulnar aspect of the lower arm and runs up the ulnar bone	18- to 24-gauge, usually over-the-needle catheter	Difficult area to access because of location Large vein, easily palpated, but moves easily ("rolling vein"); stabilize with traction during venipuncture. Often available after other sites have been exhausted.
Accessory Cephalic		
Branches off the cephalic vein along the radial bone	18- to 22-gauge, usually over-the-needle catheter	Medium to large size and easy to stabilize May be difficult to palpate in persons with large amounts of adipose tissue. Valves at cephalic junction may prohibit cannula advancement. Short length may prohibit cannula use.
Upper Cephalic		
Radial aspect of upper arm above the elbow	16- to 20-gauge, over-the-needle catheter	Difficult to visualize May be good site for confused patients because it is less visible and thus subject to less patient manipulation

> Table 6-2	SELECTING AN INSERTION SITE FOR SUPERFICIAL VEINS OF DORSUM OF HAND AND ARM—cont'd	
Vein and Location	**Insertion Device**	**Considerations**
Median Antebrachial		
Extends up the front of the forearm from the median antecubital veins	18- to 24-gauge, usually over-the-needle catheter	*Avoid* because area has many nerve endings and infiltration occurs easily.
Median Basilic		
Located in antecubital fossa; branch of median cubital vein that angles toward basilic vein	18- to 22-gauge, over-the-needle catheter	Should be reserved for blood draws for laboratory analysis only, unless an emergency situation Uncomfortable placement site because arm is extended in unnatural position Area difficult to splint with arm board
Median Cubital		
Communication of cephalic and basilic veins in antecubital fossa	16- to 22-gauge, over-the-needle catheter	Same as above

🔲 Approaches to Venipuncture: Phillips 16-Step Peripheral-Venipuncture Method

Performing a successful venipuncture requires mastery and knowledge of infusion therapy as well as psychomotor clinical skills. The Phillips 16-step venipuncture method, outlined in Table 6-3 and explained in detail in this chapter, is an easy-to-remember step approach for beginning practitioners.

Guidelines supporting safety and evidence-based practice are available from the Occupational Safety and Health Administration (OSHA) and the Centers for Disease Control and Prevention (CDC) (O'Grady et al., 2011; Siegel et al., 2007). The Infusion Nurses Society (INS) Standards of Practice (2011a) also provide recommendations for evidence-based practices related to infusion nursing. As a nurse initiating infusion therapy, be aware of these standards as well as those of your own institution.

NOTE > Current INS (2011a) standards have been integrated throughout the 16 steps.

> Table 6-3   **PHILLIPS 16-STEP PERIPHERAL-VENIPUNCTURE METHOD**

Precannulation

1. Check the LIP orders
2. Hand hygiene
3. Equipment collection and preparation
4. Patient assessment, psychological preparation, patient identification
5. Site selection and vein distention

Cannulation

6. Attention to pain management
7. Catheter selection
8. Gloving
9. Site preparation
10. Vein entry, direct versus indirect
11. Catheter stabilization and dressing management

Postcannulation

12. Labeling
13. Equipment disposal
14. Patient education
15. Rate calculations
16. Documentation

Precannulation

Before initiating the I.V. cannulation, you must follow steps 1 through 5: check the order from the licensed independent practitioner (LIP) (e.g., physician/ nurse practitioner), practice hand hygiene, prepare the equipment, assess and prepare the patient, and select the vein and the site of insertion.

Step 1: Authorized Prescriber's Order

An order by a licensed independent practitioner is required to initiate infusion therapy. The order should be clear, concise, and complete. It is also essential that the nurse understand the rationale for the order before proceeding.

NOTE > The use of electronic order entry has reduced the risk for transcription errors.

All parenteral solutions should be checked against the authorized prescriber's order. The order should include:
- Date and time of the day
- Infusate (medication/solution)
- Route of administration
- Dosage

- Volume to be infused
- Rate of infusion
- Duration of infusion
- Signature of authorized prescriber

INS Standard The nurse should accept verbal orders from an LIP only when necessary. The nurse should adhere to a standard "read-back" process when accepting verbal or telephone orders from an LIP (INS, 2011a, p. S15).

Step 2: Hand Hygiene

Appropriate and adequate hand hygiene is one of the most important steps in reducing the risk for vascular access device-related infections. The 2011 CDC guidelines for preventing vascular catheter-related infections (O'Grady et al., 2011) provide specific directions for hand hygiene, stating that it should be performed both before and after palpating catheter insertion sites and inserting, replacing, accessing, repairing, or dressing an intravascular catheter (see Chapter 2 for more information).

Step 3: Equipment Collection and Preparation

In preparation for PIV placement and delivery of a primary or secondary solution:

- Gather ordered medication/solution, appropriate administration set, catheters, stabilization device, dressing, gloves, and skin antiseptic solution. There are many prepackaged PIV start kits on the market that provide the advantage of all/most of the supplies in clean packaging.
- Inspect the infusate container at the nurses' station, in the clean utility, or in the medication room. In today's practice, two systems are available: glass system and plastic system (rigid or soft). Note that glass systems are used infrequently and primarily with medications that can be absorbed by plastic.

To check the glass system:

- Hold the container up to the light to inspect for cracks as evidenced by flashes of light. Glass systems are crystal clear.
- Rotate the container and look for particulate contamination and cloudiness.
- Inspect the seal and check the expiration date.

To check a plastic system:

- The outer wrap of the plastic system should be dry.
- Gently squeeze the soft plastic infusate container to check for breaks in the integrity of the plastic; squeeze the system to detect pinholes.
- Inspect the solution for any particulate contamination. Check the expiration date.

If the order is for an intermittent infusion device:
■ Gather catheters, skin antiseptic solution, stabilization device, gloves, and dressing, along with a prefilled syringe of sodium chloride for PIV catheter flushing.

Choose the correct administration set to match the solution delivery system. For the closed glass system, a vented administration set must be used; for the plastic system, a nonvented set should be used (see Chapter 5 for more detailed information on I.V. equipment). It is wise to **"spike"** the solution container and **"prime"** the administration set in the clean utility area or nurses' station to detect defective equipment before taking equipment into the patient care area. Spiking and priming are shown in Figure 6-5.

Step 4: Patient Identification, Patient Assessment, and Psychological Preparation

Before assessing the patient, patient identification is critical. The 2013 National Patient Safety Goals by the Joint Commission (2013) state that the nurse must use at least two patient identifiers (neither to be the patient's room number) whenever providing treatments or procedures. Examples of patient identifiers include name, an assigned identification number, and birth date.

Selection of the vascular access device and insertion site requires integration and synthesis of data obtained from the patient assessment and the specific infusion therapy prescribed. Selection of the most appropriate

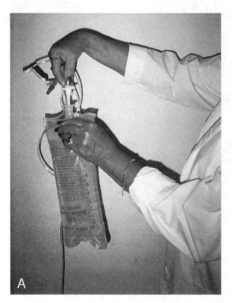
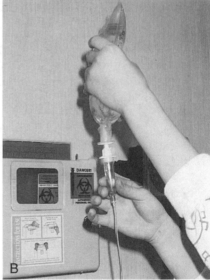

Figure 6-5 ■ *A,* Spiking. *B,* Priming plastic system.

vascular access device requires collaboration with input from the LIP, nurse, patient, and caregiver. It is important to use step 4 to gather the necessary information needed to perform a successful venipuncture and infusion therapy.

Patient education is imperative prior to PIV placement and should address the purpose of placement and what to expect in terms of the procedure. Instruct the patient regarding the type of medication/solution ordered by the LIP and why it was ordered, any mobility limitations, and signs and symptoms of potential complications. Evaluate the patient's psychological preparedness for the PIV procedure before venous access. The nurse should consider aspects such as autonomy, handedness, and independence along with invasion of personal space when I.V. placement is necessary. Often the patient has a fear of pain associated with venipuncture or the memory of a previously negative encounter related to necessity of the therapy. Make sure to assess and document fears and preferences related to pain management.

It is important to make sure that the patient is in a comfortable position, that privacy is ensured, and that the environment is conducive for the nurse to maintain aseptic technique and place the PIV. Good lighting for venous assessment and PIV placement is essential. In alternative care settings, such as the home, creating a good environment can be challenging. Often, the kitchen table works well because there is often good lighting and the surface can be cleaned for placement of supplies.

Step 5: Site Selection and Vein Dilation

SITE SELECTION

Site selection is based on a thorough assessment of the patient's condition, age, diagnosis, vascular condition, history of previous access devices, and type and anticipated duration of therapy. It is important to remember that certain therapies are not appropriate for peripheral-short catheters. These include continuous vesicant therapy, parenteral nutrition, infusates with a pH less than 5 or greater than 9, and infusates with an osmolarity greater than 600 mOsm/L (INS, 2011a, p. S37).

According to the INS Standards of Practice (2011a), the following should be taken into consideration during site selection when placing the short peripheral catheter.

1. In adults, veins that should be considered include those on the dorsal and ventral surfaces of the upper extremities.
   For pediatric infusion, additional site selection can include the veins of the scalp and lower extremities (see the section in this chapter on pediatric PIV techniques).
2. Routinely initiate venipuncture in the distal areas of the upper extremities; subsequent cannulation should be made **proximal** to the previously cannulated site.

3. Consideration should be given to use of visualization technologies that aid in vein identification, such as **transillumination** or near infrared technology (discussed later in this chapter and also in Chapter 5).
4. Areas to avoid include:
   a. Veins of the lower extremities; these should not be used in the adult population because of risk of embolism and thrombophlebitis
   b. Compromised veins, such as those that are hard and sclerosed
   c. Areas of venipunctures with subsequent injury to the vein
   d. Areas of flexion, such as the wrist or elbow, because of increased risk of infiltration and phlebitis; in the case of the antecubital fossa, PIV placement interferes with blood sampling and may prevent the use of those veins if a peripherally inserted central catheter (PICC) or **midline catheter** is required.
   e. Veins in the lateral surface of the wrist above the thumb for approximately 4–5 inches because of the potential for nerve damage
   f. The ventral surface (inner aspect) of wrist because of pain on insertion and possible nerve damage
   g. The affected extremity when there is evidence of cellulitis, presence of an arteriovenous fistula, history of lymph node dissection (e.g., breast surgery), affected extremity from a stroke, or history of radiation therapy to that side

When there has been an inadvertent infiltration or extravasation of infusate(s), there should be further assessment to determine the type of infusate, pH and osmolarity, estimated volume of the infusate, vein condition, and appropriateness of a PIV for the infusion therapy. Some additional considerations include the following:

1. Blood pressure cuffs or tourniquets should not be used during periods of infusion on an extremity with an indwelling PIV catheter.
2. Although PIVs are not used routinely for blood drawing and evidence is limited regarding the impact of dwell time with blood sampling, laboratory test results have shown PIVs to be reliable for many routine blood tests, including coagulation studies. Use of PIVs for blood draws, and thus avoidance of venipuncture for blood draws, should be considered for pediatric patients, those who require multiple laboratory tests, those with risk for bleeding, and those with difficult vascular access (INS, 2011a, p. S78).

Additional information must be considered before initiation of infusion therapy and is part of step 4 in completing a thorough assessment.

Patient assessment should be ongoing and requires the nurse to evaluate and use critical thinking skills to achieve positive patient outcomes.

The following factors help nurses make appropriate choices for site selection and should be part of step 1 in the nursing process—assessment.

1. *Type of solution*: When administering irritating fluids, such as certain antibiotics and potassium chloride, select a large vein in the forearm to initiate this therapy.

2. *Condition of the vein*: A soft, straight vein is the ideal choice for venipuncture. Palpate the vein by moving the tips of the fingers down the vein to observe how it refills. The dorsal metacarpal veins in elderly patients are a poor choice because blood extravasation (i.e., hematoma) occurs more readily in small, fragile veins. When a patient is hypovolemic, peripheral veins collapse more quickly than larger veins.
   Avoid:
   ■ Bruised veins
   ■ Red, swollen veins
   ■ Veins near previous site of phlebitis and infiltration
   ■ Sites near a previously discontinued site

3. *Duration of therapy*: Long courses of infusion therapy make preservation of veins essential. Start at the best, lowest vein. Use the hand only if a nonirritating solution is being infused. Perform venipuncture distally, with each subsequent puncture *proximal* to previous puncture and alternate arms.
   Avoid:
   ■ A joint flexion
   ■ A vein too small for cannula size

4. *Cannula size*: Small-**gauge** catheters take up less space in the vein, allowing for blood flow around the catheter; they also cause less trauma when inserted. If a larger-gauge catheter is required, as in emergency situations or blood transfusions, a larger vein should be chosen. In general, for most applications, a 20- to 24-gauge catheter is selected. For more viscous solutions such as blood, an 18- to 20-gauge catheter may be selected, although smaller catheters are used with children. For neonates, 24-gauge catheters are used; for children, 22- to 24-gauge catheters are most often used (Frey & Pettit, 2010).

5. *Patient age*: Infants do not have the accessible sites that older children and adults have because of the infants' increased body fat. Veins in the hands, feet, and antecubital region may be the only accessible sites. Veins in elderly persons are usually fragile, so approach venipuncture gently and evaluate the need for a tourniquet.

6. *Patient preference*: Consider the patient's personal feelings when determining the catheter placement site. Evaluate the extremities, taking into account the dominant hand.

7. *Patient activity*: Ambulatory patients who use crutches or a walker will need cannula placement above the wrist so that the hand can still be used.

8. *Presence of disease or previous surgery*: Patients with vascular disease or dehydration may have limited venous access. Avoid phlebitis-infiltrated sites or sites of infection. If a patient has a condition with poor vascular venous return, the affected side **must be avoided**. Examples of such conditions are cerebrovascular accident, mastectomy, amputation, orthopedic surgery of the hand or arm, and plastic surgery of the hand or arm.

9. *Presence of shunt or graft*: Do not use a patient's arm or hand that has a patent graft or shunt for dialysis.

10. *Patients receiving anticoagulation therapy*: These patients have a propensity to bleed. Local ecchymoses and major hemorrhagic complications can be avoided if the nurse is aware that the patient is taking anticoagulant drugs. Precautions can be taken when initiating infusion therapy. Venous distention can be accomplished with minimal tourniquet pressure. Use the smallest catheter that will accommodate the vein and deliver the ordered infusate. The dressing must be removed gently using alcohol or adhesive remover. On discontinuation of infusion therapy for patients on anticoagulation therapy, direct pressure should be applied over the site for at least 10 minutes.

 NURSING FAST FACT!

If the veins are fragile or if the patient is taking anticoagulants, avoid using a tourniquet; constricted blood flow may overdistend fragile veins, causing vein damage, vessel hemorrhages, or subcutaneous bleeding.

11. *Patient with allergies*: Determine whether a patient has allergies. For example, iodine allergies must be identified because iodine is contained in some products used for skin antisepsis (povidone iodine). Other allergies of concern to delivery of safe patient care include allergies to lidocaine, medications, foods, animals, latex, and environmental substances.

Table 6-4 gives tips for selecting veins for peripheral infusions.

 NURSING FAST FACT!

Always question the patient regarding allergies before administering medications, especially those given by intravenous route. Ask patients about any history of latex allergy.

> Table 6-4   TIPS FOR SELECTING VEINS

- A suitable vein should feel relatively smooth and pliable, with valves well spaced.
- Veins will be difficult to stabilize in a patient who has recently lost weight.
- Debilitated patients and those taking corticosteroids have fragile veins that bruise easily.
- Sclerotic veins are common among narcotics addicts.
- Sclerotic veins are common among the elderly population.
- Patients who require frequent infusions are often knowledgeable about which of their veins are good for venipuncture.
- Start with distal veins and work proximally.
- Veins that feel bumpy (like running your finger over a cat's tail) usually are thrombosed or extremely valvular.

CULTURAL AND ETHNIC CONSIDERATIONS: PERFORMING INFUSION THERAPY

Transcultural nursing emerged as a specialty field for nursing with the establishment of the Transcultural Nursing Society in 1975; however, it is an expectation that <u>every</u> nurse will use transcultural knowledge to deliver culturally sensitive care free of inherent biases based on gender, race, and religion. The American Nurses Association (ANA) Standards of Care address culture as follows:

• Under Standard 3 Outcomes Identification, one of the competencies states "derives culturally appropriate expected outcomes from the diagnoses" (ANA, 2010, p. 35).

• Under Standard 5 Implementation, one of the competencies addresses health-care delivery sensitive to needs of consumers, "with particular emphasis on the needs of diverse populations" (ANA, 2010, p. 38).

A formal assessment tool, the TransCultural Nursing Assessment Tool, is available online (www.culturediversity.org/assmtform.htm). It organizes an assessment into six cultural phenomena that are evident in all cultural groups:

1. Communication: Language, voice quality, pronunciation, use of nonverbal communication
2. Space: Comfort in conversation, proximity, body movement, perception of space
3. Social organization: Ethnicity, family role function, work, leisure, church, friends
4. Time: Definitions, social/work time, time orientation
5. Environmental control: Health practices, values, definition of health and illness
6. Biological variations: Skin color, body structure, nutritional preferences

In preparing to perform care for patients from different cultures, it is important to remember the following (ANA, 2010; Campinha-Bacote, 2011; Douglas et al., 2011; INS, 2011a, p. S16; Neel, 2010):

• Learn as much as possible about the patient's cultural customs and beliefs. Encourage the patient to share cultural interpretations of health, illness, and health care.

Continued

- Plan care based on cultural assessment and communicated needs.
- Identify sources of discrepancy between the patient's and your own concepts of health and illness and recognize that they may not be the same.
- Understand that respect for the patient and his or her communication needs is central to the therapeutic relationship.
- Ask permission before you touch the patient.
- Provide resources for translation and interpretation and learn how to effectively work with translators.
- Provide written materials (e.g., patient educational tools, pain scales) in the patient's preferred language.
- Be alert to words the patient seems to understand and use them frequently.
- Keep messages simple and repeat them.
- Avoid using technical medical terms and abbreviations

Vein Distention

Most often a tourniquet is used to promote venous distention both as part of the venous assessment process and then in actual preparation for venipuncture. Factors affecting the capacity for dilation are blood pressure, presence of valves, sclerotic veins, and multiple previous I.V. sites. Table 6-4 gives tips for dilating veins.

Methods to promote venous distention include:

1. *Gravity*: Position the extremity lower than the heart for a minute or two.
2. *Clenching/pumping fist*: Instruct the patient to open and close his or her fist. Squeezing a rubber ball or rolled washcloth works well.
3. *Stroking the vein*: Lightly stroke the vein downward or use light tapping with index finger to cause dilation of vein.
4. *Warm compresses*: Apply warm towels to the extremity for 7 to 10 minutes. Use of warming is a low-cost intervention that has been shown to improve PIV placement rate (Crowley et al., 2011).

EBP In a randomized trial, patients were assigned to either active warming with a carbon fiber heating mitt or passive insulation (mitt heater not activated). Significant findings included a decrease in the time required to insert the PIV and a decrease in the number of PIV attempts with active warming (Lenhardt et al., 2002). Another randomized controlled trial involving outpatient oncology patients compared dry heat to moist heat, finding that dry heat was 2.7 times more likely to result in successful PIV insertion. Dry heat also took less time and was more comfortable (Fink et al., 2009).

5. *Blood pressure cuff*: This is an excellent choice for vein dilation. Pump the cuff up slightly (e.g., about 30 mm Hg). This method prevents constriction of the arterial system.

 NURSING FAST FACT!

> When using a blood pressure cuff, care must be exercised not to start the I.V. too close to the cuff, which causes excessive back pressure.

6. *Tourniquet*: Apply the tourniquet 5 to 6 inches above the venipuncture site. It is important that the tourniquet be applied to impede venous flow but not arterial flow; an arterial pulse should be easily palpable distal to the tourniquet (INS, 2011a, p. S36). Tourniquets should be applied loosely or not used at all in patients who are at risk for bleeding, who have fragile skin/veins, or who have compromised circulation (INS, 2011a).

 NURSING FAST FACT!

> Tourniquets shall be single-patient use, and material should be considered based on potential latex allergy (INS, 2011a, p. S36).

7. *Phillips multiple tourniquet technique*: Apply additional tourniquets to increase the oncotic pressure and bring deep veins into view. This technique is useful for patients with extra adipose tissue, although ultrasonography is becoming more prevalent and is very useful for obtaining successful venous access in obese patients. Table 6-5 lists the steps for the technique, and Figure 6-6 shows a picture of a multiple tourniquet.
8. *Visualization technology (transillumination)*: Transillumination is simply defined as shining a light through tissues (Hadaway, 2010b). A small, portable battery-operated device is available for imaging subsurface veins and some structures; this side-transillumination method shines light into the skin from outside the field of view so that the light is pointed toward the center at a depth of approximately 2 cm. Figure 6-7 shows techniques for transillumination. The depth of visualization of veins is between 3 and 6 mm depending on the color of the light used. Advantages to such a device include vein location in darker-skinned and obese patients and in children. Table 6-6 provides information on how to use a transilluminator or penlight.
9. *Visualization technology (near infrared light)*: Another product used is a viewing headset that uses near infrared imaging to visualize

> Table 6-5 **PHILLIPS MULTIPLE TOURNIQUET TECHNIQUE**

- Assess patient's arms for appropriate vascular access. Explain reasons for use of multiple tourniquet technique and that some pressure discomfort may be felt for a short period of time. Verify the patient's understanding of the explanation.
- Place one tourniquet high on the arm for 2 minutes and leave in place. The arm should be stroked downward toward the hand.
- After 2 minutes, place a second tourniquet at midarm just below the antecubital fossa for 2 minutes. By increasing the oncotic pressure inside the tissue, blood is forced into the small vessels of the periphery.
- The practitioner should assess for collateral circulation. If soft collateral veins do not appear in the forearm, a third tourniquet may be placed near the wrist.
- Tourniquets must not be left on longer than 6 minutes.
- *Use Phillips multiple tourniquet technique*: If the peripheral vessels are hard and sclerosed because of a disease process, personal misuse, or frequent drug therapy, venous access is difficult.

Note: The Phillips multiple tourniquet technique helps novices learn the differences between collateral veins and sclerosed vessels. Usually, veins appear in the basilic vein of the forearm and the hands when this approach is used.

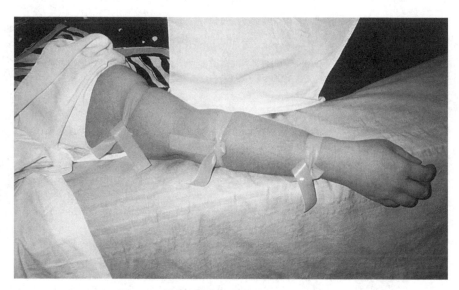

Figure 6-6 ■ Phillips tourniquet technique.

veins. Advantages include a hands-free device and the ability to better view veins in patients who are darker-skinned or obese and have compromised veins. It also offers the advantage of being able to visualize venous flow (Fig. 6-8).

10. *Visualization technology (ultrasound)*: Ultrasonography uses sound waves to locate human bodily structures. The use of ultrasound

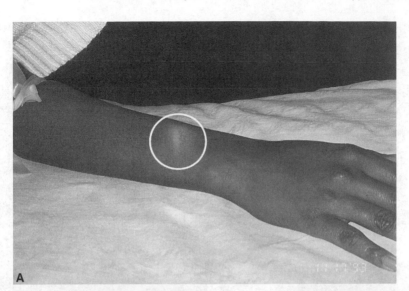

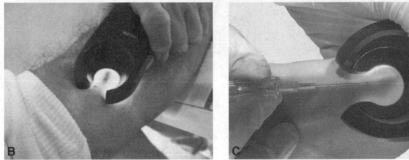

Figure 6-7 ■ Transillumination techniques. *A*, Tangential lighting using flashlight to illuminate veins of dark skin individual. *B*, Veinlite LED-assisted vein finder. *C*, Veinlite LED-assisted vein finder. (Courtesy of Translite LLC, Sugar Land, TX.)

> Table 6-6   **TRANSILLUMINATION**

- Take precautions in patients with alterations in skin surfaces caused by lesions, burns, or a disease process. Patients with altered skin integrity are often photosensitive and need additional protection of their already damaged tissue. This indirect lighting does not flatten veins or cause damage to the skin.
- Use a light directed toward the side of the patient's extremity to illuminate the blue veins and provide a guide for venipuncture.
- Refer to manufacturer's guidelines for specific product use.
- Turn down the light in the room.
- Use penlight on the side of the forearm to illuminate any veins.

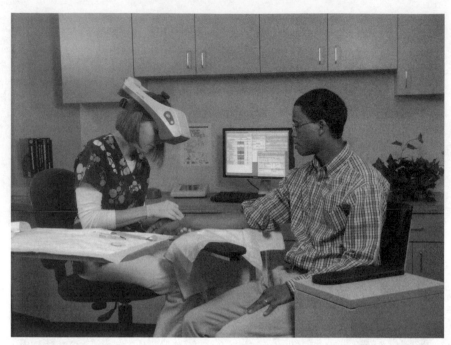

Figure 6-8 ▪ Near-infrared imaging to visualize vein using Veinsite. (Courtesy of VueTek Scientific, Gray, ME.)

for placement of central vascular access devices is standard practice. Nursing use of ultrasound for placement of PIV catheters is an emerging and increasing practice. Although most of the literature addresses use by emergency department nurses, use in other hospital units is increasing. In a quality improvement project, use of ultrasound for PIV placement on a medical–surgical unit resulted in a 20% decrease in the number of PICC placements (Maiocco & Coole, 2012). Venous access is generally difficult in obese patients, and use of ultrasound is associated with improved success rate in this special patient population (Houston, 2013) (see also Chapter 5).

EBP Evidence-based practice guidelines from the Emergency Nurses Association (Crowley et al., 2011) recommend the use of ultrasound-guided PIV placement in both adult and pediatric patients with difficult venous access. The technique can be effectively performed by nurses, physicians, and emergency department technicians.

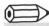 *NURSING FAST FACT!*

To enhance vein location, use adequate lighting. Bright, direct overhead examination lights may have a "washout" effect on veins. Instead, use side lighting, which can add contour and "shadowing" to highlight the skin color and texture and allow visualization of the vein shadow below the skin.

 CULTURAL AND ETHNIC CONSIDERATIONS: SKIN COLOR

Skin color is a significant biological variation in terms of infusion nursing practice. When caring for patients with highly pigmented skin, establish the baseline color with good lighting.

Table 6-7 presents a summary of tips for the difficult venous access.

Cannulation

Cannulation involves steps 6 through 11: Paying attention to pain management, selecting the appropriate catheter, gloving, preparing the site, direct or indirect entry into the vein, stabilizing the catheter, and managing the dressing.

Expected outcomes in relation to appropriate site placement include the following:

- The site must tolerate the rate of flow (e.g., high flow rates, use larger veins).
- The site must be capable of delivering the medications or solutions ordered.
- The site must tolerate the gauge of cannula needed.
- The patient must be comfortable with the site chosen.
- The site must be one that least limits the patient's activities of daily living.
- The site must be one with reduced risk for complications (e.g., avoid areas of flexion).

> Table 6-7 | **TECHNIQUES TO ASSIST WITH DIFFICULT VENOUS ACCESS**

- Alterations in skin surfaces: Use tangential lighting.
- Hard sclerosed vessels: Use multiple tourniquet technique.
- Obesity: Use ultrasonography to locate and cannulate veins, use 2-inch catheter and lateral veins, and/or consider Phillips multiple tourniquet technique.
- Edema: Displace edema with digital pressure.
- Fragile veins: Maintain traction using one-handed technique. Be gentle.

Step 6: Attention to Pain Management

Reducing pain during PIV placement is an important aspect of infusion nursing practice. Patient satisfaction is maximized and fear and anxiety are reduced when pain management is addressed. The INS Standards (2011a, p. S43) state that local anesthetic agents should be a consideration. Local anesthetic agents include intradermal injections (e.g., lidocaine), iontophoresis, pressure-accelerated lidocaine, and topical transdermal agents. Additional interventions include cognitive behavioral strategies such as distraction and positioning.

NOTE > The duration required for anesthetic agents varies depending on the agent used.

Intradermal Injections

Accepted forms of intradermal anesthesia used with I.V. insertion include lidocaine and bacteriostatic normal saline with a benzyl alcohol preservative. The benzyl alcohol is an opium alkaloid that possesses antiseptic and anesthetic properties. Although often used as an inexpensive anesthetic, bacteriostatic normal saline was found to be inferior in terms of local anesthesia compared with lidocaine in two randomized controlled trials led by nurses (Burke et al., 2011; Ganter-Ritz, Speroni, & Atherton, 2012). Lidocaine has been used in clinical practice since 1948 and is one of the safest anesthetics. Lidocaine is an amide that works by stopping impulses at the neural membrane. The anesthetized site is numb to pain, but the patient perceives touch and pressure and has control of his or her muscles. The anesthetic becomes effective within 15 to 30 seconds and lasts 30 to 45 minutes. Lidocaine can cause a slight burning sensation with initial needle insertion; when the lidocaine is buffered with sodium bicarbonate, this discomfort is reduced. However, buffered lidocaine is not commercially available and must be compounded by the pharmacy, which makes it more costly (Ganter-Ritz, Speroni, & Atherton, 2012). The nurse must have knowledge of the actions of and side effects associated with lidocaine. A history of previous allergies precludes the administration of lidocaine.

The process of using 1% lidocaine (without epinephrine, buffered lidocaine preferred) before venipuncture is as follows:

1. Review the authorized prescriber's order or the clinical procedure in the facility for use of lidocaine prior to venipuncture.
2. Check for patient allergy and lidocaine sensitivity.
3. Verify patient's identity using two independent identifiers.
4. Select the appropriate arm for infusion therapy, apply the tourniquet, and select a suitable vein.
5. Draw up 0.3 mL of 1% lidocaine in a 1-mL TB syringe.

6. Don gloves.
7. Prep the site with antiseptic solution (e.g., chlorhexidine/alcohol for 30 seconds) and allow the site to dry.
8. Reapply the tourniquet. The vein should be fully dilated, pulled taut by stretching, and stabilized while the local anesthetic is administered.
9. Insert the needle **bevel** up at a 15- to 25-degree angle.
10. Inject the lidocaine intradermally into the side of the vein forming a wheal next to the desired insertion site.
11. Withdraw the needle. Allow 5 to 10 seconds for the anesthetic to take effect.
12. Continue with Phillips step 7 in starting the I.V. (Fig. 6-9).

> EBP In a double-blind, randomized controlled trial of 256 surgical patients, 1% lidocaine, buffered 1% lidocaine, and bacteriostatic normal saline were administered before PIV placement. Statistically significant findings included the following: the most tolerable anesthetic solution (in terms of pain from the intradermal injection) was buffered 1% lidocaine; and both buffered 1% lidocaine and 1% lidocaine were more efficacious (defined as less pain with PIV placement) compared to the bacteriostatic normal saline (Ganter-Ritz, Speroni, & Atherton, 2012).

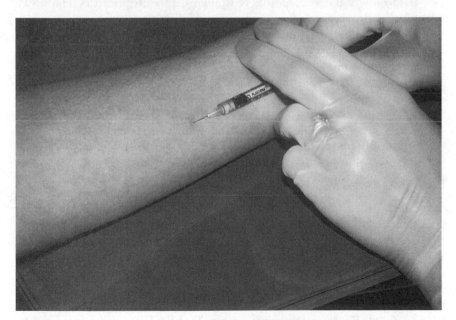

Figure 6-9 ■ Intradermal lidocaine administered before venipuncture using 0.1 to 0.2 mL of 1% lidocaine and a tuberculin syringe entering the skin at a 15- to 25-degree angle.

Transdermal Anesthetics

Topical analgesic creams and patches are available by prescription (e.g., EMLA, which contains lidocaine and prilocaine) and over the counter (e.g., ELA-Max). Although transdermal creams are effective, the disadvantage is the time duration until an anesthetic effect (up to 1 hour).

Follow these steps when applying a transdermal cream (INS, 2011b):

1. Check for allergies to lidocaine.
2. Don gloves and use clean technique.
3. Prepare the intended venipuncture site by washing with mild soap and water.
4. Apply an amount of cream according to the manufacturer's directions.
5. Place a transparent dressing over the cream.
6. Leave the dressing in place for the recommended time period (usually 30–60 minutes).
7. Remove the occlusive dressing, if one is used; remove the cream by wiping with a clean gauze or tissue. Perform any additional skin preparation or cleaning.

Iontophoresis

Iontophoresis refers to the use of a small external electric current to deliver water-soluble, charged drugs into the skin.

The following are key points with regard to iontophoresis (Hadaway, 2010b):

■ The anesthetic medication (usually lidocaine and epinephrine) is impregnated into a pad and applied to the skin over the intended venipuncture site.
■ Another pad is adhered to the skin near the medication-impregnated pad.
■ Electrodes may be preattached to the pads or attached separately; they are disposable and discarded after use.
■ Iontophoresis can cause skin irritation or burns.
■ The anesthetic effect lasts approximately 10 minutes.

Behavioral Interventions

The literature addresses behavioral interventions, particularly in the pediatric population. These include optimal timing and appropriate format and content of information presented based on developmental level. Providing information too early may increase anxiety. It is important to involve parents in the procedure; provide distraction and address positioning of infants and young children; have the pediatric patient face the parent; and secure and swaddle the infant or young child in position (Cohen, 2008). The use of sucrose water (2 mL of 25% sucrose solution by syringe or on a pacifier) is an evidence-based intervention to decrease pain from acute procedures (Cohen, 2008).

Step 7: Catheter Selection

PIV catheters are available in a variety of gauge sizes and lengths. Recommendations include using the smallest gauge and length appropriate for the prescribed therapy (INS, 2011a). Small-gauge catheters take up less space in the vein, allowing for blood flow around the catheter; they also cause less trauma when inserted (Perucca, 2010). If a larger-gauge catheter is required, as with emergent care or blood transfusions, a larger vein should be chosen. In general, for most applications, a 22- or 24-gauge catheter is selected. For more viscous solutions such as blood, an 18- or 20-gauge catheter may be selected, although smaller catheters are used with children. For neonates, 24-gauge catheters are used; for children, 22- to 24-gauge catheters are most often used (Frey & Pettit, 2010).

Additional criteria include the following:

■ Determine resources available to care for device (acute care facility, home care, or long-term care).

■ A midline catheter is considered when the duration of therapy is anticipated to last beyond 6 days (O'Grady et al., 2011).

INS Standard The catheter selected shall be of the smallest gauge and length with the fewest number of lumens and shall be the least invasive device to accommodate the prescribed therapy (INS, 2011a, p. S37).

Only safety-engineered PIV catheters should be used (see Chapter 5 for catheter choice and sizes). The choice of catheter depends on the purpose of the infusion and the condition and availability of the veins.

Most hospitals, clinics, and home care agencies have policies and procedures for the selection of catheters. Table 6-8 lists the recommended gauges and color codes for catheters. Of note, short peripheral catheters are color coded according to an international standard; midline and central vascular access devices are not.

> Table 6-8   **RECOMMENDED GAUGES**

Gauges	Color Code
16-gauge for trauma	16-gauge: gray
18- to 20-gauge for infusion of hypertonic or isotonic solutions with additives	18-gauge: green 20-gauge: pink
18- to 20-gauge for blood administration	18-gauge: green 20-gauge: pink
22- to 24-gauge for pediatric patients, older adult patients	22-gauge: blue 24-gauge: yellow
24- to 26-gauge for neonates	24-gauge: yellow 26-gauge: violet

The tip of the catheter should be inspected for integrity before venipuncture. Note the presence of burrs on the needle, peeling of catheter material, or other abnormalities.

Step 8: Gloving

The CDC (O'Grady et al., 2011) recommends wearing clean gloves during PIV catheter placement, making sure that the intended insertion site is not touched after skin antisepsis.

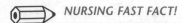 *NURSING FAST FACT!*

> *Latex and the powder used in the gloves are associated with potentially severe allergic reactions in susceptible persons. Avoid using this material if you have experienced any reactions to their use. (For more information on latex allergy, see Chapter 2 under occupational risks.)*

> **INS Standard** Standard precautions shall be used and appropriate personal protective equipment (e.g., gloves) shall be worn during all infusion procedures that will potentially expose the nurse to blood and body fluids (INS, 2011a, p. S25).

Step 9: Site Preparation

Several steps are involved in site preparation. If the site is visibly dirty, the skin should be washed with soap and water. If there is excess hair at the site, hair can be clipped using a scissors or disposable head surgical clippers. Shaving is not recommended because of the potential for **microabrasions**, which increase the risk of infection.

One of the most critical steps in reducing the risk of infection is site preparation using an antiseptic solution. Skin preparation is important because bacteria on the skin at the insertion site can travel along the external surface of the catheter during PIV catheter insertion. According to the CDC (O'Grady et al., 2011), acceptable antiseptics for PIV skin antisepsis are 70% alcohol, tincture of iodine, and an iodophor or chlorhexidine/alcohol solution. Chlorhexidine/alcohol solution is becoming the standard of practice and is the antiseptic agent preferred by the INS (2011a); unlike the other antiseptic agents, it has a residual effect on the skin for up to 48 hours. It is important that the skin is allowed to fully dry prior to venipuncture. If not, antiseptic can be tracked into the vein during insertion, which can cause phlebitis or vein inflammation (as discussed in Chapter 9). Allow to air dry; never blow on, fan, or wipe the site!

NOTE > Antiseptics should be provided in a single-unit use package.

Povidone-iodine is applied using swab sticks in a concentric circle beginning at the venipuncture site and moving outward. It must remain on the skin for 2 minutes or longer and be completely dry for adequate antisepsis (INS, 2011b). Chlorhexidine/alcohol preparations are applied using a back-and-forth method for at least 30 seconds and allowed to dry (Fig. 6-10).

NOTE > Alcohol **should not** be applied after the application of povidone-iodine preparation because alcohol negates the effects of povidone-iodine.

NOTE > The use of chlorhexidine preparations in infants younger than 2 months is not recommended given the lack of research supporting its safety and efficacy in this patient population (O'Grady et al., 2011; INS, 2011a).

Step 10: Vein Entry

Gloves should be donned before venipuncture and kept on until after the cannula is stabilized. Gloves should be removed only after the risk of exposure to body fluids has been eliminated. Venipuncture can be performed using a direct (one-step) or indirect (two-step) method. The direct method is appropriate for small-gauge needles and for fragile hand veins or rolling veins. It carries an increased risk of causing a hematoma. The indirect method can be used for all venipunctures. Procedures Display 6-1 at the end of this chapter describes the steps to initiate a peripheral-short infusion by a direct or an indirect technique.

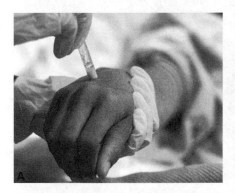
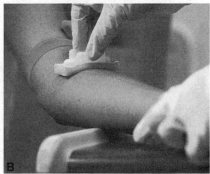

Figure 6-10 ■ Skin antisepsis prior to peripheral intravenous catheter placement. *A*, Chloraprep Sepp, which contains 0.67 mL of 2% chlorhexidine gluconate and 70% alcohol. *B*, Chloraprep Frepp, which contains 1.5 mL. (Courtesy of Carefusion, San Diego, CA.)

Traction is important to maintain stability of the vein in either a direct or an indirect approach (Fig. 6-11). Figures 6-12 and 6-13 show diagrams of insertion of a catheter into a vein, threading the cannula (catheter) into the vein, and removing the stylet.

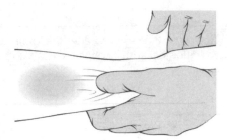

Figure 6-11 ■ Application of traction to the skin.

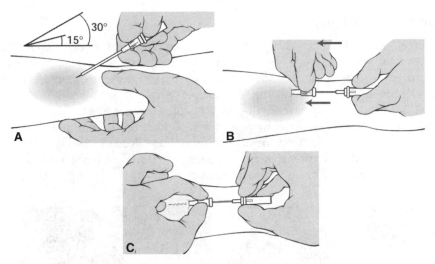

Figure 6-12 ■ *A*, Insertion of needle at a 30-degree angle through skin. *B*, Threading catheter into vein. *C*, Removing stylet from catheter.

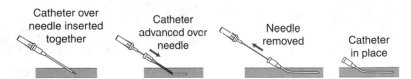

Catheter over needle inserted together

Catheter advanced over needle

Needle removed

Catheter in place

Figure 6-13 ■ Steps in insertion of an over-the-needle catheter once through the skin into the vein.

TROUBLESHOOTING TIPS

Common reasons for failure of venipuncture include:
- Failure to release the tourniquet promptly when the vein is sufficiently cannulated
- Use of a "stop and start" technique by beginners who may lack confidence; this tentative approach can injure the vein, causing bruising.
- Inadequate vein stabilization. Not using traction to hold the vein causes the stylet to push the vein aside.
- Failure to recognize that the catheter has gone through the opposite vein wall
- Stopping too soon after insertion so that only the stylet, not the catheter, enters the lumen (intima) of the vein. Blood return disappears when the stylet is removed because the catheter is not in the lumen.
- Inserting the cannula too deeply, below the vein. This is evident when the catheter will not move freely because it is imbedded in fascia or muscle. The patient also complains of severe discomfort.
- Failure to penetrate the vein wall because of improper insertion angle (too steep or not steep enough), causing the catheter to ride on top of or below the vein

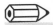 *NURSING FAST FACT!*

Only two attempts at venipuncture are recommended because multiple unsuccessful attempts cause unnecessary trauma to the patient and limit vascular access (INS, 2011a). If a nurse has made two unsuccessful attempts, the nurse with the best skills should evaluate the patient's veins and further attempts at PIV insertion be made only if venous access is believed to be adequate (Perucca, 2010).

 NURSING FAST FACT!

When aseptic technique is compromised (e.g., in an emergency situation), the cannula is also considered compromised and a new catheter should be placed as soon as possible and within 48 hours (INS, 2011a).

Safety features on all active safety catheters must be activated according to the manufacturer's recommendations (Fig. 6-14). Recognize that passive safety catheters do not require any activation because the safety features are automatic.

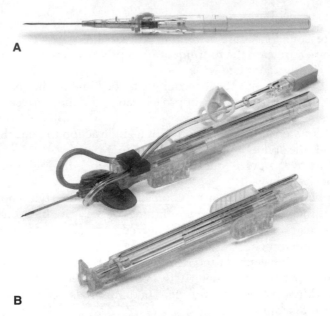

A

B

Figure 6-14 ■ *A*, BD Insyte Autoguard BC Shielded I.V. catheter provides blood control during insertion; needle safety system button. (Courtesy of BD Medical, Sandy, UT.) *B*, NovaCath has a passive safety mechanism, fully encapsulates the needle, and provides blood control during insertion and throughout the dwell time; eliminates need for external add-on device. (Courtesy of Tangent Medical, Ann Arbor, MI.)

Step 11: Catheter Stabilization and Dressing Management

Catheter Stabilization

Stabilization of movement at the catheter hub is recognized as an important intervention in increasing the dwell time for PIV catheters and reducing the risk for phlebitis, infection, catheter migration, and catheter dislodgement. Many nurses equate stabilization with application of a dressing and tape; however, use of a stabilization device is the preferred method (INS, 2011a, p. S46). Some devices consist of an adhesive pad and a mechanism for holding the catheter to the pad, thus controlling movement at the insertion site (Fig. 6-15). In a randomized controlled trial, a platform PIV catheter (essentially a "winged" catheter) in combination with an I.V. securement transparent dressing performed as well as an adhesive pad device (Bausone-Gazsa, Lefaiver, & Walters, 2010).

A stabilization device used with a PIV catheter is attached at the time of catheter placement and removed when the catheter is discontinued. It is important that the PIV catheter is stabilized in a manner that does not interfere with visualization and evaluation of the site.

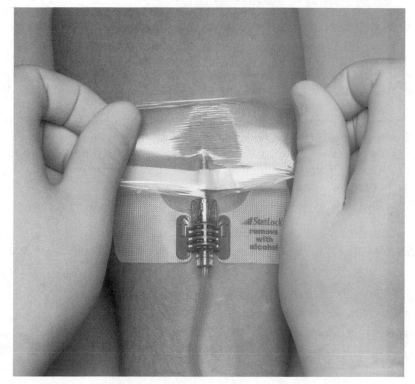

Figure 6-15 ■ StatLock stabilizing a peripheral I.V. catheter. (© 2013 C.R. Bard, Inc. Used with permission.)

ADD-ON DEVICES

With PIV catheters, typical add-on devices include extension sets, T ports, and J loops. In general, the use of add-on devices should be minimized because their use may increase the risk for accidental disconnections or misconnections (INS, 2011a, p. S31). However, advantages to their use include an easier transition from a continuous to an intermittent infusion because a needleless connector can be easily attached to the extension with less movement at the catheter site. Policies and procedures regarding add-on devices and junction securement should be in place as part of the implementation of practice guidelines in each organization. All add-on devices should be of luer-lock design to ensure a secure junction (INS, 2011a, p. S31).

JOINT STABILIZATION AND SITE PROTECTION

As previously addressed, areas of joint flexion should be avoided with PIV placement. However, there are times when this is not possible. In such cases, the joint should be stabilized with an arm board or splint (INS, 2011a, p. S47). Any joint stabilization device should be applied in a manner that allows ongoing visual assessment of the catheter and vein path. Arm boards may be flat or contoured to fit the extremity and should be padded for comfort. They should support the area of flexion to assist in maintaining a functional position. If tape is used, it should not obstruct the view of the catheter insertion site or impair circulation. When an arm board is used, additional assessment should address skin inspection for any signs of breakdown (INS, 2011a, p. S48).

Site protection refers to the methods used to prevent accidental catheter dislodgement. Site protection methods are recommended particularly for pediatric patients or for those with cognitive limitations who may be more likely to touch or manipulate the catheter or dressing. Hiding or disguising the site may decrease the risk of catheter loss. Figure 6-16 shows an example of a site protection product.

NOTE > If an arm board is used for the purpose of stabilizing an area of flexion, it is not considered a restraint.

Dressing Management

There are two methods for dressing management: (1) a gauze dressing secured with tape and (2) a transparent semipermeable membrane (TSM) dressing. A sterile gauze dressing can be applied aseptically with its edges

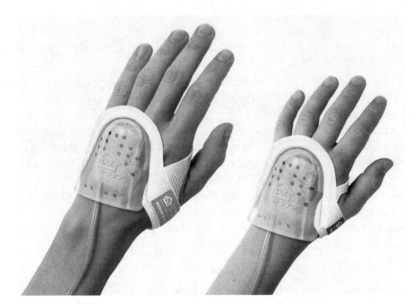

Figure 6-16 ■ I.V. House UltraDressing, which consists of flexible fabric with thumb holes and a polyethylene dome that wraps around the patient's hand after an I.V. is started. This prevents accidental snagging of the loop or catheter hub. (Courtesy of I.V. House, Inc., Chesterfield, MO.)

secured with tape. The dressing and catheter should be replaced together, unless the integrity of the dressing is impaired; then removal of the dressing with replacement of a new sterile TSM dressing is required. Do not use ointment of any kind under a TSM dressing. The TSM dressing should be applied only to the cannula hub and wings.

To apply a TSM dressing:

1. Cleanse the area of excess moisture after venipuncture.
2. Center the transparent dressing over the cannula site and partially over the hub.
3. Press down on the dressing, sealing the catheter site.
4. A piece of tape can be added to loop the administration set tubing, securing it to the skin below the TSM dressing (Fig. 6-17).

 NURSING FAST FACT!

> Do not put tape over the TSM dressing because it will be difficult to re-move the dressing if it needs to be changed because of a break in the integrity of the dressing.

Advantages of TSM dressings include the following: they allow continuous inspection of the site, and they are more comfortable than gauze and tape.

INS Standard Routine site care and dressing changes are not performed on short peripheral catheters unless the dressing is soiled or is no longer intact (INS, 2011a, p. S63).

Given the longer dwell times with PIV catheters, there is a lack of guidance on the use of gauze and tape dressings. With central venous access devices (CVADs), gauze and tape dressings are changed every 2 days so that the nurse can visualize the site and perform site care to reduce skin flora. Figure 6-18 shows a PIV site being dressed with a TSM dressing.

Postcannulation

Step 12: Labeling

For peripheral infusions, labels need to be applied to three areas: the insertion site, the tubing, and the solution container, which can be time stripped.

1. The venipuncture site should be labeled on the side of the transparent dressing or across the hub. Do not place the label over the site because this obstructs visualization of the site. Include the following on the insertion site label (INS, 2011b):
   ■ Date and time
   ■ Gauge and length of the catheter (e.g., 20-gauge, 1-inch)
   ■ The nurse's initials

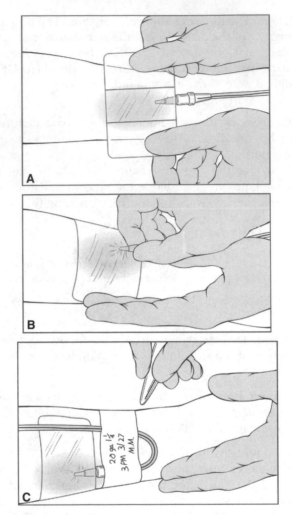

Figure 6-17 ■ *A* and *B*, Steps in applying transparent semipermeable dressing directly over the I.V. catheter hub and insertion site. *C*, Label site below transparent semipermeable membrane dressing.

2. Label the administration set with date and time according to organizational policy and procedure so that nurses on subsequent shifts will be aware of when the tubing must be changed.
3. Labeling the solution container with a strip of tape or a preprinted strip is still practiced in some areas of the country. Place a time strip on all parenteral solutions. The time strip should contain the name of the solution and additives, the initials of the nurse, and the time the solution was started if included in the policy and procedure of the institution.

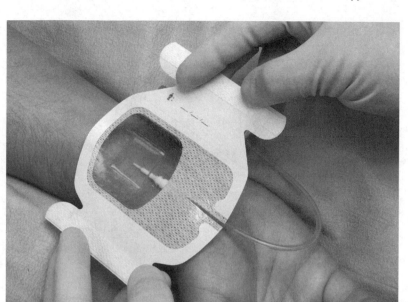

Figure 6-18 ■ Applying a Tegaderm CHG dressing over a peripheral intravenous catheter. (Courtesy 3M Medical Division, St. Paul, MN.)

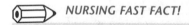 **NURSING FAST FACT!**

Time strips are helpful as a quick method to visually assess whether the solution is on schedule. They are not used in all institutions.

Step 13: Equipment Disposal

All blood-contaminated sharps must be discarded in nonpermeable, puncture-resistant, tamper-proof biohazard containers (U.S. Department of Labor, n.d.). All devices should have engineered sharps injury protection mechanisms, and these mechanisms should be activated before disposal (INS, 2011a, p. S28). Nonsharp items exposed to blood also should be discarded in a biohazard container. Figure 6-19 shows examples of tamper-proof biohazard containers.

Step 14: Patient Education

The nurse has a responsibility to educate the patient, caregiver, or legally authorized representative about the prescribed infusion therapy. The plan of care as part of the nursing process includes developing a plan for teaching and implementing the plan under interventions. Documentation of teaching is a mode of communication among the members of the health

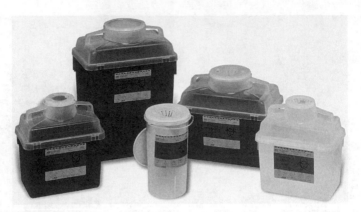

Figure 6-19 ■ Tamper-proof biohazard containers. (Courtesy of BD Medical, Sandy, UT.)

team. The nurse must document, as part of intervention, the education of the patient or the caregivers.

INS Standard The nurse shall educate the patient, caregiver, or legally authorized representative about the prescribed infusion therapy and plan of care, including, but not limited to, the purpose and expected outcomes and/or goals of treatment, infusion therapy administration, infusion device–related care, potential complications or adverse effects associated with treatment or therapy, and risks and benefits (INS, 2011a, p. S16).

 NURSING FAST FACT!

Attention should be given to age, developmental (psychosocial as well as psychomotor) and cognitive levels, and cultural and linguistic sensitivity.

Patient education begins before initiation of infusion therapy with discussion of potential complications with risks and benefits of therapy. Once the catheter is stabilized and the dressing applied, the following information should be included in education and documented:
- Limitations on movement or mobility
- Alarms if an electronic infusion device (EID) will be used
- Need to notify and call nurse if the venipuncture site becomes tender or sore or if redness or swelling develops (Gorski, Hallock, Kuehn, et al. 2012)
- Routine check of the venipuncture site by the nurse

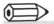 *NURSING FAST FACT!*

> *It is important to validate the patient's understanding and ability to perform infusion-related self-care procedures. Written and verbal instructions should be documented.*

Step 15: Rate Calculations

Infusions are delivered over a specific period of time. Calculating the proper infusion rate for medication and solution delivery is critical. All infusions should be monitored frequently for accurate flow rates and complications associated with infusion therapy.

NOTE > Practice problems are included in the chapter along with extra practice problems on Davis*Plus*.

Refer to Worksheet 6-2.

The following presents the basic formulas for calculation of drip rates of intravenous solutions.

PRIMARY AND SECONDARY INFUSIONS

The ability to calculate infusion rates is essential in many clinical environments. The nurse must determine the manner in which the infusion is to be administered. While most infusions are delivered via an EID, others may be delivered via a gravity infusion. When administering a gravity infusion, the rate of infusion is calculated in drops per minute. Factors to include in learning accurate rate calculations include:

1. **Drop factor** of tubing
2. Authorized prescriber's hourly rate
3. Whether an EID will be used to deliver the infusion

DROP FACTOR OF TUBING

For **macrodrop** sets:

To calculate the drip rate correctly, note the drop factor of the administration set. This is usually located on the side, front, or back of the administration package. Drop factors provided by the administration set for macrodrop tubing are as follows:

Primary (macrodrop) sets:
- 10 drops = 1 mL
- 15 drops = 1 mL
- 20 drops = 1 mL

Use macrodrop sets whenever (1) a large amount of fluid is ordered to be infused over a short period of time or (2) the microdrips per minute are too many, making counting too difficult.

Formula for I.V. Flow Rates Using Drops per Minute

After the drop factor of the tubing and the amount of solution to be infused are known, the following formula can be used to calculate the drop rate per minute:

$$\text{mL per hour} \times \text{drops per mL (drop factor [DF])} \div \text{time (minutes)}$$
$$= \text{drops per minute}$$
$$\text{Formula:} \frac{\text{mL/hr} \times \text{DF}}{\text{minutes}} = \text{drop (gtt)/min}$$

Macrodrop Infusion.
Example: Orders are for 125 mL/hr and the primary tubing selected has a drop factor of 15. Two steps are needed.

$$\text{Formula:} \frac{\text{mL/hr} \times \text{DF}}{\text{minutes}} = \text{gtt/min}$$
$$\text{Step 1:} \frac{125 \times 15}{60} = \text{gtt/min}$$
$$\text{Step 2:} = 31 \text{ gtt/min}$$

Microdrop Sets. Special administration sets such as pediatric (**microdrop**) sets and transfusion administration sets are available. All manufacturers of microdrip sets are consistent in having 60 drops = 1 mL.

Pediatric (microdrop) sets:
■ 60 drops _____ 1 mL

Use microdrop sets whenever (1) the I.V. is to be administered over a long period of time, (2) a small amount of fluid is to be administered, or (3) the macrodrops per minute are too few.

Microdrop Infusion. When using a microdrip (pediatric tubing) that is 60 drops/mL, the drops per minute equal the milliliters per hour, so only one step is needed.

Example: The LIP orders 35 mL of 0.45% sodium chloride solution per hour for a 2-year-old girl. You would set up your rate calculation as follows, using only one step.

$$\text{Formula:} \frac{\text{mL/hr} \times \text{DF}}{\text{minutes}} = \text{gtt/min}$$
$$\text{Step 1:} \frac{35 \times 60}{60} = \text{gtt/min} = 35 \text{ gtt/min}$$

NOTE > Table 6-9 gives a conversion chart for rate calculation.

> Table 6-9   **CONVERSION CHART: RATE CALCULATION**

Order (mL/hr)	10 Drops/mL	15 Drops/mL	20 Drops/mL	60 Drops/mL
		Drop Factors		
10	2	3	3	10
15	3	4	5	15
20	3	5	7	20
30	5	8	10	30
50	8	13	17	50
75	13	19	25	N/A
80	13	20	27	N/A
100	17	25	33	N/A
120	20	30	40	N/A
125	21	31	42	N/A
150	25	38	50	N/A
166	27	42	55	N/A
175	29	44	58	N/A
200	33	50	67	N/A
250	42	63	83	N/A
300	50	75	100	N/A

Microdrip tubing is not appropriate for rates greater than 50 mL/hr.

INTERMITTENT MEDICATION OR SOLUTION CALCULATIONS

Secondary infusions to be given in less than 1 hour are usually medications that have been added to small amounts of I.V. fluid (usually 50–150 mL). The rate of I.V. administration must be adjusted during the administration to the time indicated by the pharmacist or pharmaceutical manufacturer. The rate of infusion of most I.V. medications is determined to prevent the possible deleterious effects of too-rapid medication delivery.

Example: Kefzol, 0.5 g in 100 mL of dextrose in water, to run intravenous piggyback (IVPB) over 30 minutes. Administration set is 20 drop factor.

$$\text{Formula: } \frac{\text{mL/hr} \times \text{DF}}{\text{minutes}} = \text{gtt/min}$$

$$\frac{100 \text{ mL} \times 20}{30} = 2000 \text{ gtt/min}$$

$$= 67 \text{ gtt/min}$$

Step 16: Documentation

After implementation of infusion therapy, the procedure should be documented in the medical records. Documentation of patient response to the procedure must be included in the patient's chart and addressed by narrative charting, by check-off format, or by the more common electronic documentation medical record. Information documented includes the status of the patient, the reason for restart, the procedure used, and comments.

Initial documentation of PIV catheter placement and infusion therapy procedure includes (INS, 2011a, p. S20):

- Date and time of insertion, number and location of attempts (e.g., anatomic descriptors, landmarks, appropriately marked drawings)
- Site preparation
- Gauge and length of device
- Infusate, dose, rate, time, route and method of administration (e.g., gravity, EID)
- Patient's specific comments related to the procedure; patient education and response
- Patient response, excessive anxiety, patient movement, or untoward response
- Signature of the nurse

Documentation should be legible, accessible to health-care professionals, and readily retrievable. With electronic health records, there are often standardized formats with drop-down options for choices. It is essential to be familiar with the organizational guidelines for infusion-related documentation.

INS Standard Documentation shall contain accurate, factual, and complete information in the patient's permanent medical record regarding the patient's infusion therapy and vascular access (INS, 2011a, p. S20).

Table 6-10 summarizes the steps in initiating peripheral infusion.

NOTE > Refer to Procedures Display 6-1 at the end of this chapter for detailed instructions on inserting an over-the-needle catheter by the direct and indirect method.

◼ Intermittent Infusion Therapy

A needleless connector is placed on the end of the PIV catheter when a continuous infusion is converted to an intermittent access. This method of intermittent access is also called a saline lock. The needleless connector is changed when the PIV catheter is removed and the site is rotated, if blood or debris is evident within the connector, and/or with contamination

> Table 6-10	SUMMARY OF STEPS IN INITIATING PERIPHERAL I.V. THERAPY

Precannula Insertion

1. Check order from LIP; confirm all parts of the order for accuracy.
2. Perform hand hygiene.
3. Equipment collection and preparation: Prepare equipment. Check for breaks in integrity and check expiration date. Spike and prime the infusion system.
4. Patient assessment, psychological preparation, and patient identification: Provide privacy.
   Explain the procedure to the patient.
   Evaluate the patient's psychological preparation for peripheral I.V. therapy by talking with patient prior to touching to assess veins. Consider autonomy, handedness, independence. Evaluate fear of pain associated with venipuncture.
5. Site selection and vein dilation:
   Assess both arms, keeping in mind the factors for vein selection.
   Make a choice whether to use a blood pressure cuff or tourniquet for dilation.
   Use other methods for venous distention, such as warm packs, gravity, tapping, multiple tourniquet, or tangential lighting if necessary.

Cannula Insertion

6. Select appropriate pain management intervention based on assessment.
7. Choose the appropriate catheter for duration of infusion and type of infusate based on facility policy and procedure. Rewash hands.
8. Don gloves, following standard precautions for exposure to blood or body fluids. Use full barrier protection if needed.
   Note: Implement anesthetic intervention per plan.
9. Prepare site with antiseptic agent and allow to air dry. Do not remove. Do not retouch.
10. Insert the over-the-needle catheter using the direct or indirect method. Thread the catheter and activate safety mechanism per manufacturer's directions to reduce risk of needlestick. Connect the catheter hub to administration set or needleless connector.
11. Stabilize the catheter hub with stabilization device. There are two methods of dressing management: (1) 2-inch × 2-inch gauze with all edges taped, change every 48 hours; or (2) transparent semipermeable membrane (TSM) dressing applied with aseptic technique and changed when catheter site is rotated, or if integrity of dressing is compromised.

Postcannula Insertion

12. Label the insertion site with cannula size, date, time, and nurse's initials; label the tubing with date and time; place time strip on solution container per organizational protocol.
13. Dispose of sharps and blood-contaminated supplies in biohazard container.
14. Explain to patient the limitations, provide information on equipment being used, and give instructions for observation of the site and signs and symptoms for patient to report.
15. Calculate drip rate: Remember when doing rate calculations that if a roller clamp or electronic controller is used, the drops per minute should be calculated based on the drop factor.
16. Document the procedure: Monitor the patient for response to prescribed therapies. Document the procedure performed, how the patient tolerated the venipuncture, and what instructions were given to the patient.

(INS, 2011a, p. S32). All needleless connectors should be of luer-lock design to reduce the risk of accidental disconnection. The PIV is "flushed" to assess catheter patency and to prevent mixing of medications and solutions that are incompatible and is "locked" with saline to maintain patency (INS, 2011a). Review flushing procedures in this chapter. Routine flushing shall be performed in the following situations:

- Administration of blood and blood components
- Blood sampling
- Administration of incompatible medications or solutions
- Administration of medication
- Intermittent therapy
- When converting from continuous to intermittent therapy

Intermittent infusion devices have both advantages and disadvantages. Figure 6-20 shows an example of a needleless connector connected to the extension tubing of the PIV catheter, which makes it an intermittent infusion device.

ADVANTAGES

- Provide access to the vascular system, allowing for greater flexibility than hanging I.V. fluids
- Allow for reduced volume of fluid administered, which can be important for cardiac patients
- May collect blood for laboratory work in some circumstances
- Provide access for delivery of emergency medications

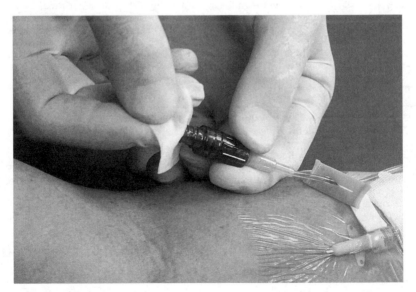

Figure 6-20 ■ Intermittent infusion device. (Courtesy of Baxter Healthcare Corp., Round Lake, IL.)

DISADVANTAGE

- May increase risk for catheter occlusion as a result of blood clot

---

NOTE > Refer to Procedures Display 6-2 at the end of this chapter for converting continuous infusion to an intermittent access device.

Midline Catheters

The midline catheter is a peripheral catheter. It is longer (up to approximately 8 inches) and is placed in the peripheral veins, generally above the antecubital fossa, with the catheter tip inserted via the basilic, cephalic, or brachial vein and the tip located below the axillary line. In infants, a midline may be placed in a scalp vein with the tip terminating in the external jugular vein. The midline catheter is an alternative to be considered between the peripheral-short catheter and a PICC.

The CDC (O'Grady et al., 2011) recommends consideration for a midline or PICC when the anticipated duration of therapy is beyond 6 days. When considering a midline catheter, the same infusate criteria apply as with short peripheral catheters: infusates with pH between 5 and 9, and osmolarity less than 600 mOsm/L. An example of appropriate use of a midline catheter is a patient who requires 3 weeks of I.V. antibiotic therapy with a medication that has a pH between 5 and 9 (e.g., ceftriaxone).

Site Selection

The three prominent antecubital veins (basilic, cephalic, median cubital) are ideal insertion sites for the midline catheter. The basilic vein is the preferred vessel because it is larger and follows a straighter path.

Patient Assessment

Before placing a midline catheter it is necessary to assess the anatomy of the patient's skin, subcutaneous tissues, and veins. Follow the criteria in step 4 of the Phillips 16-step method for initiating a short-peripheral catheter to guide assessment. Because of variations in patient size and vessel anatomy, it is recommended that the arm be premeasured.

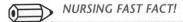 *NURSING FAST FACT!*

Optimal catheter tip location is below axillary level. Using a measuring tape, measure from the intended insertion site to the axilla and write down the distance.

INS Standard Midline catheters should be removed if the tip location is no longer appropriate for the prescribed therapy (INS, 2011a, p. S57).

NOTE > The key to successful delivery of infusion therapy is early vascular access assessment and placement of the most appropriate device for the patient and the intended infusion therapy.

■ Peripheral Infusion Site Care and Maintenance (Peripheral-Short and Midline Catheters)

The Nursing Process for Patients Receiving Peripheral Infusion

The nursing process is central to nursing actions in any setting because it helps the nurse to organize thought processes for clinical decision making and problem solving. Use of the nursing process framework (assessment, diagnosis, outcomes identification, planning, interventions, and evaluation) is beneficial for both the patient and the nurse because it helps ensure that care is planned, individualized, and reviewed over the period of time that the nurse and patient have formed a professional relationship.

Monitoring of the patient should include assessment of the PIV site and the surrounding area, flow rate, clinical data, patient response, and adherence to prescribed therapy. The INS (Gorski, et al., 2012) published a position paper providing guidance for the frequency of assessing the short PIV catheter as follows:

- At least every 4 hours for alert and oriented adult patients who are receiving nonirritant/nonvesicant infusions for any signs of problems such as pain, swelling, or redness at the site tissue.
- Every 1 to 2 hours for critically ill patients, for adult patients who have cognitive/sensory deficits or who are receiving sedative-type medications and are unable to notify the nurse of any symptoms, and for patients in whom PIVs are placed in a high-risk location (e.g., external jugular, area of flexion).
- Every hour for pediatric and neonatal patients.

Information that is obtained by monitoring should be communicated to other health-care professionals responsible for the patient's care by documentation. Observation of the patient and the delivery of infusion therapy provide data for nursing interventions. Assessment and key nursing interventions are presented under *Nursing Points of Care: Adult Peripheral Infusions.*

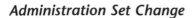

Administration Set Change

Frequency of administration set changes is the same for short-peripheral catheters and midline catheters.

CONTINUOUS INFUSIONS

The primary and secondary *continuous* administration sets and add-on devices should be replaced no more frequently than at 96-hour intervals; however, should the peripheral I.V. catheter be removed and replaced, the administration set is always replaced (O'Grady et al., 2011; INS, 2011a, p. S55).

> **INS Standard** All administration sets shall be of luer-lock design to ensure a secure junction (INS, 2011a, p. S55).

PRIMARY INTERMITTENT INFUSIONS

Primary intermittent administration sets should be changed every 24 hours (INS, 2011a, p. S55). More frequent changes are required because of increased risk for contamination at the male luer end of the administration set when intermittent infusions are disconnected and reconnected repeatedly. In other words, there is no longer a closed I.V. system. It is imperative that the male luer end of the tubing be aseptically maintained after each use.

> **INS Standard** A new sterile, compatible covering device should be aseptically attached to the end of the administration set after each use. The practice of attaching the exposed end of the administration set to a port on the same set ("looping") should be avoided (INS 2011a, p. S56).

NOTE > Administration sets used to administer blood components or lipid emulsions are discussed in Chapters 11 and 12.

Catheter Removal Criteria

All vascular access devices, including PIV catheters and midline catheters, should be removed if evidence of a complication (e.g., signs of phlebitis or infiltration) is seen, when therapy is discontinued, and when the device is no longer necessary. Traditional practice with adult patients directed that the short PIV catheter be routinely removed and replaced based on how long it was in place (e.g., every 96 hours). A major change with the 2011 INS Standards is to rotate the site based on clinical indications rather than a specific time frame. Clinical indications include assessment of the patient's condition and access site, skin and vein integrity, length and type of prescribed therapy, venue of care, and integrity and patency of the catheter (INS, 2011a, p. S57). The primary reference used to support site rotation based on clinical indications was a Cochrane systematic review of the literature (Webster et al., 2010). In the review, five randomized controlled trials that compared routine PIV catheter removal with removal only when clinically indicated were included in the analysis of 3408 trial participants, which found no conclusive evidence of benefit for routine PIV catheter site rotation.

INS Standard A peripheral-short catheter placed in an emergency situation where aseptic technique has been compromised shall be replaced as soon as possible and no later than 48 hours (INS, 2011a, p. S49).

NOTE > Refer to Procedures Display 6-4 at the end of this chapter for discontinuation of a PIV catheter.

Peripheral Flushing and Locking Standards for Intermittent Infusion Devices

The terms *flushing* and *locking* are commonly used yet sometimes misunderstood. Catheters are *flushed* after each intermittent infusion to clear any medication from the catheter and to prevent contact between incompatible medications or I.V. solutions. When not properly flushed, a precipitate can form, essentially blocking the catheter. Catheters are flushed with preservative-free 0.9% sodium chloride. Catheter *locking* refers to the solution left instilled in the catheter to prevent occlusion in-between intermittent infusions.

In 2008, the INS released "Flushing Protocols," a tool to give recommendations for flushing/locking solutions and frequency for all vascular access devices based on the type of infusion:

■ Flush peripheral catheters (short) with a minimum of 2 mL of 0.9% preservative-free sodium chloride (USP) before and after administration of medication and lock PIV catheters with 2 mL of 0.9% preservative-free sodium chloride at least every 12 hours if the catheter is not in use (INS, 2008).

■ Flush midline peripheral catheters with a minimum of 3 mL of 0.9% preservative-free sodium chloride (USP) before and after administration of medication and lock catheter with 3 mL of 10 units/mL heparin at least every 12 hours if the catheter is not in use (INS, 2008).

NOTE > This is called the *SASH method:* Saline—(clear catheter and check patency)—Administer medication—Saline (clear medication)—Heparin (administer 3 mL/10 units heparin/mL).

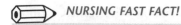

 NURSING FAST FACT!

> Some medications are incompatible with 0.9% sodium chloride. In this case, 5% dextrose in water is used for flushing, followed by normal saline and/or a heparin solution. Dextrose should not be left in the catheter lumen because it provides nutrients for growth of bacteria (INS, 2011a, p. S60).

 NURSING FAST FACT!

> ***Push–pause method versus consistent smooth flushing technique:*** Many recommend use of a rapid succession of push–pause–push–pause movements exerted on the plunger of the syringe barrel during flushing. Theoretically, this recreates a turbulence within the catheter lumen that causes a swirling effect to move any debris (residues of fibrin or medication) attached to the catheter lumen. However, no research supports the push–pause method of flushing (Macklin, 2010). Excessive turbulence could also potentially cause damage to the tunica intima. The issue of flushing technique (push–pause) versus a smooth injection of the flush solution is an area of controversy and differences in practice. Research is needed to establish the most effective flushing procedure.

NOTE > Refer to Procedures Display 6-3 at the end of this chapter for flushing technique and protocols.

Needleless Connectors

Needleless connectors (see Chapter 5) are connected to the hub of the PIV catheter or the midline and are designed to accommodate the tip of a syringe or I.V. tubing for catheter flushing or intermittent administration of solutions into the vascular system.

Important issues related to needleless connectors include frequency of device change and maintenance of aseptic technique when accessing the needleless connector for infusion, flushing, and locking. The needleless connector is changed on a regular basis as follows: when the I.V. tubing is changed, if residual blood is present in the device, and whenever the integrity is compromised or contamination is suspected (INS, 2011a). Manufacturer's guidelines and organizational policies will provide further guidance on frequency of change, including whether the device should be changed after blood withdrawal for laboratory tests.

Failure to disinfect the needleless connectors for flushing or medication administration is a significant problem. The Institute for Safe Medication Practices (ISMP, 2007) highlighted the problem of failing to disinfect the needleless connector when accessing the infusion for flushing or medication administration, thus increasing the risk for contamination and potential catheter-associated bloodstream infection. The Joint Commission includes the following in its 2013 National Patient Safety Goals: "use a standardized protocol to disinfect catheter hubs and injection ports prior to accessing the port."

The INS (2011a) recommends either 70% alcohol (i.e., typical alcohol "wipes") or greater than 0.5% chlorhexidine solution as acceptable antiseptics for needleless connector disinfection. Many nurses are familiar with the "scrub the hub" mantra, emphasizing the importance of cleansing with friction and not just a quick "wipe." The nurse should scrub the hub and the threads on the needleless connector. Guerin et al. (2010) incorporated a 15-second alcohol scrub as part of a postinsertion CVAD "care bundle" that resulted in further infection rate reduction where the central line insertion bundle was already consistently practiced. Of note, there are emerging technology solutions to infection concerns. There are needleless connectors that are designed with silver and chlorhexidine microbial barriers built into the device. There are also plastic caps, "alcohol caps," which are attached to the needleless connector. The needleless connector is continually protected until the cap is removed, and the step of scrubbing the needleless connector is not necessary.

Follow these steps every time the needless connector is accessed:

1. Perform proper hand hygiene.
2. Disinfect needleless connector with each access using 70% alcohol or 3.1% chlorhexidine/70% alcohol for 15 seconds using friction (twisting motion) (strongly recommended).
3. Let the alcohol/chlorhexidine dry (kills bacteria).

EBP A significant decrease in pediatric bloodstream infections occurred when an organization switched from alcohol to 2% chlorhexidine/alcohol for needleless connector and catheter hub disinfection on a stem cell transplant unit (Soothill et al., 2009). The Pediatric Vascular Access Network recommends allowing a 15-second scrub to dry completely before access (Pedivan, 2010).

EBP In a study that included both a clinical phase, tested on patients, and an in-vitro test, scrubbing the needleless connector for five seconds followed by a 5 second dry time resulted in adequate disinfection. Of note, this was tested on a split septum needleless connector and cannot be generalized to other types of connectors (see Chapter 5) (Rupp et al., 2012).

NOTE >   Refer to Procedures Display 6-3 at the end of this chapter for a
         peripheral-short flush procedure.

Nursing Plan of Care
ADULT PERIPHERAL INFUSION

Nursing Assessments
- Interview the patient regarding previous experiences with venipunctures, including pain issues.
- Review the purpose of the infusion and patient diagnosis.
- Assess venipuncture sites, taking into consideration the physical condition of sites, any disease processes, and cultural issues.
- Review laboratory test results, vital signs, and continued need for PIV catheter.
- Check solution container and administration set for solution clarity, system integrity, and proper labeling.
- Be alert for signs/symptoms of complications/adverse reactions.

Key Nursing Interventions
Verify the authorized prescriber's written or electronic orders for infusion therapy.
1. Educate the patient about the procedure before initiation of therapy.
2. Maintain standard precautions.
3. Adhere to hand hygiene practices.
4. Use strict aseptic technique during insertion and maintenance of the cannula.
5. Determine compatibility of all infusion fluids and additives by consulting the appropriate literature.
6. Select and prepare the EID as indicated.
7. Choose an appropriate size catheter for delivery of infusion.
8. Apply the catheter stabilization device.
9. Maintain the integrity of I.V. equipment.
10. Document the procedure and observations of the site.

AGE-RELATED CONSIDERATIONS
Pediatric Peripheral Infusion Therapy
Physiological Characteristics
A neonate is a child in the period of extrauterine life up to the first 28 days after birth. Low-birth-weight and premature infants have decreased energy stores and increased metabolic needs compared with full-term, average-weight newborns.

Whereas the adult body consists of approximately 60% water, the infant body consists of 70% to 80% water, and infants have proportionately more water in the extracellular compartment than do adults (Doellman, 2014).

Continued

Therefore, any depletion in these water stores may lead to dehydration. As an infant becomes older, the ratio of extracellular to intracellular fluid volume decreases.

Although infants have relatively greater circulating blood volume per unit of body weight compared to adults, the absolute blood volume is small, which makes infants more vulnerable to hypovolemia (Frey & Pettit, 2010). Immature and inefficient kidneys lead to excretion of more water than in older pediatric patients, and renal function does not reach maturity until the end of the second year (Doellman, 2014). Any condition that interferes with normal water and electrolyte intake or produces excessive water and electrolyte losses will result in more rapid depletion of water and electrolyte stores in an infant than it will in an adult.

Young children have immature homeostatic regulating mechanisms that need to be considered when water and electrolyte replacement is needed. Renal function, acid–base balance, body surface area differences, and electrolyte concentrations all must be taken into consideration when planning fluid needs.

The buffering capacity to regulate acid–base balance is lower in newborns than in older children. Neonates, with an average pH of 7.30 to 7.35, are slightly more acidotic than adults (Doellman, 2014). The base bicarbonate deficit is thought to be related to high metabolic acid production and renal immaturity.

The integumentary system in neonates is an important route of fluid loss, especially in illness. This must be considered when determining fluid balance in infants and young children because their body surface areas are greater than those of older children and adults. Any condition that produces a decrease in intake or output of water and electrolytes affects the body fluid stores of the infant. Because the gastrointestinal (GI) membranes are an extension of the body surface area, relatively greater losses occur from the GI tract in sick infants.

Plasma electrolyte concentrations do not vary strikingly among infants, small children, and adults. The plasma sodium concentration changes little from birth to adulthood. Potassium and chloride concentrations are higher in the first few months of life than at any other time. Magnesium and calcium levels both are low in the first 24 hours after birth. The serum phosphate level is elevated in the early months of infancy, which contributes to a low calcium level. Newborn infants are vulnerable to disrupted calcium homeostasis when they are stressed by illness or by an excess phosphate load and are at risk for hypocalcemia (Doellman, 2014).

Physical Assessment

A physical assessment of pediatric patients should be performed before I.V. therapy is initiated. Table 6-11 lists the components of a pediatric assessment. Risk factors that must be considered during the assessment phase include prematurity, catabolic disease state, hypothermia, hyperthermia, metabolic or respiratory alkalosis or acidosis, and other metabolic abnormalities.

> Table 6-11	COMPONENTS OF THE PEDIATRIC PHYSICAL ASSESSMENT

Measurement of head circumference (up to 1 year)
Height or length
Weight
Vital signs
Skin turgor
Presence of tears
Moistness and color of mucous membranes
Intake and urinary output
Characteristics of fontanelles
Level of child's activity related to growth and development

Site Selection

When selecting the venipuncture site, keep in mind that the main goal of infusion therapy is to provide the treatment with safety and efficiency while meeting the child's emotional and developmental needs.

Consider the following factors before selecting a site for venipuncture:
• Age of the child
• Size of the child
• Condition of veins
• Objective of the infusion therapy (hydration, administration of medication, etc.)
• General patient condition
• Mobility and level of activity of child
• Gross and fine motor skills (e.g., sucks fingers, plays with hands, holds bottle, draws)
• Sense of body image
• Cognitive ability of the child (i.e., can understand and follow directions)

Peripheral Sites

Peripheral routes for pediatric I.V. therapy include scalp veins and the veins in the dorsum of the hand, forearm, and foot. Table 6-12 compares selected insertion sites.

SCALP VEINS

The major superficial veins of the scalp can be used. Scalp veins can be used in children up to age 18 months (Frey & Pettit, 2010); after that age, the hair follicles mature and the epidermis toughens. Four scalp veins are used most commonly for I.V. access: temporal, frontal, posterior auricular, and occipital (Fig. 6-21). Of note, scalp veins do not contain valves (Doellman, 2014).

 NURSING FAST FACT!

The choice of a scalp vein for placement of I.V. therapy is often traumatic for the parents because removal of hair may have cultural and religious significance. In addition, maintaining patency of this site can be difficult at times.

Continued

> Table 6-12	**PEDIATRIC INFUSION SITES**		
Veins and Site	**Age Appropriate**	**Advantages**	**Disadvantages**
Scalp			
Superficial temporal (front of ear) Frontal (middle of forehead) Occipital Posterior auricular	Infant <18 months of age	Highly visible Easily accessed and monitored Veins readily dilate Keeps feet and hands free No valves	Hair must be trimmed or clipped Infiltrates easily Difficult to stabilize device Increase familial anxiety May have cultural issues
Lower Extremities			
Leg: Saphenous Foot: Metatarsal	Infant: Used before crawling and walking	Large vessels Readily dilate Hands kept free Easily restrained/ splinted	Decreased mobility Located near arterial structures Difficult to observe/ palpate in chubby infants Risk of phlebitis is increased
Hand			
Metacarpal	All ages	Easily accessible/ visible May accommo- date a larger gauge Distal location May not require splinting	Uncomfortable Difficult to anchor/ stabilize May impede child's activities (thumbsucking, schoolwork) Difficult to observe/ palpate in chubby infants/toddlers Difficult to observe/ palpate in chubby toddlers
Forearm			
Cephalic Basilic Median antebrachial	All ages	Same as for hand Keeps hands free	Difficult to observe/ palpate in chubby toddlers

The I.V. catheter must be placed in the direction of blood flow to ensure that the I.V. fluid will flow in the same direction as the blood returning to the heart. In the scalp, venous blood generally flows from the top of the head down.

NOTE > Shaving is not recommended; if necessary, clip the hair on infants.

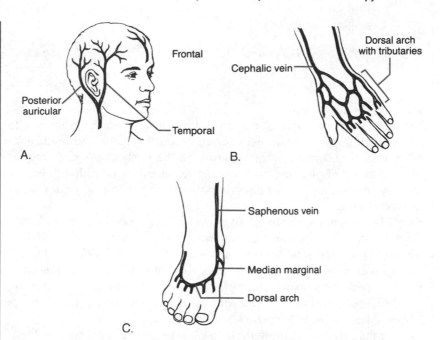

Figure 6-21 ■ *A*, Superficial veins of scalp. *B*, Dorsum of hand. *C*, Foot.

CULTURAL AND ETHNIC CONSIDERATIONS: USING SCALP VEINS

People in the Hmong culture believe that the spirit (soul) of the child can be released from the head. Be sure to check with an elder family member before choosing a site for venipuncture (Giger & Davidhizar, 2004; Munoz & Luckmann, 2005).

DORSUM OF THE HAND AND FOREARM

Because the veins over the metacarpal area are mobile and not well supported by surrounding tissue, the limb must be immobilized with a splint and taped before cannulation. This site can be used in children of all ages.

The antecubital fossa should not be routinely used for peripheral I.V. access as it is an area of flexion with an increased risk for infiltration. It should be reserved for blood drawing and may be used in emergency situations for vascular access.

LOWER EXTREMITIES

Lower extremity sites are used as venipuncture sites for infants before they can crawl and walk. The curve of the foot, especially around the ankle, makes entry and cannula advancement difficult. The veins used are the metatarsal, saphenous, median, and marginal dorsal arch.

Continued

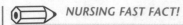 *NURSING FAST FACT!*

The foot should be secured on a padded board with a normal joint position.

Selecting the Equipment
The nurse must be aware of the special needs of pediatric patients when selecting appropriate equipment for administering fluids and medication. When choosing administration equipment, the safety of the child requires that the activity level, age, and size of the patient be considered. For safe delivery of I.V. therapy in pediatric patients, the following equipment is recommended:
• An EID for administration of therapy; tamper-proof features as well as variable pressure limits and alarms should be present (Doellman, 2014)
• A solution container with a volume based on the age, height, and weight of the patient and containing no more than 24-hour volume requirements
• Special pediatric equipment, such as controlled-volume sets (50-, 100-, 150-mL) for pediatric patients with infusion rates less than 100 mL per hour unless an EID will be used
• Plastic fluid containers (preferable to glass because of possible breakage)
• Microdrip tubing (60 gtt/min)
• Non-DEHP (di[2-ethylhexyl] phthalate) I.V. containers and administration sets to prevent toxicity (INS, 2011a, p. S6)
• A 0.2-micron air-eliminating filter set (Fig. 6-22) is available for neonates and infants to provide 96-hour bacterial and associated endotoxin retention for patient protection.
PIV catheter sites are monitored at least every hour or more frequently, depending on the patient's age and size or type of therapy (Gorski, et al., 2012).

Catheter Selection
Catheter choice depends on the site selected. In children, peripheral over-the-needle–type catheters are preferred (22- to 26-gauge). A 19- to 27-gauge scalp vein (butterfly) needle is easy to insert and can be used, but it has the risk of infiltrating easily and can be used only with single, one-time short infusions. For neonates, 24- to 26-gauge needles are used; for children, 22- to 24-gauge needles are most common. These catheters are also easier to stabilize. Use a small-size, short-length catheter appropriate for the prescribed therapy (INS, 2011a).

Equipment
• A child's I.V. container should contain no more than 24-hour volume requirements.
• A volume-controlled chamber (VCC) (metered volume containers may be used for hourly rates of less than 100 mL/hr).
• A 0.2-micron air-eliminating and particulate-retentive filter may be used for neonates and infants (Fig. 6-22).

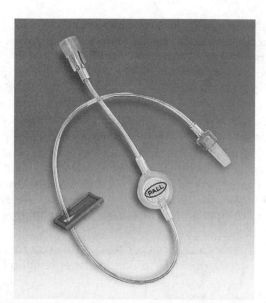

Figure 6-22 ■ 0.2 Micron air-eliminating filter set. (Provided compliments of Pall Corporation, 2013.)

NOTE > Fill the cylinder with enough fluid to prime the tubing plus fluid for a *maximum* of 2 hours.

• All infusion administrative equipment should be of luer-lock design.
• All EIDs should have safety features including anti–free-flow protection alarms, lockout protection to prevent tampering, and dose error reduction systems (INS, 2011a, p. S34).

Venipuncture Techniques
The methods for venipuncture are the same for children as for adults; a direct or indirect method can be used. Keep in mind the following safety guidelines when setting up an I.V. for a child.

Tips
The following tips on technique are unique to pediatric patients:

1. Venipuncture should be performed in a room separate from the child's room. The child's room is his or her "safe space." Always have extra help.
2. For the scalp vein position, the head is in a dependent position.
3. Use developmentally supportive measures to minimize stress, such as a pacifier, talking softly, swaddling, or avoiding sudden moves (Doellman, 2014).
4. A smaller tourniquet is preferred for neonates and pediatric patients.
5. Infants should be covered with a blanket to minimize cold stress. If the dorsum of the hand is used, place the extremity on an arm board before venipuncture.

Continued

6. A flashlight or transilluminator device placed beneath the extremity helps to illuminate tissue surrounding the vein; the veins are then outlined for better visualization

7. Warm hands by washing them in warm water before gloving.

8. Minimizing pain during venipuncture is a goal of nursing care. Involve parents in the procedure; provide distraction and address positioning of infants and young children; have the pediatric patient face the parent; and secure and swaddle the infant or young child in position (Cohen, 2008). The use of sucrose water (2 mL of 25% sucrose solution by syringe or on a pacifier) is an evidence-based intervention to decrease pain from acute procedures (Cohen, 2008). Consider use of a topical anesthetic cream, and apply up to 1 hour before venipuncture.

9. Stabilize the catheter with manufactured stabilization devices, sterile tapes, or surgical strips.

10. Use only hypoallergenic or paper tape. When you are ready to remove the tape, apply warm water so that the tape will lift off easily.

NOTE > Use colored stickers or drawings on the I.V. site as a reward. **Always have extra help.**

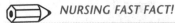 *NURSING FAST FACT!*

    When securing a child's extremity to an arm board, use clear tape for visualization of the I.V. site and digits or skin immediately adjacent to the site.

Stabilizing and maintaining the patency of I.V. cannula sites can be a challenge. Poorly secured I.V. access sites may result in dislodgements or infiltrations requiring I.V. restarts. Products are available to protect pediatric I.V.s while maintaining visualization, such as a clear, one-piece unit (Fig. 6-23).

For children, illness and hospitalization constitute major life crises. Children are vulnerable to the crises of illness and hospitalization because stress represents a change from the usual state of health and environmental routine and because children have a limited number of coping mechanisms to resolve the stressful events.

Children's understanding of, reaction to, and methods of coping with illness or hospitalization are influenced by the significance of individual stressors during each developmental phase. The major stressors are separation, loss of control, and bodily injury.

Site Care and Maintenance

Inspect and monitor the vascular access device, connections, infusate prescribed, and pump functions including flow rate. Perform site checks

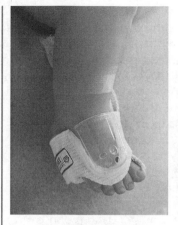 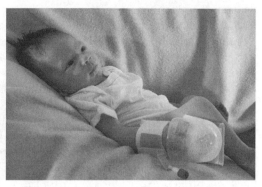

Figure 6-23 ■ IV House Ultradressing Pediatric. (Courtesy of IV House, Inc., Chesterfield, MO.)

minimally every hour (Gorski, et al., 2012). Assess the range of motion of the cannulated extremity, taking into consideration the child's developmental age. Monitor the patient's overall response to therapy. Remove and replace peripheral-short catheters based on clinical condition of the site and not on time frame (INS, 2011a).

Flushing Protocols
Flushing protocols have recently been developed by the INS for adult as well as pediatric patients. Table 6-13 gives flush standards for peripheral-short and midline catheters in children.

> Table 6-13 | **FLUSHING GUIDELINES FOR PEDIATRIC PATIENTS**

Peripheral I.V. catheters with approximate priming volume (APV) of 0.05–0.07 mL have the following guidelines for flushing:

Locking Device

NICU patient: 1 mL of preservative-free saline every 6 hours
Pediatric patient: 1–3 mL preservative-free saline every 8 hours
■ Medication pre- and post-administration: two times the volume of the administration tubing and add-on set

Midline Flushing Standards (Fr = French)

3 Fr: 0.16 APV
4 Fr: 0.19 APV
5 Fr: 0.22 APV

■ 2 Fr: 1 mL preservative-free saline + 10 units/mL heparin every 6 hours
■ 2.6 Fr and larger: 2–3 mL preservative-free saline + 10 units/mL of heparin every 12 hours
■ Medication pre- and post-administration: two times administration tubing and add-on set volume

Source: INS (2008), with permission.

Continued

Medication Administration

Delivering medication to children requires that the nurse have expert knowledge of the techniques for the delivery of medication and for the calculation of formulas. Most infusion complications in pediatric patients are attributed to dosing, fluid administration, or both. A nurse administering infusion therapy to pediatric patients must possess the knowledge necessary to verify, calculate, administer, and accurately control the rate of the prescribed therapy.

Strategies for safe delivery of medications to children include:

• Monitor weight accurately. Include weight changes in shift reports.
• Perform staff competency checks annually in weighing children, using scales on the unit.
• Collaborate with biomedical engineers regarding the frequency of quality assurance and calibration checks of scales.
• Require nurses to verify accuracy of dose recommendations and calculations on the original drug and I.V. fluid prescription forms.
• Acquire current medication manuals that provide necessary information for safe administration of I.V. medications.
• Develop charts of frequently used drugs that provide practical information on medication concentrations, drug dosing, and administration requirements.

NOTE > Pediatric medication calculations and formulas are discussed in Chapter 7, with worksheets. Calculating drug dosages by body weight, body surface area, and intermittent infusion by VCC also is discussed in Chapter 7, along with formulas.

Four methods are used to deliver intravenous medications and solutions to the pediatric patient: I.V. push or bolus, VCC, retrograde method, and syringe pump.

NOTE > The child's developmental stage is an important factor to consider when planning to administer medications.

I.V. Push or Bolus

Direct I.V. push delivers small amounts of medication over a short period of time, usually 5 minutes or less. The advantages of this method are its speed, the presence of the nurse during the complete administration of the medication, and the immediate assessment of response to the drug. Risks include speed shock when medications are given too rapidly (see Chapter 9).

Metered Volume Chamber Sets

Metered volume chamber sets are often used with children for safety in delivery of medication and solutions, although the increasing use of EIDs and syringe pumps has reduced their usage (Hadaway, 2010b). The administration set is used with a 250- to 500-mL solution container to ensure decreased risk of fluid overload. This method allows a limited amount of fluid to be available to the patient because the chamber is filled with only 1 to 2 hours' duration of the prescribed fluid volume. Frequent monitoring and refilling of the VCC by the nurse are required. Metered volume chamber sets are also used for intermittent medication infusion when the primary solution is compatible with the medication.

Retrograde Infusions

Retrograde infusion is an alternative to drug administration by syringe pumps. It is used in the general pediatric area and less often in the neonatal intensive care units (Frey & Pettit, 2010). A specific retrograde administration set is required for this purpose. The tubing volume varies but generally holds less than 1 mL. An access port is located at each end of the tubing. Use the following steps for retrograde infusion:

1. Attach the retrograde tubing and prime along with the primary administration set. The tubing functions as an extension set when it is not used to administer medication.
2. To administer the medication, attach a medication-filled syringe to the port proximal to the patient and connect an empty syringe to the port most distal from the patient.
3. Make sure the clamp between the port and the child is closed, and then inject the medication distally up the tubing (this prevents your patient from receiving medication as a bolus dose). The fluid in the retrograde tubing is displaced upward into the tubing and the empty syringe.
4. Remove both syringes and open the lower clamp. The medication is then infused into the patient at the prescribed rate by the EID.

Syringe Pump

The fourth method of infusing drugs is the syringe pump, which is the method of choice for administering most medications greater than 2 mL in volume and those that cannot be administered by the I.V. push method. Many new pumps on the market contain safety features (see Chapter 5 for a discussion of infusion equipment).

NOTE > Parenteral nutrition and transfusion therapy are also frequently administered to pediatric patients. Special considerations for the delivery of blood products and parenteral nutrition are discussed in Chapters 11 and 12.

Alternative Administration Routes

Alternative routes for administration of infusion therapy in pediatric patients include intraosseous and umbilical veins and arteries. These routes are addressed in Chapter 10.

Continued

NURSING POINTS OF CARE
PEDIATRIC PERIPHERAL INFUSION

Nursing Assessments
- Interview the patient's parents/caregiver for the patient's current health status.
- Measure height and weight for calculation of body surface area and drug dosages.
- Identify the developmental level.
- Identify the purpose of the infusion.

Key Nursing Interventions
1. Maintain standard precautions.
2. Monitor
   a. Intake and output
   b. I.V. site minimally every hour
   c. Fluid overload
   d. Alterations in vital signs
3. Explain the procedure and equipment and the rationales for treatment to the parents and child if appropriate.
4. Provide opportunities for non-nutritive sucking in infants.
5. Encourage parents to provide daily care of the child.
6. Maintain the daily routine during hospitalization.
7. Provide a quiet, uninterrupted environment during nap time and nighttime as appropriate.
8. Use appropriate equipment for delivery of safe infusions (VCC, EID, syringe pump for small volumes).
9. Calculate drug dosage correctly and double-check the dosage calculation with another health-care provider (e.g., nurse, pharmacist) before administration.
10. Follow best practices for use of safety equipment in delivery of medications and solutions to pediatric patients.

Peripheral Infusion Therapy in the Older Adult
As with the pediatric patient, care of the older adult has become an area of specialty nursing that requires special approaches to infusion-related care. Consider the following statistics (Department of Health & Human Services, Administration on Aging, 2011):
- In the United States, there were 39.6 million persons 65 years or older in 2009 (the latest year for which data are available), representing 12.9% of the U.S. population (about one in every eight Americans).

- By 2030, there will be about 72.1 million older persons, more than twice their number in 2000.

Persons older than 65 years represented 12.4% of the population in the year 2000 but are expected to grow to 19% of the population by 2030.

Physiological Changes

The skin is one of the first systems to show signs of the aging process. The epidermis and dermis are visible markers of aging and greatly affect the placement of peripheral catheters. The most striking change is an approximately 20% loss in thickness of the dermal layer, which results in the paper-thin appearance of aging skin (Baranoski et al., 2012). This also results in decreased pain perception, which potentially makes older patients less likely to feel and report pain with infiltration or phlebitis. **Purpura** and ecchymoses may appear as a result of the greater fragility of the dermal and subcutaneous vessels and the loss of support for the skin capillaries. Minor trauma can easily cause bruising.

A common symptom in older people is pruritus or "itchiness." Dryer skin may result from atrophy of sweat glands in the dermal layer as well as from medications and should be considered when preparing the patient for parenteral therapy.

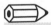 *NURSING FAST FACT!*

> *Alcohol, when used in skin antisepsis, will add to the drying effect on the skin.*

The dermis becomes relatively dehydrated and loses strength and elasticity. This layer has underlying papillae that hold the epidermis and dermis together; thus, as a person ages, the older skin loosens. Older skin has decreased flexibility of collagen fibers, increased fragility of the capillaries, and fewer capillaries (Fig. 6-24).

 ### Websites

Hartford Institute for Geriatric Nursing: http://consultgerirn.org
American Geriatrics Society: www.americangeriatrics.org

Venipuncture Techniques

Special venipuncture techniques are required to successfully place and maintain infusion therapy in older patients. Changes in the intimal layers of the vein result in increased resistance and decreased compliance of veins and arteries. The elastic fibers progressively straighten, fray, split, and fragment. There is an increase in the density and amount of collagen fibers in the vessel walls, along with decreasing elasticity of these walls. The potential complications associated with trauma, surgery, and illness in the

Continued

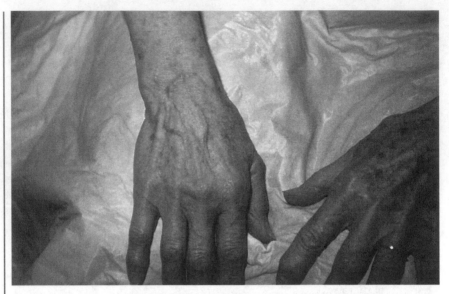

Figure 6-24 ■ Fragile veins.

older adult, along with the physiological changes previously addressed, require that nurses be knowledgeable about aging changes and their implications on nursing practice. Because the older adult patient may be at greater risk for potential complications related to infusion therapy, frequent monitoring is required. For example, even small infiltrations can lead to significant complications (Fabian, 2010).

Vascular Access Device Selection
Consider the skin and vein changes of older adults before initiating a PIV. Also consider catheter design and gauge size.

 NURSING FAST FACT!

> *To reduce insertion-related trauma, use a 22- to 24-gauge catheter.*

 NURSING FAST FACT!

> *To prevent fluid overload, use an EID when appropriate. Because of the fragile nature of the veins of elderly patients, be aware of the potential complications associated with pressures generated from mechanical infusion devices (see Chapter 5 for a discussion of safety features associated with programmable pumps).*

Selecting a Vein

Selecting a vein can be a challenge for nurses caring for the older adult. Initial venipuncture should be in the most distal portion of the extremity, which allows subsequent venipunctures to move progressively upward. However, in older adults, the veins of the hands may not be the best choice for the initial site because of the loss of subcutaneous fat and thinning of the skin. Physiological changes in the skin and veins must be considered when a site is selected. Areas for PIV access should have adequate tissue and skeletal support. Avoid flexion areas and areas with bruising because the oncotic pressure is increased in these areas and causes vessels to collapse.

Use a tourniquet to help distend and locate appropriate veins but avoid applying it too tightly because it can cause vein damage when the vein is punctured. Alternatively, a blood pressure cuff may be used, and, in some cases, a tourniquet may not be needed for venous access. During venous distention, palpate the vein to determine its condition. Veins that feel ribbed or rippled may distend readily when a tourniquet is applied, but these sites are often impossible to access and cause pain to the patient. Table 6-14 summarizes tips for use with fragile veins.

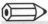 *NURSING FAST FACT!*

> Place a tourniquet over a gown or sleeve to decrease the shearing force on fragile skin.

Valves become stiff and less effective with age. Bumps along the vein path (i.e., valves) may cause problems during attempts at vein access. Venous circulation may be sluggish, resulting in slow venous return, distention, venous stasis, and dependent edema. A catheter may not thread into a vein with stiff valves.

Small surface veins appear as thin tortuous veins with many bifurcations. Appropriate catheter gauge and length selection is critical to successful I.V. access placement in these veins.

> Table 6-14 | **TIPS FOR THE OLDER ADULT WITH FRAGILE VEINS**

The following tips are for patients with fragile veins (age or disease process related):
- To prevent hematoma, avoid overdistention of the vein with tourniquet or blood pressure cuff; may not need to use tourniquet.
- Avoid multiple tapping of the vein.
- Use the smallest gauge catheter for the therapy prescribed.
- Lower the angle of approach into the vein.
- Pull the skin taut and stabilize the vein throughout venipuncture.
- Use the one-handed technique: Advance the catheter off the stylet into the vein.
- Use warm compress to dilate vein if needed. Be aware that the older adult is more sensitive to heat.

Continued

Cannulation Techniques

In elderly patients, stabilization of the vein is critical. The vessels may lack stability as a result of the loss of tissue mass and may tend to roll. Techniques to perform a venipuncture in elderly patients include:

1. Use of traction by placing the thumb directly along the vein axis about 2 to 3 inches below the intended venipuncture site. The palm and fingers of the traction hand serve to hold and stabilize the extremity. Using the index finger of the hand, provide traction to further stretch the skin above the intended venipuncture site. Maintain traction throughout venipuncture.

2. Insert the catheter, using either the direct or indirect technique. When the direct technique is used, insert the catheter at a 20- to 30-degree angle in a single motion, penetrating the skin and vein simultaneously. Do not stab or thrust the catheter into the skin, which could cause the catheter to advance too deeply and accidentally damage the vein. Use the indirect method (two-step) for patients with small, delicate veins. An alternative method is to have another nurse apply digital pressure with the hand above the site of venipuncture and release it after the vein has been entered.

NURSING POINTS OF CARE
OLDER ADULT PERIPHERAL INFUSION

Nursing Assessments
- Interview the patient regarding previous experiences with venipuncture.
- Review the purpose of the infusion and patient diagnosis, history, or comorbidities.
- Assess venipuncture sites, taking into consideration the physical condition of the skin, any disease processes, and cultural issues.
- Review trends in vital signs.

Key Nursing Interventions
1. Maintain aseptic technique and standard precautions.
2. Use appropriate techniques to dilate veins that maintain the integrity of the skin (consider blood pressure cuff).
3. Explain procedures, keeping in mind sensory or auditory deficits.

Home Care Issues

Peripheral I.V. catheters are generally indicated for short-term infusion therapy (7–10 days) or intermittent infusions (e.g., monthly infusion) of nonirritating drugs and fluids. Home care issues related to the initiation and maintenance of peripheral I.V. administration include technical procedures, such as infusion administration and site rotation, as well as monitoring for expected effects and potential adverse reactions.

- The patient who is receiving infusions via a PIV catheter in the home setting presents a unique situation because the nurse is only in the home intermittently. Patient safety is an important aspect of home care. The patient and caregiver must be motivated, willing, and able to participate in the care and monitoring of the PIV catheter and the infusion (Gorski, et al., 2012). With every home visit, the nurse assesses the I.V. site, but this becomes the patient's/caregiver's responsibility between the nurse's home visits. Patient education is critical. Information must include (Gorski, et al., 2012):
  - What to look for: Redness, tenderness, swelling, site drainage
  - Check site at least every 4 hours during waking hours
  - Ways to protect site during sleep and activity
  - How to stop infusion if signs and symptoms are present
  - To promptly report to the home care organization's 24-hour contact numbers

    The degree of technical procedures that the patient is expected to learn and perform depends on his or her cognitive ability, willingness to learn, and the specific technique being taught. In some cases, the patient/caregiver may actually self-administer the infusions; in other cases, the nurse administers each dose. For a patient/caregiver who self-administers PIV infusions, teaching will address administration sets, setting up and monitoring infusion pumps, and adhering to aseptic technique with all procedures. Challenges in the home setting include:

- The nurse may have to adapt to poor lighting, homes that are not clean, disorganized environments, and pets. It is important to establish a safe place for storage of supplies and a safe and efficient space for infusion administration. Many times the kitchen table is a good place because it has a cleanable surface and good lighting.
- Territoriality (i.e., the need for space) serves four functions: security, privacy, autonomy, and self-identification. People tend to generally feel safer in their own territory because it is arranged and equipped in a familiar manner.

    Most people believe that there is a degree of predictability associated with being in one's own personal space and that this degree of predictability is hard to achieve elsewhere (Giger & Davidhizar, 2004).

Pediatric Patients in the Home

The home care environment must be assessed to be sure that infusion therapy can be carried out safely. In the home, children are more mobile and active.

Continued

Home Care Issues—cont'd

The parents must be educated about the use and care of therapy and accept involvement in and responsibility for the treatment regimen.

• Focus on the psychosocial and developmental needs of the child and family in planning home infusion therapy.
• The best infusion device is one that is portable and easy for the child and family to operate. A syringe pump and disposable elastomeric infusion devices are examples of easy-to-use equipment.
• Keep in mind that parents need support from a home care agency.
• Identify alternate caregivers.

Older Adult Patients in the Home

Educating older adults on the administration of home infusion therapy can present challenges. The patient may be less ready to adapt to environmental changes, especially those related to independence.

Infusion therapy administration teaching requires patience, attention to patient understanding, and step-by-step approaches. All equipment should be user friendly. Written teaching materials and video programs can be helpful. Procedural demonstrations, including return demonstrations, are necessary parts of infusion therapy teaching.

• Evaluation of language or cultural differences can dramatically affect understanding of necessary health-care concepts.
• Sensory changes (e.g., vision, hearing, manual dexterity) occur with aging. Observe the patient while he or she is working with various devices to ensure proficiency. Ensure good lighting when performing infusion therapy and when evaluating the PIV catheter site. Consider ways to simplify the procedure if the patient has functional limitations. For example, elastomeric infusion devices are more expensive, and some organizations may try to use a more cost-effective method, such as a simple gravity drip infusion. However, changing to the elastomeric device, which is very easy to use, may result in patient independence and reduce the need for frequent nursing visits.

 NURSING FAST FACT!

■ *The home care nursing staff is responsible for routine restarts of PIV or blood draws. (In some areas, home laboratory services are also available for routine phlebotomy for needed laboratory studies.)*
■ *The principal diagnosis is critical for medical reimbursement, and the record must reflect total patient care, including the assessment, care plan, evaluations, implementation of care, and outcomes.*

Patient Education

Adult Patients

- Instruct on the purpose of I.V. therapy.
- Educate regarding limitations of movement.
- Instruct to notify the nurse if pump alarm sounds.
- Instruct to report discomfort at the infusion site.

Pediatric Patients

Education of the family, including the child when appropriate, should cover the following:

- Child's participation in sports with the catheter in place
- Purpose of I.V. therapy
- Instruction on equipment
- Verbal and written instructions on who, when, where, and how to call for assistance in an emergency or with significant concerns about infusion therapy
- Instruction materials tailored to age and comprehension level
- Documentation should include the responses of the patient's family and caregiver to teaching. All infusion therapy modalities should be explained to all those involved in patient care.

🔲 Nursing Process

The nursing process is a six-step process for problem solving to guide nursing action (see Chapter 1 for details on the steps of the nursing process related to vascular access). The following table focuses on nursing diagnoses, nursing outcomes classification (NOC), and nursing interventions classification (NIC) for peripheral infusion therapy in adults and pediatric patients. Nursing diagnoses should be patient specific and outcomes and interventions individualized. The NOC and NIC presented here are suggested directions for development of specific outcomes and interventions.

Nursing Diagnoses Related to Peripheral Infusion Therapy In Adults and Children	Nursing Outcomes Classification (NOC)	Nursing Interventions Classification (NIC)
Infection, risk for, related to: Inadequate acquired immunity; inadequate primary defenses (broken skin, traumatized tissue); inadequate secondary defenses; increased environmental exposure to pathogens; immunosuppression; invasive procedures	Immune status: Infection control, risk control, risk detection	Infection control and infection protection
Knowledge deficit related to: Cognitive limitation; information misinterpretation; lack of exposure; lack of interest in learning; lack of recall; unfamiliar with information resources regarding peripheral infusion therapy	Knowledge regarding health behavior, health resources, infection control, medication, personal safety, treatment procedures	Teaching: Disease process, reasons for infusion therapy, treatment
Mobility, physical, impaired related to: Activity intolerance; altered cellular metabolism; prescribed movement restrictions secondary to I.V. therapy; cognitive impairment; cultural beliefs regarding age-appropriate activity	Mobility, self-care: Activities of daily living (ADLs); ambulation; transfer performance	Joint mobility, positioning, ambulation
Injury risk for related to: Disturbed sensory perception—the older adult; chemical (pharmaceutical agents); staffing patterns; mode of transport; physical (arrangement of infusion equipment)	Personal safety behavior, risk control, safe home environment, knowledge of fall prevention	Health education, environmental management, fall prevention
Skin integrity impaired risk for: External: Extremes of age; mechanical factors; physical immobilization	Immobility consequences: Physiological, tissue integrity	Positioning: Pressure prevention, skin surveillance
Anxiety, related to: Behavioral: Restlessness, expressed concerns Affective: Apprehensive; distressed; fearful; painful procedure Physiological: Increased perspirations, trembling, voice quivering	Anxiety level, anxiety self-control, coping	Anxiety reduction strategies for parents and child
Diversional activity deficit related to: Environmental lack of diversional activity—age appropriate	Play participation, social involvement	Recreational play therapy—age appropriate
Family process interrupted related to: Shift in health status of family member; situation transition secondary to hospitalization	Family coping, family social climate, family functioning	Family integrity promotion, family process maintenance, family therapy, support system enhancement

Nursing Diagnoses Related to Peripheral Infusion Therapy In Adults and Children	Nursing Outcomes Classification (NOC)	Nursing Interventions Classification (NIC)
Fear related to: Loss of control, pain, autonomy, independence, competence, self esteem; language barrier; separation from support system; unfamiliar with environmental experiences	Fear self-control	Anxiety reduction, coping enhancement and security enhancement strategies
Parenting, impaired related to: Infant/child: Illness; separation anxiety Social: Change in family unit; lack of social support networks; lack of transportation; poverty; role strain	Family functioning, parent–infant attachment; role, safe home environment, social support; coping; family social climate; role performance	Family support, infant–parenting promotion, spiritual support, environmental management (safety); infant care; role enhancement; treatment; teaching

Sources: *Ackley & Ladwig (2011); Bulechek et al. (2013); Moorhead, Johnson, & Maas (2013).*

Chapter Highlights

- The first step is an understanding of the anatomy and physiology of the venous system. The five "layers" pertinent to performing venipuncture include the two skin layers (epidermis, dermis) and the three layers of the vein (tunica adventitia, tunica media, tunica intima).
- A working knowledge of the veins and nerves in the hand and forearm is vital so that the practitioner can successfully locate an acceptable vein for venipuncture and cannula placement. Keep in mind the type of solution, condition of vein, duration of therapy, patient age, patient preference, patient activity, presence of disease, previous surgery, presence of shunts or grafts, allergies, and medication history.
- The steps in placing a catheter that can support infusions via a PIV are as follows:

Precannulation

- Step 1: Check the order.
- Step 2: Perform hand hygiene.
- Step 3: Gather and prepare equipment.
- Step 4: Assess the patient and his or her psychological preparedness; verify patient identity.
- Step 5: Select the site and dilate the vein.

Cannula Placement

- Step 6: Attention to pain management
- Step 7: Appropriate catheter selection
- Step 8: Gloving

- Step 9: Site preparation
- Step 10: Vein entry
- Step 11: Catheter stabilization and dressing management

Postcannulation

- Step 12: Labeling
- Step 13: Equipment disposal
- Step 14: Patient education
- Step 15: Rate calculation
- Step 16: Documentation
- PIV catheters used for intermittent infusions are locked every 12 hours.
- Options for pain management include lidocaine and transdermal creams. Use of behavioral strategies should also be considered, especially with pediatric patients.
- Rate calculations: To calculate drop rates of gravity infusions, I.V. nurses must know (1) the drop factor of the administration set and (2) the amount of solution ordered.

Macrodrip Sets

- 10 gtt _____ 1 mL
- 15 gtt _____ 1 mL
- 20 gtt _____ 1 mL

NOTE > For transfusion administration sets, usually 10 gtt _____ 1 mL.

Microdrip Sets

- 60 gtt _____ 1 mL

Pediatric Infusion Therapy

- Children are not small adults. Physiological differences must be kept in mind, with particular focus on total body weight (85%–90% water), heat production (increases caloric expenditure by 7% for each degree of temperature), and immature renal and integumentary systems, which are important in regulating fluid and electrolyte needs.
- Physical assessment of a pediatric patient includes measuring the head circumference (for patients up to 1 year of age) and checking height or length, vital signs, skin turgor, presence of tears, moistness and color of membranes, urinary output, characteristics of fontanelles, and level of child's activity.
- Peripheral routes include the four scalp veins, dorsum of the hand and forearm, and lower extremities prior to walking age.

- Selection of PIV equipment must keep in mind the patient's safety, activity, age, and size.
- Needle selection depends on the age of the child: 22- to 26–gauge
- Use small volumes of solutions (250 or 500 mL). Use a VCC and, when indicated, infusion pumps.
- Always have extra help when starting an I.V. in a child, such as another nurse or having the parent hold the child in the lap.
- Perform venipuncture in a separate room, use a pacifier for neonates and infants, warm your hands before applying gloves, and use stickers or drawing as rewards.
- Delivery of medications to children can be by intermittent infusion, retrograde infusion, or syringe pump.

The Older Adult

- Physiological changes include decreased renal function; decreased drug clearance; increased risk for infection as a result of immune system changes; cardiovascular changes, including altered elasticity of the vein walls; skin losses; subcutaneous support; and thinning of skin (Smith & Cotter, 2012).
- Assessment includes skin turgor, temperature, rate and filling of veins in hand or foot, daily weight, intake and output, postural blood pressure, swallowing ability, and functional assessment of patient's ability to obtain fluids if not NPO.
- Venipuncture techniques should take into consideration the skin and vein changes of elderly persons. Use small-gauge catheters, use a blood pressure cuff, or place a loose tourniquet over clothing. Use warm compresses to visualize veins. Consider microdrip administration sets.

■■ Thinking Critically: Case Study

A 20-year-old obese African American man is readmitted to the hospital with a diagnosis of osteomyelitis. The patient is to be medically managed with I.V. antibiotics for 4 to 6 weeks and receive a diet high in protein and hydration.

Case Study Questions
1. *Decide which access devices should be used to initiate therapy, and give the rationale.*
2. *What should be taken into consideration during assessment of venous access sites?*
3. *What equipment might help you with a successful venipuncture?*

 Media Link: Answers to the case study and more critical thinking activites are provided on Davis*Plus*.

WORKSHEET 6-1
SUPERFICIAL VEINS OF THE UPPER EXTREMITIES

WORKSHEET 6-1 ANSWERS

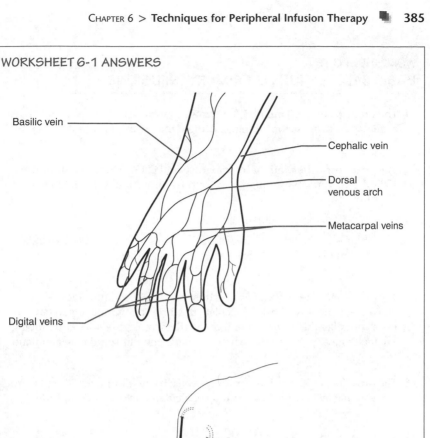

Basilic vein

Cephalic vein

Dorsal venous arch

Metacarpal veins

Digital veins

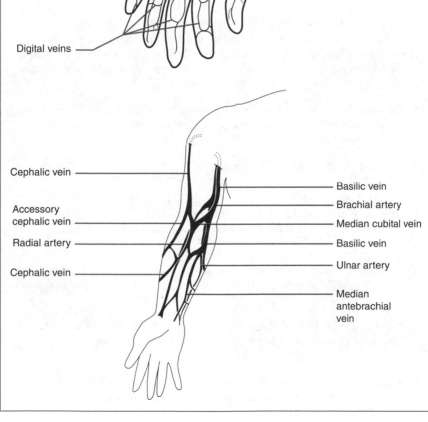

Cephalic vein

Accessory cephalic vein

Radial artery

Cephalic vein

Basilic vein

Brachial artery

Median cubital vein

Basilic vein

Ulnar artery

Median antebrachial vein

WORKSHEET 6-2
BASIC CALCULATION OF PRIMARY INFUSIONS

1. The order reads 1000 mL of 5% dextrose in water at 125 mL/hr. You have available 20 drop factor tubing. Calculate the drops per minute.

2. The order is for 1000 mL of 5% dextrose and 0.45% sodium chloride at 150 mL/hr. You have available 15 drop factor tubing. Calculate the drops per minute.

3. The order is for 250 mL (1 unit) of packed cells over 2 hours. Remember, blood tubing is always 10 drop factor. Calculate the drops per minute.

4. The order is for 45 mL/hr of 5% dextrose and 0.45% sodium chloride solution on an 8-month-old baby. Calculate the drops per minute if you have to use a controller that is drops per minute. (Remember, use microdrop tubing.) What else must you consider when administering this solution to an infant?

5. The order reads 3000 mL of a multiple electrolyte fluid over 24 hours. You have available 20 drop factor tubing. Calculate the drops per minute.

Intermittent I.V. Drug Administration

6. A fluid challenge of 250 mL of 0.9% sodium chloride over 45 minutes is ordered. You have 20 drop factor tubing available. Calculate the drops per minute in order to accurately deliver the 250 mL over 45 minutes.

7. Administer 50 mg of vinblastine sulfate diluted in 50 mL of 0.9% sodium chloride over 15 minutes. You have available a 15 macrodrop infusion set.

8. Administer 500 mg of acyclovir in 100 mL of 5% dextrose in water over 1 hour. You have available a macrodrop 20 gtt infusion set.

9. Administer trimethoprim—sulfamethoxazole 400 mg in 125 mL of dextrose in water over 90 minutes. You have available a microdrop set and a macrodrip 15 gtt infusion set.

10. At 12 noon you discover that an infusion set that was to deliver 100 mL per hour from 7 a.m. to 5 p.m. has 400 mL left in the infusion bag. Recalculate the infusion using a 10 drop macrodrop infusion set.

ANSWERS TO WORKSHEET 6-2
USING FORMULA OR RATIO/PROPORTION

1. Formula: $\dfrac{mL/hr \times DF}{minutes} = gtt/min$

   Step 1: $\dfrac{125 \times 20}{60} = gtt/min$

   Step 2: $\dfrac{125}{3} = $ **42 gtt/min**

2. Formula: $\dfrac{mL/hr \times DF}{minutes} = gtt/min$

   Step 1: $\dfrac{150 \times 15}{60} = gtt/min$

   Step 2: $\dfrac{150}{4} = $ **38 gtt/min**

3. Formula: $\dfrac{mL}{hours} = mL/hr$

   Step 1: $250 \div 2 = 125\ mL/hr$

   Formula: $\dfrac{mL/hr \times DF}{minutes} = gtt/min$

   Step 2: $\dfrac{125 \times 10}{60} = gtt/min$

   Step 3: $\dfrac{125}{6} = $ **21 gtt/min**

4. Formula: $\dfrac{mL/hr \times DF}{minutes} = gtt/min$

   Step 1: $\dfrac{45 \times 60}{60} = $ **45 gtt/min**

Only one step is needed for microdrop infusions.
When using 60 gtt tubing, gtt/min = amount of hourly infusion volume.
In addition, pediatric solutions and medications should be checked by another registered nurse. Of note, standards for double-checking in the home care setting have not been established. Options include a call to the pharmacy to verbally read the prescription or educating the caregiver (e.g., parent) about the procedure. Use a volume-controlled chamber (VCC) and limit the primary bottle to a 500-mL container.

5. Formula: $\dfrac{mL}{hours} = mL/hr$

   Step 1: $\dfrac{3000}{24} = 125\ mL/hr$

Continued

Formula: $\dfrac{mL/hr \times DF}{minutes} = gtt/min$

Step 2: $\dfrac{125 \times 20}{60} = gtt/min$

Step 3: $\dfrac{125}{6} = $ **42 gtt/min**

6. Formula: $\dfrac{mL/hr \times DF}{minutes} = gtt/min$

Step 1: $\dfrac{250 \times 20}{45} = gtt/min$

Step 2: $\dfrac{250 \times 4}{9} = $ **111 gtt/min**

7. Formula: $\dfrac{mL/hr \times DF}{minutes} = gtt/min$

Step 1: $\dfrac{50 \times 15}{15} = $ **50 gtt/min**

8. Formula: $\dfrac{mL/hr \times DF}{minutes} = gtt/min$

Step 1: $\dfrac{100 \times 20}{60} = gtt/min$

Step 2: $\dfrac{100}{3} = $ **33 gtt/min**

9. Formula: $\dfrac{mL/hr \times DF}{minutes} = gtt/min$

Step 1: $\dfrac{125 \times 15}{90} = gtt/min$

Step 2: $\dfrac{125}{6} = $ **21 gtt/min**

10. Formula: $\dfrac{mL}{hours} = mL/hr$

Step 1: $\dfrac{400}{5} = 80\ mL/hr$

Formula: $\dfrac{mL/hr \times DF}{minutes} = gtt/min$

Step 2: $\dfrac{80 \times 10}{60} = gtt/min$

Step 3: $\dfrac{80}{6} = $ **13 gtt/min**

Post-Test

1. The layer of the vein that contains smooth muscle, fibrous tissue, and nerve fibers for vasoconstriction and vasodilation is the:
   a. Tunica media
   b. Tunica adventitia
   c. Tunica intima
   d. Hypodermis

2. The vein that follows the radius side of the forearm is the:
   a. Metacarpal
   b. Cephalic
   c. Basilic
   d. Median cubital

3. PIV therapy labels should be applied to:
   a. Catheter site, tubing, and solution container
   b. Tubing, solution container, and chart
   c. Solution container, catheter site, and patient's armband

4. Which of the following infusate characteristics is appropriate for infusion through a PIV catheter?
   a. Osmolarity >600 mOsm/L
   b. pH = 6
   c. pH = 4
   d. pH = 10

5. Which of the following areas for peripheral venous access should be avoided in an adult patient?
   a. Mid-forearm
   b. Inner aspect of wrist
   c. Dorsum of the hand
   d. Upper forearm

6. In a dark-skinned person, a good method for locating an accessible vein is:
   a. Multiple tourniquets
   b. Tangential lighting
   c. Direct overhead lighting
   d. Light application of a tourniquet

7. Which of the following is the most appropriate cannula size for use on a 2-month-old infant?
   a. 18-gauge, over-the-needle catheter
   b. 23- to 25-gauge scalp vein needle
   c. 16-gauge scalp vein needle
   d. 22- to 24-gauge, over-the-needle catheter

8. The most appropriate equipment for an infant receiving I.V. fluids includes:
   a. Microdrip tubing connected to a 50-mL infusate container
   b. Microdrip volume-controlled cylinder (VCC) attached to a 250-mL infusate container
   c. Macrodrip tubing connected to a VCC
   d. Any tubing or container provided it is regulated with an electronic infusion device

9. Which of the following are techniques to dilate a vein for venipuncture in the older adult with fragile veins? (*Select all that apply.*)
   a. Apply the tourniquet loosely over the patient's sleeve.
   b. Apply multiple tourniquets.
   c. Use digital pressure to enhance vein filling.
   d. Use warm compresses before venipuncture.

10. The preferred antiseptic solution for skin antisepsis is:
   a. Povidone iodine
   b. Tincture of iodine
   c. 70% alcohol
   d. Chlorhexidine/alcohol

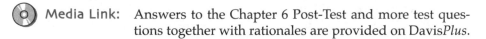 Media Link: Answers to the Chapter 6 Post-Test and more test questions together with rationales are provided on Davis*Plus*.

■ References

Ackley, B. J., & Ladwig, G. B. (2011). *Nursing diagnosis handbook: An evidence-based guide to planning care* (9th ed.). St. Louis, MO: Mosby Elsevier.

American Nurses Association (ANA). (2010). *Nursing: Scope and standards of practice* (3rd ed.). Silver Spring, MD: author.

Baranoski, S., Ayello, E. A., Tomic-Canic, M., & Levine, J. M. (2012). Skin: An essential organ. In S. Baranoski & E. A. Ayello (Eds.), *Wound care essentials: Practice principles* (3rd ed) (pp. 58-82). Philadelphia: Lippincott Williams & Wilkins.

Bausone-Gazsa, D., Lefaiver, C. A., & Walters, S. A. (2010). A randomized controlled trial to compare the complications of 2 peripheral IV catheter stabilization systems. *Journal of Infusion Nursing, 33*(6), 371-384.

Bulechek, G. M., Butcher, H. K., Dochterman, J. M., & Wagner, C. M. (2013). *Nursing interventions classification (NIC)* (6th ed.). St. Louis: MO: Mosby Elsevier.

Burke, S. D., Vercler, S. J., Bye, R. O., Desmond, P. C., & Rees, Y. W. (2011). Local anesthesia before IV catheterization. *American Journal of Nursing, 111*(2), 40-45.

Campinha-Bacote, J. (2011). Delivering patient-centered care in the midst of a cultural conflict: The role of cultural competence. *The Online Journal of Issues in Nursing, 16*(2), Manuscript 5. Retrieved from www.nursingworld.org/

MainMenuCategories/ANAMarketplace/ANAPeriodicals/OJIN/
TableofContents/Vol-16-2011/No2-May-2011/Delivering-Patient-Centered-
Care-in-the-Midst-of-a-Cultural-Conflict.html (Accessed December 26, 2012).

Cohen, L. L. (2008). Behavioral approaches to anxiety and pain management for
pediatric venous access. *Pediatrics, 122,* S134-S139.

Crowley, M., Brim, C., Proehl, J., Barnason, S., Leviner, S., Lindauer, C., ...Williams,
J. (2011). Emergency nursing resource: Difficult venous access. Retrieved
from www.ena.org/practice-research/research/CPG/Documents/
DifficultIVAccessCPG.pdf (Accessed December 30, 2012).

Department of Health & Human Services, Administration on Aging. (2011).
Aging statistics. Retrieved from http://www.aoa.gov/aoaroot/aging_
statistics/index.aspx (Accessed December 29, 2012).

Doellman, D. (2014). Pediatrics. In M. Alexander, A. Corrigan, L. Gorski & L.
Phillips (eds). Core Curriculum for Infusion Nursing (4th ed) (pp. 192-234).
Philadelphia: Lippincott, Williams & Wilkins.

Douglas, M. K., Pierce, J. U., Rosenkoetter, M., Pacquiao, D., Callister, L. C.,
Hattar-Pollara, M., ... Purnell, L. (2011). Standards of practice for culturally
competent nursing care: 2011 update. *Journal of Transcultural Nursing, 22*(4),
317-333.

Fabian, B. (2010). Infusion therapy in the older adult. In M. Alexander, A.
Corrigan, L. Gorski, J. Hankins, & R. Perucca (Eds.). *Infusion nursing: An
evidence-based practice* (3rd ed.) (pp. 571-582). St. Louis: Saunders/Elsevier.

Fink, R. M., Hjort, E., Wenger, B., Cook, P. F., Cunningham, M., Orf, A.,... Zwink,
J. (2009). The impact of dry versus moist heat on peripheral IV catheter
insertion in a hematology-oncology outpatient population. *Oncology
Nursing Forum, 36*(4), E198-E204.

Frey, A. M., & Pettit, J. (2010). Infusion therapy in children. In M. Alexander,
A. Corrigan, L. Gorski, J. Hankins, & R. Perucca (Eds.). *Infusion nursing: An
evidence-based practice* (3rd ed.) (pp. 550-570). St. Louis: Saunders/Elsevier.

Ganter-Ritz, V., Speroni, K. G., & Atherton, M. (2012). A randomized double-
blind study comparing intradermal anesthetic tolerability, efficacy, and
cost-effectiveness of lidocaine, buffered lidocaine, and bacteriostatic normal
saline for peripheral intravenous insertion. *Journal of Infusion Nursing, 35*(2),
93-99.

Giger, J. N., & Davidhizar, R. E. (2004). *Transcultural nursing: Assessment and
intervention* (4th ed.). St. Louis, MO: C.V. Mosby.

Gorski, L, Hallock, D., Kuehn, S. C., Morris, P., Russell, J., & Skala, L. (2012). INS
position paper: Recommendations for frequency of assessment of the short
peripheral catheter site. *Journal of Infusion Nursing, 35*(5), 290-292.

Guerin, K., Wagner, J., Rains, K., & Bessesen, M. (2010). Reduction in central line
associated bloodstream infections by implementation of a postinsertion care
bundle. *American Journal of Infection Control, 38*(6), 430-433.

Hadaway, L. (2010a). Anatomy and physiology related to infusion therapy.
In M. Alexander, A. Corrigan, L. Gorski, J. Hankins, & R. Perucca (Eds.).
Infusion nursing: An evidence-based practice (3rd ed.) (pp. 139-177). St. Louis:
Saunders/Elsevier.

Hadaway, L. (2010b). Infusion therapy equipment. In M. Alexander, A. Corrigan,
L. Gorski, J. Hankins, & R. Perucca (Eds.). *Infusion nursing: An evidence-based
practice* (3rd ed.) (pp. 391-436). St. Louis: Saunders/Elsevier.

Houston, P. A. (2013). Obtaining vascular access in the obese patient population. *Journal of Infusion Nursing, 36*(1), 52-56.

Infusion Nurses Society (INS). (2008). *Flushing protocols.* Norwood, MA: Author.

INS. (2011a). Infusion nursing standards of practice. *Journal of Infusion Nursing, 34*(1S), S1-S110.

INS. (2011b). *Policies and procedures for infusion nursing.* Norwood, MA: Author.

Institute for Safe Medication Practices (ISMP). (2007). Failure to cap IV tubing and disconnect IV ports place patients at risk for infections. July 26, 2007. Retrieved from www.ismp.org/newsletters/acutecare/articles/20070726.asp (Accessed January 17, 2011).

Lenhardt, R., Seybold, T., Kimberger, O., Stoiser, B., & Sessler, D. I. (2002). Local warming and insertion of peripheral venous cannulas: Single blinded prospective randomized controlled trial and single blinded randomized crossover trial. *British Medical Journal, 325*(7361), 409-410.

Macklin, D. (2010). Catheter management. *Seminars in Oncology Nursing, 26*(2), 113-120.

Maiocco, G., & Coole, C. (2012). Use of ultrasound guidance for peripheral intravenous placement in difficult-to-access patients. *Journal of Nursing Care Quality, 27*(1), 51-55.

Masoorli, S. (2007). Nerve injuries related to vascular access insertion and assessment. *Journal of Infusion Nursing, 30*(6), 346-350.

Moorhead, S., Johnson, M., Maas, M., & Swanson E. (2013). *Nursing outcomes classification* (NOC) (5th ed.). St. Louis, MO: Mosby Elsevier.

Munoz, C., & Luckmann, J. (2005). *Transcultural communication in nursing* (2nd ed.). Clifton Park, NY: Thomson Delmar Learning.

Neel, E. K. (2010). Health assessment. In A. G. Perry & P. A. Potter (Eds.). *Clinical nursing skills & techniques* (pp. 106-171). St. Louis, MO: Mosby Elsevier.

O'Grady, N. P., Alexander, M., Burns, L. A., Dellinger, E. P., Garland, J., Heard, S. O., ...the Healthcare Practices Advisory Committee (HICPAC). (2011). Guidelines for the prevention of intravascular catheter-related infections, 2011. *American Journal of Infection Control, 39*(4 Supp), S1-S34. Available at www.cdc.gov/hicpac/pdf/guidelines/bsi-guidelines-2011.pdf (Accessed September 15, 2012).

Pedivan. (2010). *Best practice guidelines in the care and maintenance of pediatric central venous catheters.* Herrman, UT: Association for Vascular Access.

Perucca, R. (2010). Peripheral venous access devices. In M. Alexander, A. Corrigan, L. Gorski, J. Hankins, & R. Perucca (Eds.). *Infusion nursing: An evidence-based approach* (3rd ed.) (pp. 456-479). St. Louis, MO: Saunders Elsevier.

Rupp, M. E., Yu, S., Huerta, T., Cavalieri, R. J., Alter, R., Fey, P. D., ... Anderson, J. R. (2012). Adequate disinfection of a split-septum needleless intravascular connector with a 5-second alcohol scrub. *Infection Control & Hospital Epidemiology, 33* (7), 661-665.

Siegel, J. D., Rhinehart, E., Jackson, M., & Chiarello, L. (2007). Guideline for isolation precautions: Preventing transmission of infectious agents in healthcare settings 2007. Retrieved from www.cdc.gov/ncidod/dhqp/hai.html (Accessed December 11, 2012).

Smith, C. M., & Cotter, V. T. (2012). Nursing standard of practice protocol: Age-related changes in health. Retrieved from http://consultgerirn.org/

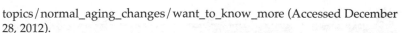

topics/normal_aging_changes/want_to_know_more (Accessed December 28, 2012).

Soothill, J. S., Bravery, K., Ho, A., Macqueen, S., Collins, J., & Lock, P. (2009). A fall in bloodstream infections followed a change to 2% chlorhexidine in 70% isopropanol for catheter connection antisepsis: a pediatric single center before/after study on a hemopoietic stem cell transplant ward. *American Journal of Infection Control* 37 (8), 626-630.

Thayer, D. (2012). Skin damage associated with intravenous therapy. *Journal of Infusion Nursing, 35*(6), 390-401.

The Joint Commission. (2013). National patient safety goals. Retrieved from www.jointcommission.org/standards_information/npsgs.aspx (Accessed October 29, 2012).

U.S. Department of Labor. (n.d.). Occupational Safety and Health Administration (OSHA). Disposal of contaminated needles and blood tube holders used for phlebotomy. Washington, DC: Author. Retrieved from http://www.osha.gov/dts/shib/shib101503.html (Accessed December 28, 2012).

Vialle, R., Pietin-Vialle, C., Cronier, P., Brillu, C., Villapadierna, F., & Mercier, P. (2001). Anatomic relations between the cephalic vein and the sensory branches of the radial nerve: How can nerve lesions during vein puncture be prevented? *Anesthesia Analgesia, 93*, 1058-1061.

Webster, J., Osborne, S., Rickard, C., & Hall, J. (2010). Clinically indicated replacement versus routine replacement of peripheral venous catheters. *Cochrane Database of Systematic Reviews, 3*, CD007798.

PROCEDURES DISPLAY 6-1

Steps for Inserting a Peripheral-Short Over-the-Needle Catheter by Direct and Indirect Methods

Equipment Needed
I.V. start kit (preferred) containing the following:
 Gloves, nonsterile
 Tourniquet
 Antiseptic solution (chlorhexidine gluconate/alcohol recommended)
 Transparent dressing
 Label
I.V. catheter (22-gauge, 20-gauge most common)
Stabilization device
Needleless connector
Extension set (optional)
Primary administration set
Prescribed infusate

Continued

PROCEDURES DISPLAY 6-1

Steps for Inserting a Peripheral-Short Over-the-Needle Catheter by Direct and Indirect Methods—*cont'd*

Delegation
This procedure can be delegated to LVN/LPN depending on the state nurse practice act for initiation of infusion therapy and agency policy.

Procedure	Rationale
1. Verify the authorized prescriber's order.	1. A written order is a legal requirement for infusion therapy.
2. Introduce yourself to the patient.	2. Establishes nurse–patient relationship
3. Check patient identity using two forms (check identification [ID] bracelet and ask patient to state name).	3. Patient Safety Goal.
4. Perform hand hygiene.	4. Single most important means of infection prevention
5. Assess patient (verify allergy status) and evaluate for psychological preparedness. Instruct patient on purpose of infusion or locking device. Apply tourniquet and evaluate both arms for best access site. Release tourniquet. Perform hand hygiene again before beginning procedure and don gloves.	5. Prepares patient for procedure. Allows for dilation of veins and assessment of both extremities. Standard precautions
6. Help patient get into a comfortable position. Place linen saver pad under arm or hand.	6. Promotes cooperation with the procedure and facilitates your ability to perform the procedure. Protects bed linens.
7. Select the site and dilate the vein.	7. Choose the most distal veins of the upper extremity on the hand and/or arm so that you can perform subsequent venipunctures proximal to the previous site. Ensures preservation of veins.

PROCEDURES DISPLAY 6-1

Steps for Inserting a Peripheral-Short Over-the-Needle Catheter by Direct and Indirect Methods—*cont'd*

Procedure	Rationale
8. Select the appropriate catheter for therapy.	8. Choose the best needle gauge for the therapy and patient age.
9. Don clean gloves. Gloves must be left on throughout the entire procedure.	9. Standard precautions
10. Prepare the site: ■ Cleanse skin with soap and water if visibly soiled ■ Remove excess hair if necessary using scissors or surgical clippers ■ Skin antisepsis with chlorhexidine: Use back and forth motion for at least 30 seconds; with povidone–iodine using a circular technique, working from insertion site outward; allow to fully dry on skin.	10. Prevents infection.
11. Reapply the tourniquet.	11. Distends veins.
12. Insert the catheter by a direct or indirect method with a steady motion using traction to maintain an anchor on the vein.	12. Anchoring the vein properly is the key to successful catheter insertion. Holding the catheter at a 20- to 30-degree angle allows you to pierce the skin without inadvertently piercing the back of the vein.
For the Direct (One-Step) Method A. Insert the catheter directly over the vein at a 20–30 degree angle B. Penetrate all layers of the vein with one motion.	Quickly passes through layers of epidermis and dermis, decreasing pain, and allows for adjustment to technique based on skin thickness.

Continued

PROCEDURES DISPLAY 6-1

Steps for Inserting a Peripheral-Short Over-the-Needle Catheter by Direct and Indirect Methods—*cont'd*

Procedure	Rationale

For the Indirect (Two-Step) Method

  A. Insert the catheter at a 30-degree angle to the skin alongside the vein; gently insert the catheter distal to the point at which the needle will enter the vein.

  B. Maintain parallel alignment and advance through the subcutaneous tissue.

  C. Relocate the vein and decrease the angle as the catheter enters the vein.

Note: Jabbing, stabbing, or quick thrusting should be avoided because such actions may cause rupture of delicate veins. For performing a venipuncture on difficult veins, follow these guidelines:

■ For paper-thin transparent skin or delicate veins: Use a small catheter (e.g., 24-gauge); use direct entry; consider not using a tourniquet (blood pressure cuff); decrease the angle of entry to 15 degrees; apply minimal tourniquet pressure.

■ For an obese patient or if you are unable to palpate or see veins, create a visual image of venous anatomy and select a longer catheter (2 inch); consider ultrasound

PROCEDURES DISPLAY 6-1

Steps for Inserting a Peripheral-Short Over-the-Needle Catheter by Direct and Indirect Methods—*cont'd*

Procedure	Rationale
guidance or use of Phillips multiple tourniquet technique.	
■ For veins that roll when venipuncture is attempted: Apply traction to the vein with the thumb during venipuncture, keeping skin taut; leave tourniquet on to promote venous distention; use a blood pressure cuff for better filling of vein; use 18-gauge catheter.	
After the bevel enters the vein and blood flashback occurs, lower the angle of the catheter and stylet (needle) as one unit and advance into the vein. After the catheter tip and bevel are in the vein, advance the catheter forward off the stylet and into the vein.	Flashback of blood indicates that the vein has been cannulated. Releasing the tourniquet restores full circulation to the patient's extremity.
After the vein is entered, cautiously advance the catheter into the vein lumen. Hold the catheter hub with your thumb and middle finger and use your index finger to advance the catheter, maintaining skin traction. A one-handed technique is recommended to advance the catheter off the stylet so that the opposite hand can maintain proper traction on the skin and maintain vein alignment. (A two-handed technique can be used, but this	

Continued

PROCEDURES DISPLAY 6-1

Steps for Inserting a Peripheral-Short Over-the-Needle Catheter by Direct and Indirect Methods—*cont'd*

Procedure	Rationale
increases the risk of vessel rupture during threading of a rigid catheter in a nonstabilized vein.) While the stylet is still partially inside the catheter, release the tourniquet. Remove the stylet and activate the safety feature of the catheter. If using a passive safety device, the safety mechanism is automatic.	
13. Connect the administration set or needleless connector with a twisting motion.	13. Secures the luer-lock and prevents leakage and contamination.
14. Stabilize the catheter with a stabilization device or apply transparent semipermeable membrane (TSM) dressing directly over the catheter and hub.	14. Prevents movement of the catheter in the vein. Prevents microorganisms from entering the catheter–skin junction.
15. Label the site with date and time; type and length of catheter; nurse's initials.	15. Legal protection of the patient and nurse
16. Dispose of all equipment in appropriate receptacle.	16. Reduces risk of exposure to blood.
17. Instruct the patient on use of an electronic infusion device (EID), what to report regarding site, and how often to expect the nurses to check the infusion site.	17. Knowledge of infusion therapy treatment assists in providing a positive outcome.
18. Calculate the infusion rate or dial appropriate rate into EID.	18. Ensure correct delivery of prescribed solution or medications.

PROCEDURES DISPLAY 6-1

Steps for Inserting a Peripheral-Short Over-the-Needle Catheter by Direct and Indirect Methods—*cont'd*

Procedure	Rationale
19. Document in the medical records: Date and time of insertion; type of device; gauge and length of catheter; solution infusing and rate of flow; any additional equipment (EID); number of attempts; condition of extremity before access; patient education, patient's response; signature.	19. Maintains a legal record and communication with the health-care team.

PROCEDURES DISPLAY 6-2

Converting a Primary Line to Intermittent Device

Equipment Needed
Needleless connector
Two prefilled syringes of 0.9% sodium chloride
Clean gloves
Alcohol

Delegation
This procedure can be delegated to a LVN/LPN who is specially trained in I.V. therapy depending on the state nurse practice act for initiation of infusion therapy and agency policy. This cannot be delegated to nursing assistant personnel.

Procedure	Rationale
1. Confirm the authorized prescriber's order to discontinue continuous infusion.	1. A written order is a legal requirement for therapy.

Continued

PROCEDURES DISPLAY 6-2

Converting a Primary Line to Intermittent Device—*cont'd*

Procedure	Rationale
2. Introduce yourself to the patient.	2. Establishes the nurse–patient relationship.
3. Perform hand hygiene.	3. Single most important means of infection prevention.
4. Verify the patient's identity using two forms of ID.	4. Patient safety
5. Help the patient get into a comfortable position that provides access to the I.V. site.	5. Promotes cooperation and facilitates the nurse's ability to perform the procedure.
6. Put on clean gloves. Remove needleless connector from the package and prime device with the first syringe of sodium chloride per manufacturer's directions. Place back in adapter sterile package.	6. Removes air from needleless connector.
7. Close the roller clamp on the administration set and turn off the electronic infusion device (EID), if appropriate.	7. Prevents loss of I.V. fluid during the procedure.
8. With your nondominant hand, apply pressure over the catheter just above the insertion site.	8. Applying pressure over the vein stops blood from flowing from the catheter as you change the administration tubing to a lock.
9. Gently detach the old tubing from the I.V. catheter. If it does not disengage easily, try gripping the catheter hub with a hemostat.	9. Prevents the catheter from becoming dislodged.
10. Quickly attach needleless connector to I.V. catheter.	10. Inserting the adapter quickly prevents blood from flowing from the I.V. catheter.

PROCEDURES DISPLAY 6-2

Converting a Primary Line to Intermittent Device—*cont'd*

Procedure	Rationale
11. Cleanse needleless connector with an alcohol pad for 15 seconds.	11. Disinfects and reduces risk for intraluminal introduction of microbes.
12. Flush the locking device with 2 mL of sodium chloride. Follow flush protocols.	12. Maintains catheter patency.
13. Discard the administration set in the appropriate container. Empty the I.V. solution in the nearest sink and discard container appropriately according to organizational procedures.	13. Standard precautions
14. Remove gloves and perform hand hygiene.	14. Standard precautions
15. Document the procedure with the date and time of conversion of primary solution infusion to locking device, amount of fluid infused, and how the patient tolerated the procedure.	15. Maintains a legal record and communication with the health-care team.

PROCEDURES DISPLAY 6-3

Flushing a Peripheral-Short I.V. Catheter

Equipment Needed
Prefilled syringe of 0.9% sodium chloride
Sharps container
Antiseptic solution: 70% alcohol

Delegation
This procedure can be delegated to an LPN/LVN who is specially trained in I.V. therapy depending on the state nurse practice act for

Continued

PROCEDURES DISPLAY 6-3

Flushing a Peripheral-Short I.V. Catheter—*cont'd*

initiation of infusion therapy and agency policy and procedure. This cannot be delegated to nursing assistive personnel.

Procedure	Rationale
1. Confirm authorized prescriber's order for flushing or follow standardized procedure for the agency.	1. A written order is a legal requirement for infusion therapy.
2. Introduce yourself to the patient.	2. Establishes the nurse–patient relationship.
3. Perform hand hygiene.	3. Single most important means of infection prevention.
4. Verify the patient's identity using two forms of ID.	4. Patient safety
5. Identify whether the needleless connector is a negative-displacement device, a positive-displacement device, or a neutral-displacement device (see note below).	5. Flushing technique varies based on category.
6. Don gloves.	6. Prevents bacterial entry into the infusion system. Standard precautions.
7. Disinfect the needleless connector with 70% isopropyl alcohol using a scrubbing motion and allow to dry. Most organizations require at least a 15-second scrub. This step may be eliminated if a protective alcohol cap has been in place over needleless connector (see Chapter 5).	7. Critical step in infection prevention. Disinfects and reduces risk for intraluminal introduction of microbes.
8. Attach prefilled syringe of 0.9% preservative-free sodium chloride to the needleless connector.	8. Maintains patency of catheter.

PROCEDURES DISPLAY 6-3

Flushing a Peripheral-Short I.V. Catheter—*cont'd*

Procedure	Rationale
9. Slowly aspirate until blood is aspirated.	9. Confirms catheter patency.
10. Flush catheter with 0.9% sodium chloride.	10. Maintains patency of catheter and prevents occlusion.
Note: There are different types of NIS devices, be sure you know which devices are used in your facility.	
10a. For negative-displacement devices: Flush all solution into the catheter lumen; maintain force on the syringe plunger as a clamp on the catheter or extension set is closed, then disconnect the syringe.	10a. Manufacturer requires "positive pressure" flushing technique to prevent reflux of blood.
10b. For positive-displacement device: Flush all solution into the catheter lumen, disconnect the syringe, then close the catheter clamp.	10b. Catheter is clamped after disconnection of the syringe.
10c. For neutral-displacement device: Flush all solution into the catheter lumen.	10c. It does not matter if the catheter clamp is closed before or after the flush procedure.
11. Document the procedure on the patient record.	11. Maintains a legal record and communication with the health-care team.

Sources: INS, 2011a; INS, 2011b.

PROCEDURES DISPLAY 6-4

Discontinuation of Peripheral-Short I.V. Catheter

Equipment Needed
Gloves
Dressing materials: 2 × 2 gauze and tape
Biohazard container

Delegation
This procedure can be delegated to an LPN/LVN who is specially trained in I.V. therapy depending on the state nurse practice act for initiation of infusion therapy and agency policy and procedure. This cannot be delegated to nursing assistive personnel.

Procedure	Rationale
1. Confirm the authorized prescriber's order for discontinuation of infusion therapy.	1. A written order is a legal requirement for infusion therapy.
2. Introduce yourself to the patient.	2. Establishes the nurse–patient relationship.
3. Perform hand hygiene.	3. Single most important means of infection prevention.
4. Verify the patient's identity using two forms of ID.	4. Patient safety.
5. Assist the patient into a comfortable position.	5. Promotes cooperation and facilitates the nurse's ability to perform the procedure.
6. Place a linen saver pad under the extremity.	6. Protects bed linens.
7. Don gloves and discontinue infusion administration if a continuous infusion is running.	7. Standard precautions Stops infusion of fluids.
8. Carefully remove the I.V. dressing, stabilization device, and tape securing the tubing.	8. Allows access for catheter removal.
9. Inspect the catheter–skin junction site.	9. Assess for signs of infection or phlebitis.
10. Apply a sterile 2 × 2 gauze pad above the I.V. insertion site and gently, using even pressure, remove catheter, directing it straight along the vein.	

PROCEDURES DISPLAY 6-4

Discontinuation of Peripheral-Short I.V. Catheter—*cont'd*

Procedure	Rationale
11. Apply pressure over site until bleeding stops, usually at least 30 seconds.	11. Prevents bleeding and hematoma formation.
12. Assess the integrity of the removed catheter. Compare length of catheter to original insertion length to ensure the entire catheter is removed.	12. Note the condition of site, including the presence of any site complications. Ensures full catheter length has been removed from the patient.
13. Dress the exit site. Secure fresh 2 × 2 gauze to the site with tape. Change dressing every 24 hours until the exit site is healed.	13. Keeps the venipuncture site clean.
14. Discard removed catheter in biohazard container, discard I.V. tubing, linen saver pad, solution container, and gloves in appropriate trash receptacle according to organizational policy.	14. Standard precautions.
15. Remove gloves and perform hand hygiene.	15. Standard precautions
16. Document date and time that I.V. therapy was discontinued. Document any complications noted and the interventions. If catheter defect is noted, report to the manufacturer and regulatory agencies.	16. Maintains a legal record and communication with the health-care team.

Sources: INS, 2011a; INS, 2011b.

Chapter **7**

Phlebotomy Techniques

To be "in charge" is certainly not only to carry out the proper measures yourself but to see that everyone else does so too; to see that no one either willfully or ignorantly thwarts or prevents such measures. It is neither to do everything yourself nor to appoint a number of people to each duty, but to ensure that each does that duty to which he is appointed.
— *Florence Nightingale 1860*

🔖 **LEARNING**   *On completion of this chapter, the reader will be able to:*
  OBJECTIVES
  1. List the various types of anticoagulants used in blood collection.
  2. Identify the tube color codes for vacuum collection.
  3. Describe phlebotomy safety supplies and equipment.
  4. Identify the various supplies that should be carried on a specimen collection tray.
  5. Identify the types of equipment needed to collect blood by venipuncture.
  6. Describe the patient identification process.
  7. List essential information for test requisitions.
  8. Identify the most common sites for venipuncture for blood collection.
  9. Describe the venipuncture procedure and steps for the evacuated tube method, winged infusion system, and syringe method.
  10. State the order of draw for collection tubes.

⧗ **GLOSSARY**

Acid–citrate–dextrose (ACD)   An anticoagulant solution available in two formulations (solution A and solution B) for immunohematology tests, such as DNA testing and human leukocyte antigen (HLA) phenotyping, which is used in paternity evaluation and to determine transplant compatibility

Anticoagulant   Substance introduced into the blood or a blood specimen to keep it from clotting

Assay   Determination of the purity of a substance or the amount of any particular constituent of a mixture

Centrifugation   The process of spinning the blood tubes at a high number of revolutions per minute.

Citrate–phosphate–dextrose (CPD)   Anticoagulant typically used for blood donations

Clinical and Laboratory Standards Institute (CLSI)   A global, non-profit, standards-developing organization comprising representatives from the profession, industry, and government.

Ethylenediaminetetraacetic acid (EDTA)   Anticoagulant additive used to prevent the blood clotting sequence by removing calcium and forming calcium slats. EDTA prevents platelet aggregation and is useful for platelet counts and platelet function tests.

Evacuated Tube System (ETS)   A closed system in which the patient's blood flows directly into a collection tube through a needle inserted into a vein.

Hemoconcentration   A decrease in the fluid content of the blood, with a subsequent increase in nonfilterable large molecule or protein-based blood components such as red blood cells

Hemolysis   The destruction of the membrane of the red blood cells

Multisample needle   Used with the evacuated tube method of blood collection. These needles are attached to a holder/adapter and allow for multiple specimen tube fills and changes without blood leakage.

Oxalates   Anticoagulants that prevent blood clotting sequence by removing calcium and forming calcium salts

Phlebotomist   Individual who practices phlebotomy

Phlebotomy   Withdrawal of blood from a vein

Point-of-care testing (POCT)   Alternate site testing (AST)—ancillary, bedside, or near patient—performed using portable or handheld instruments.

Syringe method   A sterile safety needle, a disposable plastic syringe, and a syringe transfer device

■ Introduction to Phlebotomy

Purpose of Phlebotomy

Blood and other specimen collections are important to the entire health assessment of the client. Laboratory analysis of a variety of specimens is used for three important purposes:

1. Obtain blood for diagnostic purposes and monitoring of prescribed treatment
2. Remove blood for transfusion at a donor center
3. Remove blood for therapeutic purposes such as treatment for polycythemia (McCall & Tankersley, 2012).

Professional Competencies

The term phlebotomist is applied to a person who has been trained to collect blood for laboratory tests that are necessary for the diagnosis and care of patients. The role of the nurse may include **phlebotomy**, along with the responsibility of preserving veins for infusion therapy (McCall & Tankersley, 2012). The nurse has the unique task of using a single venipuncture to permit both the withdrawal for blood and the initiation of an infusion, thereby preserving veins. Table 7-1 lists the duties and responsibilities of the nurse or phlebotomist. Usually a **phlebotomist** or blood collector must complete a phlebotomy program.

Advances in laboratory technology are making **point-of-care testing (POCT)** more common. As many health professionals are being cross-trained to perform phlebotomy, the term "phlebotomist" is being applied to anyone who has been trained to collect blood specimens. The nurse performing phlebotomy procedures or the phlebotomist must have the knowledge base listed below to perform blood withdrawal procedures safely. Certification is evidence that an individual has mastered fundamental competencies of a technical area. Examples of national agencies that certify phlebotomists along with the title and corresponding initials awarded are listed as follows:

American Medical Technologists (AMT)—Registered Phlebotomy Technician
American Certification Agency—Certified Phlebotomy Technician (CPT)
American Society for Clinical Pathology—Phlebotomy Technician (PBT)
American Society for Clinical Laboratory Sciences (ASCLS)
Clinical and Laboratory Standards Institute (CLSI)
National Center for Competency Testing (NCCT)

> Table 7-1   **DUTIES OF THE NURSE OR PHLEBOTOMIST**

1. Prepare patients for blood collection procedures.
2. Collect routine skin puncture and venous specimens for testing.
3. Prepare specimens for transport.
4. Maintain standard precautions.
5. Maintain confidentiality.
6. Perform quality control checks while performing clerical, clinical, and technical duties.
7. Transport specimens to the laboratory.
8. Comply with all procedures instituted in the procedure manual.
9. Perform laboratory computer operations.
10. Collect and perform point-of-care testing.
11. Perform quality control checks on instruments.
12. Process specimens and perform basic laboratory tests.

National Accrediting Agency for Clinical Laboratory Sciences
  (NAACLS)
The Joint Commission (TJC)

Professional competencies include the following areas:
- Demonstrates knowledge of:
  - Basic anatomy and physiology
  - Medical terminology
  - Potential sources of error
  - Safety measures and infection control practices
  - Standard operating procedures
  - Fundamental biology
- Selects appropriate:
  - Courses of action
  - Quality control procedures
  - Equipment/methods and reagents
  - Site for blood collection
- Prepares patient and equipment.
- Evaluates:
  - Specimen and patient situations
  - Possible sources of error and inconsistencies

INS Standard Phlebotomy and blood sampling via vascular access
devices (VADs) shall be performed based on the order for laboratory tests by a licensed independent practitioner (LIP) in accordance
with organizational policies, procedures, and/or practice guidelines.
The nurse shall be competent in performing phlebotomy procedures
(Infusion Nurses Society [INS], 2011a, p. S78).

 NURSING FAST FACT!

*The National Patient Safety Goals 2013 (NPSGs) for clinical laboratory
include the following:*

1. *Identify patients correctly. Use at least two ways to identify patients when
   providing laboratory services.*
2. *Improve staff communication. Quickly get important test results to the right staff
   person.*
3. *Prevent infection. Use the hand-cleaning guidelines from the Centers for Disease
   Control and Prevention or current World Health Organization hand hygiene
   guidelines.*

Health-Care Worker Preparation

All health-care workers must be familiar with current recommendations
and hospital policies for handling blood and body fluids. All specimens
should be treated as if they are hazardous and infectious.

NOTE > Review Chapter 2: Infection Prevention

Before performing any type of specimen collection, the nurse or phlebotomist should have gathered the necessary protective equipment, phlebotomy supplies, test requisitions, writing pens, and appropriate patient information. Table 7-2 gives a list of supplies that should be included on a blood collection tray.

■ Equipment for Blood Collection

Supplies for Venipuncture

Supplies for venipuncture differ according to the method used (i.e., syringe method, **evacuated tube system [ETS]**). All methods of venipuncture involve the use of disposable gloves, a tourniquet, biohazard bags, vein-locating devices (options), alcohol pads or disinfectants, cotton balls, bandages or gauze pads, glass microscope slides, needles, syringes or evacuated tube holders, pen, and watch (see Table 7-2).

Vacuum (Evacuated) Tube Systems

Venipuncture with an ETS is the most direct and efficient method for obtaining a blood specimen. It is a closed system in which the patient's blood

> Table 7-2   **BLOOD COLLECTION TRAY CONTENTS**

Equipment carriers: Hand-held carriers or phlebotomy carts
Gloves: Nonsterile, disposable latex, nitrile, neoprene, polyethylene, and vinyl exam
    gloves are acceptable. *Note:* A good fit is essential.
Marking pen or pencil
Watch
Antiseptics: Routine blood collection is 70% isopropyl alcohol; chlorhexidine gluconate or
    povidone-iodine is used for higher degree of antisepsis (for blood culture collection and
    blood gas collection).
Hand sanitizers: Alcohol-based hand sanitizers
Gauze pads/cotton balls (2 × 2 gauze pads)
Bandages (latex-free): Adhesive bandages to cover site after bleeding stopped.
Paper, cloth, or knitted tape for use over cotton balls.
Needles and sharps disposal containers
Vacuum tubes containing anticoagulants
Safety holders for vacuum tubes (single-use disposable)
Needles for vacuum tubes and syringes
Tourniquets (latex, nonlatex)
Safety lancets
Microcollection blood serum separator tubes
Vein locating device (optional)

Source: McCall & Tankersley (2012).

flows through a needle inserted into a vein and directly into a collection tube without being exposed to the air or outside contaminants. The system allows for multiple tubes to be collected with a single venipuncture. Evacuated tube systems are available from several manufacturers. Figure 7-1 shows traditional components of an evacuated tube system.

The ETS requires three components: tube holders, multisample needles, and evacuated tubes.

> **NURSING FAST FACT!**
>
> According to Occupational Safety and Health Administration (OSHA) regulations, if the needle does not have a safety feature, the equipment it will be used with (e.g., tube holder, syringe) must have a safety feature to minimize the chance of an accidental needlestick (OSHA, 2003).

Tube Holders

The tube holder is a clear plastic, disposable cylinder with a small threaded opening at one end where the needle is screwed in and a large

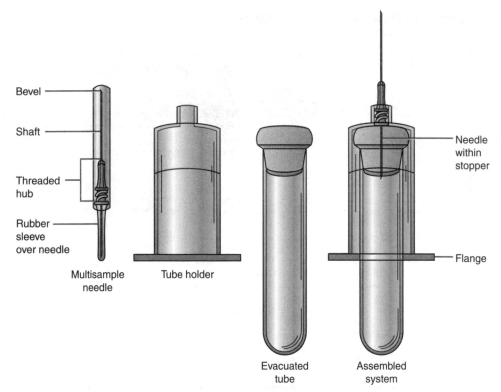

Bevel

Shaft

Threaded hub

Rubber sleeve over needle

Multisample needle

Tube holder

Evacuated tube

Assembled system

Needle within stopper

Flange

Figure 7-1 ▪ Traditional components of an evacuated tube system.

opening at the other end where the collection tube is placed. Holders are typically available in several sizes (McCall & Tankersley, 2012).

NOTE > OSHA regulations require that the tube holder with needle attached be disposed of as a unit after use and never removed from the needle and reused (OSHA, 2003).

Multisample Needles

The ETS system needles are called **multisample needles** because they allow multiple tubes of blood to be collected during a single venipuncture. They are threaded in the middle and have a beveled point on each end. The threaded portion screws into a tube holder. The end of the needle that pierces the vein is longer and has a longer bevel. The shorter end penetrates the tube stopper during specimen collection. It is covered by a sleeve that retracts as the needle goes through the tube stopper so that blood can flow into the tube (McCall & Tankersley, 2012).

Evacuated Tubes

Vacuum tubes may contain silicone to decrease the possibility of **hemolysis**. Tubes have premeasured amounts of vacuum to collect a precise amount of blood. It is imperative that the expiration date be checked before using any blood collection tube. The tubes are available in different sizes (1.8–15 mL) and can be purchased in glass or unbreakable plastic. Vacutainer system tubes are color coded according to the additive contained within the tube. The tubes are specifically designed to be used directly with chemistry, hematology, or microbiology instrumentation. The tube of blood is identified by its barcode and is pierced by the instrument probe. Some of the sample is aspirated into the instrument for analyses.

 NURSING FAST FACT!

Use of closed systems minimizes laboratory personnel's risk of exposure to blood. The expiration dates of tubes must be monitored carefully.

Evacuated tubes can also be used for transferring blood from a syringe into the tubes. The syringe needle is simply pushed through the top of the tube, and blood is automatically pulled into the tube because of the vacuum. Place the vacuum tube in a rack before pushing the needle into the tube top. A safety syringe shielded transfer device needs to be used to prevent possible exposure to the patient's blood. Figure 7-2 shows an example of a safety feature.

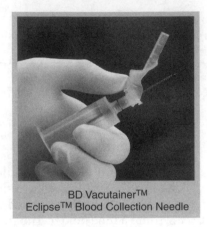

BD Vacutainer™
Eclipse™ Blood Collection Needle

Figure 7-2 ■ BD Vacutainer Eclipse™ blood collection safety needle. (Courtesy of Becton Dickinson, Franklin Lakes, NJ.)

Evacuated Tube Types

Evacuated tubes are used with both the ETS and the syringe method of obtaining blood specimens. Evacuated tubes fill with blood automatically because there is a vacuum in them.

Additive Tubes

Most ETS tubes contain some type of additive. An additive is any substance placed within a tube other than the tube stopper. Additives have one or more specific functions, such as preventing clotting or preserving certain blood components.

Anticoagulants

Most clinical laboratories use serum, plasma, or whole blood to perform various **assays**. Many coagulation factors are involved in blood clotting, and coagulation can be prevented by the addition of different types of **anticoagulants**. These anticoagulants often contain preservatives that can extend the metabolism and life span of the red blood cell. Figure 7-3 shows examples of Vacutainer tubes.

Coagulation of blood can be prevented by the addition of one of the following: **oxalates**, citrates, **ethylenediaminetetraacetic acid (EDTA)**, or heparin. These four anticoagulants are the most common. Oxalates, citrates, and EDTA prevent coagulation of blood by removing calcium and forming insoluble calcium salts. They cannot be used in calcium determinations; however, citrates are frequently used in coagulation blood studies. EDTA prevents platelet aggregation and is used for platelet counts

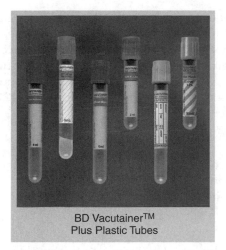

BD Vacutainer™
Plus Plastic Tubes

Figure 7-3 ■ BD Vacutainer™ plastic tubes. (Courtesy of Becton Dickinson, Franklin Lakes, NJ.)

and platelet function tests. Heparin prevents blood clotting by inactivating the blood clotting chemicals thrombin and thromboplastin.

NOTE > CLSI recommends spray-dried EDTA for most hematology tests because liquid EDTA dilutes the specimen and results in lower hemoglobin values (McCall & Tankersley, 2012).

⊳ *NURSING FAST FACT!*

It is important to choose the correct anticoagulant tube for a specific laboratory assay, along with using the correct amount or dilution of anticoagulant in the blood specimen.

⊳ *NURSING FAST FACT!*

Vigorous mixing or an excessive number of inversions can activate platelets and shorten clotting times.

Special-Use Anticoagulants

Acid–citrate–dextrose (ACD) is available in two formulations for immunohematology tests, such as DNA testing, and human leukocyte antigen (HLA) phenotyping used in paternity evaluation.

Citrate–phosphate–dextrose (CPD) is used in collection units of blood for transfusion.

Sodium polyanethol sulfonate (SPS) prevents coagulation by binding calcium. It is used for blood culture collection because, in addition to being an anticoagulant, it reduces the action of a protein called complement, which destroys bacteria, slows phagocytosis, and reduces the activity of certain antibiotics. SPS tubes have yellow stoppers and require eight inversions to prevent clotting (McCall & Tankersley, 2012).

Color Coding

Tube stoppers are color coded. Evacuated tubes are referred to as red tops, green tops, and so forth. For most tubes, the stopper color identifies a type of additive placed in the tube by the manufacturer.

Red-Topped Tubes

Red-topped tubes that are glass indicate a tube without an anticoagulant; therefore, blood collected in this tube will clot. The plastic red-topped tubes have a clot activator (silica). The red/light gray plastic tubes do not have an additive and are used as discard tubes only. The red/black (tiger) tubes have clot activator and gel separator for chemistry.

Royal Blue-Topped Tubes

Royal blue-topped tubes are used to collect samples for nutritional studies, therapeutic drug monitoring, and toxicology. The royal blue-topped tube is the trace element tube. The royal blue-topped tube with a lavender label has EDTA added; the green label has sodium heparin added. According to the Center for Phlebotomy Education, when using an ETS system, royal blue tops for trace element studies should be collected separately to avoid even the smallest amount of carryover (CLSI, 2007a).

Yellow-Topped Tubes

Yellow-topped tubes are used for blood cultures. The blood must be collected in a sterile container (vacuum tube, vial, or syringe) under aseptic conditions. The plastic tubes contain SPS for the microbiology tubes and ACD used specifically for yellow-topped tubes for blood band and immunohematology.

 NURSING FAST FACT!

Clotted specimens should not be shaken.

Green-Topped Tubes

The anticoagulants sodium heparin and lithium heparin are found in green-topped vacuum tubes. The green/gray (light green) tubes also have a gel separator.

Gray-Topped Tubes

Gray-topped vacuum tubes usually contain either potassium oxalate and sodium fluoride or sodium fluoride and EDTA. This type of collection tube is used primarily for glycolytic inhibition tests. Gray-topped tubes are not used for hematology studies.

Light Blue-Topped Tubes

Tubes with light blue tops contain sodium citrate and are used for coagulation procedures. The sodium citrate comes in a concentration of 3.2% or 3.8%. It is preferable to use the 3.2% concentration to reduce false-negative or false-positive results.

Mottled-Topped, Speckled-Topped, and Gold-Topped Tubes

These tubes contain a polymer barrier that is present at the bottom of the tube. The specific gravity of this material lies between the blood clot and the serum. During **centrifugation**, the polymer barrier moves upward to the serum–clot interface where it forms a stable barrier, separating the serum from fibrin and cells.

Pink- or Lavender-Topped Tubes

Lavender- or pink-topped tubes contain EDTA. They are also used for hematology and blood banking.

Orange- or Gray-/Yellow-Topped Tubes

Orange- or gray-/yellow-topped tubes contain thrombin for chemistry.

Tan Glass- or Tan Plastic-Topped Tubes

Glass tan-topped tubes contain sodium heparin; plastic tan-topped tubes contain EDTA. Figure 7-4 shows an illustration of a tube guide.

Expiration Dates

Manufacturers guarantee reliability of the additive and the tube vacuum until the expiration date printed on the label, providing the tubes are handled properly and stored between 4°C and 25°C.

With the use of plastic tubes, very few tubes are additive free. Even serum tubes need an additive to promote clotting if they are plastic. A few nonadditive red-topped tubes are still in existence, but most are in the process of being discontinued for safety reasons (McCall & Tankersley, 2012).

Syringe Systems

The evacuated tube system is the preferred method of blood collection, but a syringe system is sometimes used for patients with small or difficult

BD Vacutainer® Venous Blood Collection
Tube Guide

Tubes with BD Hemogard™ Closure	Tubes with Conventional Stopper	Additive	Inversions at Blood Collection*	Laboratory Use
Gold	Red/Black	• Clot activator and gel for serum separation	5	For serum determinations in chemistry. May be used for routine blood donor screening and diagnostic testing of serum for infectious disease.** Tube inversions ensure mixing of clot activator with blood. Blood clotting time: 30 minutes.
Light Green	Green/Gray	• Lithium heparin and gel for plasma separation	8	BD Vacutainer® PST™ Tube for plasma determinations in chemistry. Tube inversions prevent clotting.
Red		• None (glass) • Clot activator (plastic)	0 5	For serum determinations in chemistry. May be used for routine blood donor screening and diagnostic testing of serum for infectious disease.** Tube inversions ensure mixing of clot activator with blood. Blood clotting time: 60 minutes.
Orange	Gray/Yellow	• Thrombin	8	For stat serum determinations in chemistry. Tube inversions ensure complete clotting, which usually occurs in less than 5 minutes.
Royal Blue		• Clot activator (plastic serum) • K_2EDTA (plastic)	8 8 0 5 8	For trace-element, toxicology, and nutritional chemistry determinations. Special stopper formulation provides low levels of trace elements (see package insert).
Green		• Sodium heparin • Lithium heparin	8 8	For plasma determinations in chemistry. Tube inversions prevent clotting.
Gray		• Potassium oxalate/ sodium fluoride • Sodium fluoride/ Na_2 EDTA • Sodium fluoride (serum tube)	8 8 8	For glucose determinations. Oxalate and EDTA anticoagulants will give plasma samples. Sodium fluoride is the antiglycolytic agent. Tube inversions ensure proper mixing of additive and blood.
Tan		• K_2EDTA (plastic)	8 8	For lead determinations. This tube is certified to contain less than .01 µg/mL (ppm) lead. Tube inversions prevent clotting.
	Yellow	• Sodium polyanethol sulfonate (SPS) • Acid citrate dextrose additives (ACD): **Solution A -** 22.0 g/L trisodium citrate, 8.0 g/L citric acid, 24.5 g/L dextrose **Solution B -** 13.2 g/L trisodium citrate, 4.8 g/L citric acid, 14.7 g/L dextrose	8 8 8	SPS for blood culture specimen collections in microbiology. Tube inversions prevent clotting. ACD for use in blood bank studies, HLA phenotyping, and DNA and paternity testing.

BD Tube Guide. Courtesy and © 2008 Becton, Dickinson and Company.

Figure 7-4 ■ Blood collection tube top guide. (Courtesy of Becton Dickinson, Franklin Lakes, NJ.)

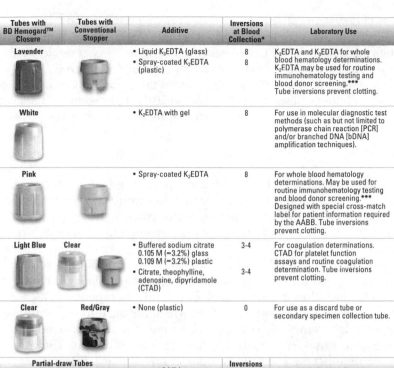

Tubes with BD Hemogard™ Closure	Tubes with Conventional Stopper	Additive	Inversions at Blood Collection*	Laboratory Use
Lavender		• Liquid K₃EDTA (glass) • Spray-coated K₂EDTA (plastic)	8 8	K₂EDTA and K₃EDTA for whole blood hematology determinations. K₂EDTA may be used for routine immunohematology testing and blood donor screening.*** Tube inversions prevent clotting.
White		• K₂EDTA with gel	8	For use in molecular diagnostic test methods (such as but not limited to polymerase chain reaction [PCR] and/or branched DNA [bDNA] amplification techniques).
Pink		• Spray-coated K₂EDTA	8	For whole blood hematology determinations. May be used for routine immunohematology testing and blood donor screening.*** Designed with special cross-match label for patient information required by the AABB. Tube inversions prevent clotting.
Light Blue	Clear	• Buffered sodium citrate 0.105 M (≈3.2%) glass 0.109 M (≈3.2%) plastic • Citrate, theophylline, adenosine, dipyridamole (CTAD)	3-4 3-4	For coagulation determinations. CTAD for platelet function assays and routine coagulation determination. Tube inversions prevent clotting.
Clear	Red/Gray	• None (plastic)	0	For use as a discard tube or secondary specimen collection tube.

Partial-draw Tubes (2 ml and 3 mL: 13 x 75 mm)	Additive	Inversions at Blood Collection*	Laboratory Use
Red	• None	0	For serum determinations in chemistry. May be used for routine blood donor screening, immunohematology testing,*** and diagnostic testing of serum for infectious disease.** Tube inversions ensure mixing of clot activator with blood. Blood clotting time: 60 minutes.
Green	• Sodium heparin • Lithium heparin	8 8	For plasma determinations in chemistry. Tube inversions prevent clotting.
Lavender	• Spray-coated K₂EDTA (plastic)	8 8	For whole blood hematology determinations. May be used for routine immunohematology testing and blood donor screening.*** Tube inversions prevent clotting.

Small-volume Pediatric Tubes (2 mL: 10.25 x 47 mm, 3 mL: 10.25 x 64 mm)	Additive	Inversions at Blood Collection*	Laboratory Use
Light Blue	• 0.105 M sodium citrate (≈3.2%)	3-4	For coagulation determinations. Tube inversions prevent clotting.

* Invert gently, do not shake

** The performance characteristics of these tubes have not been established for infectious disease testing in general; therefore, users must validate the use of these tubes for their specific assay-instrument/reagent system combinations and specimen storage conditions.

*** The performance characteristics of these tubes have not been established for immunohematology testing in general; therefore, users must validate the use of these tubes for their specific assay-instrument/reagent system combinations and specimen storage conditions.

BD Tube Guide. Courtesy and © 2008 Becton, Dickinson and Company.

Figure 7-4—cont'd

veins. This system consists of a sterile syringe needle called a hypodermic needle and sterile plastic syringe with a Luer-Lok™ tip. A newer syringe system component is an OSHA-required syringe transfer device. This device is used to transfer blood from the syringe into ETS tubes.

The barrel of the syringe is marked with graduated measurements, usually milliliters. Sizes range from 0.2 to 50.0 mL; however, for specimen collection purposes, 5- to 20-mL syringes are most often used.

Needles

The gauge and length of a needle used on a syringe or vacuum tube are selected according to the specific task. Most multisample needles come in 1- or 1.5-inch lengths. Syringe needles come in many lengths; however, 1 and 1.5 inches are most commonly used for venipuncture. Butterfly needles are typically 1/2 to 3/4 inch long. Some of the new safety needles come in slightly longer lengths to accommodate resheathing features. The needle gauges include 18-gauge needles, which are used for collecting donor units of blood and therapeutic phlebotomy, and smaller 21- or 22-gauge needles, which are used for collecting specimens for laboratory assays. The 21-gauge, 1-inch-long needle is considered the standard needle for routine venipuncture. The 22-gauge multisample needle is used on older children and adult patients with small veins or for syringe draws on difficult veins. The 23-gauge butterfly is used on infants and children and for difficult hand veins of adults. Needles are sterile and packaged by vendors in sealed shields that maintain sterility.

Different types of needles are used with vacuum collection tubes and the holder to allow for multiple tube changes without blood leakage within the plastic holder. The multisample needle has a rubber cover over the tube-top puncturing portion of the needle; this cover creates a leakage barrier. The single-sample needle is usually used for collecting blood with a syringe.

Winged Infusion Set

The winged infusion set or butterfly needle is the most commonly used blood collection set for small or difficult veins. The system consists of a 1/2- to 3/4-inch stainless steel needle permanently connected to a 5- to 12-inch length of tubing with either a Luer attachment for syringe use or a multisample Luer adapter for use with the evacuated tube system. Figure 7-5 shows an example of a blood collection butterfly collection set.

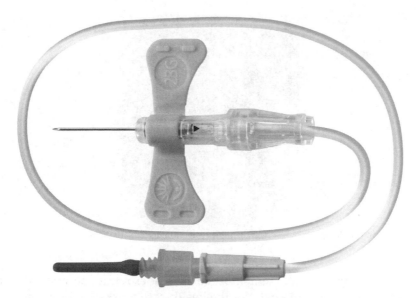

Figure 7-5 ■ BD Vacutainer Push Button blood collection set. (Courtesy of Becton Dickinson, Franklin Lakes, NJ.)

 NURSING FAST FACT!

The first tube collected with a butterfly will underfill because of the air in the tubing.

Microcollection Equipment

Lancets

Skin puncture blood collecting techniques are used on infants. Skin puncture collection is indicated for adults and older children when they are severely burned or have veins that are difficult to access because of their small size or location. The volume of plasma or serum that generally can be collected from a premature infant is approximately 100 to 150 μL, and about two times that amount can be taken from a full-term newborn. Figure 7-6 shows an example of a microcollection lancet.

Lancets for these sticks are available for two different incision depths, depending on the needs of the infant. The teal-colored Becton Dickinson (BD) Quikheel™ lancet has a depth of 1.0 mm and width of 2.5 mm, and the purple-colored Quikheel Preemie lancet has a preset incision depth of

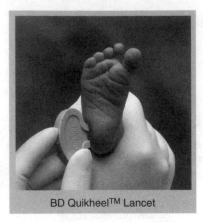

BD Quikheel™ Lancet

Figure 7-6 ■ BD Quikheel™ microcollection lancet. (Courtesy of Becton Dickinson, Franklin Lakes, NJ.)

0.85 mm and width of 1.5 mm. Most lancet blades retract permanently after activation to ensure safety for the health-care worker.

 NURSING FAST FACT!

> *The recommended penetration depth of the lancet is no more than 2.0 mm on the heel.*
>
> *The CLSI/NCCLS recommends a penetration depth of no more than 2.0 mm on heel sticks to avoid penetrating the bone (CLSI, 2007b). Refer to Age-Related Considerations for more CLSI guidelines on pediatric blood collection.*

■ Blood Collection Procedure

Blood collection includes obtaining serum, plasma, or whole blood from the patient. Serum consists of plasma minus fibrinogen and is obtained by drawing blood in a dry tube and allowing it to coagulate. A majority of the diagnostic tests require serum. Plasma consists of stable components of blood minus cells. Anticoagulant tubes are used to prevent blood from clotting. Whole blood is required in many tests, such as complete blood count and bleeding times.

When preparing for blood collection, the health-care worker carries out essential steps to ensure a successful blood specimen collection. The CLSI has recommendations for safe blood collection. These steps may vary in individual facilities depending on the characteristics of their patient populations. Some steps may be carried out simultaneously. The recommended steps include:

1. Review the test requisition.
2. Assess the patient and identify the patient using two identifiers (2013 NPSGs).
3. Approach the patient.

4. Select a puncture site.
5. Select and prepare equipment and supplies.
6. Prepare the puncture site.
7. Choose a venipuncture method.
8. Collect the samples in the appropriate tubes and in the correct order.
9. Label the samples.
10. Assess the patient after withdrawal of the blood specimen.
11. Consider any special circumstances that occurred during the phlebotomy procedure.
12. Assess criteria for sample recollection or rejection.
13. Dispose of equipment in sharps or biohazard containers.
14. Transport the specimen to the laboratory.

Test Requisition

Laboratory tests must be ordered by a qualified health-care practitioner. Test requisitions can be manual, three-part paper based, or computer generated, which are more common in today's medical settings. The computer requisitions contain the actual labels that are placed on the specimen tubes immediately after collection. With computer-generated requisitions, the phlebotomist is typically required to write the time of collection and his or her initials on the label after collection. Both the manual and computer requisitions may contain a barcode.

A barcode requisition contains a series of black stripes and white spaces of varying widths that correspond to letters and numbers. The stripes and spaces are grouped together to represent patient names, identification number, or laboratory tests. The requisition should contain the following information (McCall & Tankersley, 2012).

- Patient's first and last names and middle initial
- Physician or authorized prescriber's name
- Patient's identification or medical record number
- Patient's date of birth
- Room number and bed (if inpatient)
- Types of test to be performed
- Date of test
- Billing information and International Classification of Diseases (ICD)-10 codes (if outpatient)
- Test status (timed, priority, fasting, etc.)
- Special precautions (potential bleeder, faints easily, latex sensitivity, etc.)

Drawing Station

A blood drawing station is a dedicated area of a medical laboratory or clinic equipped for performing phlebotomy. In addition, blood is often collected from the patient in the acute care hospital at the bedside. A phlebotomy chair should be used at drawing stations where the patient sits during the blood collection procedure. Most have adjustable armrests that lock in place to prevent the patient from falling should he or she faint (Figure 7-7).

Assessment and Identification

The nurse or phlebotomist must be aware of the physical or emotional disposition of the patient, which can have an impact on the blood collection process. Cues that can help in the phlebotomy process include the following (McCall & Tankersley, 2012):

- Diet: It is important to note whether or not the patient has been fasting.
- Stress: A patient who is excessively anxious or emotional may need extra time.
- Age: The elderly may have more difficult or frail veins from which to choose for the venipuncture site. A pediatric patient often needs additional support for venipuncture.
- Weight: An obese patient may require special equipment, such as a large blood pressure cuff for the tourniquet or a longer needle to penetrate the vein.

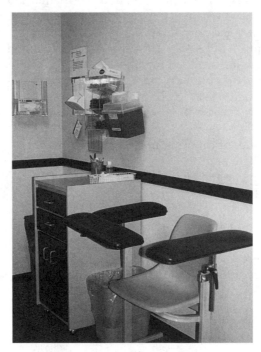

Figure 7-7 ■ Blood drawing chair.

Patient Identification Process

TJC (2013) NPSGs require at least two patient identifiers (neither to be the patient's room number) whenever taking blood samples or administering medications or blood products. This will reliably identify the individual as the person for whom the service or treatment is intended; second, it will match the service or treatment to that individual.

Before any specimen collection procedure, the patient must be correctly identified by using a two-step process:

1. Ask the patient to state his or her first and last names.
2. Confirm a match between the patient's response, the test requisition, and some form of identification, such as hospital identification bracelet, driver's license, or another identification card.

NOTE > A hospitalized patient should always wear an identification bracelet indicating his or her first and last names and a designated hospital number.

Patients in outpatient clinics usually have the same procedures as inpatient clients, with use of an identification bracelet or predistributed identification card before any specimens are collected.

NURSING FAST FACT!

Technology has advanced such that many hospitals have one- and two-dimensional barcode technologies that enable more information to be encoded. Barcodes tend to be very accurate and cost effective for larger organizations. Specimen labels are now barcoded (Figure 7-8).

Blood specimen collection for blood banking, such as typing and crossmatching, may require additional patient identification procedures and armband application.

Care must be taken in identification of emergency room patients. Often when patients come to the emergency room, they are unconscious and/or unidentified. Each hospital has policies and procedures for dealing with these cases; they usually include assigning the patient an identification tag with a hospital or medical record number.

NOTE > Never attempt to collect a blood specimen from a sleeping patient. Such an attempt may startle the patient and cause injury to the patient or the phlebotomist.

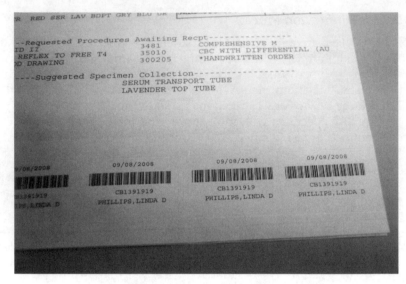

Figure 7-8 ■ Sample barcode.

Hand Hygiene/Gloving

Follow standard precautions by using alcohol-based hand sanitizer before donning gloves for the procedure. When using hand sanitizers, it is important to use a generous amount and allow the alcohol to evaporate to achieve proper antisepsis. Don nonsterile gloves.

Venipuncture Site Selection

Position the patient with his or her arm extended downward in a straight line from the shoulder to the wrist and not bent at the elbow. In the outpatient setting, blood is drawn with the patient sitting up in a special blood drawing chair.

The tourniquet is applied 3 to 4 inches above the intended venipuncture site. The tourniquet should be tight enough to slow venous flow without affecting arterial flow. If a patient has prominent visible veins, tourniquet application can wait until after the site is cleansed and before insertion of the needle.

The most common site for venipuncture is the antecubital area of the arm, where the median cubital veins lie close to the surface of the skin (Figure 7-9). The median cubital vein is most commonly used; the cephalic vein lies on the outer edge of the arm, and the basilic vein lies on the inside edge. The health-care practitioner should palpate the veins to determine the size, angle, and depth of the vein. The patient can assist in the process by closing his or her fist tightly (McCall & Tankersley, 2012).

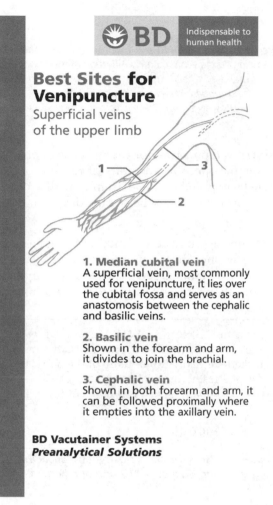

Figure 7 9 ■ Best sites for venipuncture. (Courtesy of Becton Dickinson, Franklin Lakes, NJ.)

The dorsal side of the hand or wrist should be used only if arm veins are unsuitable. Hand veins or the veins on the dorsal surface of the wrist are preferred over foot or ankle veins because coagulation and vascular complications may occur in the lower extremities, especially in diabetic patients. Position patients with hand well supported on the bed, a rolled towel, or an armrest.

INS Standard The nurse should select an appropriate vein for phlebotomy. The most common veins include the median cubital, the cephalic, and the basilica veins in the antecubital area (INS, 2011a, p. S78).

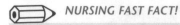 *NURSING FAST FACT!*

> ■ *Never draw above an infusing I.V.; this can alter the test results.*
> ■ *Use caution during venipuncture. Although nerve damage during venipuncture is rare, it has been known to occur as a result of excessive needle probing and sudden movement of the patient.*
> ■ *Never heat towels or washcloths in a microwave oven.*

INS Standard Venipuncture for the purpose of phlebotomy should be drawn from the opposite extremity of an infusion. Should venipuncture be required on the extremity with a VAD infusion, it should be performed in a vein below the device or infusion (INS, 2011a, p. S78).

The venipuncture site may be warmed to facilitate vein prominence. A surgical towel or washcloth warmed to about 42°C and then wrapped around the site for 3 to 5 minutes can increase skin temperature. Encasing the towel or washcloth in a plastic bag or wrap helps to retain heat.

NOTE > According to CLSI Standard H3-A5, an attempt must have been made to locate the median cubital on both arms before considering an alternate vein. Also, because of the possibility of nerve injury and damage to the brachial artery, the basilic vein should not be chosen unless **no** other vein is prominent (CLSI, 2007a).

 NURSING FAST FACT!

> *If the patient has sensitive skin or dermatitis, apply the tourniquet over a dry washcloth or gauze wrapped around the arm or a hospital gown sleeve.*

Preparation of the Venipuncture Site

Once the site is selected, the site should be prepped with 70% isopropyl alcohol or chlorhexidine (ChloraPrep®) and allowed to dry. Alcohol is not recommended for use when obtaining a specimen for blood alcohol level determination. Chlorhexidine is recommended; however, check the institutional policy.

Povidone-iodine (Betadine) or chlorhexidine is usually used for drawing blood for blood gas analysis and blood cultures. Remove excess povidone-iodine from the skin with sterile gauze after prepping because iodine can interfere with some laboratory tests. Cleanse the site with a circular motion, starting at the point where you expect to insert the needle and moving outward in ever-widening concentric circles until a 2- to 3-inch area is prepped (McCall & Tankersley, 2012).

NURSING FAST FACT!

> *Do not touch the prepared venipuncture site after prepping. The alcohol should be allowed to dry (30–60 seconds). Do not fan the site with your hand or blow on it to hasten drying time.*

Equipment Preparation and Venipuncture Technique

Place all collection equipment and supplies within easy reach, typically on the same side of the patient's arm as your free hand during venipuncture.

 NURSING FAST FACT!

> *Do not place the phlebotomy tray on the patient's bed or any other place that could be considered contaminated.*

Once the venipuncture site is prepped and the tourniquet reapplied, the health-care worker may hold the patient's arm below the site, pulling the skin tightly with the thumb (traction) to anchor the vein.

 NURSING FAST FACT!

> *For safety do not use a two-finger technique (also called "C") in which the entry point of the vein is straddled by the index finger above and the thumb below. If the patient pulls the arm back when the needle is inserted, there is a possibility that the needle may recoil as it comes out of the arm and spring back into the phlebotomist's index finger.*

A safety syringe, butterfly, or Vacutainer system can be used for venipuncture. The needle should be lined up with the vein and inserted smoothly and quickly at approximately a 15- to 30-degree angle with the skin. The needle should be inserted with the bevel side upward and directly above a prominent vein or slightly below the palpable vein. Sometimes a slight "pop" can be felt when the needle enters the vein. The tourniquet can be released immediately after blood begins to flow so that blood that is **hemoconcentrated** is not collected. When a tourniquet is placed on the patient, the tourniquet pressure forces low molecular compounds and fluid to move into the tissues from the intravascular space. Large molecules such as cholesterol and proteins cannot move through the capillary wall, and their blood levels increase as the tourniquet remains on the arm. In addition, the longer the tourniquet remains on the arm, the greater the amount of potassium leakage from tissue cells into the blood, which increases the chances of a false blood potassium level reading.

NURSING FAST FACT!

> ■ It is recommended that the tourniquet be released as the last tube is fill-
> ing but always before the needle is withdrawn from the arm.
> ■ If the patient continues to bleed, the health-care practitioner should ap-
> ply pressure until the bleeding stops.

Evacuated Tube System Equipment Preparation and Venipuncture Technique

Select the appropriate ETS tubes based on requisition. Check the expiration date on each of the tubes. Tap additive tubes lightly to dislodge any
additive that may be adhering to the tube stopper. Inspect the seal of the
needle and discard if broken. Twist the needle cover apart to expose the
short or back end of the needle that is covered by a retractable sleeve.
Screw this end of the needle into the threaded hub of an ETS tube holder.
Place the first tube in the holder and use a slight clockwise twist to push
it onto the needle just far enough to secure it from falling out but not far
enough to release the tube vacuum (Figure 7-10).

 NURSING FAST FACT!

> ■ For beginners it is easier not to try to balance the tube in the holder
> before venipuncture. Access the vein and then pick up the tube and
> push it onto the inner needle.
> ■ Vigorous handling of the blood tubes and sluggish propulsion of blood
> into the tube can cause hemolysis and separation of cells from liquid,
> which can affect the test results.
> ■ Some health-care workers use the dominant hand to change tubes
> while using the other hand to keep the needle apparatus steady.

See Procedures Display 7-1 at the end of this chapter for steps in performing the evacuated tube blood collection method.

When multiple sample tubes are to be collected, each tube should be
gently removed from the Vacutainer holder and replaced with the next
tube. Experienced health-care workers are able to mix a full tube in one
hand while holding the needle apparatus with the other hand. Multiple
tubes can be filled in less than 1 minute if the needle remains stable in the
vein and the vein does not collapse. The holder must be securely held
while the tubes are being changed so that the needle is not pushed further
into or removed from the vein.

After collection of the blood and removal of the last tube, the entire
needle assembly should be withdrawn quickly. Safety devices should be
activated immediately, depending on the manufacturer's specifications.

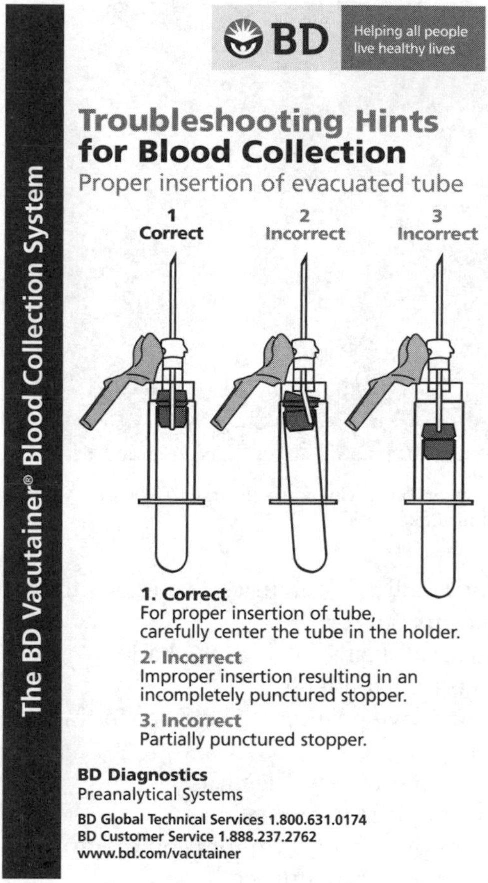

Figure 7-10 ■ Proper insertion of needle into Vacutainer holder. (Courtesy of Becton Dickinson, Franklin Lakes, NJ.)

Winged Infusion Set Equipment Preparation and Venipuncture Technique

The 23-gauge winged set is most commonly used. Select the type of butterfly needle set, either one with a hub to attach a syringe or a hub with a multisample Luer adapter that can be threaded onto an ETS tube holder (Figure 7-11). Verify the sterility of the needle packaging before aseptically opening it. Attach the butterfly to the evacuated tube holder or syringe. Select small-volume tubes because larger tubes may collapse the vein or cause hemolysis of the specimen. When using a butterfly needle on a hand vein, insert it into the vein at a shallow angle between 10 and 15 degrees. Use a 15- to 30-degree angle for an antecubital vein.

A winged infusion system can be used for particularly difficult venipunctures. This method is now used with safety equipment to

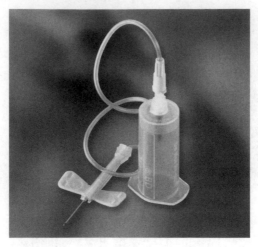

Figure 7-11 ■ Insertion of winged needle into ETS holder. (Courtesy of Becton Dickinson, Franklin Lakes, NJ.)

decrease the risk of needlestick injuries to the health-care worker. This method is sometimes useful for:

- Patients with small veins, such as the hand
- Pediatric or geriatric patients
- Patients in restrictive positions (i.e., those in traction or with severe arthritis)
- Patients with numerous needlesticks
- Patients with fragile skin and veins
- Patients undergoing short-term infusion therapy
- Patients who are severely burned

The needles range from 1/2 to 3/4 inch in length and from 21 to 25 gauge in diameter. Attached to the needle is a thin tubing with a Luer adapter at the end, which can be used on a syringe or an evacuated tube system from the same manufacturer.

 NURSING FAST FACT!

Because the tubing contains air, it will underfill the first evacuated tube by 0.5 mL. This affects the additive-to-blood ratio. A red-topped nonadditive tube should be filled before any tube with additives is filled.

Health-care workers should be extra cautious when they are removing the needle from the patient to activate the safety device that is built into the system. Use of the winged infusion or butterfly system requires training and practice. Failure to activate the safety devices correctly as described by the manufacturer may result in a higher incidence of needlestick injuries. Figure 7-12 shows the steps for push-button winged needle

BD Vacutainer® Push Button Blood Collection Set
In-Vein Needle Activation at the Push of a Button

General Use and Disposal (See package insert for detailed directions for use.)

 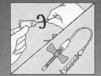 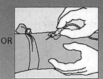

1a. Peel back packaging at arrow so that the back end of the wing set is exposed.

1b. With thumb and middle finger, grasp the rear barrel of the wingset and remove from package. Be careful to avoid activating the button.

2. CAUTION - Never use a blood collection set without a holder or syringe attached.

Assemble to BD Vacutainer® One Use Holder or BD Syringe. (Disregard this step if pre-attached holder is used.)

3a. With thumb and index finger, grasp the wings together and access vein using standard needle insertion technique.

3b. If preferred by your institution, the body of the device can be held, instead of the wings, during insertion.

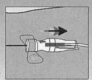 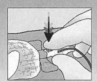

4. Proper access to the vein will be indicated by the presence of "flash" directly behind and below the button.

5a. The device is designed to be activated while the needle is still in the patient's vein. Place your gauze pad or cotton ball on the venipuncture site. Allow gauze pad or cotton ball to cover nose of front barrel. Following the collection procedure, **and while the needle is still in the vein, grasp the body** with the thumb and middle finger. Activate the button with the tip of the index finger.

5b. To ensure complete and immediate retraction of device, make sure to keep fingers and hands away from the end of the blood collection set during retraction. Do not impede retraction.

6. Apply pressure to the venipuncture site in accordance with your facility's protocol.

Ordering Information

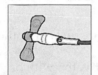

7. Confirm that the needle is in the shielded position prior to disposal.

8. Discard the entire shielded blood collection set and holder into an approved sharps disposal container.

Facility Reference Number	BD Reference Number	Needle Gauge	Wing Color	Tubing Length	Configuration	Packaging
BD Vacutainer® Push Button Blood Collection Sets with Pre-Attached Holder						
367352	21			12"	with holder	20/Box 100/Case
368656	23			12"	with holder	20/Box 100/Case
BD Vacutainer® Push Button Blood Collection Sets						
367338	21			7"	with luer	50/Box 200/Case
367344	21			12"	with luer	50/Box 200/Case
367326	21			12"	without luer	50/Box 200/Case
367336	23			7"	with luer	50/Box 200/Case
367342	23			12"	with luer	50/Box 200/Case
367324	23			12"	without luer	50/Box 200/Case
367341	25			13"	with luer	50/Box 200/Case
367323	25			12"	without luer	50/Box 200/Case
BD Vacutainer® One Use Holder						

Facility Reference Number	BD Reference Number	Description		Packaging
364815		One Use Holder		250/Bag 1,000/Case

BD Global Technical Services: 1.800.631.0174
vacutainer_techservices@bd.com
BD Customer Service: 1.888.237.2762
www.bd.com/vacutainer

CAUTION:
Handle all biologic samples and blood collection "sharps" (lancets, needles, luer adapters, and blood collection sets) in accordance with the policies and procedures of your facility. Obtain appropriate medical attention in the event of any exposure to biologic samples (e.g., through a puncture injury) since samples may transmit viral hepatitis, HIV (AIDS), or other infectious diseases. Utilize any safety-engineered feature if the blood collection device provides one. Discard all blood collection "sharps" in biohazard containers approved for their disposal.

BD, BD Logo and all other trademarks are property of Becton, Dickinson and Company. © 2006 BD
05.06 VS7104-3

BD

Helping all people
live healthy lives

BD Diagnostics
Preanalytical Systems
1 Becton Drive
Franklin Lakes, NJ 07417
www.bd.com/vacutainer

Figure 7-12 ■ Vacutainer push-button winged needle blood collection set steps. (Courtesy of Becton Dickinson, Franklin Lakes, NJ.)

blood collection. See Procedures Display 7-2 at the end of this chapter for steps on using winged needle system for blood collection.

Syringe Equipment Preparation and Venipuncture Technique

Select a syringe and needle size compatible with the size and condition of the patient's vein and the amount of blood to be collected. Open the needle package aseptically and then attach the syringe. A blood specimen collected in a syringe will have to be transferred to ETS tubes.

When using the **syringe method**, follow the same approach to needle insertion as the one used for the evacuated tube method. Once the needle is in the vein, the syringe plunger can be drawn back gently to avoid hemolysis of the specimen until the required volume of blood has been withdrawn. The health-care worker must be careful not to withdraw the needle from the vein while pulling back on the plunger.

 NURSING FAST FACT!

- *Turn the syringe so that the graduated markings are visible.*
- *See Procedures Display 7-3 at the end of this chapter for steps on the syringe method of blood collection.*

Order of Tube Collection

The Clinical and Laboratory Standards Institute (CLSI, 2007) recommends the following specific order when collecting multiple tubes of blood via the evacuated method or the syringe transfer method:

1. Blood culture tubes (yellow top), or blood culture vials or bottles
2. Coagulation tubes (light blue top)
3. Serum tube red-topped with or without clot activator, with or without gel. Heparin tubes (green) or plasma separator tubes (PSTs) (green and gray, light green plastic)
4. EDTA tubes (lavender or pink)
5. Glycolytic inhibitor (glucose) tubes (gray)

Table 7-3 gives the order of draw for multiple tube collections.

Yellow, Light Blue, Red, Green, Lavender/Pink, and Gray Tops

- Be meticulous about time, type of test, and volume of blood required.
- Always draw blood cultures first to decrease the possibility of bacterial contamination.
- When drawing just coagulation studies for diagnostic purposes, it is preferable that at least one other tube of blood be drawn before the coagulation test specimen. This diminishes contamination

> Table 7-3	ORDER OF DRAW FOR MULTIPLE TUBE COLLECTIONS	
Collection Tube	**Mix by Inverting**	**Color**
Blood cultures— Sodium polyanethol sulfonate (SPS)	8–10 times	Yellow
Coagulation citrate tubes	3–4 times	Light blue
Serum tube (glass)	None for glass	Red
Plastic clot activator tubes	5 times for plastic	Red or red/gray rubber Gold plastic
Plasma separator tubes (PSTs) with gel separator/heparin	8–10 times	Green/gray Light-green plastic
Heparin tube	8–10 times	Green
EDTA tube	8–10 times	Lavender or pink
Oxalate/fluoride tubes	8–10 times	Gray

Note: Always follow your facility's protocol for order of draw.

with tissue fluids, which may initiate the clotting sequence. Usually a nonadditive red top is used.

- Coagulation tubes should be mixed as soon as possible after collection.
- Minimize the transfer of anticoagulants from tube to tube by holding the tube horizontally or slightly downward during blood collection.
- When a large volume (more than 20 mL) of blood has been drawn using a syringe, there is a possibility that some of the blood may be clotted.
- If two syringes of blood have been withdrawn, CLSI (2007a) recommends taking blood from the second syringe for coagulation studies.
- Watch the "fill" rate and volume in each tube; evacuated tubes with anticoagulants must be filled to the designated level for the proper mix of blood with the anticoagulant.

NOTE > Partial fill tubes are available when it is suspected that the blood specimen will not be adequate.

Fill and Mix of Tubes

If the tube contains an additive, mix it by gently inverting it three to eight times depending on the type of additive and the manufacturer's recommendations as soon as it is removed from the tube holder. Nonadditive tubes do not require mixing.

NOTE > Do not shake or vigorously mix blood specimens because this can cause hemolysis.

Remove the last specimen tube from the holder before removing the needle from the vein. Gently but quickly remove the needle. After collection of the blood, the entire blood collection assembly should be withdrawn quickly. Safety devices should be activated immediately, depending on the manufacturer's specifications.

A dry sterile gauze or cotton ball should be applied with pressure to the puncture site for several minutes or until bleeding has stopped. Keep the patient's arm straight or elevate it above the heart, if possible. A pressure bandage should be applied and the patient instructed to leave it on for at least 15 minutes.

Disposal of Equipment

All contaminated equipment should be discarded into appropriate containers. Paper and plastic wrappers can be thrown into a wastebasket. Needles and lancets should be placed into a sturdy puncture-proof disposable container following OSHA guidelines.

Any items, such as cotton or gauze, that have been contaminated with blood should be discarded in biohazard disposal containers following standard precautions.

Specimen Identification and Labeling

Specimens should be labeled immediately at the patient's bedside or ambulatory setting. Some laboratories require labels to be placed so that the label does not obscure the entire specimen. If using preprinted computer or barcode label, write the date, time, and your initials on the label immediately after withdrawal from the tube. Any handwritten labeling must be done with permanent ink pen and provide the following information:

- Patient's full name
- Patient's identification numbers
- Date and time of collection
- Health-care worker's initials
- Patient's room number, bed assignment, or outpatient status are optional information.

Postprocedure Patient Care

Once the last tube has been removed from the holder, fold a clean gauze square into fourths or use a cotton ball and lightly apply for venipuncture site. Do not press down until the needle is removed. Activate the safety feature of the needle according to the manufacturer's recommendations. Apply pressure to the site for 3 to 5 minutes or until the bleeding stops. Do not ask the patient to bend his or her arm.

 NURSING FAST FACT!

> *Folding the arm back at the elbow to hold pressure or keeping the gauze in place after a blood draw actually increases the chance of bruising by keeping the wound open or disrupting the platelet plug when the arm is lowered (McCall & Tankersley, 2012).*

Apply adhesive bandage (or tape and folded gauze or cotton ball) over the site. If the patient is allergic to adhesive bandage, use paper tape and gauze. Instruct the patient to leave the bandage on for a minimum of 15 minutes, after which it should be removed to avoid irritation. Instruct an outpatient not to carry a purse or other heavy object for 1 hour.

 NURSING FAST FACT!

> *Failure to apply pressure or applying inadequate pressure can result in leakage of blood and hematoma formation.*
> *It is acceptable to have the patient hold pressure while you label the tubes providing the patient is fully cooperative.*

Transport of the Specimen to the Laboratory

All specimens should be transported to the laboratory or designated pickup site in a timely fashion. The phlebotomist is typically responsible for verifying and documenting collection by computer entry or manual entry in a log book (McCall & Tankersley, 2012).

 NURSING FAST FACT!

> *If the specimen cannot be transported to the laboratory within a reasonable time or if analysis is delayed, arrange for proper storage to prevent deterioration or contamination that can cause inaccurate results (Van Leeuwen, Poelhuis-Leth, & Bladh, 2012).*

NURSING POINTS OF CARE
COLLECTION OF BLOOD SPECIMENS

Focus Assessment
- Assess the patient's understanding of the blood test.
- Assess the patient's degree of anxiety about the procedure.
- Assess the infant's or child's need for restraint and reassurance.
- Ensure that food, fluid, and medication restrictions have been followed.
- Verify the patient's identity using two identifiers.
- Assess both median antecubital sites for the appropriate venipuncture site.

Key Nursing/Phlebotomist Interventions
1. Select appropriate evacuated tubes, winged set, or syringe.
2. Ensure the collected sample is valid by applying the tourniquet appropriately. Avoid possible invalid testing caused by prolonged use of tourniquet, excessive suction on the syringe, or vigorous shaking of specimen in a tube.
3. Use aseptic technique.
4. Apply adhesive bandage after bleeding has stopped.
5. Provide support to the client if the puncture is not successful and another must be performed to obtain the blood sample.
6. Check the venipuncture site after 5 minutes for hematoma formation.
7. If the client is immunosuppressed, check the puncture site every 8 hours for signs and symptoms of infection.
8. Document in the patient medical record; include the amount of blood used for sampling and patient's response to the procedure (INS, 2011b).
9. Instruct the patient to leave the bandage over the site for a minimum of 15 minutes.

Complications

Hematoma

Hematoma formation is the most common complication of venipuncture. It is caused by blood leaking into the tissues during or after venipuncture and is identified by rapid swelling at or near the venipuncture site. Presence of a hematoma makes the site unacceptable for subsequent venipunctures.

If a hematoma forms during blood collection the draw should be discontinued, and pressure must be held over the site for 2 minutes. Cold compresses can be used for large hematomas to reduce swelling. Figure 7-13 shows an example of hematoma formation after venipuncture.

Situations that can trigger hematoma formation:
- Use of excessive or blind probing to locate a vein
- Inadvertent arterial puncture
- The vein is fragile or too small for the needle size.
- The needle penetrates all the way through the vein.
- The needle is only partly inserted into the vein.
- The needle is removed while the tourniquet is still on.
- Pressure is not adequately applied following venipuncture (McCall & Tankersley, 2012)

NOTE > Ice can be applied for the first 24 hours to help manage discomfort. After 24 hours, heat or warm moist compresses can help reabsorb accumulated blood (McCall & Tankersley, 2012).

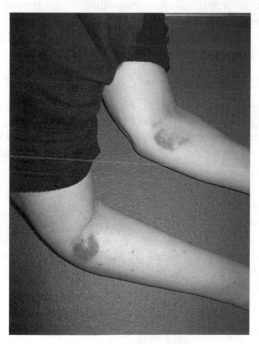

Figure 7-13 ■ Hematoma resulting from multiple attempts at blood draw.

Iatrogenic Anemia

Blood loss as a result of blood removal for testing is called iatrogenic blood loss. Removing blood on a regular basis or in large quantities can lead to iatrogenic anemia in some patients, especially infants.

INS Standard Only the volume of blood needed for accurate testing should be obtained. Phlebotomy contributes to iron deficiency and blood loss in neonates and critically ill patients (INS, 2011a, p. S78).

Infection

Although rare, infection at the site of venipuncture can occur. The risk of infection can be minimized by use of proper aseptic technique, hand hygiene, and gloves.

Nerve Injury

Nerves and veins lie close to each other in the arms. Improper vein selection can lead to nerve injury if the needle is inserted too deeply or quickly. Movement by the patient as the needle is inserted can also cause nerve injury. Blind probing while attempting venipuncture can lead to injury of a main nerve. The consequences of nerve injury may be minor or major. Minor nerve injury results in the formation of a traumatic neuroma (an unorganized mass of nerve fibers) at the point of needle contact. Should the needle actually tear the nerve fibers, complex regional pain syndrome (CRPS) may result (Massorli, 2007).

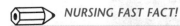 NURSING FAST FACT!

Extreme burning or pain, electric shock sensation, numbness of the arm, and pain that radiates up or down the arm are all signs of nerve involvement. Remove the needle immediately. Applying an ice pack to the site can help reduce inflammation associated with nerve involvement (McCall & Tankersley, 2012).

Vein Damage

Numerous venipunctures in the same area over an extended period of time can cause a buildup of scar tissue and increase the difficulty of performing subsequent venipunctures. Blind probing and improper technique when redirecting the needle can also damage veins and impair patency (McCall & Tankersley, 2012).

AGE-RELATED CONSIDERATIONS

The Pediatric Client

Collection of blood by venipuncture from infants and children may be necessary for tests that require large amounts of blood (e.g., crossmatching and blood cultures).

- Venipuncture in children younger than age 2 year should be limited to superficial veins. The accessible veins of infants and toddlers are veins of the antecubital fossa and forearm.
- Heel stick: Capillary collection is normally recommended for pediatric patients, especially newborns and infants up to 12 months. Venipuncture is done in the area of the heel where there is little risk of puncturing the bone. According to CLSI, the only safe area of the heel is the plantar surface of the heel, medial to an imaginary line extending from the middle of the great toe to the heel or lateral to an imaginary line extending from between the fourth and fifth toes to the heel (Fig. 7-14).
- CLSI/NCCLS (2007b) infant capillary puncture precautions include:
  - Do not puncture earlobes.
  - Do not puncture deeper than 2.0 mm.
  - Do not puncture through previous puncture sites.
  - Do not puncture the area between the imaginary boundaries.
  - Do not puncture the posterior curvature of the heel.
  - Do not puncture in the area of the arch and any other areas of the foot.
  - Do not puncture severely bruised areas.
- Removal of large quantities of blood at once or even small quantities on a regular basis can lead to anemia. Removing more than 10% of an infant's blood volume at one time can lead to shock and cardiac arrest. Most facilities have limits on the amount of blood that can be removed per draw. Many facilities do not allow more than 3% of a

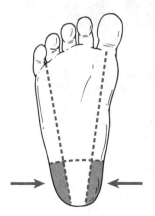

Figure 7-14 ■ Appropriate site for heel puncture on infant.

Continued

child's blood volume to be collected at one time and no more than 10% in 1 month.

NOTE > CLSI (2007a) recommends that procedures be in place to monitor the amounts of blood drawn from pediatric, geriatric, and other vulnerable patients to avoid phlebotomy-induced anemia.

INS Standard For the pediatric patient, the amount of blood obtained for laboratory assay should be documented in the patient's medical record (INS, 2011a, p. S78-79).

- Interventions to ease pain include the use of EMLA cream, oral sucrose, and pacifiers for infants and toddlers.
- Selecting the method of restraint is important when dealing with infants and children to ensure their safety. A newborn or young infant can be wrapped in a blanket, but physical restraint is often required for older infants, toddlers, and younger children. Older children can sit by themselves in the blood drawing chair, but a parent or another phlebotomist should help steady the arm.

NOTE > Never tell a child that it won't hurt. Instead, say that it may hurt just a little bit, but it will be over quickly.

EBP The use of 12% to 24% solution of oral sucrose has been shown to reduce the pain of procedures such as heel puncture and venipuncture in infants up to 6 months of age. A 24% solution of sucrose can be administered by dropper, nipple, or oral syringe, or on a pacifier, provided it will not interfere with the sample to be collected. Sucrose nipples or pacifiers are available commercially. The sucrose must be given to the infant 2 minutes before the procedure (Gradin, Ericksson, Holmqvist, Holstein, & Schollin, 2002).

The Older Adult

Physical effects of aging, such as skin changes, hearing and vision problems, and mobility issues often related to a disease process, require expert skills from a phlebotomist.

- Blood vessels lose elasticity and become more fragile and more likely to collapse, resulting in an increased chance of bruising and failure to obtain blood.
- Hearing-impaired patients may strain to hear and have difficulty answering questions and understanding instructions.

- The phlebotomy area should have adequate lighting without glare. The patient may require assistance to the drawing chair or escort to the restroom. Provide instructions in large print.
- Slower nerve conduction may lead to slower learning, slower reaction times, and diminished perception of pain, which could lead to an increase in injuries. Approach the patient in a calm, professional manner.
- Effects of the disease process may affect blood collection. Patients who have coagulation disorders who take blood thinning medications are at risk for hematoma formation or uncontrolled bleeding at the blood collection site. Patients with Parkinson's disease may have difficulty with tremors and movement of the hands, which can make blood collection difficult.
- Poor nutrition can intensify the effects of aging on the skin, affect clotting ability, and contribute to anemia.
- If the patient is in a wheelchair and cannot be transported to the laboratory drawing chair, it is safest and easiest to draw blood from the patient in the wheelchair by supporting the arm on a pillow or on a special padded board placed across the arms of the chair (McCall & Tankersley, 2012).

NOTE > Never use force to extend a patient's arm or open a hand because this can cause pain and injury.

 NURSING FAST FACT!

The safest and easiest way to draw blood from a patient in a wheelchair is by supporting the arm on a pillow or on a special padded board placed across the arms of the chair.

 Home Care Issues

A home care phlebotomist must have exceptional phlebotomy, interpersonal, and organizational skills; be able to function independently; and be comfortable working in varied situations. The physical setting can affect the collection of blood in the home care setting. If specimens are to be collected in homes, the procedures are similar and key points are listed.

- Obtain necessary supplies, including venipuncture supplies, blood collection tubes, a biohazard container for disposal, and a specimen transport container, and bring to the home.
- Perform hand hygiene: Wash hands before and after phlebotomy; most often, alcohol-based hand gel is used.
- Identify the patient: Use at least two patient identifiers.
- Carefully inspect the area after the procedure to ensure that all trash and used supplies have been properly discarded before leaving the home environment.

Continued

* Label specimens and place in leak-proof containers.
* Ensure that specimens are transported at appropriate temperatures.
* Reinforce patient education.

Patient Education

The first and last steps of phlebotomy procedures are to prepare the patient for the procedure. Pretesting explanation to the patient or caregiver follows essentially the same pattern for all sites and types of studies and includes:

■ Explain the purpose of the test.
■ Describe the procedure, including site and method.
■ Describe any sensations, including discomfort and pain, that the patient may experience during the specimen collection procedure.

NOTE > Cultural and social issues, as well as concern for modesty, are important in providing psychological support.

■ Instruct regarding pretesting preparations related to diet, liquids, medications, and activity as well as any restrictions.
■ Identify any anxiety related to test results. Encourage the patient to ask questions and verbalize his or her concerns.
■ Educate regarding any limitations of movement.
■ Instruct the patient to notify the nurse if the puncture site begins to bleed after the pressure dressing is applied.
■ Instruct the patient to notify the nurse if the puncture site becomes red or warm to the touch, or if pain develops (Van Leeuwen, Poelhuis-Leth, & Bladh, 2012).

▪ Nursing Process

The nursing process is a five- or six-step process for problem-solving to guide nursing action (see Chapter 1 for details on the steps of the nursing process related to vascular access). The following table focuses on nursing diagnoses, nursing outcomes classification (NOC), and nursing interventions classification (NIC) for patients requiring laboratory analysis. Nursing diagnoses should be patient specific and outcomes and interventions individualized. The NOC and NIC presented here are suggested directions for development of specific outcomes and interventions.

Nursing Diagnoses Related to Management of Venipuncture for Laboratory Analysis	Nursing Outcomes Classification (NOC)	Nursing Interventions Classification (NIC)
Infection, risk for related to: Invasive procedure	Infection control risk detection and control	Infection control, infection protection
Knowledge deficit related to: Information misinterpretation; lack of exposure; unfamiliarity with information resources (phlebotomy lab analysis)	Health resources; infection management, personal safety, treatment procedures(s)	Teaching: Purpose of phlebotomy and laboratory tests
Skin integrity impaired related to: External: interruption in barrier protection—venipuncture	Tissue integrity: skin, primary intention	Venipuncture site care; skin surveillance
Tissue integrity impaired related to: Mechanical wound care factors—arterial puncture	Tissue integrity: skin and wound healing	Skin care; skin surveillance

Sources: Ackley & Ladwig (2011); Bulechek, Butcher, Dochterman, & Wagner (2013); Moorhead, Johnson, Maas, & Swanson, 2013.

Chapter Highlights

- Specimens incorrectly acquired, labeled, or transported by the nurse can cause the laboratory tests to be useless or even cause harm to the patient.
- The nurse performing phlebotomy procedures must have the following knowledge base to perform blood withdrawal procedures safely: knowledge of basic anatomy and physiology, medical terminology, sources of error, safety measures and infection control practices, fundamental biology, quality control procedures, equipment and methods, and sites for blood collection.
- A two-step process must identify the patient: Ask the patient's name and confirm the match among patient response, test requisition, and ID bracelet.
- The vacuum (evacuated) tube system includes the evacuated sample tube, the double-pointed needle, and the plastic holder.
- Vacuumized tubes for blood include those without additives and those with anticoagulant additives.
- Safety syringes should be used when the syringe method of blood collection is used.
- The antecubital area is the most frequently used area for blood collection. The dorsal side of hand or wrist should be used only if the arm veins are unsuitable.

- The tourniquet should be released once blood begins to flow into the tube (no longer than 1 minute) to prevent hemoconcentration of the blood specimen.
- The order of tube draw is blood culture tubes (yellow), then plain tubes (nonadditives), coagulation tubes (light blue), additive tubes (green), EDTA (purple), and then oxalate/fluoride (gray top).

■■ Thinking Critically: Case Study

A 70-year-old Hmong, non–English-speaking woman was admitted to an acute care hospital accompanied by her husband, who had limited English language ability. On admission her physician had ordered a series of blood tests. When the health-care worker arrived to collect blood for laboratory tests, she introduced herself and asked the patient her name. The patient did not respond and looked perplexed.

Case Study Questions
1. What should the health-care worker do next?
2. What do TJC Patient Safety Goals state regarding patient identification?
3. What other factors need to be considered in this scenario (i.e., safety, ethics, legal)?

 Media Link: Answers to the case study and more critical thinking activities are provided on Davis*Plus*.

Post-Test

1. Which of the following anticoagulants is found in a green-topped collection vacuum tube?

   a. EDTA
   b. Sodium citrate
   c. Sodium heparin
   d. Ammonium oxalate

2. The color coding for tubes indicates the:

   a. Length of needle needed to access the tube
   b. Manufacturer
   c. Additive contained within the tube
   d. Amount of blood necessary to fill the tube

3. From the following list of tubes, which would be the first tube to be used in the evacuated tube system?

   a. Lavender-topped tube
   b. Yellow-topped tube
   c. Light blue-topped tube
   d. Red-topped tube

4. What causes evacuated tubes to fill with blood automatically?

   a. Tube vacuum
   b. Pressure created by application of the tourniquet
   c. Venous pressure
   d. Fist pumping by the patient

5. The most common site for venipuncture is in which of the following areas?

   a. The dorsal side of the wrist
   b. The antecubital fossa of the arm
   c. Hand veins
   d. The heel

6. Blood collection tubes are labeled:

   a. Before the collection
   b. Immediately after specimen collection
   c. After all draws are completed
   d. Whenever it is convenient for the phlebotomist

7. Which of the following tubes contain an anticoagulant additive? (*Select all that apply.*)

   a. Lavender
   b. Pink
   c. Green
   d. Red

8. In which of the following situations may the use of a winged needle system be beneficial? (*Select all that apply.*)

   a. Heel puncture
   b. Veins in the hand
   c. Geriatric patients
   d. Central line blood collection

9. Which of the following solutions is used most frequently as a prep solution for venipuncture for lab collection for blood chemistry?

   a. 70% Isopropyl alcohol
   b. Povidone-iodine
   c. 2% Iodine
   d. Acetone

10. What is the minimum amount of time a pressure bandage should be left in place after a venipuncture for blood collection?
    a. 5 minutes
    b. 10 minutes
    c. 15 minutes
    d. 30 minutes

Media Link: Answers to the Chapter 7 Post-Test and more test questions together with rationales are provided on DavisPlus.

References

Ackley, B. J., & Ladwig, G. B. (2011). *Nursing diagnosis handbook: An evidence-based guide to planning care* (9th ed.). St. Louis, MO: Mosby Elsevier.

Bulechek, G. M., Butcher, H. K., Dochterman, J. M., & Wagner, C. M. (2013). *Nursing interventions classification (NIC)* (6th ed.). St. Louis MO: Mosby Elsevier.

Clinical and Laboratory Standards Institute (CLSI). (2007a). *Procedures for the collection of diagnostic blood specimens by venipuncture. Approved standard H3-A5* (5th ed.). Wayne, PA: CLSI/NCCLS.

CLSI. (2007b). *Procedures for the collection of capillary blood specimens. Approved standard H4-A6* (6th ed.). Wayne, PA: CLSI/NCCLS.

Gradin, M., Eriksson, M., Holmqvist, A., Holstein, A., & Schollin, J. (2002). Pain reduction at venipuncture in newborns; oral glucose compared with local anesthetic cream. *Pediatrics, 110,* 1053-1057.

Infusion Nurses Society (INS). (2011a). Infusion nursing standards of practice. *Journal of Infusion Nursing, 34*(IS), S77-S79.

INS. (2011b). *Policies and procedures for infusion nursing* (4th ed.). Norwood MA: Author.

Massorli, S. (2007). Nerve injuries related to vascular access insertion and assessment. *Journal of Infusion Nursing, 30*(6), 346-350.

McCall, R. E., & Tankersley, C. M. (2012). *Phlebotomy essentials* (5th ed.). Philadelphia: Lippincott Williams & Wilkins.

Moorhead, S., Johnson, M., Maas, M., & Swanson, E. (2013). *Nursing outcomes classification (NOC)* (5th ed.). St. Louis, MO: Mosby Elsevier.

Occupational Safety and Health Administration (OSHA). (2003). Disposal of contaminated needles and blood tube holders used for phlebotomy. Safety and Health Information Bulletin. Retrieved from www.osha.gov/dts/shib/shib101503.html (Accessed December 12, 2012).

The Joint Commission (TJC). (2013). National patient safety goals. Retrieved from www.jointcommission.org/standard-information/npsgs.aspx (Accessed September 26, 2013).

Van Leeuwen, A. M., Poelhuis-Leth, D. J., & Bladh, M. L. (2012). *Davis's comprehensive handbook of laboratory and diagnostic tests with nursing implications* (5th ed.). Philadelphia: F. A. Davis.

PROCEDURES DISPLAY 7-1

Collection of Blood in Evacuated Tube System

Equipment Needed
Gloves, nonsterile
Tourniquet
Sharps container
Waste receptacle
Collection vials or tubes
Vacutainer tube holder
Evacuated tube system (ETS) needle
Labels (barcoded) for tubes
Transport container
Site disinfectant (70% alcohol, chlorhexidine gluconate, or povidone-iodine)
Gauze pads or cotton ball
Tape

Delegation
This procedure can be delegated to a phlebotomist.

Procedure	Rationale
1. Review the test request.	1. A test request is reviewed for completeness, date and time of collection, status, and priority. A written order is a legal requirement for blood analysis.
2. Approach, identify, and prepare the patient. Introduce yourself to the patient. Use two identifiers to verify patient identity. Place the patient in a position of comfort and safety, arm extended and in a dependent position if possible if in a hospital bed. Use a drawing chair in outpatient setting. Explain the procedure to the patient. Verify diet restrictions and latex sensitivity.	2. Establishes the nurse–patient relationship. The Joint Commission (2013) safety goal recommendation. Explaining the procedure reduces anxiety. Test results can be meaningless or misinterpreted and patient care compromised if diet requirements have not been followed. Exposure to latex can trigger a life-threatening reaction.

Continued

PROCEDURES DISPLAY 7-1

Collection of Blood in Evacuated Tube System—cont'd

Procedure

3. Arrange all supplies in an accessible place so that reaching for equipment is minimized. Line up tubes in the order of draw.

4. Hand hygiene procedure/ don gloves; use alcohol-based product.

5. Apply tourniquet 3–4 inches above intended site, locate the vein, usually the antecubital fossa, usually the median cubital. Release the tourniquet.

6. Cleanse the area with approved antiseptic, using a circular or back-and-forth technique. Allow the skin to air dry or blot with sterile gauze.

7. Select the appropriate equipment for the size, condition, and location of the vein. Prepare while the site is drying. Attach a needle to an ETS holder. Put the first tube in the holder at step 7 or wait until after needle entry (step 10).

8. Reapply the tourniquet.

9. Apply traction to the skin of the forearm, below the intended venipuncture site, to stabilize the vein. Hold the vacuum tube assembly between the thumb and last

Rationale

3. Having all equipment at hand will save time and lessen patient anxiety.

4. Good hand hygiene is the single most important means of preventing the spread of infection. According to OSHA, bloodborne pathogen (BBP) standard gloves must be worn.

5. A tourniquet placed 3–4 inches above the antecubital area dilates the veins and makes them easier to see, feel, and enter with a needle.

6. Avoids contaminating the specimen with bacteria picked up by the needle. Letting the site dry naturally permits maximum antiseptic action.

7. Ensures successful blood draw and accuracy of test results.

8. Allows for dilation of vein.

9. Anchors the skin so that the needle enters easily and with less pain; keeps vein from rolling.

PROCEDURES DISPLAY 7-1

Collection of Blood in Evacuated Tube System—cont'd

Procedure

Rationale

three fingers of your dominant hand. Rest the backs of these fingers on the patient's arm. The free index finger rests against the hub of the needle and serves as a guide. With the needle held at an angle of 15–30 degrees to the arm and in line with the vein, insert the needle into the vein, with the bevel up.

10. Once you feel that you are in the vein, change your grip: The hand that was stabilizing the vein in place should now hold the hub firmly, while the index and third finger of the dominant hand grip the tube. This will prevent movement of the needle. Now use your thumb to gently but firmly push the tube onto the needle. This will allow the vacuum to pull blood into the tube.

10. Blood will not flow until the needle pierces the tube stopper.

11. Fill the additive tubes until the vacuum is exhausted and mix them immediately on removal from the holder using 3–10 gentle inversions (depending on the type and manufacturer). Follow the order of draw. If more than one tube is to be drawn, pull the filled tube out of the hub very gently with the hand that pushed it in.

11. Ensures correct blood-to-additive ratio.

Continued

PROCEDURES DISPLAY 7-1

Collection of Blood in Evacuated Tube System—cont'd

Procedure	Rationale
12. When the last tube of blood is drawn, remove it from the hub. Release the tourniquet during filling of the last tube, then gently remove the needle from the arm and place a cotton ball or small gauze pad over the puncture site. Ask the patient to put pressure on the area if appropriate.	12. Prevents hematoma formation.
13. Activate the safety feature on the needle	13. OSHA standard
14. Label all samples at the bedside.	14. Prevents mislabeling errors.
15. Examine the patient's arm to verify bleeding has stopped on the skin surface. If bleeding has stopped, apply bandage and advise patient to keep it in place for a minimum of 15 minutes.	15. Prevents hematoma formation and bleeding.
16. Dispose of used and contaminated materials in biohazard container and sharps container.	16. OSHA requirement
17. Remove gloves and sanitize hands.	17. Removing gloves in an aseptic manner and washing or decontaminating hands are infection control precautions.
18. Transport specimen to the laboratory.	18. Prompt delivery to the laboratory protects specimen integrity.

Sources: INS (2011b); McCall & Tankersley (2012).

PROCEDURES DISPLAY 7-2

Collection of Blood Using a Winged or Butterfly Collection Set

Equipment Needed
Gloves, nonsterile
Tourniquet
Sharps container
Waste receptacle
Butterfly (winged) needle with safety feature
Evacuated tube system (ETS) tube holder
Blood collection tubes
Labels (barcoded) for tubes or permanent marking pen
Transport container
Site disinfectant (70% alcohol, chlorhexidine gluconate, or povidone-iodine)
Gauze pads or cotton ball
Tape

Delegation
This procedure can be delegated to a phlebotomist.

Procedure	Rationale
1. Review the test request.	1. A test request is reviewed for completeness, date and time of collection, status, and priority. A written order is a legal requirement for blood analysis.
2. Approach, identify, and prepare the patient. Introduce yourself to the patient. Use two identifiers to verify patient identity. Place the patient in a position of comfort and safety, arm extended and in a dependent position if possible if in hospital bed. Use a drawing chair in the outpatient setting.	2. Establishes the nurse–patient relationship. The Joint Commission (2013) safety goal recommendation. Explaining the procedure reduces anxiety. Test results can be meaningless or misinterpreted and patient care compromised if diet requirements have not been followed. Exposure to latex can trigger a life-threatening reaction.

Continued

PROCEDURES DISPLAY 7-2

Collection of Blood Using a Winged or Butterfly Collection Set—cont'd

Procedure	Rationale
Explain the procedure to the patient. Verify diet restrictions and latex sensitivity.	
3. Arrange all supplies in an accessible place so that reaching for equipment is minimized. Line up tubes in the order of draw.	3. Having all equipment at hand will save time and lessen patient anxiety.
4. Hand hygiene procedure/don gloves; use an alcohol-based product.	4. Good hand hygiene is the single most important means of preventing the spread of infection. According to OSHA, BBP standard gloves must be worn.
5. Apply tourniquet 3–4 inches above intended site, locate the vein, usually the median antecubital fossa. Release the tourniquet.	5. A tourniquet placed 3-4 inches above the antecubital area dilates veins and makes them easier to see, feel, and enter with a needle.
6. Cleanse the area with approved antiseptic, using a circular or back-and-forth technique. Allow the skin to air dry or blot with sterile gauze.	6. Avoids contaminating the specimen with bacteria picked up by the needle. Letting the site dry naturally permits maximum antiseptic action.
7. Select the appropriate equipment for the size, condition, and location of the vein. Prepare while the site is drying. Attach the butterfly to an ETS holder. Grasp the tubing near the needle end and run your fingers down its length, stretching it slightly to help keep it from coiling back up. Position the first tube in the holder now or wait until vein entry.	7. Ensures successful blood draw; first step in accuracy of test results.

PROCEDURES DISPLAY 7-2

Collection of Blood Using a Winged or Butterfly Collection Set—cont'd

Procedure	Rationale
8. Reapply the tourniquet.	8. Dilates vein
9. Apply traction to the skin of the forearm, below the intended venipuncture site, to stabilize the vein. Hold the wing portion of the butterfly between your thumb and index finger or fold the wings upright and grasp them together. Cradle the tubing and holder in the palm of your dominant hand or lay it next to the patient's hand. Uncap and inspect the needle for defects and discard if flawed.	9. Anchors the skin so that the needle enters easily and with less pain; keeps the vein from rolling.
10. Insert the needle into the vein at a shallow angle between 10 and 15 degrees. A flash or small amount of blood will appear in the tubing when the needle is in the vein. Slightly thread within the lumen of the vein.	10. Winged needles can pierce the vein, causing a hematoma. Thread the needle carefully in the vein. Flash of blood indicates vein entry.
11. Establish blood flow by placing the tube in the holder and pushing it part way onto the needle with a clockwise twist. Grasp the holder flange with your middle and index fingers, pulling back slightly to keep the holder from moving, and push the tube onto the needle with your thumb. Release the tourniquet.	11. Blood will not flow until the needle pierces a tube stopper. Release of tourniquet allows blood flow to normalize.

Continued

PROCEDURES DISPLAY 7-2

Collection of Blood Using a Winged or Butterfly Collection Set—cont'd

Procedure	Rationale
12. Maintain the tubing and holder below the site and positioned so that the tubes fill from the bottom up to prevent reflux. Fill additive tubes. Immediately upon removal use 3–10 gentle inversions (depending on type and manufacturer) to prevent clot formation. Follow CLSI order of draw.	**12.** Ensures correct blood-to-additive ratio.
13. Place a clean gauze over the site. Apply pressure after the needle is removed from the hub. Ask the patient to put pressure on the area if appropriate.	**13.** Prevents hematoma formation.
14. Activate the safety feature on the needle.	**14.** OSHA standard to prevent needlestick injuries.
15. Label all samples at the bedside.	**15.** Prevents mislabeling errors.
16. Examine the patient's arm to verify that bleeding on the skin surface has stopped. If bleeding has stopped, apply bandage and advise patient to keep it in place for a minimum of 15 minutes.	**16.** Prevents hematoma formation and bleeding.
17. Dispose of used and contaminated materials in a biohazard container and sharps container.	**17.** OSHA requirement
18. Remove gloves; sanitize hands using alcohol-based product for 15 seconds.	**18.** Removing gloves in an aseptic manner and washing or decontaminating hands are infection control precautions.

PROCEDURES DISPLAY 7-2

Collection of Blood Using a Winged or Butterfly Collection Set—cont'd

Procedure	Rationale
19. Transport the specimen to the laboratory.	19. Prompt delivery to the laboratory protects specimen integrity.

Sources: INS (2011b); McCall & Tankersley (2012).

PROCEDURES DISPLAY 7-3

Collection of Blood Using the Syringe Method

Equipment Needed
Gloves, nonsterile
Tourniquet
Sharps container
Waste receptacle
Syringe
Syringe needle
Evacuated tube system (ETS) tubes
Labels (barcoded) for tubes or permanent marking pen
Transport container
Site disinfectant (70% alcohol, chlorhexidine gluconate, or povidone-iodine)
Gauze pads
Tape

Delegation
This procedure can be delegated to a phlebotomist.

Procedure	Rationale
1. Review the test request.	1. A test request is reviewed for completeness, date and time of collection, status, and priority. A written order is a legal requirement for blood analysis.

Continued

PROCEDURES DISPLAY 7-3

Collection of Blood Using the Syringe Method—cont'd

Procedure	Rationale
2. Approach, identify, and prepare the patient. Introduce yourself to the patient. Use two identifiers to verify patient identity. Place the patient in a position of comfort and safety, arm extended and in a dependent position if possible if in hospital bed. Use a drawing chair in an outpatient setting. Explain the procedure to the patient. Verify diet restrictions and latex sensitivity.	2. Establishes the nurse–patient relationship. The Joint Commission (2013) safety goal recommendation. Explaining the procedure reduces anxiety. Test results can be meaningless or misinterpreted and patient care compromised if diet requirements have not been followed. Exposure to latex can trigger a life-threatening reaction.
3. Arrange all supplies in an accessible place so that reaching for equipment is minimized. Line up tubes in the order of draw.	3. Having all equipment at hand will save time and lessen patient anxiety.
4. Hand hygiene procedure/don gloves; use an alcohol-based product.	4. Good hand hygiene is the single most important means of preventing the spread of infection. According to OSHA, BBP standard gloves must be worn.
5. Apply the tourniquet 3–4 inches above intended site, locate the vein, and release tourniquet. *Note:* The vein used most frequently is the median antecubital fossa.	5. A tourniquet placed 3–4 inches above the antecubital area; it dilates the veins and makes them easier to see, feel, and enter with a needle.
6. Cleanse the area with approved antiseptic using a circular or back-and-forth technique. Allow the skin to air dry or blot with sterile gauze.	6. Avoids contaminating the specimen with bacteria picked up by the needle. Letting the site dry naturally permits maximum antiseptic action.

PROCEDURES DISPLAY 7-3

Collection of Blood Using the Syringe Method—cont'd

Procedure	Rationale
7. Select the appropriate equipment for the size, condition, and location of the vein. Prepare while site is drying. Select a syringe needle according to the size and location of the vein; select the appropriate size syringe and tube size. Attach the needle to the syringe; do not remove the cap at this time. Hold the syringe as you would an ETS tube holder.	7. Ensures accuracy of test results. First step in accuracy of test results.
8. Reapply the tourniquet.	8. A tourniquet aids in dilation of vein.
9. Apply traction to the skin of the forearm, below the intended venipuncture site, to stabilize the vein. Hold the syringe in your dominant hand as you would an ETS holder. Place your thumb on top near the needle end and fingers underneath. Uncap and inspect the needle for defects and discard if flawed.	9. Facilitates venipuncture and placement of the needle correctly in the vein.
10. Ask the patient to make a fist, line the needle up with the vein, and insert it into the skin using a smooth forward motion. Stop when you feel a decrease in resistance, often described as a "pop," and press your fingers into the arm to anchor the holder.	10. Anchoring stretches the skin so that the needle enters smoothly with less pain.

Continued

PROCEDURES DISPLAY 7-3

Collection of Blood Using the Syringe Method—cont'd

Procedure

11. Establishment of blood flow is normally indicated by blood in the hub of the syringe. Release the tourniquet and have the patient open his or her fist.

12. Fill the syringe.

13. Place a folded gauze square over the site or cotton ball and apply pressure immediately after the needle is removed.

14. Discard the needle, fill the tubes, discard the syringe, and add the transfer device. An ETS tube is placed in the transfer device in the order of draw and pushed onto the internal needle until the stopper is pierced. Blood from the syringe is then safely drawn into the tube. Several tubes can be filled as long as there is enough blood in the syringe.

Rationale

11. Allows blood flow to return to normal and helps prevent hemoconcentration. (According to CLSI Standard H3-A5, the tourniquet should be released as soon as possible after blood begins to flow and should not be left on longer than 1 minute.)

12. Venous blood will not automatically flow into a syringe. It must be filled by slowly pulling back on the plunger with your free hand.

13. Prevents damage to vein and hematoma formation.

14. The needle must be removed and discarded in a sharps container so that a transfer device for filling the tubes can be attached to the syringe. A transfer device greatly reduces the chance of accidental needlesticks and confines any aerosol or spraying that may be generated as the tube is removed.

PROCEDURES DISPLAY 7-3

Collection of Blood Using the Syringe Method—cont'd

Procedure	Rationale
15. After use, discard the syringe and transfer device unit in a sharps container.	15. OSHA standard to prevent needlestick injuries.
16. Label all samples at the bedside.	16. Prevents mislabeling errors.
17. Examine the patient's arm to verify bleeding has stopped on the skin surface. If bleeding has stopped, apply bandage and advise the patient to keep it in place for a minimum of 15 minutes.	17. Prevents hematoma formation and bleeding.
18. Dispose of used and contaminated materials in a biohazard container and sharps container.	18. OSHA requirement
19. Remove gloves and sanitize hands.	19. Removing gloves in an aseptic manner and washing or decontaminating hands are infection control precautions.
20. Transport the specimen to the laboratory.	20. Prompt delivery to the laboratory protects specimen integrity.

Sources: INS (2011b); McCall & Tankersley (2012).

Chapter **8**

Techniques for Initiation and Maintenance of Central Vascular Access

Never keep a patient a day longer in hospital than absolutely necessary.
—*Florence Nightingale, 1863*

LEARNING OBJECTIVES *On completion of this chapter, the reader will be able to:*

1. Define terms related to central vascular access devices (CVAD).
2. Compare and contrast advantages and disadvantages of different types of CVADs.
3. Discuss risks and benefits of CVADs.
4. Identify tip location for a properly placed CVAD.
5. Discuss evidence-based practices related to care and maintenance of CVADs.
6. Describe options in the types of dressings used in protecting the CVAD site.
7. Discuss aspects of CVAD care and maintenance aimed at reducing risk for bloodstream infection.
8. Discuss advantages and disadvantages of withdrawing blood for laboratory studies via a CVAD.

GLOSSARY

Anthropometric measurement Measurement of the size, weight, and proportions of the human body

Biocompatibility The quality of not having a toxic or injurious effect on biological systems

Central vascular access device (CVAD) Catheter inserted into the central circulation for infusion therapy, the tip located in the lower $1/3$ of the superior vena cava. CVADs are commonly referred to as "central lines."

Distal   Farthest from the heart; farthest from the point of attachment; below previous site of cannulation

External jugular   Peripheral vein located on the exterior aspect of the neck

Implanted vascular access port   A type of CVAD; surgically placed and consisting of a catheter attached to a reservoir (port) and placed completely underneath the skin and accessed using a noncoring needle

Lymphedema   Swelling of an extremity caused by obstruction of lymphatic vessels

Nontunneled central vascular access device   A short-term type of CVAD that is inserted directly through the skin, usually via the subclavian or internal jugular vein

Peripherally inserted central catheter (PICC)   A type of CVAD; catheter inserted above the antecubital fossa and threaded into the superior vena cava via the cephalic, basilic, or median veins

Polyurethane   Medical-grade resins, widely varying in flexibility, used in chemical-resistant coatings and adhesives for making catheters for venous access

Port, distal   Catheter lumen opening located farther from the catheter tip. **Proximal**   Lumen opening closest to catheter tip.

Silicone elastomer   A polymer of organic silicone oxides, which may be a liquid, gel, or solid depending on the extent of polymerization; used in surgical implants, a coating on the inside of glass vessels for blood collection. Some VADs are made of silicone elastomer.

Trendelenburg position   in which the head is lower than the feet; used to increase venous distention

Subcutaneously tunneled catheter   A CVAD that is surgically placed and tunneled in the subcutaneous tissue between the entrance and exit sites. A synthetic cuff attached to the catheter lies in the subcutaneous tissue along the tunnel tract.

Valsalva maneuver   The process of making a forceful attempt at expiration with the mouth, nostrils, and glottis closed

Vascular access device (VAD)   Access device inserted into a main vein or artery, or bone marrow; used primarily to administer fluids and medication, monitor pressure, and collect blood

■ General Overview of Central Vascular Access Devices

The first step in provision of infusion therapy is selection and placement of the best type of **vascular access device (VAD)** to meet the patient's needs. A variety of factors guide the decision-making process, such as the characteristics of the prescribed infusate, expected duration of treatment, integrity of the patient's veins, and patient preference. As discussed in Chapter 6, the peripheral I.V. catheter is often the first choice for short-term (i.e., usually less than 1 week) infusion needs. A midline peripheral I.V. catheter might be best if therapy is anticipated to last between 1 and 4 weeks. A peripheral I.V. catheter is associated with fewer risks and complications compared to a **central vascular access device (CVAD)**. However, characteristics of the infusate (e.g., acidic or alkaline pH, hyperosmolar solution) or other patient factors may make a peripheral catheter an inappropriate choice, even if short-term infusion therapy is planned. A CVAD then becomes the necessary choice. Specific guidelines indicating need for a CVAD rather than peripheral I.V. catheters include:

- Medications or solutions with osmolarity greater than 600 mOsm/L
- Parenteral nutrition (PN) formulations with dextrose concentration greater than 10%
- Medications or solutions with pH less than 4 or greater than 9
- Vesicant infusions
- Prolonged duration of therapy (more than 6 days) when a midline catheter is not an appropriate choice (Infusion Nurses Society [INS], 2011a).

A CVAD is defined by placement of the catheter tip in the central vasculature, specifically located in the lower superior vena cava (SVC), near its junction with the right atrium (INS, 2011a, p. S45). Of note, CVADs are commonly called "central lines" or "central venous catheters."

The goal of VAD selection and placement should be to deliver safe, efficient therapy that maximizes the patient's quality of life, with minimal risk of complications. Once the decision is made to place a CVAD, there remain more choices. There are four main types of CVADs:

1. The **nontunneled CVAD** is a percutaneously placed catheter that is usually placed by way of the subclavian or internal jugular vein. This type of CVAD is indicated for short-term needs and used primarily in the acute care setting.
2. The **peripherally inserted central catheter (PICC)** is the most common type of CVAD used in all settings, including acute care, long-term care, outpatient, and home care. The PICC may be placed for short-term or longer-term (generally less than 1 year) infusion therapy needs.
3. The **subcutaneously tunneled catheter** is a surgically placed CVAD that is indicated for long-term infusion needs, such as chemotherapy administration or PN.
4. The **implanted vascular access port** is also a surgically placed CVAD consisting of a catheter attached to a reservoir ("port"). It is placed completely underneath the skin.

In this chapter, anatomy related to CVAD placement, appropriate device selection, and care and maintenance are explored.

▪ Anatomy of the Vascular System

The anatomy and physiology of the upper extremity venous system, arm, and axilla are important for the infusion nurse to understand before placement of a CVAD. Important veins to central vascular access include the basilic, cephalic, axillary, subclavian, internal and **external jugular**, right and left innominate (brachiocephalic) veins, and SVC.

Venous Structures of the Arm

The superficial veins of the upper extremities lie in the superficial fascia; they are visible and palpable. Superficial veins include the cephalic and the basilic veins, which originate from the dorsal venous network on the back of the hand. In the antecubital fossa, the cephalic and basilic veins are connected by the median cubital vein.

The cephalic vein ascends along the outer border of the biceps muscle to the upper third of the arm. It passes in the space between the pectoralis major and deltoid muscles and the clavicle. In this area of depression, the vein passes into the axilla by penetrating the deep fascia inferior to the clavicle. Normally, the cephalic vein turns sharply (90 degrees) as it pierces the clavipectoral fascia and passes beneath the clavicle. Near its termination, the cephalic vein may bifurcate into two small veins, one joining the external jugular vein and one joining the axillary vein. Valves are located along the course of the cephalic vein (Drake, Vogl, & Mitchell, 2010).

The basilic vein is larger than the cephalic vein. From the posterior–medial aspect of the forearm, it passes upward in a smooth path along the inner side of the biceps muscle and then becomes the axillary vein. The origins of these veins in the lower arm are most often used for short-term peripheral devices. Above the antecubital fossa, these veins are appropriate for the placement of PICCs and peripherally implanted ports.

Valves are present in the venous system until approximately 1 inch before the formation of the brachiocephalic vein. The presence of valves within veins helps to prevent the reflux of blood and is especially important in the lower extremities, where venous return is working against gravity (Fig. 8-1).

Venous Structures of the Chest

The main venous structures of the chest include the subclavian, internal and external jugular, and brachiocephalic veins (formerly called the innominate veins), and the SVC. Large veins in the head, neck, and chest do not have valves. Gravity helps blood to flow properly from the head and neck, and negative intrathoracic pressure promotes flow from the head, neck, and inferior vena cava.

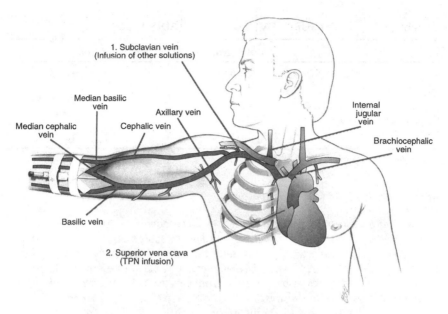

1. Subclavian vein
(Infusion of other solutions)

Median basilic
vein

Axillary vein

Internal
jugular
vein

Median cephalic
vein

Cephalic vein

Brachiocephalic
vein

Basilic vein

2. Superior vena cava
(TPN infusion)

Figure 8-1 ▪ Veins of the arm and chest. (Courtesy of Medivisuals, Dallas, TX.)

The subclavian vein extends from the outer border of the first rib to the sternal end of the clavicle and measures about 4 to 5 cm in length. The right brachiocephalic vein measures about 2.5 cm, and the left brachiocephalic vein measures about 6 to 6.5 cm. The external jugular lies on the side of the neck and follows a descending inward path to join the subclavian vein along the middle of the clavicle. The internal jugular vein descends first behind and then to the outer side of the internal and common carotid arteries; it joins the subclavian vein at the root of the neck.

The right brachiocephalic (innominate) vein is about 1 inch long and passes almost vertically downward to join the left brachiocephalic (innominate) vein just below the cartilage of the first rib. The left brachiocephalic vein is about 2.5 inches long and is larger than the right vein. It passes from left to right in a downward slant across the upper front of the chest. It joins the right brachiocephalic vein to form the SVC. The SVC receives all blood from the upper half of the body. It is composed of a short trunk 2.5 to 3.0 inches long in an average adult. It begins below the first rib close to the sternum on the right side, descends vertically slightly to the right, and empties into the right atrium of the heart. The right atrium receives blood from the upper body via the SVC and from the lower body via the inferior vena cava. The venae cavae are referred to as the great veins. Table 8-1 summarizes the **anthropometric measurements** of the upper extremity veins.

> Table 8-1	MEASUREMENTS OF VEINS (ADULT)	
Vein	**Length (cm)**	**Diameter (mm)**
Cephalic	35–38	4-5
Basilic	24	8
Axillary	13	16
Subclavian	6	19
Right brachiocephalic	2.5	19
Superior vena cava	7–9	20

Source: Bullock-Corkhill (2010).

 NURSING FAST FACT!

> *Blood flow in the SVC in the average adult is approximately 1.5 to 2.5 L/min. Poiseuille's law (fourth power law) states that flow through a single vessel is most affected by the vessel diameter, and as vessel diameter increases, the flow rate increases by a factor of 4. For example, when the diameter doubles, flow rate increases 16 times; when the diameter increases by 4, the flow rate increases 256 times. The amount of blood flow in the veins follows this law:*
> *Cephalic and basilic veins: 45–95 mL/min*
> *Subclavian veins: 150–300 mL/min*
> *SVC: 2000 mL/min*

■ Assessment and Device Selection

When the decision is made to place a CVAD, a number of factors are considered when selecting the most appropriate type of CVAD. Factors include the type of prescribed therapy, anticipated duration of treatment, vascular integrity, patient preferences, and ability and resources available to care for the device (INS, 2011a, p. S37). Using a VAD selection algorithm along with a thorough patient assessment can help with device selection (Fig. 8-2).

The various features of CVADs were discussed in Chapter 5. A CVAD with the least number of lumens should be selected for the patient's infusion therapy. There is more manipulation and catheter access with multilumen catheters, which increases the risk for bloodstream infection. However, patients who require multiple medications and fluids, such as the critically ill, will likely need a multilumen catheter. Patients who require ongoing testing involving contrast media (i.e., computed tomographic [CT] scans) may benefit from a power injectable CVAD, which can tolerate the high pressures required for rapid injection of contrast material. Antimicrobial impregnated CVADs are used routinely by some organizations as an infection prevention measure.

Physical factors considered during assessment including the suitability of target vessels in terms of size and patency, presence of other devices,

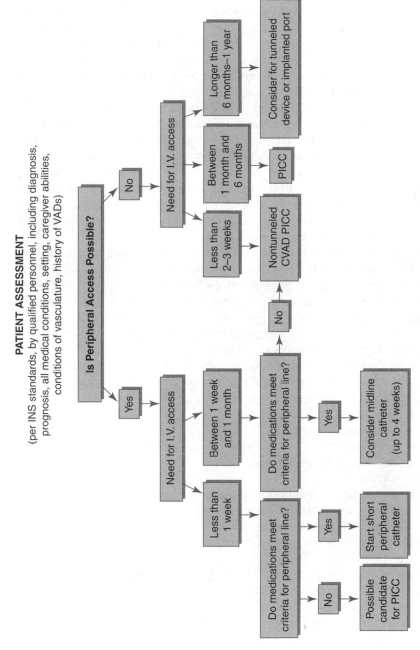

PATIENT ASSESSMENT
(per INS standards, by qualified personnel, including diagnosis, prognosis, all medical conditions, setting, caregiver abilities, conditions of vasculature, history of VADs)

Is Peripheral Access Possible?

Medication criteria: Final osmolarity < 600 mOsm/L, pH between 5.0 and 9.0, non-vesicant.

Figure 8-2 ■ Venous access device selection algorithm.

and inspection of skin for breaks in integrity. The vein must be large enough to accommodate the selected VAD to minimize the risk of phlebitis and thrombosis. The smallest device in the largest vein allows for better hemodilution of the infusate and better blood flow around the catheter. The presence of a pacemaker requires special consideration. Pacemakers are usually placed on the left side of the chest or abdomen, and, when present, the opposite side is preferred for CVAD placement. If a CVAD must be placed on the same side as the pacemaker, a PICC is a better and safer choice (INS, 2011a, p. S45).

Patient preference and lifestyle should be evaluated. This is especially important when the intended infusion therapy will extend beyond the acute care setting and the patient will be sent home with the CVAD in place. For PICCs, placement in the nondominant arm should be considered. The patient's lifestyle is an important consideration in choosing an implanted versus an external device. Take into consideration activity restrictions, maintenance requirements, body image distortion, and ease of use. The patient's usual occupational and recreational activities need to be included in the assessment process.

The ability of the patient or designated caregiver to manage day-to-day CVAD care and infusions should be assessed before device selection and placement. Important considerations include the ability to see, hear, perform fine motor tasks, read and understand written instructions, and emotionally cope with the demands of site care and therapy. In addition, the home environment and caregiver support for patients who will transition from acute care to home care should be evaluated.

The nursing process related to assessment for CVAD placement, communication of the plan, and ongoing monitoring and evaluation includes:

- Systematic assessment of:
  - Patient health problems
  - Previous I.V. complications
  - Purpose, nature, and duration of I.V. therapy
  - Patient needs/preferences
- Planning
  - Discussion of recommendations and plan with patient and family
  - Discussion of multidisciplinary plan
- Evidence of communication of decision to health-care team
- Evidence of ongoing assessment of the CVAD site, patency, and need for catheter
- Assessment for potential complications and assessment of response to the infusion therapy, including evidence of side effects/adverse reactions and actions taken

Therapeutic indications for CVAD placement include:

- Administration of chemotherapy
- Administration of PN
- Administration of blood products

- Administration of medications
- Intravenous fluid administration
- Monitoring of central venous pressure (CVP)
- Performance of plasmapheresis
- Performance of hemodialysis

Conditions that Limit Central Vascular Access Device Placement

Clinical conditions such as coagulopathy, venous stenosis, acute thrombosis, and local skin infection at the insertion site are factors that may affect the decision-making process as to the best CVAD option. For example, a PICC may be the best choice for patients with bleeding disorders. Any abnormalities should be considered as part of the risk-to-benefit ratio prior to CVAD placement. Conditions that may limit VAD site placement are listed in Table 8-2.

> Table 8-2	CONDITIONS AFFECTING VASCULAR ACCESS DEVICE SITE PLACEMENT
Previous Surgical Interventions	Lymph node dissections Subclavian vein stenting or resection Vena cava filters Myocutaneous flap reconstruction Skin grafts Previous vein harvesting Presence of arteriovenous (A-V) grafts and hemodialysis fistulas Presence of intravascular stents
Cutaneous Lesions in Proximity to VAD Exit or Puncture Site	Herpes zoster and skin tears Malignant cutaneous lesions Bacterial or fungal lesions and nonintact skin Burns Extensive scarring or keloids
Disease Process or Conditions	Severe thrombocytopenia (<50,000 platelets) Other coagulopathy (e.g., hemophilia, idiopathic thrombocytopenia purpura) Concurrent anticoagulation therapy Lymphedema Allergies Extremity paraplegia Pre-existing vessel thrombosis or stenosis
Other Considerations	Site within current radiation port Devices near exit site (e.g., tracheostomy) Morbid obesity Patient inability to position desired site for placement Patient inability to tolerate insertion procedure

Catheter Materials

Most CVADs are made of thermoplastic urethane (**polyurethane**) or **silicone elastomers**. There is also the emergence of newer catheter materials, which reduce the risk of thrombus formation. Important characteristics of CVADs include biocompatibility and tensile strength. Catheters must be very strong yet remain soft and pliable while they are indwelling. Tensile strength is measured in pounds of force per square inch (psi) and allows the material to resist breaking under high loads. Ultimate elongation is usually measured as the relative change in length of a catheter that has been placed under load, to the breaking point. Catheters possessing elongation psi of 400% to 700% usually are very pliable, making them ideal for vascular placement. Less pliable catheters are easier to insert; however, they can create intravascular irritation leading to phlebitis.

All catheters, whether they are used for short- or long-term access, should be radiopaque, which allows for location of the catheter/fragment in the event of a catheter fracture or embolus. All catheter material is tested for **biocompatibility**, which includes cytotoxicity, risk of allergic reactions, hemocompatibility, potential for causing inflammation, and other toxicities (Hadaway, 2010).

Polyurethane

Polyurethane catheters are the most commonly used catheters because of the material's versatility, malleability (i.e., tensile strength and elongation characteristics), and biocompatibility. Polyurethane is composed of alternating groups of soft segments and hard segments that provide the strength and flexibility needed for a catheter (Hadaway, 2010). Polyurethane catheters do not have any plasticizers or other harmful additives that can be readily extracted. Because of their tensile strength, catheters made of polyurethane can be made with thinner walls and larger internal catheter lumen diameters, which allow for greater blood flow. Polyurethane is stiffer than silicone, which makes threading of the catheter easier, yet once inside of the body, it becomes softer and more flexible, which reduces irritation to the intimal layer of the vein.

An important potential problem with polyurethane catheters is that when they are exposed to alcohol, the alcohol can act as a solvent. The concern is with the increasingly more common use of ethanol (instead of heparin) locks to reduce risk of bloodstream infections (discussed in Chapter 12). Clinical data addressing the effect of ethanol on polyurethane is conflicting (Maiefski, Rupp, & Hermsen, 2009). The manufacturers' instructions for use should always be reviewed and followed.

Silicone Elastomers

Silicone elastomer materials used for catheters are soft and pliable and cannot be inserted by the conventional over-the-needle technique. They are inserted through an introducer (Hadaway, 2010). Because of its soft, flexible nature, silicone is less likely to damage the intima of the vein wall and is reported to cause less fibrin adherence and thus decrease the risk of thrombosis or occlusion. Subcutaneously tunneled catheters, implanted ports, and some PICCs are made of this biocompatible material. The catheter walls are thicker to achieve adequate strength as a CVAD. Silicone catheters are not affected by alcohol, and ethanol locks have been efficacious in infection prevention in these catheters (Maiefski et al., 2009).

Antimicrobial Catheters

Certain catheters are coated or impregnated with antimicrobial or antiseptic agents, which decrease the risk for catheter-associated bloodstream infection. The coated catheters currently available include:

- Chlorhexidine/silver sulfadiazine: A combination of chlorhexidine/ silver sulfadiazine on the external luminal surface, and a second-generation catheter with a coating on the internal surface extending into the extension set and hubs
- Minocycline/rifampin: Impregnated catheter on both the external and internal surfaces
- Platinum/silver: Because of studies showing no difference between this and nonimpregnated catheters, no current recommendations can be made according to the Centers for Disease Control and Prevention (CDC) (O'Grady et al., 2011).

NOTE > Most of the studies involving antimicrobial-/antiseptic-impregnated catheters have been conducted using triple-lumen, noncuffed catheters in place less than 30 days in adults. All catheters that are impregnated currently are approved by the Food and Drug Administration (FDA) for patients weighing more than 3 kg (O'Grady et al., 2011).

NOTE > Potential development of resistant organisms is a concern with these catheters.

CDC Guideline: Use a chlorhexidine/silver sulfadiazine or minocycline/ rifampin–impregnated CVAD in patients whose catheter is expected to remain in place >5 days if, after successful implementation of a comprehensive strategy to reduce rates of central-line associated bloodstream infections (CLABSIs), the CLABSI rate is not decreasing (O'Grady et al., 2011).

Catheter Valves

Some CVADs have built-in catheter valves that reduce the risk for blood reflux into the catheter and thus reduce the risk for catheter occlusion. The first valved catheter, which was developed in the 1980s, has a valve located on the catheter wall near the catheter tip. The catheter tip is closed and the valve opens during infusion and during aspiration. There are also catheters with valves located inside the catheter hub (Fig. 8-3). In terms of catheter care, valved catheters can be locked with 0.9% sodium chloride rather than heparin according to the manufacturer's instructions for use.

Multilumen Central Vascular Access Devices

Catheters are available with single, double, triple, and quadruple lumens. The diameter of each lumen varies, allowing for the administration of hypertonic or viscous solutions. The lumens are available in several sizes. The lumens of the catheter may have staggered locations near the catheter tip, or they may exit at the same place at the end of the catheter tip (Figs. 8-4, 8-5b). With staggered locations, the lumens will be labeled, for example, proximal, **distal**, and medial lumen (see Fig. 8-5). Because blood flow in the SVC is great (about 2000 mL/min), the likelihood of incompatible fluids administered simultaneously via a multilumen catheter mixing and precipitating is not likely. It is important to refer to each particular manufacturer's

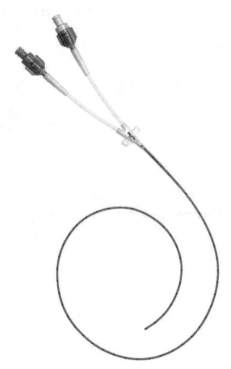

Figure 8-3 ▪ BioFlo PICC made of a thromboresistant material that is blended into the polyurethane and resistant to accumulation of blood. Also contains a valve located in the catheter hub. (Courtesy of Angiodynamics, Marlborough, MA.)

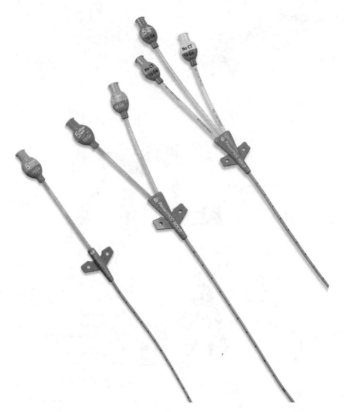

Figure 8-4 ■ Power PICC Solo*2 catheters, single, double, and triple lumen; valve located in catheter hub. (©2013 C. R. Bard, Inc. Used with permission.)

information to ascertain which of their lumens is the largest if rapid administration is needed. Multiple-lumen CVADs allow for a dedicated port for blood sampling. Example of lumen sizes and indications for a four-lumen nontunneled CVAD are as follows:

- **Distal port 16 gauge**: CVP monitoring and high-volume or viscous fluids, colloids, medications (distal port is the largest lumen), administration of blood or CVP monitor
- **Medial port 18 gauge**: Reserved for PN; medication only if PN not ordered
- **Proximal port 18 gauge**: Blood sampling, medications, or blood component administration
- **Fourth port 18 gauge**: Infusion of fluids or medications

Catheter Gauge

The outer diameter of a catheter is usually used to indicate catheter size. French size is calculated by multiplying the outer diameter in millimeters

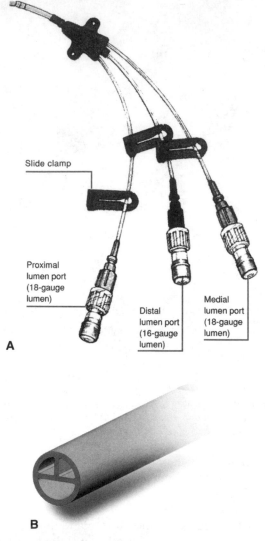

Slide clamp

Proximal
lumen port
(18-gauge
lumen)

Distal
lumen port
(16-gauge
lumen)

Medial
lumen port
(18-gauge
lumen)

A

B

Figure 8-5 ■ *A,* Injection ports of the triple-lumen catheter include the proximal lumen port, distal lumen port, and medial lumen port. The distal port (middle line) is usually the largest of the three lines. *B,* Cross section of a triple-lumen catheter without staggered openings. (©2013 C. R. Bard, Inc. Used with permission.)

times three. Gauge size is most often used for short peripheral catheters, lumen sizes for multilumen catheters, and introducers. Gauge and French sizes do not evenly convert. The gauge of a catheter influences flow rate. Silicone catheters tend to be smaller gauge than those made of polyurethane and have slower flow rates. Gauge depends in part on the type of material from which the catheter is made. The sizes of PICCs range from 1.1 French (neonate) to 7 French. Nontunneled catheters are available in sizes from 5 to 12 French.

It is very important to consider catheter size in relation to the blood vessel that will be cannulated. The catheter selected should be of the smallest gauge and length needed to accommodate the prescribed therapy (INS, 2011a, p. S37). Large-gauge catheters take up more space in the vein. Presence of the catheter in the vein decreases blood flow and can potentially create venous stasis and lead to catheter-associated venous thrombosis, a complication more common than infections. Larger catheters are associated with increased risk for this complication (see Chapter 9). In an experimental study, researchers demonstrated that fluid flow is dramatically decreased by insertion of a centrally located obstruction (i.e., a catheter). Assuming that blood flow behaves in a similar way to that shown in experimental models, PICCs in particular may substantially decrease venous flow rates by as much as 93% (Nifong & McDevitt, 2011)! The researchers state that choosing the smallest catheter size is probably a controllable risk factor for catheter-associated venous thrombosis.

 NURSING FAST FACT!

> *Equivalent gauge and French sizes of common central venous catheters are as follows:*
>   *23 ga = 1.9 Fr*
>   *20 ga = 2.7 Fr*
>   *18 ga = 3.8 Fr*
>   *16 ga = 5.0 Fr*
>   *14 ga = 6.3 Fr*
> *Information about the flow rates for catheters can be found in the manufacturer's specifications.*

Power Injectable Central Vascular Access Devices

Power injectable catheters can tolerate the high pressures required for rapid injections of contrast materials used in radiological studies such as CT scans. There are power injectable catheters for all categories of CVADs, including implanted vascular access ports. These types of CVADs are commonly used by acute care organizations. From a general care and management standpoint, care of a power injectable CVAD is the same as for a nonpower catheter. However, there may be potential confusion and risk if a nonpower injectable catheter is used for that purpose, thus increasing the risk of catheter rupture. When planning to use a CVAD for power injection, power injection capability should be identified at the time of access and immediately prior to power injection. This is particularly important with implanted ports because there is no reliable external method to determine the type of port. Some power injection–capable ports have unique characteristics that can be identified by palpation, but palpation should not be the only identification method used. It is recommended that at least two identification methods be used, including presence of identification cards, wristbands, or keychains provided by the manufacturer, review of operative procedure documentation, and palpation of the port (INS, 2011a, p. S50).

There is risk for serious injury when VADs not designed to tolerate high pressures are used for power injection of contrast media. The FDA (2013) has received over 250 adverse event reports in which VADs ruptured when used with power injectors to administer contrast media as part of CT or magnetic resonance imaging studies. Ruptured devices included CVADs, small-gauge peripheral catheters, implanted ports, extension tubing, and intravenous administration sets. Adverse events included device fragmentation, embolization or migration that required surgical intervention, extravasation of contrast media, loss of venous access requiring device replacement, and contamination of the room and personnel with blood and contrast media. Recommendations to prevent VAD rupture include the following:

1. Check the labeling of each VAD for its maximum pressure and flow rate. If none is provided, assume the device is NOT intended for power injection and do not use.
2. Know the pressure limit setting for the power injector and how to adjust it.
3. Ensure that the pressure limit set for the power injector does not exceed the maximum labeled pressure for the VAD (FDA, 2013).

Vascular Access Teams

Specially trained I.V. teams have demonstrated unequivocal effectiveness in reducing VAD-related infections associated with VADs (O'Grady, et al., 2011). Based on well-designed studies, the CDC strongly recommends the following:

■ Designate only trained personnel who demonstrate competence for the insertion and maintenance of peripheral and central intravascular catheters.
■ Educate health-care personnel regarding the indications for intravascular catheter use, proper procedures for the insertion and maintenance of intravascular catheters, and appropriate infection control measures to prevent intravascular catheter-related infections (O'Grady et al., 2011).

Furthermore, as part of the 2013 National Patient Safety Goals, The Joint Commission (2013) requires education about CVAD-related infections when personnel is hired, annually thereafter, and when involvement in such procedures is added to the clinician's responsibilities. The use of consistent, dedicated teams has improved patient safety, decreased multiple insertion attempts, and improved outcomes. Early vascular access is an important component of many teams' responsibilities and involves assessing the patient's needs for vascular access when he or she is admitted to the hospital. For example, the pain and potential complications caused by multiple attempts at short-term peripheral venous access are prevented when a CVAD is placed because it best met the patient's needs. In another example, inappropriate PICC placement was decreased when use of ultrasound for peripheral I.V. placement by a specially trained team of nurses resulted in a 20% decrease in the number of PICC line placements (Maiocco & Coole, 2012). Some teams perform all PICC insertions, conduct daily surveillance of each catheter and dressing, perform dressing changes, troubleshoot catheter problems, provide formal and informal staff education, and conduct outcome monitoring. Other teams may limit interventions to only CVAD placement while the general nursing staff performs care and management of the catheter. In a white paper, INS (Hadaway, Dalton, & Mercanti-Erieg, 2013) defines an infusion team as a group of nursing personnel centrally structured within an acute health facility charged with the shared mission of outcome accountability for the delivery of infusion therapy.

> EBP A hospital achieved 7 years of no PICC-associated bloodstream infections. This is attributed to a safety-first organizational culture and an innovative catheter bundle that not only addresses the central line insertion bundle but also focuses on postinsertion care and maintenance by a dedicated vascular access team (Harnage, 2012).

> EBP A group of clinical nurse specialists (CNSs) organized and implemented strategies beyond the central line bundle. The infection rate in the critical care unit (CCU) setting decreased from a high of 1.5 infections per 1000 catheter-days to zero for over 1 year (Richardson & Tjoelker, 2012).

> EBP In a study of nurse-led CVAD placement in three Australian hospitals, CVADs placed included PICCs, nontunneled CVADs, and dialysis catheters. There were minimal complications among the 760 catheters placed by the nurse teams. Insertion-related complications included one pneumothorax and one arterial puncture (Alexandrou et al., 2012).

◼ Nontunneled Central Vascular Access Devices and Peripherally Inserted Central Catheters

Nontunneled Catheters

The nontunneled CVAD is a short-term device intended to be used for several days and primarily placed and used in an acute care setting. These devices are available as single- or multiple-lumen (two-, three-, or four-lumen) catheters and are most often made of polyurethane.

The nontunneled catheter is usually placed at the bedside. It is inserted via the subclavian, internal jugular, or femoral veins. In fact, they are often referred to by their insertion site rather than the term nontunneled, for example, "subclavian line" or "jugular" or "IJ" (internal jugular). Site selection for nontunneled catheter placement is an important issue related to the risk for catheter-associated bloodstream infection. In fact, the density of skin flora at the catheter insertion site is a major risk factor for infection (O'Grady et al., 2011). The femoral site should be avoided because of its higher colonization rates and higher risk for catheter-associated venous thrombosis compared to the subclavian or internal jugular sites. Furthermore, the risk for infection related to femoral placement is increased in obese patients.

CDC Guideline: Use a subclavian site, rather than a jugular or a femoral site, in adult patients to minimize risk for nontunneled CVAD placement (O'Grady et al., 2011).

Patients with renal disease present with special issues. Because these patients may ultimately require long-term venous access for hemodialysis, vein preservation is critical. The preference for vascular access in this population is an arteriovenous fistula (American Nephrology Nurses Association, 2013). In contrast to the situation in the majority of patients, subclavian vein catheterization should be *avoided* in patients with renal disease (American Nephrology Nurses Association, 2009). Subclavian vein catheterization is associated with central venous stenosis, which may preclude the use of the entire ipsilateral arm for vascular access.

> **INS Standard** The nurse should be knowledgeable about vein preservation techniques for patients who are likely to need vascular access for hemodialysis (INS, 2011a, p. S51).

Insertion Issues

CVADs are usually inserted by a physician, but increasingly nurses with specialty training and education are also placing nontunneled CVADs. Strict technique is maintained during the procedure. The central line bundle (discussed in Chapter 2) is the standard of care for CVAD placement. It includes adherence to the following evidence-based actions during placement: hand hygiene, maximal sterile barrier precautions during insertion, chlorhexidine skin antisepsis, and avoidance of the femoral site. Adherence to the central line bundle along with the presence of an observer to ensure adherence to critical actions via a checklist during each insertion is one of the top 10 patient safety strategies strongly encouraged by the Agency for Healthcare Research and Quality (AHRQ, 2013). The CVAD placement procedure is stopped for any breaches in technique that occur (INS, 2011a, p. S45).

NURSING FAST FACT!

> *Maximal sterile barrier precautions require the inserter of the CVAD to wear a mask, cap, sterile gown, and sterile gloves. Furthermore, the patient is covered with a large, sterile drape (head-to-toe) during catheter placement.*

Use of Ultrasound Guidance

Ultrasound should be used during placement to identify blood vessels, increase success rates, and decrease insertion-related complications such as inadvertent puncture of an artery. Use of real-time ultrasound with CVAD placement is also one of the top 10 patient safety strategies (AHRQ, 2013).

Improvements in ultrasound portability and transducer ability have greatly enhanced its viability for VAD placement. Ultrasound guidance for CVAD insertion is being implemented at all levels of practice for both nurses and physicians and is now the standard of care for all CVAD placements, including PICCs (Fig. 8-6).

Catheter Placement

The patient is placed in the supine or **Trendelenburg position** with a rolled bath blanket or towel between his or her shoulders; such positioning reduces the risk of air embolism during the procedure. The patient may be instructed to perform a **Valsalva maneuver** during the venipuncture procedure to reduce the risk for air embolism. The nontunneled catheter is inserted via either of the following methods:

■ Modified Seldinger technique (MST): Using ultrasound to locate the vein, venipuncture is made using a metal finder needle; a guidewire is inserted several inches into the vein through the needle; the guidewire is secured to prevent embolism and the needle is removed; a dilator and introducer sheath is threaded over the

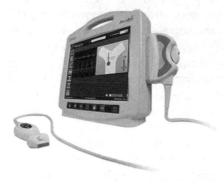

Figure 8-6 ■ SiteRite ultrasound system. (©2013 C. R. Bard, Inc. Used with permission.)

guidewire and advanced into the skin (the opening of the skin may be slightly enlarged with a scalpel to accommodate the dilator) and into the vein; the guidewire and dilator are removed; and the catheter is threaded into the introducer and advanced to the SVC. The sheath is then withdrawn, broken, and peeled apart (Bullock-Corkhill, 2010; Hadaway, 2010).

■ Seldinger technique: Similar to the MST using a metal finder needle and guidewire; however, the catheter is advanced over the guidewire and into the vein, and the guidewire is then removed from the catheter hub. A larger guidewire is required (completely different from one used for MST; guidewires are not interchangeable), and careful control is needed to prevent embolization of the guidewire (Hadaway, 2010).

Following placement, the catheter is secured, preferably using a stabilization device rather than sutures, and a sterile transparent dressing is placed over the site.

 NURSING FAST FACT!

After insertion of the catheter, final verification must be performed before any infusion. Chest x-ray confirmation is the most common method for verification and should occur before the administration of vesicant chemotherapy and whenever tip location is questioned. After placement, the catheter can be maintained as a closed patent device with a needleless connector and heparinized while the catheter tip location is verified by radiological examination.

Peripherally Inserted Central Catheters

The PICC is the most commonly placed CVAD. The increasing use of PICCs has been challenged in the literature, especially when used in hospitalized patients with difficult venous access (Chopra, Flanders, & Saint, 2012). PICCs are also associated with a higher risk of venous thrombosis compared to other types of CVADs (Chopra et al., 2013). (Catheter-associated venous thrombosis is addressed in Chapter 9). As with any CVAD, there are risks and complications, and the decision for placement should be based on clear need for the catheter. The least invasive device needed to accommodate and manage the infusion therapy should be selected (INS, 2011a).

PICCs are made of silicone elastomers or polyurethane, and they may have one, two, or three lumens. Dual-lumen PICCs are commonly inserted; they allow for administration of multiple medications. As with nontunneled catheters, PICCs are often placed at the bedside. The PICC is placed in an insertion site above the antecubital fossa and threaded to the central location in the SVC. Veins considered for cannulation via a PICC include the basilic, median cubital, cephalic, and brachial veins (see Fig. 8-1).The basilic vein is the most desirable because it is the largest vein and the pathway in the upper arm to the thorax is a direct route with less obstructions (Bullock-Corkhill, 2010). Veins considered for PICC placement in pediatric patients include the temporal vein and posterior auricular vein in the head; the saphenous veins of the legs may also be used (INS, 2011a, p. S41). Selection of the external jugular site for PICC placement is indicated for emergent access when other veins cannot be accessed. This site can be used for high-pressure injection through catheters rated for this use; and CVP monitoring may be performed through these catheters (INS, 2008a).

When assessing potential sites, areas to avoid include those with pain on palpation, compromised veins, the upper extremity on the side of previous axillary node dissection, after previous radiation therapy, if **lymphedema** is present, or the affected side after stroke (INS, 2011a). The risk for infection is increased when lymph nodes are removed. Recall from Chapter 2 that lymph fluid is filtered at the lymph nodes, which remove foreign material such as bacteria. Patients who have paralysis from strokes have increased risk for venous thrombosis because of venous stasis from lack of skeletal muscle compression (Nifong & McDevitt, 2011).

As with nontunneled CVADs placed via the subclavian vein, PICCs are not recommended for use in patients with chronic renal disease because of a high incidence of upper-extremity thrombosis (American Nephrology Nurses Association, 2009).

Insertion Issues

PICCs are frequently placed by specialized nurse teams who have completed education and demonstrated competency. Alternatively, in some organizations, PICCs are placed in the interventional radiology suite by radiologists. The central line bundle, as discussed earlier, is followed by PICC placement. PICCs should be inserted with ultrasound guidance, which allows visual inspection of the vasculature and assessment of the size and location of the vessel.

> **INS Standard** Ultrasound technology should be used when inserting PICC and percutaneous (nontunneled) CVADs to increase success rates and decrease insertion-related complications (INS, 2011a, p. S45).

Indications for Peripherally Inserted Central Catheter Use

PICCs are designed for delivery of infusion therapies extending beyond 6 days to several months, with some PICCs having been documented with a dwell time of more than 1 year.

PICCs may be indicated when pre-existing illness prevents the placement of a nontunneled CVAD (low platelet count, neutropenia, inability to tolerate Trendelenburg position for placement of the device).

Advantages

1. Peripheral insertion eliminates the potential complication of pneumothorax or hemothorax.
2. Decreased risk of air embolism because of the ease of maintaining the insertion site below the heart and a small diameter.
3. Decreased pain and discomfort associated with frequent venipunctures with peripheral I.V. catheter placement.
4. Is cost effective and time efficient.
5. Is appropriate for home I.V. therapy.
6. Appropriate for individuals of all ages.
7. May be used for laboratory draws.
8. Can be removed by a registered nurse (RN) who has been educated on the procedure.

Disadvantages/Risks

1. Daily or weekly care is required.
2. Consistent flushing after infusions and blood draws is necessary to prevent clotting of the catheter.
3. Difficulty in obtaining blood samples with small-lumen PICCs.
4. Contraindicated in patients whose lifestyles or occupations involve being in water; those with pre-existing skin infections in the arm; those with anatomic distortions related to injury, surgical dissection, or trauma; and those with coagulopathies.
5. Potential for CVAD-related complications such as catheter-associated venous thrombosis and catheter occlusion (see Chapter 9).

Catheter Placement

The patient is placed in the supine position for PICC placement. Most PICCs require premeasurement so that the PICC can be trimmed to the appropriate length needed to reach the SVC from the insertion site. Anthropometric measurements are used to calculate catheter length. A close estimation is achieved by measuring from the insertion site to the right sternal notch and then to the third intercostal space; this correlates with the distance from the insertion site to the SVC (Bullock-Corkhill, 2010). The most common insertion method used for PICC insertion is the MST described earlier.

Increasingly, technology systems that can locate the catheter tip immediately after insertion are being used. The use of electrocardiographic (ECG) tracing may be the most reliable way to accurately locate the catheter tip position. Simply described, this method involves placement of electrodes on the patient, a metal connection between the PICC and the ECG device, and monitoring of the ECG as the PICC is threaded through the veins. As the catheter tip passes the sinoatrial node, the P wave of the ECG increases in voltage and has an upward spike (Hadaway, 2010). Use of such technology may replace the need for chest x-ray film to verify catheter tip placement; however, the current gold standard for tip placement remains the chest radiography.

INS Standard Tip location of a CVAD shall be determined radiographically or by other approved technologies prior to initiation of infusion therapy (INS, 2011a, p. S44).

Catheter Removal

The CVAD should be removed when it is no longer needed. Because the very existence of the CVAD is a risk factor for catheter-associated bloodstream infection, daily review of catheter necessity and prompt removal when it is no longer needed is a component of the central line bundle. The risk of bloodstream infection is increased as catheter duration is extended. Catheter removal when it is no longer needed is equally applicable in other settings.

Nurses can remove nontunneled catheters and PICCs as long as there are organizational procedures in place. An order is always obtained. Potential complications associated with CVAD removal include air embolism, catheter embolism, and excessive bleeding. Minimize the risk of air embolism by positioning the patient in a supine position, and instruct the patient to perform the Valsalva maneuver while the catheter is being withdrawn. Digital pressure should be applied to the puncture site until hemostasis is achieved, and an occlusive dressing is always placed over the insertion site after removal. The recommended procedure is presented in Procedures Display 8-4 at the end of this chapter.

Particularly with PICCs, resistance during removal is also possible. When the PICC is pulled through the vein during removal, an irritation can cause a venospasm, often the cause of resistance during removal. A blood clot around the catheter and within the vein is a rare cause of removal resistance. Patient anxiety may contribute to the problem (Gorski, Perucca, & Hunter, 2010). It is important to never pull against resistance because catheter breakage and catheter embolism, or vein wall damage, can occur. If resistance is present, the following interventions may be helpful:

- Use of a warm compress to dilate the vein proximal to the exit site
- Use of relaxation techniques
- Hand and arm exercises
- Reattempt removal after a short or intermediate time period

Figure 8-7 shows an algorithm for a "stuck" PICC catheter. If such interventions do not work, the patient should be sent to the interventional radiology suite for evaluation and catheter removal. The following should be documented in relation to catheter removal:

- Catheter length and integrity
- Site appearance

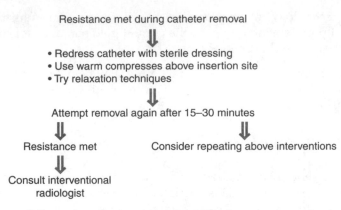

Resistance met during catheter removal

⇓

• Redress catheter with sterile dressing
• Use warm compresses above insertion site
• Try relaxation techniques

⇓

Attempt removal again after 15–30 minutes

⇓   ⇓

Resistance met   Consider repeating above interventions

⇓

Consult interventional
radiologist

Figure 8-7 ■ Algorithm for a "stuck" peripherally inserted central catheter.

■ Application of dressing
■ Patient response to the procedure.

After catheter removal, the site should be assessed every 24 hours until the site is epithelialized.

Risks and Complications

The risks and complications associated with CVADs are discussed in Chapter 9. During insertion of the CVAD via the subclavian vein, risks include pneumothorax, hemothorax, and chylothorax. Although a pneumothorax used to be one of the more common insertion-related complications, it is rare today because standard practice includes the use of ultrasound to guide all CVAD placements. Additional potential complications include nerve damage, cardiac dysrhythmias (as a result of myocardial wall irritation from a guidewire or catheter that entered the right atrium), malposition of the catheter, air/catheter embolism, phlebitis, bloodstream infection, catheter-associated venous thrombosis, and air embolism. With PICCs, nerve damage is related to the median nerve, which lies parallel and medial to the brachial artery in the antecubital space. On the lateral side, the lateral cutaneous nerve is proximal to the cephalic vein. Because of the close proximity of these nerves, damage is a risk during PICC insertion.

⬥ *NURSING FAST FACT!*

If the patient complains of pain in the shoulder, neck, or arm at the insertion site, catheter placement should be checked by radiographic examination at any time during the course of therapy. These may be signs of catheter-associated venous thrombosis.

NURSING POINTS OF CARE
NONTUNNELED CVADS AND PICCS: INSERTION AND PLACEMENT

Nursing Assessments
- Identify prescribed therapy and expected duration of therapy.
- Obtain health history (including history of previous VAD placements).
- Identify patient preferences.
- Assess for suitability of target vessels; evaluate for size (the vein must be large enough to accommodate the selected VAD to minimize the risk of phlebitis and thrombosis).
- Assess for skin lesions, presence of a pacemaker, or other implanted device.
- Obtain baseline vital signs.

Key Nursing Interventions
1. Select proper type of CVAD and insertion site.
2. Insert CVADs only when medically necessary.
3. Have all supplies needed for catheter insertion at the bedside before starting insertion.
4. Adhere to central line bundle during insertion.
   a. Hand hygiene
   b. Maximum sterile barrier precautions
   c. Skin antisepsis using chlorhexidine/alcohol
   d. Avoidance of femoral site
   e. Time-out called if proper procedures are not followed (then start again)
5. Obtain order to remove catheter when it is no longer medically necessary.
6. Document the following:
   a. Patient education and response to teaching
   b. Performance of procedure
   c. Patient response
   d. Type of CVAD/insertion site location
   e. Description of the insertion site
   f. Condition of catheter tract and surrounding tissue
   g. Type of I.V. site dressing
   h. Patient response to catheter and patient education

■ Long-Term Central Vascular Access Devices

Subcutaneously Tunneled Catheters

The need for prolonged central venous access and a method to decrease potential infection from the skin exit site resulted in the development of the subcutaneously tunneled CVAD. It was originally developed by Dr. Broviac in 1973 for patients requiring long-term PN and later modified by Dr. Hickman to meet the needs of patients undergoing bone marrow transplant. These long-term catheters can remain in place for years.

The tunneled catheter is considered a long-term catheter for patients who require lifelong or long-term infusion therapy such as PN or chemotherapy. Tunneled catheters may also be placed for apheresis procedures, for example, when a patient requires stem cells for bone marrow transplant. There are also tunneled catheters used for hemodialysis.

The catheter is "tunneled" in the subcutaneous tissue between an "entrance" and an "exit" site. The exit site is where the catheter extrudes, usually in the lower area of the chest. The entrance site is where the catheter enters the venous circulation, generally in the area of the clavicle, and will appear as an incision (Fig. 8-8). A synthetic "cuff" attached to the catheter lies in the subcutaneous tissue along the tunnel tract; the cuff can be seen on the photograph of a tunneled catheter (Fig. 8-9). Over time, the tissue attaches to the cuff to stabilize the catheter and hold it in place. This cuff is located approximately halfway between the entrance and exit sites. It becomes embedded with fibroblasts within 1 week to 10 days after insertion, which reduces the chances for accidental removal and minimizes the risk of ascending bacterial infection. Within 7 to 10 days of catheter insertion, scar tissue grows onto the cuff, anchoring the catheter and preventing microorganisms from migrating up the tunnel. The tunneling/cuff also serves to seal the path from the exit site to the vein, which reduces the risk of bloodstream infection. After the site is well healed, the

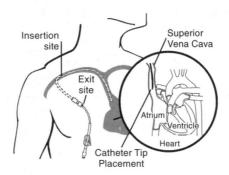

Figure 8-8 ■ Diagram of subcutaneously tunneled catheter placement. (©2013 C. R. Bard, Inc. Used with permission.)

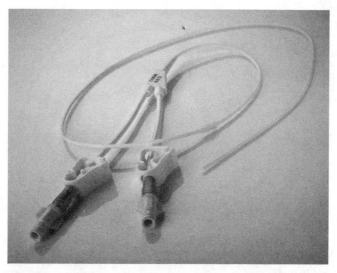

Figure 8-9 ■ Subcutaneously tunneled catheter. (Permission for use granted by Cook Medical Incorporated, Bloomington, IN.)

tunneled catheter is difficult to dislodge and may be managed without a dressing (Bullock-Corkhill, 2010). Surgeons, radiologists, and specialist advanced practice nurses place tunneled catheters.

Tunneled catheters are often made of silicone elastomers, but they may also be made of polyurethane. They may be single lumen or have multiple lumens with varying diameters.

ADVANTAGES

1. Potentially repairable if catheter cracks/tears
2. Low risk of catheter-associated bloodstream infection
3. May remain in place for months to years
4. May not require dressing after tunnel track is well healed

DISADVANTAGES

1. More costly surgical placement and removal (compared to nontunneled CVADs/PICCs)
2. External catheter requires long-term maintenance and attention
3. Body image concerns

Insertion of Tunneled Catheters

Subcutaneously tunneled catheters are inserted with the patient under local or general anesthesia. The catheter can be inserted using MST, as previously discussed, or by a cutdown technique.

During insertion, the venipuncture site is typically made at a point near the subclavian (Fig. 8-10) or internal jugular vein. Using a tunneler

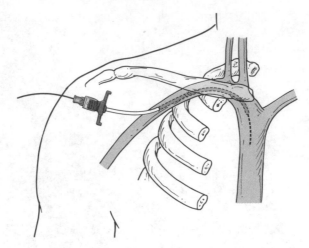

Figure 8-10 ■ Subclavian insertion site for a tunneled catheter.

(a small pencil-like device), a subcutaneous tunnel from the venipuncture site down the chest wall is created leading to an exit site somewhere on the chest. The tunnel may be from 2 to 12 inches long (Hadaway, 2010). The catheter is attached to the tunneler and drawn through the subcutaneous tissue, and the catheter is passed through an introducer and placed in the SVC (Fig. 8-11). The catheter may be sutured to the skin at the catheter exit site; these sutures are removed in 10 to 14 days (Fig. 8-9). A dressing is applied over the catheter insertion site after catheter placement.

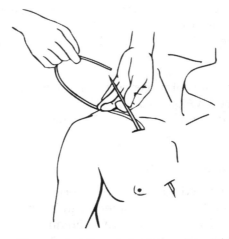

Figure 8-11 ■ Diagram of creation of subcutaneous tunnel. (©2013 C. R. Bard, Inc. Used with permission.)

NURSING POINTS OF CARE
SUBCUTANEOUSLY TUNNELED CATHETERS

- Subcutaneously tunneled catheters are long-term catheters, and patients or their caregivers will learn to care for their catheter independently.
- The catheter may or may not require clamping between infusions; if an open-ended catheter is used, clamp it at all times. This is a safety issue because if the needleless connector accidentally disconnects, there is risk of air embolism. If the catheter has an integral valve in the catheter tip or hub, a clamp is not necessary, and the catheter will not come with a clamp. It is always important to refer to the manufacturer's directions regarding care and management issues.
- Keep all sharp objects away from the catheter. Never use scissors or pins on or near the catheter.
- If the catheter leaks or breaks, take a nonserrated (without teeth) clamp and clamp the catheter between the broken area and the exit site. Cover the broken part with a sterile gauze bandage and tape it securely. Do not use the catheter. Notify the licensed independent practitioner (LIP) (e.g., physician, nurse practitioner, physician assistant).
- Protect the catheter when the patient is showering or bathing by covering the entire catheter with transparent dressing or clear plastic wrap. There are also specific products for this use. Cover the connections and protect hub connections from water contamination.
- A dressing is not required on well-healed catheters.

Complications Associated with Tunneled Catheters

 NURSING FAST FACT!

Refer to Chapter 9 for general complications associated with CVADs, both local and systemic.

Implanted Ports

The implanted port is another type of long-term CVAD that has been used for vascular access since the 1980s. Originally, implanted ports were targeted in oncology patients who required frequent intermittent vascular access for chemotherapy administration. This is still a common indication for implanted port use. Other patient populations include those with intermittent long-term infusion needs, such as patients with hemophilia, cystic fibrosis, and sickle cell disease, and patients who desire a completely implanted device despite daily use, for example, the patient on PN who wants to be able to swim. The implanted port provides safe and reliable vascular access and offers patients improved body image, reduced maintenance, and potentially a better quality of life compared to the external CVAD.

The implanted port is a surgically placed and completely implanted CVAD that is placed in the operating room or in the interventional radiology suite. The port consists of a silicone catheter attached to a reservoir or ("port"), which is made of titanium or plastic (Figs. 8-12, 8-13). The center of the port is covered with a dense silicone septum. The port septum is accessed using a noncoring needle. Most ports can tolerate up to 2000 needle punctures, and the manufacturer's directions will provide specific information about port access. Most often, ports are located in the chest; however, there are "peripheral" ports where the port body is located in the antecubital area. Despite its name, the peripheral port is a CVAD with the catheter threaded through a vein of the upper arm and the tip located in the SVC. When the port is not accessed for use, the only external evidence is a small protrusion in the skin. Port care is minimal, usually requiring only monthly access for flushing if the port is not being actively used.

Figure 8-14 shows additional examples of various ports. There are ports available with two lumens. Of note, there are also ports with catheters

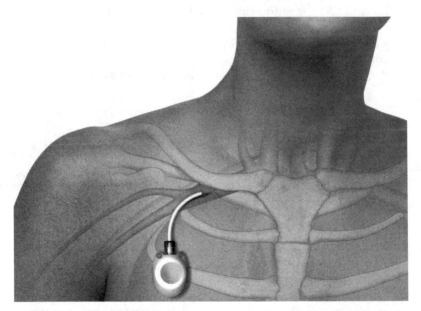

Figure 8-12 ■ Example of port placement in chest. (©2013 C. R. Bard, Inc. Used with permission.)

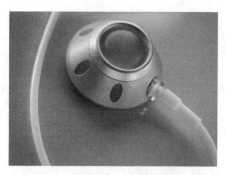

Figure 8-13 ■ Example of an implanted venous access port. (Permission for use granted by Cook Medical Incorporated, Bloomington, IN.)

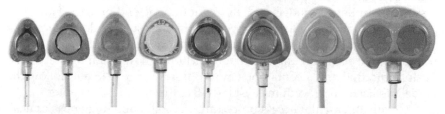

Figure 8-14 ■ Examples of implanted vascular access ports. (©2013 C. R. Bard, Inc. Used with permission.)

placed and located in the hepatic artery, the epidural space, and the peritoneum. These are briefly addressed in Chapter 10. The nurse must be aware and knowledgeable about the type of implanted port before accessing for an infusion.

ADVANTAGES

1. Low risk of catheter-associated bloodstream infection
2. Minimal maintenance required; no dressing unless being actively used for infusion
3. Monthly heparinization required for maintenance
4. May remain in place for months to years
5. Improved body image; no external evidence of port other than small "bump"
6. Few limitations on patient activity; ability to swim when not accessed

DISADVANTAGES

1. More costly device and placement
2. Requires use of a noncoring needle to access the port
3. Pain during needle insertion may be an issue for some patients
4. Minor surgical procedure is necessary to remove the device.

Insertion

The port is usually inserted in the operating room or interventional radiology suite. The surgeon makes an incision in the upper to middle chest, usually near the collarbone, to form a pocket to house the port. The silicone catheter is inserted via cutdown into the SVC; the port is then placed in the subcutaneous fascia pocket. The port contains a reservoir leading to the catheter. The incision for the port pocket is sutured closed, and a sterile dressing is applied. The port requires a dressing until it heals. This area should be monitored until the incision has healed, about 10 days to 2 weeks after insertion.

Accessing the Port

Implanted port access is a skill that must be validated with a competency assessment. Simulation models are helpful for training and practice. However, ports can be challenging to access because of issues such as deep placement and, it is necessary to have a skilled preceptor observe a nurse's first-time port access. To access an implanted port, including how to administer an I.V. push medication and a continuous infusion, see Figure 8-15 and follow the guidelines listed in Procedures Display 8-5 at the end of this chapter.

As with all vascular access procedures, proper hand hygiene is critical. Accessing the port requires adherence to aseptic technique (i.e., wearing a mask and sterile gloves). Should the patient require a continuous infusion via the implanted port, the noncoring needle can be left in place for up to 7 days and covered with a dressing (INS, 2011a). A transparent dressing can be left in place with the needle and changed every 7 days. If a gauze dressing is used, it must be changed every 48 hours. Some nurses may use a gauze dressing under the transparent dressing to stabilize the access needle; if it does not obscure the catheter–skin junction, the dressing is not considered a gauze dressing and can be changed at least every 7 days (INS, 2011a, p. S50). If the port is not routinely used, it can be flushed monthly using flushing protocol. Table 8-3 lists flushing protocols.

> **INS Standard** Noncoring safety needles shall be used to access an implanted vascular access port (INS, 2011a, p. S50).

Some patients may require attention to pain management during port access. It is important that the nurse explore patient preferences and feelings related to access. Most often, topical analgesic creams or patches are used, such as prescription EMLA (contains lidocaine and prilocaine) or an over-the-counter anesthetic cream (e.g., ELA-Max). Although transdermal creams are effective, the disadvantage is the time duration to gain an anesthetic effect, which can be up to 1 hour.

Follow these steps when applying a transdermal cream (INS, 2011b):

1. Check for allergies to lidocaine.
2. Don gloves and use clean technique.

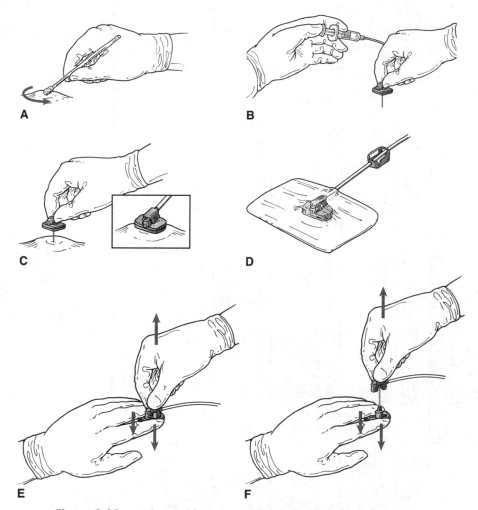

Figure 8-15 ■ Accessing the port wearing gloves. Also wear a mask during port access: *A*, Prep the port site. *B*, Prime the port and extension tubing with 0.9% sodium chloride. *C*, Insert the noncoring needle into the port septum; use nondominant forefinger and thumb to stabilize the port during access (not shown). *D*, Cover with transparent dressing. Deaccessing the port: *E*, Press down and pull straight up. *F*, Engage the safety device according to manufacturer's instructions to decrease risk of accidental needlestick.

3. Prepare the intended venipuncture site by washing with mild soap and water.
4. Apply an amount of cream according to manufacturer's directions.
5. Place a transparent dressing over the cream.
6. Leave in place for recommended time period (usually 30–60 minutes).

> Table 8-3   FLUSHING PROTOCOLS

Device	Intermittent Flushing	Flushing with No Therapy	Heparin Locking	Blood Draws	Blood Product Administration	Parenteral Nutrition Administration
Nontunneled	Minimum of 5 mL	Nonvalved: At least every 24 hours Valved: At least weekly	5 mL of 10 units/mL heparin	Predraw 5 mL Postdraw 10 mL	Preadmin 5 mL Postadmin 10 mL	Minimum of 5 mL
PICC	Minimum of 5 mL	Nonvalved: At least every 24 hour Valved: At least weekly	5 mL of 10 units/mL heparin	Predraw 5 mL Postdraw 10 mL	Preadmin 5 mL Postadmin 10 mL	Minimum of 5 mL
Tunneled	Minimum of 5 mL	Nonvalved: At least 1–2 times per week Valved: At least weekly	5 mL of 10 units/mL heparin	Predraw 5 mL Postdraw 10 mL	Preadmin 5 mL Postadmin 10 mL	
Port	Minimum of 5 mL	Accessed: Nonvalved: At least 1–2 times per week Valved: At least weekly Deaccessed: At least monthly	3–5 mL of 100 units/mL heparin	Predraw 5 mL Postdraw 10 mL	Preadmin 5 mL Postadmin 10 mL	

NOTE: Always use a 10-mL syringe for all flushing of CVCs.
NOTE: Use single-use preservative-free 0.9% sodium chloride flushes.
Source: Flushing Protocols (INS, 2008c), with permission.

7. Remove the occlusive dressing, if one was used. Remove the cream by wiping with a clean gauze or tissue. Perform any additional skin preparation or cleansing at this time prior to port access.

Other pain management strategies include distraction or relaxation techniques and use of ice over the port site for several minutes before site preparation and access (Gorski et al., 2010).

Deaccessing an Implanted Port

After performing hand hygiene, nonsterile gloves are worn and the dressing is removed. The port is stabilized using the thumb and forefinger of the nondominant hand. The needle device is grasped with the dominant hand and removed following the directions of the safety needle. It is very important that the nurse understand the safety mechanism when removing the noncoring needle. When it is removed from the port the needle often may "pull," and there is risk of rebound and accidental needlestick to the nurse's fingers during the removal process should the safety features not be engaged.

INS Standard Aseptic technique, including the use of sterile gloves, should be used when accessing an implanted port (INS, 2011a, p. S50).

Refer to Procedures Display 8-6 at the end of this chapter for full instructions on deaccessing an implanted port.

Complications Associated with Implanted Ports

The same complications associated with all CVADs can occur with implanted ports (see Chapter 9 for CVAD complications). Extravasation of vesicant medications can occur if the needle is not in place through the septum of the port and the position is not confirmed, or if the needle dislodges. Patients and nurses must always verify placement by ensuring the ability to easily aspirate blood and ensuring there is no swelling or discomfort during flushing or infusion. The needle should be secured before initiating the infusion and the site observed for signs such as swelling or the presence of pain or burning.

Table 8-4 compares CVADs, with advantages and disadvantages of each.

■ Care and Maintenance

Assessment

Assessment, including the CVAD site, catheter patency, and catheter need, is an important aspect of catheter care and maintenance and is critically

> Table 8-4 ▮ **COMPARISON OF CENTRAL VENOUS CATHETERS**

Type and Use	Available Features	Advantages	Disadvantages
Nontunneled CVAD	Material: Polyurethane (most common), silicone elastomer Antimicrobial coating or impregnated Single or multiple (2–4) lumens Valved or nonvalved Power injectable	Inserted at bedside Less expensive than subcutaneously tunneled or implanted port Can be removed by nurse Can be exchanged over guidewire	Short-term device (usually days) Increased risk for infection compared to peripheral I.V. catheter or long-term CVADs Need to protect from water
PICC	Material: Polyurethane (most common), silicone elastomer Single or multiple (2–3) lumens Valved or nonvalved Power injectable	Short-term (days) to longer-term device (weeks to months) Inserted at bedside Less expensive than subcutaneously tunneled or implanted port Can be removed by nurse Can be exchanged over guidewire	Lower risk of insertion-related complications Maintenance care required Location in arm may be challenging to manage long term Need to protect from water
Subcutaneously Tunneled CVAD	Material: Silicone elastomer (most common), polyurethane Single or multiple (2–4) lumens Valved or nonvalved Power injectable	Low risk for infection Repairable May remain in place for months to years May not require dressing after tunnel tract is well healed Decreased care and maintenance costs	More costly device and surgical placement Removed per LIP
Implanted Ports	Material: Catheter: Silicone elastomer or polyurethane Port: Titanium, stainless steel, plastic Single or double Valved or nonvalved Power injectable	Low risk for infection May remain in place for months to years Decreased care and maintenance costs Monthly maintenance locking No activity restrictions Improved body image	More costly surgical placement and removal Requires noncoring needle to access Pain during needle insertion may be an issue for some patients, although anesthetic options are available

important to ensuring positive patient outcomes. Assessment related to the CVAD site should include:

- Signs of local infection, such as erythema, drainage, swelling, and induration
- For patients with subcutaneously tunneled CVADs or implanted ports, the tunnel tract or port area is assessed for pain, tenderness, or edema.
- Signs of catheter-associated venous thrombosis, including swelling in the arm, shoulder, chest, or neck; pain along the extremity, in the shoulder, chest, neck, jaw, or ear; or dilated collateral veins over the arm, neck, or chest on the placement side of the CVAD (see Chapter 9)
- Presence of fluid leakage at the insertion site that might be indicative of a crack in the catheter or possible thrombotic problems
- Patient complaints of pain or evidence of pain or tenderness when the area is gently palpated
- Integrity of the dressing and the stabilization device/method used
- Evidence of outward migration of the catheter. The external length of the CVAD extruding from the site should be measured at the time of placement so that any suspected catheter migration can be objectively validated by subsequent measurements.
- Catheter patency: Each lumen of a patent CVAD should be easy to flush (i.e., without any resistance) and should yield a free, flowing blood return with aspiration.

Beyond assessment of the CVAD site, vital signs and a general head-to-toe assessment should be performed. Laboratory test results should be checked for abnormalities, for example, an increase in the white blood cell count may be indicative of infection. Finally, the need for the central line is reviewed as part of the assessment process. To summarize, positive outcomes include:

- The catheter exit site is clean and free of blood or drainage, erythema, and edema; the dressing is intact; and there is no pain or evidence of thrombosis.
- The CVAD flushes easily and yields a blood return with aspiration.

Abnormalities (including signs and symptoms) are reported to the LIP. Frequency of site assessment is dependent on the patient's condition, organizational policies, and the health-care setting. In most hospitals, CVAD site assessment is done at least every 8 hours. For patients with long-term CVADs in alternative settings such as long-term care facilities, the site should be checked at least daily and possibly more often, based on how often the CVAD is being used for infusion therapy. For home care patients, the site should be assessed by the nurse at every home visit, and patients should be taught to inspect their site at least every day (Gorski, 2010).

INS Standard Catheter–skin junction sites should be visually inspected or palpated through the intact dressing daily for tenderness (INS, 2011a, p. S64).

Site Care and Dressing Changes

Site care is performed regularly in conjunction with dressing changes for external CVADs, which include PICCs, nontunneled, and subcutaneously tunneled catheters. Regular site care is required to cleanse the skin and reduce the presence of microorganisms on the skin around the catheter insertion site, which are a potential source of catheter-associated bloodstream infection. The basic steps included in site care and dressing changes include:

- Removal of the old dressing and stabilization device, if used
- Cleansing the skin using an acceptable antiseptic
- Assessing the condition of the insertion site, surrounding skin, and catheter (as outlined in the previous section)
- Replacing the stabilization device and dressing

The preferred skin antiseptic agent for ongoing site care is chlorhexidine alcohol (INS, 2011a; O'Grady et al., 2011), except for children younger than 2 months of age (addressed later in Age-Related Considerations). Although chlorhexidine is preferred due to its residual antimicrobial activity, other acceptable solutions include 1% to 2% tincture of iodine, povidone-iodine, and 70% alcohol (INS, 2011a; O'Grady et al., 2011).

When applying chlorhexidine, a back-and-forth scrubbing method using friction for at least 30 seconds is recommended. This is based on the original research used to validate the use of chlorhexidine (INS, 2011a). It is important to allow the antiseptic to fully dry before replacing the dressing.

For patients who are sensitive or allergic to chlorhexidine or alcohol and for children younger than 2 months of age, povidone-iodine is considered an acceptable disinfectant. To be most effective, povidone-iodine requires at least 2 minutes of contact on the skin (INS, 2011b; O'Grady et al., 2011; Pedivan, 2010). It is applied using swab sticks. Each swab stick of povidone-iodine is applied in a concentric circle beginning at the catheter insertion site, then moving outward. It is important to recognize that the practice of applying povidone-iodine is based on "traditional" practice rather than research. This is certainly an area of practice that lacks evidence and needs research to validate the procedure. Povidone-iodine should not be removed with alcohol after application.

Use of a central line dressing kit is recommended because it standardizes the dressing change procedure and improves time efficiency by eliminating the need to gather individual supplies (Fig. 8-16) (Gorski, et al., 2010).

For newly placed subcutaneously tunneled CVADs, the dressing change procedure is the same as for nontunneled CVADs or PICCs. Once

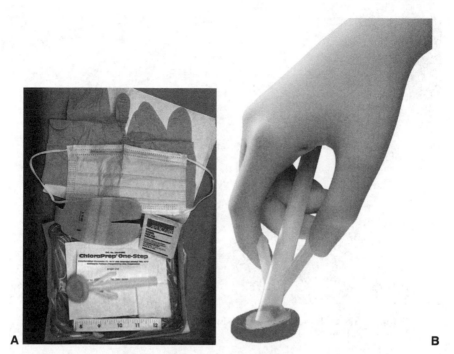

A   B

Figure 8-16 ■ *A,* Example of a dressing kit. (Courtesy of Mark Hunter.)
B, Skin antisepsis prior to CVAD placement and with routine site care using
Chloraprep® 3 mL applicator. (Courtesy of Carefusion, San Diego, CA.)

the tunnel is healed, a dressing may not be required. If the patient is not immunosuppressed and healing at the insertion site is complete, site care may be limited to daily inspection and cleansing with soap and water while the patient is bathing (Gorski et al., 2010). Should a patient with a long-term subcutaneously tunneled catheter, managed at home without a dressing, be admitted to the hospital, organizational policies may require a dressing because of the increased risk for infection in the inpatient setting.

Options for catheter dressings include the transparent semipermeable membrane (TSM) dressing or the gauze and tape dressing. Advantages to TSM dressings include continuous visual inspection of the catheter site and cost effectiveness because of less frequent dressing changes. Gauze dressings may be appropriate for the patient who experiences site drainage, perspires excessively, or has sensitivity to TSM dressings (Figs. 8-17, 8-18, and 8-19). TSM dressings are replaced when they are damp, loosened, or soiled or at least every 7 days (O'Grady et al., 2011). Gauze dressings should be changed every 48 hours (2 days) or if the site requires visual inspection (INS, 2011a, p. S44; O'Grady et al., 2011).

A chlorhexidine-impregnated dressing is often placed around the catheter exit site before placement of the transparent dressing. One dressing consists of a small foam disc impregnated with chlorhexidine gluconate. The

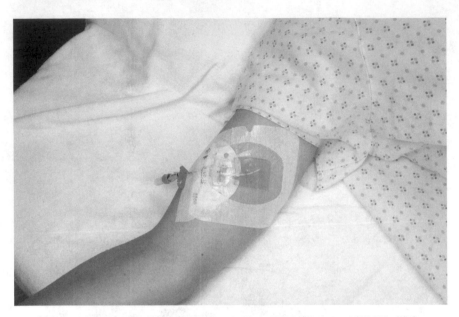

Figure 8-17 ▪ Tegaderm CHG dressing over PICC. (Courtesy of 3M Medical Division, St. Paul, MN.)

dressing has a small slit, which allows it to be positioned around and under the VAD (Fig. 8-20). The chlorhexidine-impregnated dressing is changed every 7 days. There are also TSM dressings with a chlorhexidine gel pad (Fig. 8-17).

The 2011 CDC guidelines recommend routine use of impregnated sponge dressings only if the organizational CLABSI rate is not decreasing despite adherence to basic prevention measures (O'Grady et al., 2011). Of note, chlorhexidine gel pad dressings were not addressed in the 2011 guidelines because of lack of studies at that time. However, many organizations do include them as part of their central line bundle. The research supporting use of chlorhexidine dressings is primarily with short-term nontunneled catheters and PICCs in acute care settings. There is wide variance in practice on use of these dressings for long-term CVAD use in home care or for patients in long-term care hospitals or nursing homes. Some organizations use these dressings around implanted port needles during the access period as well.

> EBP In a randomized controlled trial involving 1636 patients and 3778 catheters in ICU patients, it was found that use of a chlorhexidine-impregnated foam dressing decreased the risk of catheter-related bloodstream infection rate by 76% despite a low baseline infection rate. In this study, it was also found that changing dressings every 7 days was found to be safe and was not inferior to dressing changes every 3 day (Timsit et al., 2009).

EBP The chlorhexidine-impregnated foam dressing covers the insertion site and does not allow continuous assessment of the site. The TSM dressing with a chlorhexidine gel pad does allow visualization of the site. In a randomized controlled trial involving 1879 patients and 413 catheters, three types of dressings were compared: a TSM dressing with chlorhexidine gel pad, a highly adhesive TSM dressing, and a standard TSM dressing. The catheter-related bloodstream infection rate was 60% lower in the chlorhexidine dressing group compared to the nonchlorhexidine dressing group (0.5 per 1000 catheter-days vs 1.3 per 1000 catheter-days) (Timsit et al., 2012).

Site care and dressing changes are performed using aseptic technique. Refer to Procedures Display 8-1 at the end of this chapter.

INS Standard The dressing should be labeled with the following information: date, and time and initials of the nurse performing dressing change (INS, 2011a, p. S64).

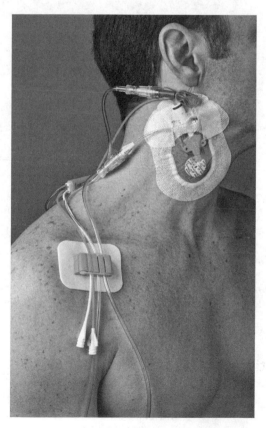

Figure 8-18 ■ SorbaView Shield Contour TSM dressing over nontunneled CVAD placed via internal jugular vein. (Courtesy of Centurion, Williamston, MI.)

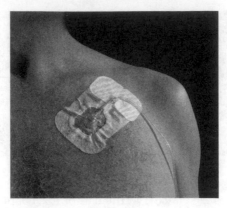

Figure 8-19 ■ SorbaView TSM dressing over accessed implanted vascular access port. (Courtesy of Centurion, Williamston, MI.)

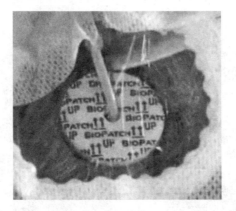

Figure 8-20 ■ Biopatch®-impregnated foam dressing around a CVAD. (Courtesy of J&J Wound Management, Division of Ethicon, Inc., Somerville, NJ.)

 NURSING FAST FACT!

When removing the old dressing, lift it from the catheter hub toward the patient's head, taking care not to pull the catheter out of the insertion site.

Administration Set Changes

Administration sets are regularly changed based on the type of infusion (continuous or intermittent) and type of infusate as follows:
   ■ Aseptic technique is adhered to at all times when changing any administration tubing.

- Primary and secondary continuous administration sets used to administer fluids other than lipids, blood, or blood products should be changed no more frequently than every 96 hours.
- Primary intermittent administration sets are changed every 24 hours (i.e., administration sets taken down after each infusion and CVAD locked between infusions). A sterile cap is placed on the male end of the administration set between infusions.
- Administration sets used to deliver PN with lipid emulsions are changed every 24 hours. If fat emulsion is piggybacked into administration sets that have been used for PN, the sets must be changed every 24 hours if running continuously or changed after each unit if running intermittently.
- Intravenous fat emulsion administration sets are changed every 24 hours.
- Administration sets and add-on filters that are used for blood and blood components are changed after administration of *each* unit or at the end of 4 hours, whichever comes first.
- Any administration set that is suspected of being contaminated or when the integrity of the product is in question should be changed (INS, 2011a, pp. S55-S56).

Flushing and Locking

As discussed in Chapter 6, catheters are *flushed* after each intermittent infusion to clear any medication from the catheter and to prevent contact between incompatible medications or I.V. solutions. If not properly flushed, a precipitate can form, essentially blocking the catheter, or thrombotic occlusion can occur as a result of blood clotting within the catheter lumen. Catheters are flushed with preservative-free 0.9% sodium chloride. Catheters are *locked* with a solution left instilled in the catheter to prevent occlusion in between intermittent infusions. In 2008, the INS released "Flushing Protocols," a tool that gives recommendations for flushing/locking solutions and frequency for all VADs based on the type of infusion.

Table 8-3 lists flushing protocols from INS (2008b). The evidence continues to emerge regarding the best locking solution and the frequency of locking; therefore, there remains variation in protocols between organizations. Also, alternative locking solutions may be used in some situations, for example, ethanol may be used in patients with a history of bloodstream infections (see Chapter 12 for discussion). Ethanol, sodium citrate, taurolidine, and ethylenediaminetetraacetate (EDTA) have been used as alternative locking solutions in patients with heparin-induced thrombocytopenia (INS, 2011a, p. S61). Such solutions must be made by a compounding pharmacy because they are not available in single-dose syringes or containers. It is important to review and follow organizational policies and procedures.

The CDC Guidelines state that antibiotic lock solutions should not be routinely used to prevent central line infections but could be used in special circumstances, such as a patient with repeated infections despite optimal maximal adherence to aseptic technique (O'Grady et al., 2011).

Low-concentration heparin is used to maintain patency of some central venous catheters. Catheters with integral valves are locked with 0.9% sodium chloride according to manufacturer's instructions. When heparin is recommended, a concentration (e.g., 10 units/mL) that does not interfere with clotting factors should be used.

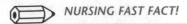 *NURSING FAST FACT!*

> *Heparin-induced thrombocytopenia is a rare but life- and limb-threatening immunological reaction caused by platelet activation resulting in a hypercoagulable state leading to arterial thrombosis as a result of heparin exposure (INS, 2011a).*

Needleless Connectors

Needleless connectors are placed on the hub of the CVAD. They are designed to accommodate the tip of the syringe or I.V. tubing for catheter flushing or I.V. administration. A review of important aspects of needleless connectors is given below (see Chapters 5 and 6 for further information):

■ There are different types of needleless connectors, including simple devices (e.g., split septum) and complex devices. Complex devices include negative, positive, and neutral needleless connectors. To reduce the risk of blood reflux and thus catheter occlusion, the nurse must understand proper flushing technique in relation to the type of needleless connector. Refer to Procedures Display 8-2 at the end of this chapter.

■ Needleless connectors are changed when the I.V. administration set is changed, if residual blood is present in the device, and whenever the integrity of the product is compromised or is suspected of being contaminated. Manufacturer's guidelines will provide further information regarding frequency of change, including whether the connectors should be replaced after blood withdrawal. Also, to prevent contamination of blood cultures drawn through a CVAD, the needleless connector is replaced before drawing the blood culture sample.

■ The needleless connector must be disinfected before any access into the CVAD. INS (2011a) recommends 70% alcohol or chlorhexidine/alcohol solution.

■ Although the optimal disinfection (i.e. "scrubbing") time is not known, many organizations use a 15-second scrub.

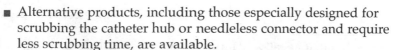

- Alternative products, including those especially designed for scrubbing the catheter hub or needleless connector and require less scrubbing time, are available.
- Protective alcohol disinfection caps are available that are placed on the needleless connector of locked CVAD lumens between infusions.

NOTE > Whenever a needleless connector is removed from a catheter, it should be discarded and a new one attached.

NOTE > Refer to the manufacturer's guidelines for specific device usage.

 NURSING FAST FACT!

If you have a multilumen catheter, remember to change the needleless connectors on all lumens.

Blood Sampling

For patients receiving infusion therapy, laboratory testing is common practice because of the patient's condition and the nature of the solutions and medications administered. Use of the VAD for blood sampling provides patient benefits such as eliminating anxiety and pain from venipuncture and decreasing patient dissatisfaction with being repeatedly "stuck." However, there are potential risks, including:

- Increased risk for occlusion, especially that associated with inadequate technique and flushing
- Increased risk for catheter-related bloodstream infection as a result of manipulation at the catheter hub
- Potential for inaccurate laboratory test results

A study examining the efficacy and safety of blood sampling through PICCs in a pediatric population did not find any significant increase in occlusion, infection, or other complications (Knue, Doellman, Rabin, & Jacobs, 2005). The INS Standards recommend making the decision to use the catheter for blood sampling based on the evaluation of risks versus benefits (INS, 2011a). Organizations should have procedures in place that address safe blood sampling via the VAD. From the INS Standards, the following issues should be considered in relation to blood draws from a CVAD (INS, (2011a, p. S79):

- Use caution when interpreting drug levels. When a questionable result is obtained (e.g., unexpected high level that would require a

medication dose change), consider the need to retest via a direct venipuncture.
- Factors that negatively influence accuracy include sampling from implanted ports, silicone catheters, which may have more of a tendency for drug adsorption to the catheter wall, and sampling from the same catheter lumen used to administer the drug.
- Avoid drawing coagulation levels from a heparinized CVAD because this practice has been associated with falsely elevated activated partial thromboplastin times (apTT), prothrombin (PT), and international normalized ratio (INR) times.

An issue not always recognized by nurses is that frequent blood sampling, whether by peripheral venipuncture or via a VAD, can contribute to iron deficiency and blood loss, especially in neonates and critically ill patients. This topic is also addressed in Chapter 11 as it relates to reducing the need for blood transfusions. Blood conservation methods include avoiding routine testing, consolidating all laboratory tests with a daily blood draw, considering the use of point-of-care testing methods (e.g., blood glucose meters), recording the volume of blood obtained, and using low-volume blood collection tubes (INS, 2011a, p. 79).

The most common method used for blood sampling is what is commonly called the "discard" method. The first aspirate of blood is discarded to reduce the risk of any drug, normal saline, or heparin interfering with the laboratory test results. Key points in obtaining blood sampling from a CVAD include:
- Stop running infusion as appropriate.
  - Of note, there is no evidence for a specific time that the infusion must be stopped. Remember from Chapter 1 that the CVAD tip is placed in the SVC where blood flow is approximately 2 L/min. When the infusion is stopped, any medication flowing from the catheter is rapidly dispersed into the central circulation.
- Flush the CVAD with 5-10 mL of 0.9% sodium chloride for injection to flush any remaining medication or fluid out of the catheter.
- Withdraw blood in an amount at least twice the catheter's priming volume or 4 to 5 mL as recommended by the INS (2011b) and discard this blood because it contains heparin and/or medication.
- Withdraw the amount of blood needed for the laboratory tests.
- Flush the CVAD with at least 10 mL of 0.9% sodium chloride for injection.

Refer to Procedures Display 8-3 at the end of this chapter for steps on drawing a blood sample from a CVAD using the discard method. Of note, another method endorsed by INS (2011a) is the push–pull or mixing method. The advantage to this method is less blood loss because there is no discarded blood. Key steps include:
- Flush the CVAD with 5 mL of 0.9% sodium chloride for injection using a 10-mL syringe.

- Aspirate 6 mL of blood (without detaching the syringe).
- Push blood back into the catheter and repeat process three times.
- Remove empty syringe; attach a new syringe or Vacutainer to obtain laboratory sample.
- Flush catheter with saline and heparinize per orders or resume infusion.

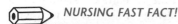 *NURSING FAST FACT!*

> *Be aware that withdrawal of blood through the CVAD can contribute to thrombotic catheter occlusion if the catheter is not flushed adequately.*

Catheter Repair

Catheter damage can occur from exerting excessive pressure while flushing or by accidental cutting from scissors or the catheter clamp. Nurses and patients with a central line must be knowledgeable about immediate actions to take in the event of catheter damage (INS, 2011a). Air can enter the catheter through the tear, causing an air embolism. Patients should be provided instructions on how to immediately clamp or fold the catheter to prevent blood loss or air embolism and informed to notify the nurse.

Some CVADs may be repairable. Catheter repair kits are available and are specific to the manufacturer and size of the catheter. Risks versus benefits must be considered when weighing the appropriateness of catheter removal versus catheter repair. Factors to consider include risk for infection from the damaged catheter, catheter type and potential for repair, expected duration of catheter need, and patient safety. Patient benefits from catheter repair include avoidance of the risk, cost, and disruption in life associated with another catheter insertion procedure; potential risks include the possibility of catheter-related bloodstream infection resulting from the damaged catheter or the catheter repair procedure (Gorski et al., 2010). The risk of catheter-associated infection is reduced by nursing competence and use of sterile technique while performing the repair.

Other options for managing a damaged or ruptured catheter include a catheter exchange procedure or insertion of a new catheter in a different site (INS, 2011a, p. S75). The catheter exchange procedure involves replacing the catheter in the same site using a guidewire; this procedure is performed under the same level of aseptic technique and following the central line insertion bundle interventions.

INS Standard Catheter damage increases the risk for catheter fracture and embolization, air emboli, bleeding, catheter lumen occlusion, and bloodstream infection. If catheter repair is chosen, it should be performed as soon as possible to reduce the risk of these complications (INS, 2011a, p. S75).

Discontinuation of Therapy

Removal of a tunneled catheter or implanted port is considered a surgical procedure and should be performed by a physician or advanced practice nurse. If a catheter-related bloodstream infection is suspected, consideration should be given to culturing the catheter and clinical assessment of the patient's condition with a possible treatment option for catheter salvage. If a catheter-related complication is suspected, the catheter should be removed after patient assessment and collaboration with the health-care team.

Table 8-5 summarizes the care and maintenance of the four types of CVADs.

> Table 8-5	SUMMARY OF CARE AND MAINTENANCE OF CENTRAL VASCULAR ACCESS DEVICES
Care/Maintenance	**Standards of Care**
Dressings	Sterile dressings should be applied and replaced routinely. Gauze dressing are replaced at least every 48 hours. TSM dressings are replaced at least every 7 days. If gauze is used in conjunction with a transparent semipermeable membrane (TSM) dressing, it is considered a gauze dressing and must be changed every 48 hours.
Administration Set Changes	Primary and secondary continuous administration sets used to administer fluids other than lipids, blood, or blood products should be changed no more frequently than every 96 hours. Primary intermittent infusion sets should be changed every 24 hours. Administration sets used to administer lipid containing parenteral nutrition (PN) solutions are changed every 24 hours. Intravenous fat emulsion administration sets are changed every 24 hours. Blood sets and add-on filters should be changed after administration of each unit or at the end of 4 hours, whichever comes first. Any administration set that is suspected of being contaminated or product whose integrity is in question should be changed.
Flushing and Locking	See Tables 8-3 and 8-6 for specific flushing guidelines. *Note:* Valved CVADs can be locked with 0.9% sodium chloride. Always use a 10-mL size syringe to reduce risk of catheter damage. *Note:* Ports when not in use do not require daily care.
Needleless Connectors	Disinfect with 70% alcohol using a twisting motion for 15 seconds before every access or use special products developed for disinfection according to manufacturer's directions. May consider use of alcohol disinfection caps on unused CVAD lumens between infusions.
Blood Sampling	Flush the catheter with 5 mL of sodium chloride predraw. Draw back 4–5 mL of blood and discard the sample. Attach a new syringe or Vacutainer and collect samples. Label all samples at the bedside.

NOTE: All add-on devices (extension tubing sets, injection caps, filters, syringes) should have luer-lock connections to reduce risk of accidental disconnection.
Source: Adapted from INS (2011a, 2011b).

> Table 8-6 **NEONATAL AND PEDIATRIC FLUSHING PROTOCOLS**

Device	Locked Device: Volume, Frequency, and Solution	Medications: Pre- and Postadministration	Blood Product Administration and Sampling Withdrawal
PICC	*2 Fr:* 1 mL NS +10 units/mL heparin every 6 hours *2.6 Fr and larger:* 2–3 mL NS +10 units/mL heparin every 12 hours	Two times administration tubing and add-on set volume	*2 Fr: Sampling and pre- and postblood administration:* 1 mL to clear the catheter, then flush with 1 mL of NS followed by locking solution until clear *2.6 Fr and larger: Sampling and pre- and post-blood administration:* 1–3 mL NS followed by locking solution or resume infusion *Withdrawal volume:* Three times administration tubing and add-on set volume
Tunneled and Nontunneled	*NICU patients:* 1–3 mL NS +10 units/mL of heparin every 12–24 hours *Pediatrics:* 2 mL NS + 10 units/mL of heparin every 24 hours	Two times administration tubing and add-on set volume	*Pre- and post-blood administration:* 1 mL NS for NICU patients and 3 mL NS for all others, followed by locking solution or resume infusion *Withdrawal volume for sampling:* Three times administration tubing and add-on set volume. *Note:* Variation in size makes it difficult to recommend one volume for all patients
Ports	*If used for more than one medication daily:* 3–5 mL NS + 10 units/mL heparin Monthly maintenance flush: 3–5 mL NS +100 units/mL of heparin	Two times administration tubing and add-on set volume	*Pre- and post-blood administration:* 3–5 mL NS followed by locking solution or resume infusion *Withdrawal volume for sampling:* Three times administration tubing and add-on set volume. *Note:* Variation in size makes it difficult to recommend one volume for all patients

NOTE: Use single-use preservative-free 0.9% sodium chloride for flushes.
NICU = neonatal intensive care unit; NS = normal saline (sodium chloride).
Source: Flushing protocols. INS (2008c), with permission.

NURSING POINTS OF CARE
CARE AND MAINTENANCE

Nursing Assessments
- Signs of local infection, such as erythema, drainage, swelling, and induration
- Patients with subcutaneously tunneled CVADs or implanted ports: Assess tunnel tract or port area for pain, tenderness, and edema
- Signs of catheter-associated venous thrombosis
- Presence of fluid leakage at the insertion site indicative of a crack in the catheter or possible thrombotic problems
- Patient complaints of pain or evidence of pain or tenderness
- Integrity of the dressing and the stabilization device/method used
- Evidence of outward migration of the catheter
- Catheter patency
- Vital signs

Key Nursing Interventions
1. Regular site care and dressing changes
   a. At least every 7 days if using a TSM dressing
   b. At least every 2 days if using a gauze dressing
   c. More often if dressing is damp, loosened, or soiled
2. For continuous infusions, change administration sets at least every 96 hours; for intermittent infusions (CVAD locked between infusions), change set every 24 hours. Replace tubing used to administer blood or blood products every 4 hours and lipids every 24 hours.
3. Flush CVAD with 0.9% sodium chloride to assess patency and to prevent contact between incompatible solutions/medications.
4. Lock unused lumens of CVAD with low-concentration heparin or 0.9% sodium chloride to maintain patency (follow organizational protocol).
5. Use a noncoring needle to access implanted ports; change the needle every 7 days if running a continuous infusion via the port.
6. For nonvalved CVADs, clamp unused lumens at all times.
7. Keep sharp objects away from the CVAD; never use scissors or pins on or near the catheter.
8. Protect CVAD when patient is showering or bathing by covering the entire catheter with transparent dressing or clear plastic wrap. Cover the connections and protect hub connections from water contamination.

9. Avoid use of blood pressure cuffs or tourniquet over the site of the PICC, but they may be placed distal to the catheter's location.
10. Document the following:
    a. Location of insertion site
    b. Assessment of the catheter and insertion site
    c. Condition of catheter tract and surrounding tissue
    d. Site care and type of I.V. site dressing
    e. Flushing/locking solutions, amount, time
    f. Administration set changes
    g. Patient response to catheter and patient education

AGE-RELATED CONSIDERATIONS
The Pediatric Patient

Pediatric Central Vascular Access
The same four categories of CVADs used in adults—nontunneled, PICCs, subcutaneously tunneled, and implanted ports—are also used for pediatric infusion therapy for similar indications. As with adults, it is important to assess the infant or child early during the hospital stay to determine the most appropriate VAD. Selection criteria include:
• Length and type of anticipated therapies
• Age and weight
• Diagnoses
• Condition of the vasculature (some children have difficult venous access which may lead to preference for a CVAD)
• Current clinical condition
• Number of different infusion therapies. A child receiving multiple medications and/or blood products will benefit from a CVAD.

Nontunneled CVADs are used for short-term access in the critically ill child. Insertion site preferences, in order of preference, safety, and accessibility, are the femoral, internal jugular, and subclavian vein (Frey & Pettit, 2010). In contrast to adults, the femoral site is not contraindicated in pediatric patients. PICCs are commonly placed in infants and children, with a lower rate of complications compared to other types of CVADs (Pedivan, 2010). PICC sites include the arm in children of all ages, and the leg, foot, or scalp/neck veins in infants. The vein of choice for the upper arm is the basilic because of the ease of threading; for the lower extremities, the saphenous vein is commonly used (Pedivan, 2010). Long-term central venous access, often with subcutaneously tunneled catheters, is an integral part of managing children with cancer, certain congenital malformations, or gastrointestinal (GI) malfunction, as well as those who need long-term access for medication or blood products. Implanted ports may be placed in children who have ongoing intermittent infusion needs, such as those with severe hemophilia requiring regular factor replacement.

Continued

In infants, the umbilical vein and artery are additional routes for venous access for the first few days after birth. The umbilical cord includes three vessels: one thin-walled vein with a large diameter lumen, and two thick-walled arteries with small diameter lumens (Frey & Pettit, 2010). The umbilical vein is preferred in emergency infusions and can be used for up to 2 weeks. Catheters placed in the vein can be also used for CVP measurement, venous blood sampling, prostaglandin administration, and exchange transfusions. The catheter tip for umbilical vein catheters is located in the inferior vena cava above the diaphragm (INS, 2011a, p. S52). The umbilical artery is used for hemodynamic monitoring, arterial blood gas measurements, and obtaining blood for other laboratory work.

CDC Guideline: Umbilical venous catheters should be removed as soon as possible when no longer needed but can be used for up to 14 days if managed aseptically. Umbilical artery catheters should be removed as soon as possible when no longer needed or when any sign of vascular insufficiency to the lower extremities is observed. Optimally, an umbilical artery catheter should not be left in place over 5 days (O'Grady et al., 2011).

The INS Standards address some specific practice criteria for infusion in the pediatric patient. In relation to CVAD use, included are:

1. The nurse shall verify that informed consent for treatment of neonatal and pediatric patients, as well as for patients deemed emancipated minors, is documented.
2. The nurse providing infusion therapy for neonatal and pediatric patients shall have clinical knowledge and technical expertise with respect to this population.
3. The nurse providing infusion therapy should have knowledge and demonstrated competency in the areas of:
   a. Anatomy and physiology related to neonatal and pediatric patients and their effect on physical assessment, VAD and non-VAD selection, insertion procedures, and use of specialized equipment.
   b. Growth and development stages
   c. Physiological characteristics and their effect on drug and nutrient selection (INS, 2011, p. S6)

Pain Management
Pain management must be considered for children who will undergo CVAD insertion and maintenance. Pain may cause short-term suffering, but there may also be long-term detrimental effects. Lasting negative effects may impact neuronal development, pain threshold and sensitivity, coping strategies, emotions, and perceptions of pain (Cohen, 2008). Patients undergoing certain vascular procedures at times may need sedation or general anesthesia. The use of transdermal anesthetics, as discussed earlier, is appropriate for children facing procedures such as implanted port access. With infants, nonnutritive sucking is an effective analgesic, especially when combined with sucrose solution (e.g., such as that given with a pacifier). Skin-to-skin contact and breast feeding are additional important and effective behavioral interventions

(Cohen, 2008). Behavioral interventions appropriate to CVAD placement also include:

- Age-appropriate and clear, nonemotive procedural information
- Training in coping skills and encouragement of skills during procedures
- Use of distraction (Cohen, 2008)

Care and Maintenance of Central Vascular Access Devices in Children

Although the preferred antiseptic for ongoing site care is chlorhexidine alcohol, the exception is for children younger than 2 months of age (INS, 2011a; O'Grady et al., 2011). However, there is evolving evidence of chlorhexidine safety and efficacy for all age groups (Pedivan, 2010). For children younger than 2 months of age, povidone-iodine is considered an acceptable disinfectant. To be most effective, povidone-iodine requires at least 2 minutes of contact on the skin (INS, 2011b; O'Grady et al., 2011; Pedivan, 2010). Povidone-iodine should not be removed with alcohol after application. An exception is with infants younger than 2 months old, for whom it is recommended that povidone-iodine be removed with sterile normal saline or sterile water to prevent absorption of the product through the skin (Pedivan, 2010).

Blood Sampling

Catheter lumens smaller than 26 gauge are too restrictive to allow blood samples. Evidence does support blood sampling through a 3 Fr PICC without a significant increase in occlusion (Knue et al., 2005).

The Older Adult

- Evaluation of a short-term versus a long-term device should be evaluated, as should the older adult's ability to care for the device. The nontunneled short-term CVC may be appropriate for several weeks of therapy.
- The patient and/or caregiver may have difficulty maintaining and coping with dressing and flushing procedures.
- Implanted vascular access port may be a better alternative because of fewer catheter care requirements.

Home Care Issues

Most patients who require home infusion therapy will have a CVAD in place rather than a peripheral I.V. catheter. CVADs are commonly used in home administration of antimicrobial medications, PN, chemotherapy, biological therapy, and other medications. The most commonly used type of CVAD is the PICC. For home care patients, the emphasis on patient education is especially strong. Home care patients will be assuming many facets of self-care related to their VAD. The INS Standards (INS, 2011a, p. S16) state that "effective patient education is critical to the safe provision of infusion therapy and in reducing the risk for infusion related complications." The patient is responsible for

Continued

living day to day with the CVAD and is likely to be participating in self-infusion of prescribed medications.

In terms of catheter management, patients need to learn how to check their catheter site daily for any signs of complications and to flush, lock, and maintain the patency of their catheter. When considering site care and dressing changes, it may or may not be appropriate to teach these procedures. If the patient has a tunneled catheter, site management is usually taught, and, as discussed earlier, regular site care and dressings may not be necessary. With implanted ports, in some cases patients will learn how to self-access the port. Although this is less common, patients who have lifelong needs for infusion therapy, such as factor replacement for hemophilia or frequent and ongoing needs for I.V. antibiotics as occurs with cystic fibrosis, often desire complete independence in their care and the advantages of a completely implanted device in between infusion needs.

For patients with a PICC, most often the home care nurse will see the patient on a weekly basis. Teaching family members PICC site care is not recommended, especially when a stabilization device is being used. There is risk of catheter dislodgement when dressings and stabilization devices are removed and replaced. A weekly visit also allows for a thorough assessment of the VAD. As stated earlier, the use of chlorhexidine dressings in home care is not consistent. The research for such dressings supports their use with short-term catheters. For long-term catheter placement, the entry of microbes via the catheter hub/needleless connector is of concern. Continued attention to disinfection of the needleless connector is critical, and consideration for the use of alcohol caps is warranted. Between scheduled home care visits, it is critical to provide patients with education addressing what symptoms to report, when and who to report them to, and the necessary telephone numbers (Gorski, 2010). Use clear and simple terms, for example: "Call your home care nurse right away if you have pain, redness, or swelling where the PICC enters your skin or if you have a fever above 100°F, chills, or weakness."

 Patient Education

Patient instructions for CVADs should include:
- Type of CVAD, purpose and description of the device
- Proper care of the device
- Precautions aimed at infection prevention and other complications, including aseptic technique and hand hygiene
- Signs and symptoms to report, such as increased temperature, discomfort, or pain
- Making sure all health-care providers use proper infection prevention methods when accessing the CVAD
- Emergency measures for clamping the catheter if it breaks (INS, 2011a, p. S16)

■ Nursing Process

The nursing process is a six-step process for problem-solving to guide nursing action (see Chapter 1 for details on the steps of the nursing process related to vascular access). The following table focuses on nursing diagnoses, nursing outcomes classification (NOC), and nursing interventions classification (NIC) for patients with central vascular access. Nursing diagnoses should be patient specific and outcomes and interventions individualized. The NOC and NIC presented here are suggested directions for development of specific outcomes and interventions.

Nursing Diagnoses Related to Central Venous Access	Nursing Outcomes Classification (NOC)	Nursing Interventions Classification (NIC)
Protection, ineffective related to: Treatments: Placement of CVAD	Health-promoting behavior; endurance	Infection prevention
Infection, risk for related to: Inadequate primary defenses (broken skin, traumatized tissue); inadequate secondary defenses (decreased hemoglobin, leukopenia); increased environmental exposure to pathogens through I.V. equipment	Infection control, risk control, risk detection	Infection control practices and infection protection
Skin integrity impaired related to: External: VAD; medications Internal: irritation for I.V. solution; inflammation; infection	Tissue integrity: Primary intention healing of VAD insertion site	Incision site care, skin surveillance; risk identification
Body image disturbance related to: Biophysical: Illness treatment: VAD	Body image, self-esteem, acceptance of health status, coping, identity	Body image enhancement
Knowledge deficit related to: Unfamiliarity with information resources (CVAD and information provided)	Knowledge of treatment regimen	Teaching: Disease process and CVC care and maintenance
Interrupted family processes related to: Shift in health status of a family member	Family coping; role performance	Family process maintenance, family therapy, normalization promotion, role enhancement, support system enhancement
Anxiety (mild, moderate, and severe) related to: Threat to change in health status or misconception regarding therapy; unmet needs	Anxiety level; coping	Anxiety reduction

Sources: Ackley & Ladwig 2011; Bulechek, Butcher, Dochterman & Wagner, 2013; Moorhead, Johnson, Maas, & Swanson, 2013.

Chapter Highlights

- Nurses must have knowledge of venous anatomy prior to initiation of, and care and maintenance of central lines.
- The decision to place a CVAD is based on a thorough assessment that includes patient health problems; patient's vascular integrity; type of prescribed infusion therapy; anticipated duration of I.V. therapy; and patient's needs/preferences with lifestyle.
- The tip of CVADs should be in the lower SVC.
- Nurses should be knowledgeable regarding CVAD features such as the type of catheter material, antimicrobial properties, presence of valves, lumen types, and power injectability.
- The central line insertion bundle is followed with CVAD insertion; this includes a checklist to ensure that all procedures are properly followed during the insertion. If there is a breach, the procedure is stopped and restarted correctly.
- Although there are no specific limitations to CVAD dwell time, when selecting a device, the following are guidelines for choosing a specific type of CVAD:
  - Nontunneled percutaneous catheters: Days to weeks, primarily in acute care settings
  - PICCs: Days to months, usually less than 1 year
  - Subcutaneously tunneled CVADs: Months to years
  - Implanted ports: Months to years
- After insertion of the central line, confirmation of proper tip location must be obtained before any infusion is administered.

Care and Maintenance Issues

- Regular site care and dressing changes are required. Site care for TSM dressings is performed at least every 7 days. Site care when using gauze dressings is at least every 2 days. The use of antimicrobial dressings on short-term catheters is associated with a decrease in risk for infection.
- Only 10 mL or larger syringes are used to flush central lines because excessive pressure from smaller-barreled syringes can damage or rupture the line.
- Nurses managing CVADs must be trained in their use; follow manufacturer guidelines; comply with agency protocols and policies; and be fully competent in the assessment, planning, intervention, and evaluation of the patient.
- Use luer-lock connections on all VADs.
- All CVADs are flushed with 0.9% sodium chloride to establish patency and between medications/solutions to prevent precipitation
- Unused lumens of CVADs are locked to maintain patency between infusions. Locking solutions include low-concentration heparin and

saline (valved catheters). Alternative solutions are considered for patients with a history of heparin-induced thrombocytopenia or frequent bloodstream infections. INS (2008b) flushing protocols are presented in Tables 8-3 and 8-4.

■ Needleless connectors must be disinfected properly before each use. Special products such as alcohol caps may be used.

■ Competency needs to be demonstrated by the nurse for accessing and deaccessing implanted ports.

■■ Thinking Critically: Case Study

As a new graduate, you have been asked to change a complicated abdominal dressing on a patient postoperatively. This patient is receiving chemotherapy via a tunneled catheter. As you are cutting off the dressing, you accidentally puncture the catheter.

Case Study Questions
1. *What do you do?*
2. *How could this have been avoided?*

Media Link: Answers to the case study and more critical thinking activities are provided on DavisPlus.

Post-Test

1. Assessment before consideration of CVAD placement in a patient should include which of the following? (*Select all that apply.*)
   a. Vascular integrity
   b. Expected duration of therapy
   c. Patient preference related to lifestyle
   d. Health history

2. An indication for placement of a CVAD is:
   a. Medication with a pH of 5
   b. Medication with a pH of 12
   c. Solution with an osmolarity of 500 mOsm/L
   d. Solution with an osmolarity of 300 mOsm/L

3. Maximal sterile barrier precautions implemented with CVAD insertion include wearing:
   a. A mask, sterile gloves, a gown, and foot covers
   b. A cap, a mask, a sterile gown, and sterile gloves
   c. Sterile gloves, a gown, and foot covers
   d. A mask and sterile gloves

4. The most desirable vein for PICC insertion is the:
   a. Cephalic
   b. Basilic
   c. Brachial
   d. Median cubital

5. An advantage to the subcutaneously tunneled catheter is:
   a. Low cost
   b. Improved body image
   c. Ease of removal by the nurse
   d. Decreased risk for bloodstream infection

6. An important risk associated with the procedure of CVAD removal is:
   a. Bloodstream infection
   b. Catheter-associated venous thrombosis
   c. Nerve damage
   d. Air embolism

7. Implanted ports, when not in use, are locked:
   a. Monthly
   b. Weekly
   c. Every 3 weeks
   d. Every 2 months

8. Advantages of the TSM dressing include:
   a. It is changed every 3 days.
   b. It is easier to visualize site.
   c. It covers up any perspiration.
   d. Patient preference

9. Chlorhexidine-impregnated dressings should be considered for use:
   a. In organizations with high infection rates
   b. On all subcutaneously tunneled CVADs
   c. On all PICCs
   d. With home care patients

10. Potential risks associated with withdrawal of blood through the CVAD include:
    a. Patient anxiety
    b. Increased risk for catheter occlusion
    c. Patient dissatisfaction
    d. Catheter dislodgement

Media Link: Answers to the Chapter 8 Post-Test and more test questions together with rationales are provided on Davis*Plus*.

■ References

Ackley, B. J., & Ladwig, G. B. (2011). *Nursing diagnosis handbook: An evidence-based guide to planning care* (9th ed.). St. Louis, MO: Mosby Elsevier.

Agency for Healthcare Research and Quality (AHRQ). (2013). Making health care safer II: An updated critical analysis of the evidence for patient safety practices—Executive report. Retrieved from www.ahrq.gov/research/findings/evidence-based-reports/ptsafetysum.html (Accessed March 29, 2013).

Alexandrou, E., Murgo, M., Calabria, E., Spencer, T. R., Carpen, H., Brennan, K., ... Hillman, K. M. (2012). Nurse-led central venous catheter insertion: Review of 760 procedures performed across three hospitals reveals a low rate of complications. *International Journal of Nursing Studies 49*, 162-168.

American Nephrology Nurses Association. (2009). Position statement: Vascular Access for Hemodialysis. Retrieved from http://www.annanurse.org/sites/default/files/download/reference/health/position/vascAccess.pdf (Accessed March 21, 2013).

American Nephrology Nurses Association. (2013). Vascular access fact sheet. Retrieved from http://www.annanurse.org/download/reference/practice/vascularAccessFactSheet.pdf (Accessed March 21, 2013).

Bulechek, G. M., Butcher, H. K., Dochterman, J. M., & Wagner, C. M. (2013). *Nursing interventions classification (NIC)* (6th ed.). St. Louis, MO: Mosby Elsevier.

Bullock-Corkhill, M. (2010). Central venous access devices: access and insertion. In M. Alexander, A., Corrigan, L. Gorski, J. Hankins, & R. Perucca (Eds.), *Infusion nursing: An evidence-based practice* (3rd ed.) (pp. 480-494). St. Louis: Saunders/Elsevier.

Chopra, V., Flanders, S. A., & Saint, S. (2012). The problem with peripherally inserted central catheters. *Journal of the American Medical Association, 308*(15), 1527-1528.

Chopra, V., Anand, S., Hickner, A., Buist, M., Rogers, M. A., Saint, S., & Flanders, S. A. (2013). Risk of venous thromboembolism associated with peripherally inserted central catheters: A systematic review and meta-analysis. *Lancet, 382*(9889) 311-325.

Cohen, L .L. (2008). Behavioral approaches to anxiety and pain management for pediatric venous access. *Pediatrics, 122*, S134-S139.

Drake, R. L., Vogl, W., & Mitchell, A. W. M. (2010). Gray's anatomy for students (2nd ed). Philadelphia: Churchill Livingstone Elsevier.

Food and Drug Administration. (2013). Reminders from FDA regarding ruptured vascular access devices from power injection. Retrieved from http://www.fda.gov/MedicalDevices/Safety/AlertsandNotices/TipsandArticleson DeviceSafety/ucm070193.htm (Accessed March 23, 2013).

Frey, A. M., & Pettit, J. (2010). Infusion therapy in children. In M. Alexander, A., Corrigan, L. Gorski, J. Hankins, & R. Perucca (Eds.), *Infusion nursing: An evidence-based practice* (3rd ed.) (pp. 550-570). St. Louis: Saunders/Elsevier.

Gorski, L. A. (2010). Central venous access device associated infections: Current evidence & recommendations. *Home Healthcare Nurse, 28*(4): 221-227.

Gorski, L., Perucca, R., & Hunter, M. (2010). Central venous access devices: care, maintenance, and potential complications. In M. Alexander, A. Corrigan,

L.Gorski, J. Hankins, & R. Perucca (Eds.), *Infusion nursing: An evidence-based practice* (3rd ed.) (pp. 495-515). St. Louis: Saunders/Elsevier.

Hadaway, L. (2010). Infusion therapy equipment. In M. Alexander, A. Corrigan, L. Gorski, J. Hankins, & R. Perucca (Eds.), *Infusion nursing: An evidence-based practice* (3rd ed.) (pp. 391-436). St. Louis: Saunders/Elsevier.

Hadaway, L., Dalton, L., & Mercanti-Erieg, L. (2013). Infusion teams in acute care hospitals: Call for a business approach. Retrieved from http://www.ins1. org/files/public/05_13_Infusion_Teams_White_Paper.pdf (Accessed June 1, 2013).

Harnage, S. (2012). Seven years of zero central-line associated bloodstream infections. *British Journal of Nursing, 21*(21), S6, S8, S10-S12.

Infusion Nurses Society (INS). (2008a). *Position paper: The role of the registered nurse in the insertion of external jugular peripherally inserted central catheters (EJ PICC) and external jugular peripheral intravenous catheter (EJ PIV).* Norwood, MA: Author.

INS. (2008b). *Flushing protocols.* Norwood, MA: Author.

INS. (2011a). Infusion nursing standards of practice. *Journal of Intravenous Nursing, 34*(1S), S1–S110.

INS. (2011b). *Policies and procedures for infusion nursing* (4th ed.). Norwood, MA: Author.

Knue, M., Doellman, D., Rabin, K., & Jacobs, B. R. (2005). The efficacy and safety of blood sampling through peripherally inserted central catheter devices in children. *Journal of Infusion Nursing, 28*(1), 3–35.

Maiefski, M., Rupp, M. E., & Hermsen, E. D. (2009). Ethanol lock technique: Review of the literature. *Infection Control and Hospital Epidemiology, 30*(11), 1096-1108.

Maiocco, G. & Coole, C. (2012). Use of ultrasound guidance for peripheral intravenous placement in difficult-to-access patients. *Journal of Nursing Care Quality, 27*(1), 51-55.

Moorhead, S., Johnson, M., Maas, M., & Swanson, E. (2013). *Nursing outcomes classification (NOC)* (5th ed.). St. Louis, MO: Mosby Elsevier.

Nifong, T. P., & McDevitt, T. J. (2011). The effect of catheter to vein ratio on blood flow rates in a simulated model of peripherally inserted central venous catheters. *Chest, 140* (1), 48-53.

O'Grady, N. P., Alexander, M., Burns, L. A., Dellinger, E. P., Garland, J., Heard, S. O., ... Healthcare Practices Advisory Committee (HICPAC). (2011). Guide-lines for the prevention of intravascular catheter-related infections, 2011. *Am J Infect Control, 39*(4 Suppl): S1-S34. Also available at http://www. cdc.gov/hicpac/pdf/guidelines/bsi-guidelines-2011.pdf (Accessed September 15, 2012).

Pedivan. (2010). *Best practice guidelines in the care and maintenance of pediatric central venous catheters.* Herrman, UT: Association for Vascular Access.

Richardson, J., & Tjoelker, R. (2012). Beyond the central line-associated bloodstream infection bundle: The value of the clinical nurse specialist in continuing evidence-based practice changes. *Clinical Nurse Specialist, 26*(4), 205-211.

The Joint Commission. (2013). National patient safety goals. Retrieved from http://www.jointcommission.org/standards_information/npsgs.aspx (Accessed March 23, 2013).

Timsit, J. F., Schwebel, C., Bouadma, L., Geffroy, A., Garrouste-Orgeas, M., Pease S., ... Dressing Study Group. (2009). Chlorhexidine-impregnated sponge and less frequent dressing changes for prevention of catheter-related infections in critically ill adults. *Journal of the American Medical Association, 301*(12), 1231-1241.

Timsit, J. F., Mimoz, O., Mourvillier, B., Souweine, B., Garrouste-Orgeas, M., Alfandari, S., ... Lucet, J. C. (2012). Randomized controlled trial of chlorhexidine dressing and highly adhesive dressing for preventing catheter-related infections in critically ill adults. *American Journal of Respiratory Critical Care Medicine, 186*(12), 1272-1278.

PROCEDURES DISPLAY 8-1

Central Vascular Access Device Dressing Change

Equipment Needed
CVAD dressing kit, which should include sterile gloves, mask, sterile drape, transparent semipermeable membrane (TSM) dressing, antiseptic solution applicators (chlorhexidine alcohol preferred)
Clean gloves
Stabilization device
Single use measuring tape

Delegation
Do not delegate to an LPN/LVN or nursing assistive personnel (NAP) unless it is part of the state nursing practice for LPN/LVN and is included in the policies and procedures for the institution. All nurses require education and competency training for CVAD care and maintenance.

Procedure	Rationale
1. Verify authorized prescriber's order and organizational procedure.	1. A written order is a legal requirement for infusion therapy. Policies and procedures provide a framework for standard of care at the institution.
2. Introduce yourself to the patient.	2. Establishes the nurse–patient relationship
3. Verify patient's identity using two forms of identification.	3. Patient safety.
4. Perform hand hygiene.	4. Single most important means of infection prevention.

Continued

PROCEDURES DISPLAY 8-1

Central Vascular Access Device Dressing Change—*cont'd*

Procedure	Rationale
5. Place sterile barrier on clean surface and open CVAD dressing kit; open stabilization device and drop onto barrier.	5. Ensures adherence to aseptic technique during site care procedure
6. Place patient in comfortable, reclining position, ensuring that site is accessible.	6. Promotes cooperation with the procedure and facilitates your ability to perform the procedure.
7. Put on mask and clean gloves (mask should be on top of sterile supplies in CVAD dressing kit).	7. Standard precautions.
8. Remove existing transparent dressing by slowly loosening it at the distal end while anchoring catheter to skin.	8. Prevents accidental dislodgement or removal of nontunneled catheter
9. Remove stabilization device per manufacturer's directions.	9. The stabilization device is removed and replaced at least every 7 days.
10. Inspect site for signs and symptoms of site infection. If present, notify the LIP.	10. Identifies complications associated with the CVAD
11. Measure and verify that external catheter length corresponds to initial placement measurement. If it does not, notify the LIP before continuing use.	11. Identifies any external catheter migration; significant migration means that catheter tip may no longer be located in the superior vena cava (SVC)
12. Remove gloves and perform hand hygiene.	12. Infection prevention
13. Don sterile gloves.	13. Aseptic technique.
14. Perform skin antisepsis. a. Chlorhexidine solution: Apply using back-and-forth motion for at least 30 seconds (preferred).	14. Ensures proper and thorough cleansing, skin antisepsis, and removal of debris. Reduces microbial growth around catheter insertion site.

PROCEDURES DISPLAY 8-1

Central Vascular Access Device Dressing Change—*cont'd*

Procedure	Rationale
b. Povidone-iodine or 70% alcohol: Apply using swab sticks in a concentric circle beginning at the insertion site, moving outward. Note that povidone-iodine must remain on the skin for at least 2 minutes or longer to dry completely for adequate skin antisepsis.	
c. *Note:* The prepped site will be approximately the size of the dressing (2–4 inches).	
15. Apply new stabilization device according to manufacturer's directions.	**15.** Reduces risk of catheter dislodgement
16. Apply a new transparent dressing over the exposed catheter, including the hub.	**16.** Occlusive dressing required for CVAD to inhibit entry of microorganisms
17. Remove gloves and discard; dispose of all used materials. Perform hand hygiene.	**17.** Infection prevention
18. Label dressing with the nurse's initials, date and time.	**18.** Maintains proper documentation and communicates dressing change information to all who care for the patient
19. Document the procedure in the patient's permanent record, including assessment data, condition of the removed dressing, appropriate intervention data, and evaluation of patient's response to the procedure.	Maintains a legal record and communication with the health-care team

Reference: INS (2011b).

PROCEDURES DISPLAY 8-2

Flushing a Central Venous Catheter

Equipment Needed

Prefilled syringe of 0.9% sodium chloride

Prefilled syringe of heparinized saline (if ordered; nonvalved CVADs)

Antiseptic solution: 70% alcohol or chlorhexidine/alcohol

Delegation

This procedure can be delegated to an LPN/LVN who is specially trained in I.V. therapy depending on the state nurse practice act for initiation of infusion therapy and agency policies and procedures. This cannot be delegated to nursing assistive personnel.

Procedure	Rationale
1. Verify authorized prescriber's order for flushing and organizational procedure.	1. A written order is a legal requirement for infusion therapy.
2. Introduce yourself to the patient.	2. Establishes the nurse–patient relationship
3. Verify the patient's identity using two forms of identification.	3. Patient safety
4. Perform hand hygiene.	4. Single most important means of infection prevention.
5. Identify whether the needleless connector is a negative-displacement device, a positive-displacement device, or a neutral-displacement device (see note under Step 10 below).	5. Flushing technique varies based on category.
6. Don gloves if according to organizational procedure; gloves not required as long as aseptic technique is followed (i.e., maintain sterility of syringe tip and no-touch to needleless connector after disinfection procedure).	6. Prevents bacterial entry into the infusion system; standard precautions

PROCEDURES DISPLAY 8-2

Flushing a Central Venous Catheter—*cont'd*

Procedure	Rationale
7. Disinfect the needleless connector with 70% isopropyl alcohol using a scrubbing motion and allow to dry. Most organizations require at least a 15-second scrub. There are also alternative specially designed scrub products that require less scrubbing time. This step may be eliminated if a protective alcohol cap has been in place over needleless connector (see Chapter 5).	7. Critical step in infection prevention. Disinfects and reduces risk for intraluminal introduction of microbes.
8. Attach prefilled syringe of 0.9% preservative-free sodium chloride to the needleless connector.	8. Maintains patency of catheter
9. Slowly pull back on syringe plunger until able to aspirate blood.	9. Confirms catheter patency
10. Flush catheter with 0.9% sodium chloride followed by heparinized saline, if ordered.	10. Maintains patency of catheter and prevents occlusion. Valved CVADs require saline only for catheter locking.

Note: There are different types of NIS devices. Be sure you know which devices are used in your facility.

a. *For negative-displacement devices:* Flush all solution into the catheter lumen, maintain force on the syringe plunger as a clamp on the catheter or extension set is closed, then disconnect the syringe.	a. Manufacturer requires "positive pressure" flushing technique to prevent reflux of blood.

Continued

PROCEDURES DISPLAY 8-2

Flushing a Central Venous Catheter—*cont'd*

Procedure	Rationale
b. *For positive-displacement device:* Flush all solution into the catheter lumen, disconnect the syringe, then close the catheter clamp.	**b.** Catheter is clamped *after* disconnection of the syringe.
c. *For neutral-displacement device:* Flush all solution into the catheter lumen; it does not matter if the catheter clamp is closed before or after the flush procedure.	**c.** Clamping sequence does not matter.
11. Document the procedure on the patient record.	**11.** Maintains a legal record and communication with the health-care team

Sources: INS (2011a, 2011b).

PROCEDURES DISPLAY 8-3

Blood Sampling from a Central Vascular Access Device (CVAD)

Equipment Needed

Clean gloves

Blood tubes for ordered tests

Vacutainer/Luer adapter device

Alcohol wipes or other disinfectant used by organization

Appropriate number of empty 10-mL syringes (if vacuum system is not used)

Two or three prefilled syringes of 10 mL preservative-free 0.9% sodium chloride

Heparin syringe, if ordered

Biohazard container

PROCEDURES DISPLAY 8-3

Blood Sampling from a Central Vascular Access Device (CVAD)—*cont'd*

Needleless connector (if organizational policy requires replacement after blood withdrawal)

Delegation
Most institutions do not have phlebotomists draw blood from a central line. This procedure cannot be delegated to an LPN/LVN or NAP. The practitioner needs competency training for central venous access care and maintenance.

Procedure	Rationale
1. Verify the LIP order for laboratory work.	1. A written order is a legal requirement for blood collection.
2. Introduce yourself to the patient.	2. Establishes the nurse–patient relationship
3. Verify patient identity using two forms of identification.	3. Patient safety
4. Perform hand hygiene.	4. Single most important means of infection prevention.
5. Gather and organize needed supplies; verify the correct blood collection tubes and line them up in appropriate sequence for obtaining blood.	5. Saves time and prevents interruption during the blood draw
6. Don gloves.	6. Standard precautions
7. If CVAD is locked (i.e., no active infusion): Disinfect needleless connector with alcohol for 15 seconds using a twisting motion; allow to dry. (*Note:* If drawing blood for blood cultures, the needleless connector is changed prior to blood draw; see procedure in Chapter 2).	7. Prevents introduction of microorganisms into the system

Continued

PROCEDURES DISPLAY 8-3

Blood Sampling from a Central Vascular Access Device (CVAD)—*cont'd*

Procedure	Rationale

8. If CVAD is in use (i.e., active infusion)
  a. Single-lumen:
    i. Stop infusion.
    ii. Close catheter clamp.
    iii. Disconnect administration set tubing from catheter hub/needleless connector.
    iv. Place sterile cap on the end of the administration set.
    v. Disinfect needleless connector with alcohol for 15 seconds using a. twisting motion; allow to dry.
  b. Multilumen:
    i. Stop all infusions.
    ii. Use the proximal lumen for blood withdrawal; if infusion running through lumen, follow steps i–v above.
	8. Prevents air entry into the circulation and thus risk for air embolism; prevents introduction of microorganisms into the system

9. Attach the 10-mL syringe of 0.9% sodium chloride, unclamp CVAD, flush CVAD, withdraw 4–5 mL of blood and discard into biohazard container.	9. Establishes catheter patency; reduces risk of inaccurate laboratory test results (e.g., elevated drug levels)
10. Disinfect needleless connector with alcohol for 15 seconds using a twisting motion; allow to dry.	10. Prevents introduction of microorganisms into the system

PROCEDURES DISPLAY 8-3

Blood Sampling from a Central Vascular Access Device (CVAD)—*cont'd*

Procedure	Rationale
11. Attach the vacuum container to the needleless connector.	
12. Insert each blood tube into the Vacutainer and allow to fill with blood in the correct sequence.	12. Obtains all required specimens
13. Disinfect needleless connector with alcohol for 15 seconds using a twisting motion; allow to dry.	13. Prevents introduction of microorganisms into the system
14. Attach the 10-mL syringe of 0.9% sodium chloride and flush CVAD.	14. Clears the CVAD of blood and reduces risk for thrombotic occlusion
15. Replace needleless connector if required by organizational policy; resume infusion as ordered or lock CVAD with prescribed heparin.	
16. Label all blood collection tubes with patient name, date and time, and your name/initials according to organizational policy; arrange for laboratory pickup or deliver blood collection tubes to the laboratory.	16. Prevents clerical errors and ensures the correct lab sample is for that particular patient
17. Dispose of used supplies in biohazard container.	17. Prevents exposure to bloodborne pathogens
18. Document the procedure in the patient's permanent record.	18. Maintains a legal record and communication with the health-care team

Sources: INS (2011a, 2011b).

PROCEDURES DISPLAY 8-4

Discontinuation of a Short-Term Vascular Access Device (Nontunneled Catheter or Peripherally Inserted Central Catheter)

Note: If a culture of the catheter tip is ordered, see Chapter 2 Procedures Display.

Equipment Needed
Gloves
Suture removal set, if appropriate
CVAD dressing kit

Delegation
This procedure **cannot** be delegated to an LPN/LVN or NAP. The practitioner needs competency training for central venous access care and maintenance.

Procedure	Rationale
1. Confirm authorized prescriber order for removal of the PICC or nontunneled catheter.	1. An order is required for discontinuation of a CVAD.
2. Introduce yourself to the patient.	2. Establishes the nurse–patient relationship
3. Verify the patient's identity using two forms of identification.	3. Patient safety
4. Elevate the bed.	4. Conducive to a successful procedure and prevents back injury to the practitioner
5. Position the patient in supine position.	5. Reduces risk for air embolism during catheter removal
6. Perform hand hygiene.	6. Single most important means of infection prevention.
7. Don gloves.	7. Standard precautions.
8. Discontinue infusion.	8. The infusion must be discontinued before removal of the catheter.

PROCEDURES DISPLAY 8-4

Discontinuation of a Short-Term Vascular Access Device (Nontunneled Catheter or Peripherally Inserted Central Catheter)—*cont'd*

Procedure	Rationale
9. Close the slide clamp on the CVAD.	9. The CVAD is no longer needed for therapy.
10. Remove the dressing and securement device and discard.	10. Removal is to be done in a manner that will not compromise the skin and cannula exit site.
11. Remove gloves and perform hand hygiene.	11. Infection prevention
12. Open central line kit and don fresh gloves.	12. Prepares for procedure; aseptic technique
13. Cleanse insertion site with chlorhexidine/alcohol or other acceptable skin antiseptic.	13. Removes any contaminants on or around the exit site that could migrate into the CVC removal site and cause contamination after the catheter is removed
14. Carefully clip and remove any sutures (if present).	14. Allows catheter removal
15. Ask patient to perform Valsalva maneuver during procedure, unless contraindicated (e.g., recent myocardial infarction, glaucoma)	15. Reduces risk of air embolism during removal
16. Place the 4 × 4 gauze over the CVAD site and hold it in place with the nondominant hand.	16. Prevents air embolism
17. Withdraw the CVAD from the vein in one smooth, steady motion; continue to hold the 4 × 4 gauze over the site. (**Do not pull** if resistance met.)	17. Reduces risk of catheter breakage and potential catheter embolism.

Continued

PROCEDURES DISPLAY 8-4

Discontinuation of a Short-Term Vascular Access Device (Nontunneled Catheter or Peripherally Inserted Central Catheter)—*cont'd*

Procedure	Rationale
18. Maintain firm pressure over the exit site until bleeding stops or for a minimum of 30 seconds.	
19. Cover the site with petroleum gauze and sterile occlusive dressing.	19. Prevents postremoval air embolism
20. Instruct the patient to remain in a recumbent position for 30 minutes.	20. Prevents postremoval air embolism
21. Leave the pressure dressing in place for 24 hours.	21. Prevents bleeding.
22. Inspect integrity of the removed CVAD. Compare length of catheter to original insertion length.	22. Ensures entire catheter has been removed
23. Dispose of all equipment in biohazard container and perform hand hygiene.	23. Prevents the spread of microorganisms
24. Document the patient's response to CVAD removal, appearance of the site, dressing regimen, condition and length of catheter, and any interventions implemented.	24. Maintains a legal record and communication with the health-care team

PROCEDURES DISPLAY 8-5

Accessing an Implanted Port

Equipment Needed
CVAD dressing kit, which should include sterile gloves, mask, sterile drape, transparent semipermeable membrane (TSM) dressing, antiseptic solution applicators (chlorhexidine alcohol preferred)
Needleless connector
Noncoring needle with extension set
Prefilled sterile syringe containing 10 mL of 0.9% sodium chloride
Chlorhexidine-impregnated foam dressing (depending on institutional policy)
Sharps container

Delegation
This procedure **cannot** be delegated to an LPN/LVN or nursing assistive personnel (NAP). The practitioner needs competency training for CVAD care and maintenance.

Pre-Procedure
Assess patient tolerance of procedure and evaluate for need for local anesthetic to reduce pain during needle insertion. For example, if using an anesthetic cream, it must be placed on the site approximately 60 minutes prior to access.

Procedure	Rationale
1. Confirm authorized prescriber's order and organizational procedure.	1. A written order is required. Organizational procedures should be followed.
2. Introduce yourself to the patient.	2. Establishes the nurse–patient relationship
3. Verify the patient's identity using two forms of identification.	3. Patient safety
4. Perform hand hygiene.	4. Single most important means of infection prevention
5. Elevate the bed level.	5. Conducive to successful access and prevents back injury to the practitioner
6. Position the patient either in a comfortable reclining position or in a chair with a pillow behind the shoulder.	6. Provides comfort for the patient and access to the port

Continued

PROCEDURES DISPLAY 8-5

Accessing an Implanted Port—*cont'd*

Procedure	Rationale
7. Palpate the area of the port.	7. Locates the port septum and increases success with port access
8. Instruct the patient to turn head away from the port site.	8. Prevents introduction of microorganisms
9. Place sterile barrier on clean surface and open CVAD dressing kit; open and drop sterile syringe, noncoring needle/extension set, and needleless connector onto sterile barrier.	9. Ensures adherence to aseptic technique during the procedure
10. Put on mask and sterile gloves; attach needleless connector to noncoring needle/extension set and prime with 0.9% sodium chloride to purge all of the air.	10. Adherence to aseptic technique; infection prevention.
11. Perform skin antisepsis by applying chlorhexidine/alcohol solution using back-and-forth scrubbing motion for at least 30 seconds.	11. Skin antisepsis is a critical step in reducing the risk for bloodstream infection.
12. Using nondominant hand to palpate and stabilize port.	12. Locates the correct position of the port septum.
13. Insert the noncoring needle perpendicular to the septum, pushing firmly through skin and septum until the needle tip contacts the back of the port (gripper style device should lie flush with the skin).	13. Accesses the port correctly

PROCEDURES DISPLAY 8-5

Accessing an Implanted Port—*cont'd*

Procedure	Rationale
14. Aspirate for blood return to confirm patency; flush with the attached 10 mL of 0.9% sodium chloride.	14. Verifies correct needle placement and patency of the port

15. If the port is to remain accessed:
  a. Stabilize noncoring needle with sterile tape; place sterile gauze to support wings if needed, making sure gauze does not obscure needle site.
  b. Cover the needle and gauze with TSM dressing.
  c. Initiate the prescribed therapy.
	15. Protect accessed port site and reduces risk of needle dislodgement.

16. If a port is to be used for intermittent infusion therapy, flush using heparin for final locking method.	

17. Document in the patient record:
  ■ Size/length of noncoring needle
  ■ Site assessment/type of dressing
  ■ Date and time of access
  ■ Presence of blood return, ease of flushing
  ■ Anesthetic methods, if used
  ■ Patient tolerance of the procedure
	17. Maintains a legal record and communication with the health-care team

Source: INS (2011b).

PROCEDURES DISPLAY 8-6

Deaccessing an Implanted Port

Needed equipment
Gloves
Sterile gauze dressing
Alcohol swabs
10 mL of sodium chloride
Two 10-mL prefilled saline syringes
10-mL syringe for 5 mL of 100 units/mL heparin
Occlusive dressing

Delegation
This procedure **cannot** be delegated to LVN/LPN or NAP. The practitioner needs competency training for central venous access care and maintenance.

Procedure	Rationale
To deaccess the needle from the port:	
1. Introduce yourself to the patient.	1. Establishes the nurse–patient relationship
2. Verify patient identity using two forms of ID.	2. Patient safety
3. Perform hand hygiene.	3. Single most important means of infection prevention
4. Put on gloves.	4. Standard precautions.
5. Disinfect the needleless connector with 70% isopropyl alcohol using a scrubbing motion and allow to dry.	5. Critical step in infection prevention
6. Attach syringe of 0.9% sodium chloride to needleless connector and flush the port.	6. Maintains the integrity of the port and prevents occlusions
7. Attach syringe of prescribed heparin and lock the port follow flushing guidelines for positive-displacement devices and negative-displacement devices.	7. Maintain patency of port between infusions.

PROCEDURES DISPLAY 8-6

Deaccessing an Implanted Port—*cont'd*

Procedure	Rationale
8. Palpate the port with nondominant hand and stabilize with thumb and index finger.	8. Reduces discomfort with deaccess procedure
9. Grasp needle with dominant hand and remove device, engaging safety mechanism.	9. Reduces risk of needlestick injury
10. Apply gauze pressure dressing to site if bleeding occurs.	10. Covers the puncture site to prevent infection
11. Discard the needle in biohazard container; remove gloves and perform hand hygiene.	11. OSHA guidelines to prevent needlestick injuries; infection control procedure
12. Document in the patient record: ■ Date and time of deaccess, gauge and length of needle ■ Presence of blood return, ease of flushing ■ Assessment of port site ■ Patient tolerance of the procedure	12. Maintains a legal record and communication with the health-care team

Source: INS (2011b).

Chapter **9**

Complications of Infusion Therapy: Peripheral and Central Vascular Access Devices

The most important practical lesson that can be given to nurses is to teach them what to observe—how to observe—what symptoms indicate improvement— what the reverse—which are of importance—which are of none—which are the evidence of neglect—and of what kind of neglect.
—*Florence Nightingale, 1859*

Chapter Contents

▪ **LEARNING** *On completion of this chapter, the reader will be able to:*
OBJECTIVES
1. Define terms related to the complications of peripheral and central vascular access devices.
2. Differentiate between local and systemic complications.
3. Identify six local complications.
4. Describe preventative interventions for local complications.
5. Document relevant information related to vascular access device-related complications.
6. List three risk factors for phlebitis.
7. Apply the Infusion Nurses Society (INS) phlebitis scale in rating the level of phlebitis.
8. Apply the INS infiltration scale in rating the degree of infiltration.
9. Describe evidence-based interventions shown to decrease risk for bloodstream infections.
10. Identify risk factors and potential consequences of circulatory overload.
11. Identify preventative interventions for the four systemic complications.
12. Identify complications and risks associated with central vascular access devices.

▧ GLOSSARY

Air embolism (venous air embolism) A sudden obstruction of a blood vessel caused by air introduced into the circulation

Catheter malposition Position of the central vascular access device tip outside the superior vena cava

Catheter occlusion Inability to infuse or inject fluid into a catheter; inability to aspirate blood from a catheter

Circulatory overload Increased blood volume, often caused by transfusions or excessive I.V. fluid administration

Ecchymosis A bruise; a "black and blue spot" on the skin caused by escape of blood from injured vessels

Embolism A sudden obstruction of a blood vessel by a clot or foreign material formed or introduced elsewhere in the circulatory system and carried to the point of obstruction by the bloodstream

Extravasation Escape of a vesicant medication/solution from the vein into the surrounding tissue

Fibrin sheath   A covering over a catheter formed by the action of thrombin on fibrinogen; the fibrin sheath can potentially grow and cover the entire catheter, potentially leading to catheter occlusion

Hematoma   A swelling comprising a mass of blood confined to subcutaneous tissue caused by break in a blood vessel

Hemothorax   Blood in the pleural cavity caused by rupture of blood vessels

Infiltration   Escape of a nonvesicant medication/solution from the vein into the surrounding tissue

Phlebitis   Inflammation of the inner layer (tunica intima) of a vein

Pinch-off syndrome   Central venous catheter placed via the subclavian vein compressed by the clavicle and the first rib; results in mechanical occlusion

Pneumothorax   The presence of air or gas in the pleural cavity between the lung and chest wall

Pulmonary edema   Accumulation of extravascular fluid in lung tissues and alveoli

Septicemia   The presence of pathogenic microorganisms in the blood

Speed shock   A systemic reaction that occurs when a substance is rapidly introduced into the circulation

Superior vena cava syndrome   Condition caused by an obstruction of blood flow through the superior vena cava

Thrombophlebitis   Venous inflammation with thrombus (clot) formation

Thrombosis   Formation or presence of a blood clot; clotting within a blood vessel that may cause interruption of blood flow

Venous spasm   Sudden constriction of the vein

Vesicant   Any medication or fluid capable of causing tissue injury, such as necrosis or tissue damage, when it escapes from the vein

Complications associated with peripheral intravenous (PIV) catheters and central vascular access devices (CVADs) are often classified according to their location. A local complication is usually seen at or near the insertion site or occurs as a result of mechanical failure. Systemic complications are those occurring within the vascular system. Systemic complications such as bloodstream infection (BSI), air embolism, and circulatory overload are very serious and can be life threatening.

■ Local Complications

Local complications of infusion therapy occur as adverse reactions or trauma to the surrounding venipuncture site. They can be recognized early by objective assessment. Assessing and monitoring are the key components of early intervention. Good venipuncture technique is one important factor related to the prevention of many local complications associated with vascular access device (VAD) placement. Local complications include hematoma, phlebitis/thrombophlebitis, infiltration/extravasation, local infection, nerve injury, and venous spasm.

Hematoma

Description and Etiology

The terms **hematoma** and **ecchymosis** are used to describe formations resulting from the infiltration of blood into the tissues at the venipuncture site. Loss of integrity in a vessel wall as a result of disease or trauma allows blood to escape into the surrounding area. This complication is often related to venipuncture technique. Patients who bruise easily can develop a hematoma from vein trauma during insertion of a large-gauge catheter used to initiate I.V. therapy. Patients receiving anticoagulant therapy and long-term steroid therapy are at particular risk for bleeding from vein trauma (Fig. 9-1).

A hematoma is caused more often by incorrect manipulation technique and rarely by spontaneous rupture of the vein. It may be caused by:
- Poor venipuncture technique in which the cannula passes through the distal vein wall
- Opening of the flow clamp for the infusion before the tourniquet is removed

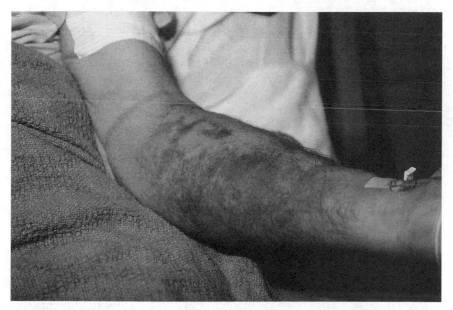

Figure 9-1 ▪ Hematoma. (Courtesy of Beth Fabian, CRNI.)

- A cannula too large for the vessel, resulting in rupture of the vein
- Pressure of the tourniquet to fragile skin

NOTE > To dilate veins in the older adult, use a blood pressure cuff or other techniques described in Chapter 6.

Signs and Symptoms

Signs and symptoms of hematoma include:
- Discoloration of the skin (i.e., ecchymoses) surrounding the venipuncture (immediate or slow)
- Site swelling and discomfort
- Inability to advance the cannula all the way into the vein during insertion
- Resistance to positive pressure during catheter flushing

Prevention

Techniques for prevention of hematoma formation include:

1. Use an indirect method rather than a direct approach for starting a PIV. This decreases the chance of piercing through the vein, which then causes seepage of blood into the subcutaneous tissue (see Chapter 6 for venipuncture techniques).
2. Use vein visualization techniques (see Chapters 5 and 6).
3. Apply the tourniquet just before venipuncture.
4. For older adult patients, patients taking corticosteroids, or patients with thin, fragile skin, use a small needle or catheter, preferably 22 or 24 gauge. Use a blood pressure cuff rather than a tourniquet to fill the vein so that you have better control of the pressure exerted on the vein; in some cases, it is best to avoid using a tourniquet.
5. Be very gentle when performing venipuncture.

 NURSING FAST FACT!

The presence of either ecchymoses or hematomas limits future use of the affected veins.

Treatment

1. Apply direct, light pressure using a sterile 2- × 2-inch gauze pad over the site for 2 to 3 minutes after catheter or needle removal.
2. Have the patient elevate the extremity on a pillow to maximize venous return.

3. Apply ice to the area to prevent further enlargement of the hematoma.

Documentation

Document presence of ecchymotic areas and nursing interventions.

Phlebitis/Thrombophlebitis

Description and Etiology

Phlebitis is an inflammation of the delicate inner lining (the tunica intima) of the vein. It is characterized by pain, inflammation, and tenderness along the vein and is a common complication associated with PIVs. Phlebitis may result in other complications such as **thrombosis** formation (**thrombophlebitis**) and potentially BSIs, although the link between phlebitis and BSIs is not well established (Hadaway, 2012; Zingg & Pittet, 2009).

Phlebitis is attributed to damage from chemical irritation, mechanical trauma, and bacteria. Chemical phlebitis results from infusate damage to the tunica intima. Certain characteristics of medications/solutions are associated with vein damage when they are administered via a PIV catheter (Infusion Nurses Society [INS], 2011a):

■ Dextrose content greater than 10%
■ Acidic or alkaline pH (i.e., <5 or >9)
■ High osmolarity (>600 mOsm/L)

Chemical damage to the vein may also result from failure to allow the skin antiseptic solution to fully dry prior to catheter insertion. Vein irritation results when the antiseptic is pulled into the vein during catheter insertion.

Mechanical vein trauma occurs when the catheter irritates or injures the endothelial cells lining the vein wall. This may occur during insertion, when a large catheter is placed in a small vein or at a point of flexion, or when a catheter lacks adequate stabilization, causing catheter movement that irritates the vein wall. During placement of a midline peripheral catheter or a peripherally inserted central catheter (PICC), mechanical phlebitis may result if the catheter is advanced too rapidly into the vein. Symptoms occur soon after placement and tend to be transient. Catheter removal is considered if the symptoms persist beyond 24 to 48 hours.

Bacteria can also cause phlebitis, and the consequences can be serious, including catheter-related bloodstream infection (CR-BSI). Bacteria may be introduced through poor aseptic technique during insertion or during catheter access or maintenance care. Phlebitis may not be evident during peripheral catheter dwell time but appear after removal. This is called "postinfusion phlebitis" and becomes apparent 48 to 96 hours after the catheter is removed. Types of phlebitis are summarized in Table 9-1.

> Table 9-1 | **TYPES OF PHLEBITIS**

Mechanical Phlebitis

Mechanical vein trauma occurs when the catheter irritates or injures the endothelial cells lining the vein wall. This may occur during insertion, when a large catheter is placed in a small vein or at a point of flexion, or when the catheter lacks adequate stabilization causing catheter movement that irritates the vein wall.

Chemical Phlebitis

Chemical phlebitis results from infusate damage to the tunica intima. Infusates with a dextrose content greater than 10%, an acidic or alkaline pH (i.e., <5 or >9), and a high osmolarity (>600 mOsm/L) cause vein damage when administered via a peripheral I.V. catheter. Also, failing to allow the antiseptic solution to fully dry prior to catheter insertion may cause irritation when antiseptic is pulled into the vein during insertion.

The type of catheter material may increase the risk of phlebitis. Several different materials are used in the manufacture of catheters. Catheters made of silicone elastomer and polyurethane have a smoother microsurface, are thermoplastic, are more hydrophilic, become more flexible than polytetrafluoroethylene (Teflon) at body temperature, and cause less venous irritation.

 NURSING FAST FACT!

Examples of three common I.V. solutions, and their pH and osmolarity:

Solution	pH	Osmolarity (mOsm/L)
5% dextrose in water	4.8	252
5% dextrose in water with 0.45% sodium chloride	4.6	406
0.9% sodium chloride	6.0	308

Bacterial Phlebitis

Bacteria can cause phlebitis, and the consequences can be serious, including catheter-related bloodstream infection. Bacteria may be introduced through poor aseptic technique during insertion, or during catheter access or maintenance care. Suppurative or purulent thrombophlebitis is characterized by the presence of purulent drainage in the vein. This serious complication is associated with bloodstream infection and requires surgical removal of the vein.

 NURSING FAST FACTS!

Hand hygiene is critical in preventing health-care–associated infections and thus bacterial phlebitis.

All equipment should be inspected for integrity, particulate matter, cloudiness, and any signs indicating a break in sterility.

When inspecting the venipuncture site, if the skin is noted to be visibly dirty, it should be washed with soap and water prior to skin antisepsis.

If there is excess hair at the site, hair can be clipped using a scissors or disposable head surgical clippers.

The skin should not be shaved because microabrasions from shaving may increase the risk of infection.

> Table 9-1	TYPES OF PHLEBITIS—cont'd

Postinfusion Phlebitis

Postinfusion phlebitis is associated with inflammation of the vein that usually becomes evident within 48–96 hours after the cannula has been removed, so the site should be monitored for that time period. On discharge, patients should be instructed on signs and symptoms of postinfusion phlebitis and who to contact if it occurs (INS, 2011a, p. S65).

Host factors that may also contribute to risk of phlebitis include fragile vessels, a predisposition toward thrombosis (hypercoagulable state), high hemoglobin levels, female gender, older age, and underlying medical disease (e.g., diabetes, infectious diseases, cancer, immunodeficiency) (Dychter, Gold, Carson, & Haller, 2012; Zingg & Pittet, 2009) (Table 9-2).

NOTE > Peripheral phlebitis can prolong hospitalization unless treated early.

INS Standard If phlebitis occurs, the nurse should determine the potential etiology of the phlebitis—chemical, mechanical, bacterial, or postinfusion phlebitis—and implement appropriate interventions for midline catheters and PICCs. Remove the short peripheral catheter (INS, 2011a, p. S65).

> Table 9-2	FACTORS INCREASING RISK FOR PHLEBITIS

1. Catheter material
   Teflon (less favorable thrombogenic properties)
2. Catheter size
   Larger-gauge catheters take up more space in the vein and allow less blood flow around catheter
3. Insertion factors
   Placed in emergency room/emergent situations
   Placed by inexperienced staff
   Placed in lower extremity
4. Increasing duration of catheter placement in adults
5. Infusate characteristics
   pH <5 or >9
   High osmolarity (>600 mOsm/L)
6. Host factors
   Fragile vessels
   Predisposition toward thrombosis (hypercoagulable state)
   High hemoglobin levels
   Female gender
   Older age
   Underlying medical disease (diabetes, infectious diseases, cancer, immunodeficiency, poor-quality peripheral veins)

Sources: Dychter et al. (2012); Zingg & Pittet, 2009.

Signs and Symptoms

Inspection of the affected site reveals a similar appearance regardless of the underlying cause (Fig. 9-2). Local signs and symptoms associated with phlebitis include:

- Redness at the site
- Site warm to touch
- Local swelling
- Palpable cord along the vein
- Sluggish infusion rate
- Possible fever

INS Standard The nurse should use a standardized phlebitis scale that is valid, reliable, and clinically feasible (see Table 9-3 for an example).

A clinically feasible calculation for the phlebitis rate is performing a point-prevalence study, which measures phlebitis at one point in time (INS, 2011a, p. S66):

$$\frac{\text{Number of phlebitis incidents} \times 100}{\text{Total number of PIV lines}} = \text{Percent of peripheral phlebitis}$$

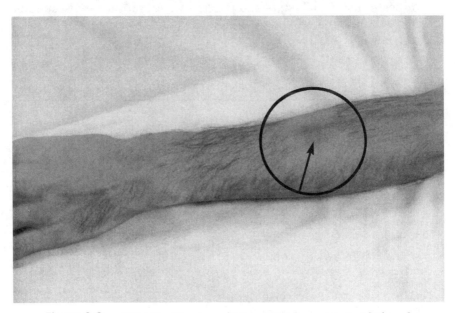

Figure 9-2 ■ Phlebitis. (Courtesy of Johnson & Johnson Medical [Ethicon], Somerville, NJ.)

> Table 9-3 | **PHLEBITIS SCALE**

Grade	Clinical Criteria`
0	No clinical symptoms
1	Erythema at access site with or without pain
2	Pain at access site, with erythema and/or edema
3	Pain at access site with erythema and/or edema, streak formation, and palpable venous cord
4	Pain at access site with erythema and/or edema, streak formation, palpable venous cord >1 inch in length, purulent drainage

Source: INS (2011a), with permission.

Prevention

The risk for phlebitis is reduced by the following:

1. Assess the appropriateness of the infusate characteristics and the duration of infusion for PIV therapy.
2. Consider a midline catheter or CVAD (e.g., PICC) for:
   a. Infusion therapies anticipated to last longer than 1 week and/or
   b. Infusates with a pH less than 5 or greater than 9, or with osmolarity greater than 600 mOsm/L, or for dextrose concentrations in excess of 10%.
3. Perform proper hand hygiene and use aseptic technique with all I.V. procedures.
4. Wear clean gloves during PIV insertion and maintain aseptic technique with catheter insertion.
5. Prepare the skin with an antiseptic and allow it to fully dry prior to catheter insertion. Do not touch skin after antisepsis.
6. Choose the smallest cannula appropriate for the infusate.
7. Infuse solutions at the prescribed rate. Do not attempt to catch up on delayed infusion time.
8. Avoid placing PIV catheters in areas of flexion (e.g., wrist). If an area of flexion must be used, use a joint stabilization device.
9. Ensure that the catheter is adequately stabilized in place to minimize catheter movement within the vein.
10. Assess the site at least every 4 hours for signs of complications, more frequently when administering irritating infusates, when the patient is sedated or has cognitive limitations and cannot report changes, and/or when the PIV is placed in a high-risk location such as an area of flexion (Gorski, Hallock, Kuehn, et al., 2012).

NURSING FAST FACT!

> Be aware that solutions that are highly acidic (pH <5), highly alkaline (pH >9), or hyperosmolar (>600 mOsm/L) or have a high dextrose concentration (>10%) are associated with a higher risk of phlebitis.

Treatment

Standard treatment of phlebitis is the application of warm compresses to the affected site. In addition, INS (2011b) recommends the following actions:

- Determine the potential etiology, whether chemical, mechanical, bacterial, or postinfusion phlebitis. Additionally, use this information in planning for ongoing venous access. For example, if the etiology is likely an irritating infusate, consider the need for an alternate plan, such as a PICC.
- Remove the PIV and replace as clinically indicated.
- Restart the infusion in the opposite extremity, using a fresh administration set.
- Monitor the site for postinfusion phlebitis for 48 hours.
- Provide patient education about postinfusion phlebitis, including instructions about its signs and symptoms, and who to contact if it occurs.

Documentation

Document the site assessment, the phlebitis rating (1, 2, 3, or 4), whether the licensed independent practitioner (LIP) was notified, and the treatment provided. Document the discontinuation of the PIV catheter and the location of the new I.V. site. Document all observable symptoms and the patient's subjective complaints, such as "feels tender to touch" and "it hurts." Document the actions taken to resolve the problem and the time of LIP notification.

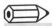 *NURSING FAST FACT!*

> If the inflammation is the result of bacterial phlebitis, a much more serious condition may develop if the patient is not treated. Untreated bacterial phlebitis can lead to septicemia.

Infiltration/Extravasation

Description and Etiology

When I.V. fluid escapes from the vein into the surrounding tissue, the complication called **infiltration** or **extravasation** has occurred. The difference between these two terms relates to the type of I.V. fluid. *Infiltration* is defined as the inadvertent administration of a *nonvesicant* medication or solution into the surrounding tissue, whereas *extravasation* is the inadvertent administration of a vesicant medication into the surrounding tissue (INS, 2011a). A **vesicant** is a medication or fluid capable of causing injury, such as necrosis or tissue damage, when it escapes from the vein.

Many antineoplastic drugs used in cancer treatment are classified as vesicants. These drugs can be divided into two categories: DNA binding and non-DNA binding. The vesicants that bind directly to the nucleic acids in DNA cause immediate damage to the tissue outside of the vein, result in a larger and deeper area of damage, and are more painful (Schulmeister, 2011). Vesicants that are non-DNA binding have an indirect effect on the tissue, are more easily neutralized, and cause less severe injuries that improve over time. Nonantineoplastic drugs (e.g., some antibiotics) can also cause depletion of intracellular enzymes that sustain cell function and lead to cellular death. Drugs that cause vasoconstriction (e.g., dopamine) can cause ischemic necrosis should they extravasate (Doellman et al., 2009).

> *EBP In an important systematic review of the literature supplemented with local data and experience, researchers identified common pediatric infusates associated with risk of tissue damage when administered peripherally (Clark et al., 2013). Characteristics of harmful infusates included extreme pH, high osmolarity, vasoactivity, and cytotoxicity. Infusates were categorized as red (higher risk), yellow (intermediate risk), or green (lower risk). Infusates in the red category included acyclovir, caffeine citrate, calcium, dextrose over 12.5% concentration, doxycycline, mannitol 20% and 25%, promethazine, potassium greater than 60 mEq/L concentration, sodium bicarbonate, sodium chloride 3% or greater, parenteral nutrition solutions with osmolarity 950 mOsm/L or greater, vasopressors (e.g., dopamine), and chemotherapy drugs.*

Both infiltration and extravasation can result in significant injury. (Fig. 9-3) The severity of damage is directly related to the type, concentration, and volume of fluid infiltrated into the interstitial tissues. Large infiltration volumes (e.g., >25–50 mL) increase the risk of tissue damage, and consultation with a plastic surgeon may be necessary (INS, 2011a, p. S67). In a review of liability claims related to PIV catheters, approximately half of the cases were related to fluid or drug infiltration/extravasation (Bhananker et al., 2009). Infiltration/extravasation may also occur with a CVAD. Some risk factors include:

- Needle dislodgement/improper needle access with implanted vascular access ports
- Deeply placed ports
- Catheter attached to an implanted port that separates or fractures internally

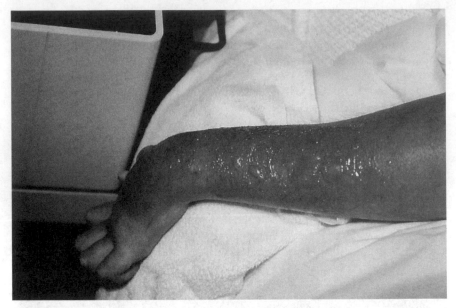

Figure 9-3 ■ Infiltration of vancomycin into subcutaneous tissue, causing blistering of skin. (Courtesy of Beth Fabian, CRNI.)

- Catheter migration and subsequent malposition into the tissue
- Loss of catheter integrity (e.g., hole/crack in the catheter)
- Presence of a fibrin sleeve along the catheter that allows the medication to back track along the fibrin sleeve back to the catheter insertion site (Faraj, Zaghal, El-Beyrouthy, & Kutoubi, 2010; Polovich, Whitford, & Olsen, 2009; Schulmeister, 2011).

Risk factors for infiltration/extravasation related to PIVs are categorized into three areas: mechanical, physiological, and pharmacological (Doellman et al., 2009). Mechanical factors include:

- Small, fragile veins/poor vein condition
- Large catheters causing mechanical friction of the vein
- Catheter dislodgement resulting from joint movement when a PIV catheter is placed in an area of flexion
- Failure to adequately stabilize catheter
- Overmanipulation of the I.V. catheter
- Multiple attempts at venipuncture or puncture of the vein wall during venipuncture
- Use of an infusion pump during infiltration or extravasation. Although infusion pumps do not cause infiltration, it is important to recognize that infusion pumps also *do not detect* infiltration. When an I.V. catheter has infiltrated, the fluid or medication will continue to infuse and worsen the problem.

Physiological factors include blood clot formation and lymphedema. For example, blood clot formation above the PIV may force the infusate into the tissue at the catheter insertion site, thereby causing infiltration.

Pharmacological factors also play an important contributing role. Medications or solutions characterized by an acidic or alkaline pH and/or high osmolarity can damage the endothelial cells of the vein, increasing the risk for venous rupture (Doellman et al., 2009). Other pharmacological factors include drugs that cause vasoconstriction, which can cause ischemic necrosis within the vein. Specific examples include dobutamine, dopamine, epinephrine, and some cytotoxic drugs (Bhananker et al., 2009; Doellman et al., 2009).

Signs and Symptoms

Assessment of the I.V. site and the venous pathway up the extremity is essential to identifying infiltration or extravasation. Early recognition of infiltration/extravasation is **vital** to limiting the volume of fluid and reducing the risk for tissue injury (INS, 2011a, p. S67). Signs and symptoms that may occur at or around the site include:

- Cool skin temperature at the PIV site
- Skin that appears blanched and taut
- Patient complaints of skin tightness, pain, burning, or discomfort
- Swelling at, above, or below the insertion site
- Decreased mobility of the extremity
- Leaking of fluid from the insertion site
- Absence of a blood return or presence of a "pinkish" blood return
- Changes in infusion flow quality

One way to assess for PIV-related infiltration is as follows. With infusion running, apply pressure 3 inches above the catheter site in front of the catheter tip with either digital pressure or use of a tourniquet. Infiltration should be suspected if the infusion continues to run. When the vein is compressed and the catheter is properly aligned in the vein, the I.V. solution will stop because of occlusion. In addition, compare both of the patient's arms when assessing for infiltration (Fig. 9-4).

Complications associated with infiltration/extravasation fall into three categories:

1. *Ulceration and possible tissue necrosis:* The severity of tissue damage depends on many variables, including the drug's vesicant potential, the amount of drug infiltrated, and the venipuncture site. Ulceration is not immediately apparent; the ulcer may actually take days or weeks to develop.
2. *Compartment syndrome:* Muscles, nerves, and vessels are in compartments confined in inflexible spaces bound by skin, fascia, and bone. When fluid inside a compartment increases, the venous end of the capillary bed becomes compressed. If vessels cannot carry away the excessive fluid, hydrostatic pressure rises, leading to

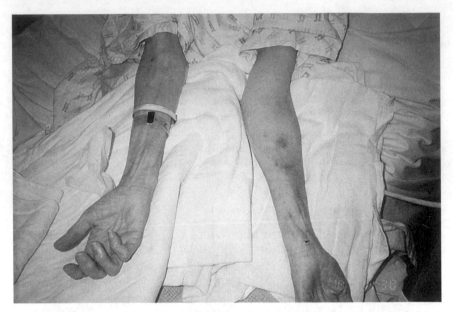

Figure 9-4 ■ Infiltration. Compare both arms when assessing for infiltration (note that the left arm is swollen compared with the right arm).

vascular spasm, pain, and muscle necrosis inside the compartment. Functional muscle changes can occur within 4 to 12 hours of injury. Within 24 hours, ischemic nerve damage can result in functional loss.

3. *Complex regional pain syndrome (CRPS)*: This may result from a severe infiltration/extravasation. It is a chronic pain condition that is believed to result from dysfunction in the central or peripheral nervous system. It is characterized by dramatic changes in the color and temperature of the skin over the affected limb or body part, accompanied by intense burning pain, skin sensitivity, sweating, and swelling. When the symptoms are clearly associated with a nerve injury, it is called CRPS II (National Institute of Neurological Disorders and Stroke, 2011). One theory is that CRPS is caused by a triggering of the immune response, which leads to the characteristic inflammatory symptoms of redness, warmth, and swelling in the affected area that represent a disruption in the healing process.

Prevention

The risk for infiltration/extravasation is reduced when risk factors are mitigated and with adequate and continuous assessment of the site.

1. Assess the appropriateness of the infusate characteristics and the duration of infusion for PIV therapy.

2. Consider a CVAD (e.g., PICC) for infusates with a pH less than 5 or greater than 9, with osmolarity greater than 600 mOsm/L, and for dextrose concentrations in excess of 10% (Fig. 9-4).

3. Avoid placing PIV catheters in areas of flexion (e.g., wrist), which increases the risk of catheter dislodgement and infiltration. If placement in an area of flexion is necessary, use of a joint stabilization device (e.g., arm board) is recommended (INS, 2011a). If used, apply it in a manner that allows visual assessment of the PIV site.

4. Any one nurse should not attempt PIV placement more than two times (INS, 2011a). After two unsuccessful attempts, the nurse with the best skills should evaluate the patient's veins. Further attempts at PIV insertion should be made only if venous access is believed to be adequate (Perucca, 2010). Multiple attempts limit future access and cause unnecessary pain and suffering. For patients with poor venous access, there should be collaboration with the LIP and I.V. team, if available, to discuss alternative options for venous access.

5. Use the smallest size and shortest length catheter to accommodate the infusion therapy.

6. Never place a new PIV proximal to a previously used site. An infusate administered below a previously used and potentially damaged vein may infiltrate into the damaged area.

7. Administer irritating infusates into large peripheral veins if a CVAD is not indicated. Avoid use of small veins in the hand or fingers.

8. Ensure that the catheter is stabilized in place to minimize catheter movement within the vein.

9. Turn patients carefully. Infiltration and swelling below the I.V. site may occur as a result of placing hands underneath the patient during turning. Occlusion or restriction of blood flow causes fluid to back up in the vessels, resulting in infiltration and dependent edema below rather than above the I.V. site (Fig. 9-5).

10. Assess the PIV site frequently (Gorski et al., 2012):
    a. At least every 4 hours in patients who are receiving a nonirritant/nonvesicant for any signs of problems, such as pain, swelling, or redness at the site tissue.
    b. Every 1 to 2 hours in critically ill patients, adult patients who have cognitive/sensory deficits or who are receiving sedative-type medications and are unable to notify the nurse of any symptoms, and in patients whose PIVs are in a high-risk location (e.g., external jugular, area of flexion)
    c. Every hour in pediatric and neonatal patients

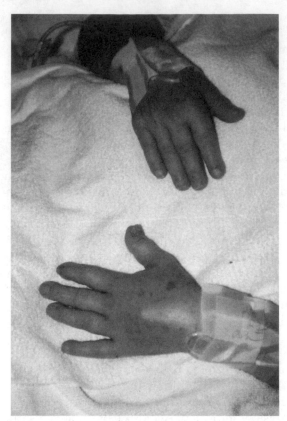

Figure 9-5 ■ Infiltration and swelling below the I.V. site occurring after hands were placed underneath the patient during turning. Occlusion or restriction of blood flow caused fluid to back up in the vessels, resulting in infiltration and dependent edema below rather than above the I.V. site. (Courtesy of Beth Fabian, CRNI.)

11. Provide patient education. Instruct patient to immediately report any pain, burning, or swelling with infusion.
12. Additional strategies for vesicant administration:
    a. Ensure knowledge and competence of nurses administering vesicants, including venipuncture skills, use of CVADs, and assessing for signs/symptoms of extravasation.
    b. Use sound decision making in relation to venous access, devices, and infusions:
       i. Do not use a site older than 24 hours.
       ii. Do not use steel needles to administer vesicants.
       iii. Use smooth, pliable veins.
       iv. Avoid injured/sclerosed veins, areas of flexion, small veins, lower extremities, and extremity with altered venous return or diminished sensation.

     v. Administer any vesicant infusion exceeding 30 to 60 minutes via a CVAD (Polovich et al., 2009)

  c. Advocate for a CVAD when administering vesicant and vasoconstrictor agents whenever possible (Gorski et al., 2012).

  d. Administer vesicants through the side arm of a free-flowing infusion of a hydration solution.

  e. Check patency before, during, and after vesicant administration.

  f. In addition to visual assessment of site, verify presence of blood return before infusion and every 5 to 10 minutes during infusion (Gorski et al., 2012; Polovich et al., 2009).

INS Standard Use of a standardized scale to assess and document infiltration/extravasation is recommended (see Table 9-4 for an example) (INS, 2011a, p. S67).

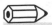 *NURSING FAST FACT!*

    Immobilized patients and patients with muscular weakness or paralysis of an extremity may have edema of an extremity that is not related to infiltration of an I.V. site. Accurate assessment of the cannula and infusion site is the key to differentiation.

> Table 9-4   **INFILTRATION SCALE**

Grade	Criteria
0	No symptoms
1	Skin blanched Edema <1 inch Cool to touch With or without pain
2	Skin blanched Edema 1–6 inches Cool to touch With or without pain
3	Skin blanched and translucent Gross edema >6 inches Cool to touch Mild to moderate pain Possible numbness
4	Skin blanched and translucent Skin tight, leaking Gross edema >6 inches Deep, pitting tissue edema Circulatory impairment Moderate to severe pain Infiltration of any amount of blood product, irritant, or vesicant

Source: INS (2011b), with permission.

Treatment

1. Stop infusion *immediately* when infiltration/extravasation is suspected. It is recommended that the PIV be left in place and an attempt made at aspirating any residual drug/I.V. fluid using a small (1–3 mL) syringe (Doellman et al., 2009; Dychter et al., 2012; INS, 2011a).
2. Notify LIP immediately of any extravasation or significant infiltration (e.g., >25 mL and/or presence of pain or numbness).
3. Use warm or cold compresses as appropriate (Doellman et al., 2009; Schulmeister, 2011). Cooling promotes vasoconstriction, which limits dispersion of the drug in the tissue. Heat promotes vasodilation, which enhances drug dispersal. Cold is recommended for extravasation of certain vesicants, contrast media, and hyperosmolar fluids. Heat is recommended for certain cytotoxic drugs, including the vinca alkaloids.
4. Elevate the infiltrated extremity. This is recommended because it promotes reabsorption of the infiltrate (Doellman et al., 2009).
5. Assess the site regularly after an infiltration/extravasation at a frequency based on the type of infusate and individual patient needs (INS, 2011a, p. S67).
6. Instruct patient to report any worsening of signs or symptoms, such as changes in extremity mobility, sensation, or elevated temperature.
7. Pharmacological antidotes may be used to treat extravasations, although this remains controversial (Doellman et al., 2009).
8. Provide written instructions on which symptoms to report to the clinician, how to manage pain, and any follow-up care.

NOTE > Do not apply excessive pressure to the area because it will disperse fluid further into surrounding tissues.

Vesicant Extravasation and Use of Pharmacological Antidotes

The use of antidotes is generally not recommended based on limited evidence of their efficacy (Doellman et al., 2009; Polovich et al., 2009). Data are primarily based on anecdotal evidence. There is one exception. In 2007 the Food and Drug Administration (FDA) approved dexrazoxane hydrochloride as the first drug to treat extravasation of an anthracycline (e.g., doxorubicin). This medication is administered as an I.V. infusion for 3 days in a large vein that is not in the area of the extravasation, and it must be started no later than 6 hours after the extravasation occurred.

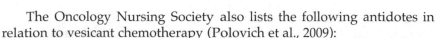

The Oncology Nursing Society also lists the following antidotes in relation to vesicant chemotherapy (Polovich et al., 2009):

- Hyaluronidase may be used in extravasation of plant alkaloids (e.g., vincristine). This enzyme increases tissue permeability and facilitates absorption. It has also been used for treatment of infiltration and extravasation of several other drugs such as nafcillin and 10% dextrose solutions (Doellman et al., 2009).
- Sodium thiosulfate is indicated for extravasation of alkylating agents (e.g., nitrogen mustard).
- Phentolamine is indicated for extravasation of vasopressors (e.g., dopamine) because it reduces local vasoconstriction and ischemia (Doellman et al., 2009).

NOTE > The goal of pharmacological antidotes is to lessen tissue injury.

EBP The importance of vigilant nursing assessment in detection of infiltration injuries was highlighted in a case study review of three infants who suffered significant infiltrations of I.V. fluids with subsequent development of compartment syndrome. Signs of infiltration included tissue blanching, decreased capillary refill time, and severely restricted active/passive range of motion of the extremity. Restricted joint movement was considered an important finding because infant "chubbiness" made swelling difficult to detect and infants cannot express specific areas of pain or discomfort. Of note, I.V. fluids were delivered via infusion pumps that did not alarm with the infiltrations. Fasciotomies were performed on all three infants with full recovery (Talbot & Rogers, 2011).

Documentation

Comprehensive documentation of an extravasation or significant infiltration event in the patient's medical record is vital for medical and legal purposes. Litigation rarely reaches a civil court until several years after the negative event. Medical record documentation is the key to understanding the events that occurred. Documentation of the infiltration/extravasation should include:

- Date/time of event
- VAD type; number/location of PIV attempts
- Presence of blood return prior to and during administration of vesicant
- Insertion site
- Fluid/medication infused and method of infusion (e.g., I.V. push)

- Patient report of symptoms
- Estimated volume of infiltration; amount of fluid aspirated
  - Estimate how much solution entered the subcutaneous tissue by noting the time of the last assessment and the first complaint, and the rate of the infusion.
- Status of circulation at, above, and below the insertion site, including skin color, capillary refill, and circumference of both extremities at the site.
- Description of the site: Anatomic location, size of infiltrated area, signs/symptoms as listed above
  - Photograph site if this is part of organizational policy
- Initial and follow-up interventions
- Notification of LIP
- Use of any antidotes, dosages, administration
- Patient education provided (INS, 2011a; Schulmeister, 2011)

Infiltrations and extravasations, especially those that cause tissue damage, should be tracked as part of the organizational quality management program.

Patients who are at high risk for extravasation injury are presented in Table 9-5.

 NURSING FAST FACT!

Never increase the flow rate to determine the infiltration of a vesicant. Assessment of the site around the catheter tip is important, as is questioning the patient about discomfort at the access site. When extravasation or infiltration is suspected, discontinue the infusion immediately. An extravasation should always result in immediate reporting and completion of an unusual occurrence report.

> Table 9-5   **FACTORS THAT INCREASE RISK FOR EXTRAVASATION INJURY**

Age

Neonate
Geriatric patient

Condition

Receiving vesicant medications/solutions
Decreased level of consciousness (e.g., anesthesia, sedation)
Patient with cognitive limitations/chronic confusion
Patients with diseases affecting blood vessels/sensation (e.g., diabetes)

Equipment

Use of infusion pumps with vesicant medications

NURSING FAST FACT!

Joint stabilization devices (e.g., splints/arm boards) should be well padded and applied so that they do not cause nerve damage, constrict circulation, or cause pressure areas. They should be removed at frequent intervals, and nurse-assisted range-of-motion exercises should be performed. Inadequate or improper use of such devices can result in pressure ulcers, circulatory constriction, and nerve injury. Policies and procedures should be established to guide their use.

INS Standard Treatment of infiltration and extravasation should be established in organizational policies, procedures, and/or practice guidelines (INS, 2011a, p. S66).

 NURSING FAST FACT!

Soft tissue damage from extravasation can lead to prolonged healing, potential infections, necrosis, multiple débridement surgeries, cosmetic disfiguration, loss of limb function, and even amputation.

Local Infection

Description and Etiology

This section is limited to the presence of signs and symptoms of a local infection at the VAD insertion site. It is important to recognize however, that the presence of a local site infection increases the risk of a BSI because microbial colonization at the site can migrate into the catheter tract and along the catheter surface, gaining access to the circulation (O'Grady et al., 2011). One of the most serious forms of PIV-related infection occurs when an intravascular thrombus surrounding the cannula becomes infected, leading to purulent drainage from the insertion site. This is referred to as suppurative or purulent thrombophlebitis (Hadaway, 2012).

INS Standard Catheter-related infection includes exit-site, tunnel, port pocket, or CR-BSI (INS, 2011a, p. S68).

Local infections at the exit site are preventable with use of hand hygiene, skin antisepsis, and aseptic technique for catheter insertion and all catheter-related care and access. Local infections may be related to:

- Lack of appropriate hand hygiene
- Inadequate skin cleansing and skin antisepsis at the time of placement
- Inadequate skin cleansing and skin antisepsis or failure to adhere to aseptic technique with implanted port access

- Failure to adhere to aseptic technique during VAD insertion and I.V. access
- Placement of catheters in emergent situations that are not changed within 48 hours
- Poor technique in maintaining and monitoring the VAD site
- Lack of catheter stabilization, which allows catheter movement and thus migration of pathogens on the skin into the catheter tract (McGoldrick, 2010)

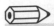 **NURSING FAST FACT!**

In any patient with an intravascular catheter who develops high-grade BSI that persists after an infected cannula has been removed, it is likely the patient has an infected thrombus in a recently cannulated vein (Maki & Mermel, 2007).

Signs and Symptoms

Signs and symptoms of local infection include:
- Redness, swelling, induration, and/or drainage at the site
- Elevated body temperature that may/may not be present and, if present, is indicative of possible systemic infection

Prevention

Techniques used to prevent local infections include the following:

1. Perform proper hand hygiene and utilize aseptic technique with all I.V. procedures.
2. Wash the patient's skin with soap and water prior to VAD placement if the site is visibly dirty.
3. Clip hair using a scissors or disposable head surgical clippers if there is excess hair at the site. Never shave because microabrasions from shaving may increase the risk of infection.
4. Apply antiseptic to the skin for the required amount of time. For example, chlorhexidine/alcohol solution (preferred antiseptic) should be applied for at least 30 seconds and allowed to fully dry.
5. Change I.V. tubing at recommended intervals:
   - Every 96 hours for continuous infusions
   - Every 24 hours for intermittent infusions via a locked VAD; place a sterile covering over the end of the tubing between infusions
   - Change the I.V. tubing whenever the PIV site is rotated or if the CVAD site changed
6. Choose the catheter type, insertion site, and technique based on which pose the lowest risk of infections for the type and duration of infusion therapy. For adult patients, the femoral site should be avoided.

7. Maintain aseptic technique during cannula insertion, during therapy, and during catheter removal.
   - CVAD placement: Use maximal sterile barrier precautions, chlorhexidine alcohol solution for skin antisepsis, and a standardized checklist to ensure adherence to aseptic technique (e.g., central line bundle as discussed in Chapters 2 and 8).
8. Assess insertion site regularly.
9. Maintain dressing. If the site is bleeding or oozing or the patient is diaphoretic, a gauze dressing is preferred.
10. Use a chlorhexidine-impregnated sponge dressing for nontunneled CVADs (O'Grady et al., 2011; Timset et al., 2009).
11. Instruct the patient to keep catheter site/dressing dry. Instruct patient on how to protect the site while bathing.
12. Disinfect needleless connector prior to each access. Scrub for at least 15 seconds and allow to dry. Alternatively, consider using an alcohol cap product that protects the connector between intermittent uses.

NOTE > See Chapter 2 for further information on infections at cannula sites.

INS Standard The infection rate should be calculated according to a standard formula (INS, 2006a, p. 56).

Calculation:

$$\frac{\text{Number of infections}}{\text{Total number of I.V. catheter-days}} \times 1000 = \text{Infection rate}/1000 \text{ catheter-days}$$

Treatment

When there is a suspected local site infection, the LIP should be immediately notified.

1. Any purulent drainage at the PIV or CVAD site should be cultured and gram stained (INS 2011a, p. S68).
2. A PIV should be removed and consideration given to culturing the catheter tip.
3. Removal of a CVAD is not recommended based on local signs and symptoms because these are not reliable indicators of a BSI (INS, 2011a).
4. Topical as well as systemic antimicrobial treatment may be indicated.
5. Cultures are obtained prior to administration of any antibiotics. It is important to follow organizational policy when obtaining any cultures to avoid contaminated specimens.

Documentation

Document the assessment of the site, culture technique, sources of culture, notification of the LIP, and any treatment initiated.

NOTE ▷ Culture technique procedures are addressed in Chapter 2.

Nerve Injury

Description and Etiology

Nerves and veins lie close to each other in the arms; therefore, inadvertent injury to a nerve during venipuncture could occur. In fact, according to an infusion nursing expert, nerve injuries are the most commonly reported insertion-related complication (Masoorli, 2007).

When planning to place a PIV, it is important to recognize that certain sites should be avoided and/or used with caution because of nerve proximity. Nerves specifically related to risk of injury with PIV placement in the arm include the radial and the median nerves.

The consequences of nerve injury may be minor or major. Minor nerve injury results in the formation of a traumatic neuroma (an unorganized mass of nerve fibers) at the point of needle contact. Should the needle actually tear the nerve fibers, CRPS may result (as discussed earlier in the section on infiltration/extravasation).

Nerve compression injury may occur as a result of infiltration or extravasation of an infusion. A compartment syndrome may occur when the I.V. fluid or medication collects in tight spaces bound by the fascia, bone, muscle, and skin. The increased pressure of the fluid decreases perfusion in the area, which can lead to irreversible nerve damage and loss of function. Early identification of infiltration/extravasation reduces such risk.

NOTE ▷ See Chapter 6 for a review of the anatomy of nerves in relation to PIV placement.

Signs and Symptoms

Signs and symptoms of direct puncture nerve injury include:
- Immediate symptoms with PIV, midline, or PICC placement, including sharp acute pain at the venipuncture site.
- Sharp shooting pain up or down the arm

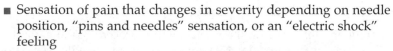

- Sensation of pain that changes in severity depending on needle position, "pins and needles" sensation, or an "electric shock" feeling
- Pain or tingling discomfort in the hand or fingertips

Monitor closely for the following signs of impending compartment syndrome as a result of a severe infiltration/extravasation, which may lead to nerve compression injury:

- Pain, pallor, paresthesia (e.g., numbness, tingling), paralysis, and/or pulselessness (Talbot & Rogers, 2011)
- Restricted joint movement and resistance to passive motion (Talbot & Rogers, 2011)

Prevention

The risk for nerve injury as a result of PIV placement is reduced when the following recommendations are followed:

1. If the patient complains of paresthesias, numbness, or tingling on catheter insertion, remove the catheter immediately and notify the LIP promptly. Rapid attention may prevent permanent injury (INS, 2011a).
2. Avoid the lateral surface of the wrist for approximately 4 to 5 inches because of the potential for nerve damage (INS, 2011a).
3. Avoid the ventral surface of wrist because of pain on insertion and possible nerve damage (INS, 2011a).
4. Avoid the antecubital area for routine PIV placement.
5. Avoid excessive probing for the vein.
6. Use no more than a 15-degree angle when inserting the PIV catheter.
7. Reduce risk for infiltration/extravasation as discussed in the section on infiltration/extravasation.

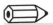 *NURSING FAST FACT!*

Avoid the wrist area. A simple landmarking technique involves placing the clinician's index, middle, and ring fingers at the crease of the wrist at the base of the thumb. This segment of the cephalic vein should be avoided! This is called the three-finger test. Venipuncture should be 2 inches above the crease of the wrist and 1 inch above the crease of the wrist of a baby (Masoorli, 2007).

NOTE > Minor nerve injury may result in scar tissue and formation of a neuroma at the point of needle contact. The patient may require months of rehabilitation. Major nerve injury, which occurs when the needle tears the nerve fibers, may result in CRPS.

Treatment: Direct Pressure Nerve Injury

1. If at any time during the venipuncture procedure the patient complains of pain, electric shock, or pins and needles sensation, stop the venipuncture immediately and withdraw the I.V. device, remove the catheter immediately, and notify the LIP promptly because rapid attention may prevent permanent injury (INS, 2011a).
2. Apply pressure to the site to prevent a hematoma.
3. Document the incident.

Treatment: Nerve Compression Injury

1. Immediately notify the LIP when compression nerve injury is suspected.
2. Discontinue the infusion.
3. Assess for swollen area for paleness and pulselessness, which indicate tissue necrosis and nerve compression injury are developing.
4. Place the affected limb at the level of the heart. Elevation is contraindicated because it decreases arterial flow (Rasul, 2011).
5. Anticipate that the patient will be taken to surgery for fasciotomy.
6. Notify supervisor of event and complete an unusual occurrence report. This type of unusual occurrence would be considered a sentinel event (see Chapter 1).

NOTE > Irreversible nerve damage begins after 6 hours of tissue hypertension (Rasul, 2011).

Documentation

Document the patient's complaints, duration of complaints, treatment, and length of time to resolve the problem. It is also important to document the time the LIP was notified. Table 9-6 provides a summary of local and systemic complications.

Venous Spasm

Description and Etiology

A spasm is a sudden, involuntary contraction of a vein or artery resulting in temporary cessation of blood flow through a vessel. **Venous spasm** can occur suddenly and for a variety of reasons. The spasm usually results from the administration of a cold infusate or an irritating solution, or from too rapid administration of an I.V. solution or viscous solution (e.g., blood product). Venous spasm may also occur during PICC or midline catheter

> Table 9-6   **LOCAL AND SYSTEMIC COMPLICATIONS OF PERIPHERAL INTRAVENOUS THERAPY**

Complication	Signs and Symptoms	Treatment	Prevention
		Local	
Hematoma	Ecchymoses Site swelling and discomfort Inability to advance catheter Resistance during flushing	Remove catheter if indicated. Apply pressure with 2- × 2-inch gauze. Elevate extremity. Cold compresses may be applied.	Use indirect method of venipuncture. Apply tourniquet just before venipuncture. Use blood pressure (BP) cuff for patients with delicate/fragile skin.
Phlebitis	Redness at site Site warm to touch Local swelling Palpable cord along vein	Discontinue catheter. Apply warm compresses.	Advocate for central vascular access device (CVAD) when infusing hyperosmolar, high/low pH, and vesicant solutions or medications. Choose smallest I.V. cannula that is appropriate for infusion. Practice hand hygiene prior to placement and I.V. access. Rotate infusion sites when signs and symptoms are present. Stabilize catheter to prevent mechanical irritation. Avoid placing peripheral intravenous (PIV) catheter in areas of flexion.

Infiltration/ extravasation	Coolness of skin around site
	Taut/blanched skin
	Edema above or below insertion site
	Back flow of blood absent
	Slowed infusion rate
	For extravasation:
	  Complaints of pain
	  Burning or stinging at insertion site
	  Blisters
		Stop infusion and remove catheter.
		Apply cool/warm compresses as indicated by type of infusate.
		Elevate extremity.
		Follow guidelines if extravasation occurs.
		Use antidote when appropriate.
		Any incident of infiltration grade 2 or greater needs unusual occurrence report.
			Advocate for CVAD when infusing hyperosmolar, high/low pH, and vesicant solutions or medications.
			Choose smallest I.V. cannula that is appropriate for infusion.
			Stabilize catheter to prevent mechanical irritation.
			Avoid placing PIV in areas of flexion.
			Do not use veins that have a previous venipuncture.

Continued

> Table 9-6	LOCAL AND SYSTEMIC COMPLICATIONS OF PERIPHERAL INTRAVENOUS THERAPY—cont'd		
Complication	Signs and Symptoms	Treatment	Prevention
		Local	
			Avoid antecubital fossa. Turn the patient carefully. Assess site frequently.
Nerve Injury	Immediate sharp pain during venipuncture Shooting pain up arm Pain or tingling in hand or fingertips	Stop venipuncture. Notify LIP. Apply pressure.	Avoid lateral surface of wrist, antecubital area, ventral surface of wrist. Avoid probing. Reduce risk for infiltration or extravasation as above. Make only two attempts.
Local Infection	Redness and swelling at site Possible exudate of purulent material	Discontinue catheter; culture site and cannula. Apply sterile dressing over the site. Administer antibiotics as ordered.	Practice aseptic technique during venipuncture and site maintenance.
Venous Spasm	Sharp pain at I.V. site associated with infusion Slowing of infusion Resistance to PICC or midline removal	Apply a warm compress to the site with infusion still running. Restart the infusion if spasm continues. Consult with interventional radiology for resistance to line removal.	Dilute medications. Keep I.V. solution at room temperature. Administer infusion at prescribed rate.
		Systemic	
Bloodstream Infection (BSI)	Fever and chills Diaphoresis Tachycardia Tachypnea Change in mental status Hypoxemia Decreased urine output Hypotension Evidence of decreased perfusion or dysfunction	Notify the LIP. Restart new I.V. system. Obtain cultures. Initiate antimicrobial therapy ordered. Monitor the patient closely.	Hand hygiene. Aseptic technique with all aspects of infusion related care. Attention to skin antisepsis prior to placement and with ongoing site care; preference to use chlorhexidine and alcohol solutions. Attention to intact dressings over VAD. Attention to needleless connector disinfection.

> Table 9-6	LOCAL AND SYSTEMIC COMPLICATIONS OF PERIPHERAL INTRAVENOUS THERAPY—cont'd		
Complication	Signs and Symptoms	Treatment	Prevention
		Systemic	
			Carefully inspect solutions. Follow standards of practice related to rotation of sites and hang time of solutions.
Circulatory Overload and Pulmonary Edema	Rapid weight gain Increase in BP, heart rate Bounding pulse Edema Intake>output Rise in central venous pressure Shortness of breath Crackles in lungs Cough Distended neck veins Restlessness and headache	Call rapid response team. Decrease I.V. flow rate. Place the patient in a high Fowler position. Keep the patient warm. Monitor vital signs. Administer oxygen as ordered. Administer drug therapy. Administer oxygen therapy.	Monitor the infusion. Maintain flow at the prescribed rate. Monitor intake and output, daily weights. Know the patient's cardiovascular history. Do not "catch up" infusions; instead, recalibrate. Use electronic infusion devices (EIDs) that have dose-error reduction systems and anti–free-flow administration sets.
Air Embolism	Light-headedness Dyspnea, cyanosis, tachypnea, expiratory wheezes, cough Mill wheel murmur, chest pain, hypotension Change in mental status, confusion coma, seizures	Call rapid response team. Place patient in Trendelenburg position. Administer oxygen as ordered. Monitor vital signs.	Remove all air from administration sets. Use luer-lock connections. Follow protocol for catheter removal.
Speed Shock	Dizziness Facial flushing Headache Tightness in chest Hypotension Irregular pulse Progression of shock	Stop infusion immediately. Call rapid response team.	Use an EID. Monitor the infusion rate. Administer I.V. push medications over appropriate time frame.

removal. Stimulation of the vein causes irritation and spasm (Macklin, 2010). Patient anxiety may also contribute to this problem (Gorski, Perucca, & Hunter, 2010). Venous spasm is related to:

■ Administration of cold infusates
■ Mechanical or chemical irritation of the intima of the vein

Signs and Symptoms

Signs and symptoms of venous spasms include:

■ Cramping or sharp pain above the I.V. site that travels up the arm caused by a piercing stream of fluid that irritates or shocks the vein wall
■ Resistance to PICC/midline catheter removal

Prevention

Venous spasm can be prevented. Techniques used to prevent vasospasm include:

1. Ensure adequate dilution of medications.
2. Administer the medication/I.V. solution at the prescribed rate.
3. Allow refrigerated medications and parenteral solutions to reach room temperature before administering them.
4. Use a fluid warmer for rapid/large-volume transfusions in accordance with organizational policies.

 NURSING FAST FACT!

If a rapid infusion rate is desired, use a larger cannula.

Treatment

1. Apply warm compresses to warm the extremity and decrease flow rate until the spasm subsides.
2. If spasm is not relieved, remove catheter and restart with a new cannula.
3. If resistance to midline/PICC removal persists, interventional radiology should be consulted for evaluation and catheter removal.

Documentation

Document the patient's complaints, duration of complaints, treatment, and length of time to resolve the problem. Also document whether the PIV catheter required replacement to resolve the problem.

Systemic Complications

Systemic complications are serious and can be life threatening. Such complications include catheter-associated BSI, circulatory overload, air embolus, and speed shock. With appropriate preventative interventions and ongoing monitoring, these complications are preventable.

Bloodstream Infection

Description and Etiology

BSI, defined as the presence of bacteria in the blood, is a serious and potentially life-threatening complication of VADs. The scope, terminology, and pathogenesis of BSIs are addressed in Chapter 2. The risk for CR-BSIs in the home is low, although there are limited current data documenting the prevalence. Prevention of CVAD-related infections is a National Patient Safety Goal for both hospitals and long-term care organizations (The Joint Commission [TJC], 2012a).

Although most of the literature is focused on BSIs associated with central VADs, BSI associated with PIV catheters is becoming a research focus. Although evidence indicates a low rate, because of the large number of PIV catheters that are used, even a low rate translates into a large number of BSIs per year (Hadaway, 2012).

The microorganisms most frequently implicated in central-line-associated bloodstream infections (CLABSIs) are coagulase-negative staphylococci, *Staphylococcus aureus*, and *Candida* (O'Grady et al., 2011). A BSI can progress to sepsis or **septicemia**, which is a systemic infection caused by pathogenic microorganisms or their toxins that can result in a profound systemic reaction (McGoldrick, 2010). Septicemia is a serious and life-threatening infection that often begins with fever, chills, tachycardia, and tachypnea. Septicemia can advance to septic shock, adult respiratory distress syndrome, and death.

Biofilm

It is recognized that all catheters form a "biofilm" on the device shortly after insertion. A biofilm is a community of microorganisms surrounded by a slime matrix that protects the bacteria from antibiotics. Biofilm development occurs when, immediately after insertion, plasma proteins attach to the catheter. Platelets and white blood cells also adhere to the catheter surface. The coagulation cascade is initiated with vessel wall injury, and, within a few hours, the catheter is coated with a **fibrin sheath** from all of these substances. Microbes from the skin and dermal layers are potentially introduced during catheter insertion; they also can gain access to the internal catheter surface during any access procedure (e.g., flushing). The microbes interact with the platelet–protein layer, and bacteria and fungi easily attach themselves to this protein layer. When these microorganisms gain access to either the internal or external surface of the catheter, they become irreversibly adherent and begin to produce a biofilm that incorporates the microorganisms, providing a protective environment (TJC, 2012a). A BSI can occur if biofilm bacteria detach from either the external or internal catheter surface. Although microorganisms that are dispersed as single cells can be killed by host defenses, a BSI can result if dissemination of the microbes is more extensive or if the host defenses are compromised (TJC, 2012a). If the biofilm is dispersed in clumps and is resistant to host defenses, infections such as endocarditis may result. Because of the presence and nature of biofilm adherence, every effort must be made to reduce the introduction of microorganisms into the catheter/bloodstream. This means practicing hand hygiene and aseptic technique during the insertion, taking care with *every* catheter access, and maintaining the device.

Catheter Management to Prevent Catheter-Related Bloodstream Infections

Catheter management to prevent infections must focus on insertion practices, care and maintenance, and appropriate use of available technologies. TJC (2012b) 2013 National Patient Safety Goals direct the organization to implement the following evidence-based interventions to reduce the risk of CLABSI. All 13 recommendations apply to hospitals. Several also apply to long-term care facilities as indicated. General recommendations are summarized in Table 9-7.

> Table 9-7	CENTRAL VENOUS CATHETER BLOODSTREAM INFECTION PREVENTION

Hand hygiene
Maximum sterile barrier precautions (sterile gowns, sterile gloves, mask, cap, patient drape) during insertion
Chlorhexidine/alcohol solution for skin antisepsis during insertion and with routine site care
Trained catheter inserters; use of ultrasound
Proper selection of type of catheter and insertion site
Insertion of catheters only when medically necessary
All materials needed for catheter insertion at bedside before starting insertion
Time-out called if proper procedures are not followed (then start over)
Use of aseptic technique during catheter manipulation (including hub/needleless connector disinfection)
Removal of catheters when no longer medically necessary
Organizational quality improvement activities including monitoring infection rates and adherence to compliance with central line bundle

CHAPTER 9 > **Complications of Infusion Therapy** ■ 573

Specific recommendations from the CDC (O'Grady et al., 2011) that support the National Patient Safety Goals are listed below each of the 13 goals:

1. Educate all staff involved in CVAD use about CLABSI and prevention on hire and annually.
   a. This recommendation applies to long-term care settings.
   b. The CDC recommends designating only trained, competent personnel to insert and maintain both peripheral and central VADs.
2. Educate patients and families about CLABSIs.
3. Implement policies and practices to reduce CLABSI risk.
   a. Use ultrasound guidance to place CVADs.
   b. Use CVAD with minimum number of ports (lumens) for management of the patient. More lumens are associated with more catheter manipulation, which increases risk of microorganisms entering the I.V. system.
   c. Do not submerge catheter or catheter site in water.
   d. Maintain aseptic technique for insertion and care of CVADs.
      i. This is also referred to as "sterile technique."
      ii. Only sterile-to-sterile contact is allowed (e.g., sterile male end of I.V. tubing to disinfected needleless connector).
   e. Replace dressings every 2 days if using gauze dressings, every 7 days if using transparent dressings.
   f. Consider use of chlorhexidine-impregnated sponge dressing for short-term CVADS in patients older than 2 months.
   g. When adherence to aseptic technique cannot be ensured (e.g., during medical emergencies), replace as soon as possible (i.e., within 48 hours).
   h. Monitor sites visually or by palpation through an intact dressing.
   i. Do not use antimicrobial ointment or creams on insertion sites because of increased risk of fungal infections and antimicrobial resistance.
4. Conduct periodic risk assessment for CLABSIs. Monitor compliance with evidence-based practices and evaluate prevention efforts.
5. Provide CLABSI infection rate data and prevention outcome measures to staff.
6. Use a catheter checklist and standardized protocol at the time of insertion.
7. Practice hand hygiene prior to catheter insertion or use.
8. Avoid the femoral site.
9. Use a standardized supply cart or kit that contains all needed supplies for insertion.

10. Use a standardized protocol for sterile barrier precautions during CVAD insertion.

11. Use an antiseptic for skin preparation during CVAD that is cited in scientific literature or endorsed by professional organizations.
    a. Prepare clean skin with >0.5% chlorhexidine/alcohol preparation before CVAD placement and during dressing changes.
    b. Allow antiseptic to fully dry prior to CVAD placement.

12. Use a standardized protocol to disinfect catheter hubs and injection ports (e.g., needleless connector) before access.
    a. This recommendation applies to long-term care as well as acute care settings.
    b. Scrub needleless connector with an appropriate antiseptic (chlorhexidine, 70% alcohol, povidone-iodine) and access only with sterile devices.

13. Evaluate all CVADs and remove them when they are no longer necessary (INS, 2011a; O'Grady et al., 2011).
    a. This recommendation also applies to long-term care settings.

Another intervention is daily bathing with chlorhexidine-impregnated washcloths. This is recommended as a special approach in organizations with high rates of infection despite adherence to basic recommendations as previously listed (Marschall et al., 2008). In a multicenter randomized trial of 7727 patients, chlorhexidine bathing compared to nonchlorhexidine bathing was associated with a 53% decrease of BSI among patients with CVADs (1.55 vs 3.30 cases per 1000 catheter-days; $P = .004$) (Climo et al., 2013). Additional infection prevention measures recommended by the CDC (O'Grady et al., 2011) and INS (2011a) include the following, which address reducing risk of infection with peripheral as well as central VADs:

- Do not place PIVs in the lower extremity in adults.
- Use a midline catheter or PICC when the duration of I.V. therapy will likely exceed 6 days.
- Replace catheters placed during an emergent situation (and thus under less than aseptic conditions) as soon as possible and no later than 48 hours.
- Remove PIVs if symptoms of phlebitis (or infection) appear.
- Maintain aseptic technique during insertion and care of all catheters.
- Use sterile gauze or a transparent, semipermeable dressing to cover catheter site.
- Do not use topical antibiotic ointments or creams on insertion sites.
- Use a sutureless securement device to reduce the risk of infection.

- Consider use of an antimicrobial or antiseptic-impregnated CVAD in adults whose catheter is expected to remain in place for longer than 5 days.
- Do not routinely use antibiotic lock solutions to prevent CR-BSI.
- Do not remove CVADs or PICCs on the basis of fever alone. Use clinical judgment.
- Only use guidewire exchanges to replace a malfunctioning nontunneled catheter if no evidence of infection is present.
- Change the needleless components at least as frequently as the administration sets.
- Minimize contamination risk by wiping the access port with an appropriate antiseptic.
- Perform admixture of all routine parenteral fluids in the pharmacy under a laminar-flow hood.
- Do not use any container of parenteral fluid that has visible turbidity, leaks, cracks, or particulate matter.
- Use single-dose vials.

> EBP A California hospital reported zero infections over 7 years among patients receiving PICCs inserted by a PICC team (Harnage, 2012). Interventions in the care bundle included 100% use of ultrasound guidance during placement, maximal barrier precautions, chlorhexidine skin preparation, use of a chlorhexidine-impregnated dressing, catheter stabilization, a neutral needleless connector, a standard flushing protocol, daily line monitoring, and great attention to RN training. The author emphasizes the need for attention to postinsertion care beyond the central line bundle, a dedicated vascular access team, and a culture of patient safety.

Signs and Symptoms

Signs and symptoms of BSI include fever, chills, backache, nausea, malaise, headache, and hypotension.

Signs and symptoms of septicemia include all those of BSI and advancing to:

- Profuse, cold sweat
- Tachycardia
- Increased respirations or hyperventilation
- Evidence of decreased perfusion or dysfunction of vital organs
- Change in mental status
- Hypoxemia (measured by pulse oximetry)
- Elevated lactate levels
- Diminished urine output
- Elevated white blood cell and absolute neutrophil counts

EBP Infections related to central venous catheters are the second most costly hospital medical error (an injury resulting from inappropriate medical care). According to a study by Shreve et al. (2010), CVAD infections have an average cost of over $83,000 per episode, and more than 90% of CVAD infections were considered the result of medical errors. The data were derived from insurance claims, and the researchers used control groups to compare the difference in cost of care between patients who did not versus those who did experience a medical error.

 NURSING FAST FACT!

Education is critical in infection prevention. Nurses must be knowledgeable about the pathogenesis of infection and consistently use evidence-based strategies for prevention.

Treatment

The steps in treating suspected BSI/septicemia include:

1. Report signs and symptoms to the LIP immediately.
2. Anticipate an order for blood cultures.
   a. Blood cultures drawn from a peripheral venipuncture and obtained from a CVAD are used to diagnose CLABSI and should be obtained within 10 minutes of each (INS, 2011b).
   b. When obtaining a blood culture specimen from a CVAD, change the needleless connector prior to obtaining the sample, disinfect the needleless connector with antiseptic solution and allow it to dry (reduces risk for contaminated specimen), and collect blood sample in the volume recommended for the culture bottles (INS, 2011a, 2011b).
3. Initially manage a suspected BSI with a CVAD (O'Grady & Chertow, 2011).
   a. In high-risk, seriously ill patients, the catheter is removed, two sets of blood cultures are recommended, antibiotic therapy is initiated, and an infectious disease expert is consulted.
   b. In patients with mild or moderate symptoms who have high-risk factors (e.g., immunosuppressed, evidence of infection at insertion site, proven bacteremia or fungemia), the CVAD is removed, two sets of blood cultures are recommended, and antibiotic therapy is initiated.
   c. In patients with mild or moderate symptoms without high-risk factors, the CVAD may not be removed, two sets of blood cultures are recommended, and antibiotic therapy initiated. The decision for CVAD removal is also based on the causative pathogen.

4. Anticipate an order for the peripheral or central catheter tip if the CVAD was removed.
5. If a peripheral cannula is in place, restart a new I.V. system in the opposite extremity. This includes changing not only the PIV but also the solution container and I.V. tubing.
6. Administer antibiotics, fluid replacement, vasopressors, and oxygen as prescribed.
7. Monitor the patient closely.
8. Anticipate possible transfer to the intensive care unit (ICU), depending on the severity of the symptoms.

Documentation

Document the signs and symptoms assessed, the time the LIP was notified, and all treatments instituted. Document the time of transfer to the ICU, the time the new I.V. infusion system was started, and how the patient is tolerating interventions.

Circulatory Overload

Description and Etiology

Circulatory overload is caused by infusing excessive amounts of isotonic or hypertonic crystalloid solutions too rapidly, failure to monitor the I.V. infusion, or too rapid infusion of any fluid in a patient compromised by cardiopulmonary or renal disease (Phillips, 2010). Circulatory overload in hospitalized patients is associated with an increased death risk (Traynor, 2012).

Pulmonary edema may result from circulatory overload when left ventricular filling pressure suddenly increases. Fluid is shifted from the pulmonary capillaries into the interstitial space and alveoli. Patients at risk for circulatory overload and pulmonary edema are those with cardiovascular disease, those with renal disease, and elderly patients. Any sodium chloride solution should be used cautiously in high-risk patients. Hypertonic sodium chloride solutions (3% and 5%) given to correct profound sodium deficits can lead to pulmonary edema and must be monitored aggressively (Phillips, 2010).

Fluid overload and pulmonary edema are related to:
- Overzealous infusion of I.V. fluids, especially those that contain sodium
- Compromised cardiovascular or renal systems

Signs and Symptoms

Signs and symptoms of circulatory overload include:
- Increase in blood pressure or heart rate, bounding pulse
- Intake > output
- Weight gain over a short period of time

- Increase in central venous pressure
- Jugular venous distention
- Cough
- Presence of edema (eyes, dependent, over sternum)
- Pulmonary edema:
  - Moist crackles in lungs
  - Severe dyspnea
  - Anxiety, restlessness
  - Blood tinged sputum
  - Pallor
  - Cyanosis
  - Hypoxia, with severe respiratory distress
  - Oxygen saturation less than 90% on room air
- Diagnostic tests: Arterial blood gases (ABGs), blood urea nitrogen (BUN), and serum creatinine to evaluate renal function; natriuretic peptide levels may be increased; chest radiograph

If the condition is allowed to persist, congestive heart failure, shock, and cardiac arrest can result.

Prevention

Techniques used to prevent circulatory overload leading to pulmonary edema include:

1. Review the patient's cardiovascular history and risk factors for circulatory overload.
2. Monitor intake and output and daily weights for all patients receiving I.V. fluids.
3. Monitor patients for signs and symptoms, especially when infusing sodium chloride solutions, and know the solution's physiological effects on the circulatory system.
4. Maintain flow at the prescribed rate.
5. Never "catch up" on I.V. solutions that are behind schedule; instead, recalculate all infusions that are not on time.
6. Report changes, including increased body weight, intake > output.
7. Use electronic infusion devices (EIDs) that have dose-error reduction systems and anti–free-flow administration sets.

Treatment

Report signs and symptoms of circulatory overload to LIP promptly. The goal of treatment is to decrease pulmonary venous and capillary pressures, improve cardiac output, and correct underlying pathology.

1. Drug therapy: Use loop diuretics to decrease pulmonary congestion. Consider vasodilators to decrease pulmonary vascular pressure (nitroprusside or nitroglycerin) and morphine sulfate to cause venous dilation.

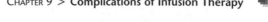

2. Administer oxygen therapy with dose titrated to patient response (intubation and mechanical ventilation may be necessary).
3. Place a pulmonary artery catheter to monitor hemodynamic status, including cardiac output.
4. Position the patient in a semi-Fowler position.
5. Monitor daily weights to monitor fluid status.
6. Obtain frequent intake and output measurements.
7. Decrease I.V. flow rate per orders.
8. Keep the patient warm to promote peripheral circulation.
9. Monitor vital signs.

Documentation

Document patient assessment, notification of LIP, and treatments instituted by LIP order. Monitor the patient and record vital signs, intake and output, and weights on an interval flow sheet.

Venous Air Embolism

Description and Etiology

Venous **air embolism** is a rare, potentially lethal, and *preventable* complication in relation to VADs. Two conditions must be present to cause a venous air embolism: direct communication between a source of air and the vasculature, and a pressure gradient favoring passage of air into the circulation (Natal et al., 2012). The pathophysiology is as follows. The entry of a bolus of air into the vascular system creates an air lock at the pulmonic valve and prevents ejection of blood from the right side of the heart. The right side of the heart overfills with blood, and the force of ventricular contractions increase in an attempt to eject blood past the occluding air pocket. These forceful contractions break small air bubbles loose from the air pocket. Minute air bubbles are subsequently pumped into the pulmonary circulation, causing even greater obstruction to the forward flow of blood as well as local pulmonary tissue hypoxia. Pulmonary hypoxia results in vasoconstriction in the lung tissue, which further increases the workload of the right ventricle and reduces blood flow out of the right heart. This leads to diminished cardiac output, shock, and death unless interventions are implemented immediately.

Small amounts of air are broken up in the capillary bed and absorbed into the circulation without symptoms. However, it has been asserted that even small bubbles of air have the potential to cross into arterial circulation and create cerebral or coronary ischemic events (Wilkins & Unverdorben, 2012). Although not current standard practice, these authors suggest consistent use of air-eliminating filters with I.V. infusion. Minimally, it is critical that air be aspirated not only from I.V. tubing but also from syringes, needleless connectors, and other add-on devices (e.g., extension tubing sets).

The risk for air embolism may be associated with the following procedures or clinical situations:
- During placement or removal of a CVAD
  - Pressure in the central veins decreases during inspiration and increases during expiration. If an opening into a central vein exposes the vessel to the atmosphere during the negative inspiratory cycle, air can be sucked into the central venous system in much the same manner that air is pulled into the lungs.
- Catheter breakage or fracture
- Presence of a persistent catheter tract following CVAD removal
- Disconnection between the catheter and the I.V. administration set or needleless connector in the absence of a catheter clamp
- Inadvertent infusion of air into the administration set
  - Failure to prime the administration set
  - Adding a new I.V. bag to a line that has run dry without clearing the line of air
  - Loose connections that allow air to enter the system

NOTE > It is estimated that 5 mL/kg of air is required for significant injury including shock and cardiac arrest (e.g., ~340 mL in a 150-pound patient); however, complications have been reported with as little as 20 mL of air injected I.V. (Natal et al., 2012).

Signs and Symptoms

Signs and symptoms of air embolism include:
- Light-headedness and weakness
- Pulmonary findings: Dyspnea, cyanosis, tachypnea, expiratory wheezes, cough, pulmonary edema
- Cardiovascular findings: Palpitations, "mill wheel" murmur; weak, thready pulse; tachycardia; tachydysrhythmias; substernal chest pain; hypotension; jugular venous distention
- Neurological findings: Change in mental status, altered speech, confusion, coma, anxiousness, seizures
- Agitation and anxiety (e.g., feelings of "impending doom") not uncommon (Cook, 2013)

If untreated, these signs and symptoms lead to hemiplegia, aphasia, generalized seizures, coma, and cardiac arrest.

Prevention

Techniques used to prevent air embolism include:
1. Prime all air from administration sets, syringes, and any add-on devices (e.g., needleless connectors, extension tubing).

2. Use only luer-lock devices within the I.V. administration set.
3. Check administration set junctions for securement, especially when getting patients out of bed.
4. Check infusion system regularly for air bubbles, an empty infusion container, leakage or disconnection, or cracks at the catheter hub.
5. Ensure that the CVAD is clamped during administration set and needleless connector changes. If no clamp is present, place patient in a position with the CVAD exit site at or below heart level and have patient perform a Valsalva maneuver during the procedure.
6. Trace all lines from the catheter hub to the fluid container to prevent missed connections.
7. Add new I.V. solution containers before the previous solution runs completely dry.
8. During CVAD removal:
   - Position patient in supine position or Trendelenburg position if tolerated
   - Instruct patient to perform Valsalva maneuver during removal unless contraindicated; if so, have patient exhale during removal
   - Remove catheter slowly and place immediate pressure over exit site until hemostasis is achieved
   - Apply an occlusive dressing with a petroleum-based ointment/gauze and cover with transparent dressing; maintain in place for at least 24 hours until epithelialization is complete
   - Have patient remain in supine position 30 minutes after removal (Cook, 2013; Gorski et al., 2010; Jurgensonn, 2010; INS, 2011b)

NOTE > The risk of venous air embolism is greater with CVADs than with PIV catheters (Jurgensonn, 2010).

 NURSING FAST FACT!

The complications of air emboli include shock, death, neurological injury, and/or myocardial infarction.

Treatment

Immediate actions are required in the event of suspected air embolism:

1. Prevent more air from entering system (clamp catheter, occlude catheter exit site).

2. Place patient in left lateral Trendelenburg position. This causes the air to rise in the right atrium, preventing it from entering the pulmonary artery.
   a. If patient cannot tolerate this position, use the left lateral decubitus (left side, head flat) position (Cook, 2013).
3. Activate code system/rapid response team.
4. Administer 100% oxygen and intubate for significant respiratory distress or refractory hypoxemia.
5. Maintain systemic arterial pressure with fluid resuscitation and vasopressors/beta-adrenergic agents if necessary.
6. Monitor vital signs.

 NURSING FAST FACT!

A pathognomonic indicator of an air embolism is a loud, churning, drum-like sound audible over the precordium, called a "mill wheel murmur." This symptom may be absent or transient.

EBP Failure to place an occlusive dressing after removal of a CVAD may have caused a patient to suffer a fatal air embolism in a case report. Steps followed in the institutional protocol included placing patient in supine position during device removal, patient holding his breath during removal, direct pressure to site, and covering site with gauze and tape. The patient then got up to dress himself in preparation for discharge and suddenly slumped over onto his bed. A disparity between procedures for CVAD removal and introducer catheter sheath removal (followed by the nurse) was identified. The authors assert the need for trustworthy and consistent policies, procedures, and protocols (Clark & Plaizier, 2011).

Documentation

Document patient assessment, nursing interventions, notification of LIP, and treatment. If emergency treatment was necessary, use an interval flow sheet to document the management of the air embolism, record interval vital signs, and indicate patient response.

Speed Shock

Description and Etiology

Speed shock is a systemic reaction that occurs when a foreign substance, usually a medication, is rapidly introduced into the circulation (Perucca, 2010). Rapid injection permits the concentration of medication in the plasma to reach toxic proportions, flooding the organs rich in blood—the heart and the brain. The vital organs, therefore, are "shocked" by a toxic dose. Syncope, shock, and cardiac arrest may result.

The causes of speed shock include:
- I.V. medications or solutions are administered too rapidly.
- The flow control clamp is inadvertently left completely open.
- The EID is programmed incorrectly.

Signs and Symptoms

Signs and symptoms of speed shock include:
- Dizziness
- Facial and neck flushing
- Patient complains of severe pounding headache
- Tightness in the chest
- Hypotension
- Irregular pulse
- Progression of shock

Prevention

Speed shock is preventable as follows:

1. Review information about drug and implications of adverse effects resulting from rapid administration.
2. Use an EID with high-risk drugs. Do not bypass the drug library or override alerts when using "smart pumps."
3. Monitor the infusion rate for accuracy before "piggybacking" in a medication.
4. Administer I.V. push medications over the appropriate time frame. Usually the label on the medication syringe will indicate the time (e.g., administer over 3–5 minutes); if not labeled, the nurse should consult with the pharmacist.

 NURSING FAST FACT!

More than 50% of nurses administered I.V. push medications incorrectly based on an assessment of technique during a competency skills day. Proper technique in I.V. push medication administration should be assessed as a nursing competency in nursing curricula (Carter, Gelchion, Saitta, & Clark, 2011).

Treatment

If you suspect speed shock, do the following:

1. Stop infusion immediately.
2. Activate code system/rapid response team.
3. Administer antidote or resuscitation medications as ordered.
4. Begin cardiopulmonary resuscitation (CPR) if cardiac arrest occurs.

NOTE > See Chapter 10 for appropriate steps in delivery of I.V. push medications.

Documentation

Document the medication or fluid administered, and the signs and symptoms. Also document the LIP notification, the treatment initiated, and the patient response.

NURSING POINTS OF CARE
PERIPHERAL INTRAVENOUS COMPLICATIONS

Nursing Assessment
- Record subjective complaints from patient regarding the I.V. site.
- Assess infusion site regularly for:
  - Signs and symptoms of complications: redness, swelling, drainage, tenderness, pain
  - Dressing integrity
  - Catheter stabilization
- Monitor intake and output.
- Assess cardiac and renal function.
- Assess for age-related risks.
- Determine baseline weight.
- Assess and monitor vital signs and pain level.
- Monitor for adverse effects.

Key Nursing Interventions
1. Determine if a drug or solution has vesicant or irritant qualities and advocate for a CVAD if appropriate.
2. Perform hand hygiene prior to and after any PIV-related care.
3. Maintain aseptic technique with PIV placement and access.
4. Maintain an occlusive dressing.
5. Administer fluids that have reached room temperature.
6. Administer I.V. medications at prescribed rate; use an EID as appropriate.
7. Perform site checks and document at regular intervals.
8. Rotate the PIV site as clinically indicated based on condition of site; remove PIV at first signs of complications.
9. Use a phlebitis scale and infiltration scale, and document.

Central Vascular Access Device Complications

Complications and risks related to CVADs include the local and systemic complications discussed so far in the chapter. Complications specifically associated with central venous catheters fall into two groups: insertion-related complications and complications associated with indwelling CVADs. CVAD malposition may occur during insertion as well as any time during the catheter dwell time. Other complications associated during the catheter dwell time include catheter occlusion, catheter-associated venous thrombosis, **pinch-off syndrome**, and **superior vena cava syndrome** (SVC syndrome).

Insertion-Related Complications

There are a number of complications that can occur during the catheter insertion procedure. Venous air embolism, venous spasm, and nerve injury are possible during catheter insertion and have been previously described. During insertion of the CVAD via the subclavian vein, the introducer may inadvertently cause trauma to the lung, veins, or thoracic duct because of the anatomic location of the subclavian vein and the lung, potentially resulting in a **pneumothorax**, **hemothorax**, or chylothorax. A pneumothorax is created by the collection of air in the pleural space. A hemothorax occurs when blood enters the pleural cavity as a result of trauma or transection of a vein during insertion. A chylothorax is a condition in which chyle (lymph) enters the pleural cavity as a result of transection of the thoracic duct on the left side.

Although a pneumothorax used to be one of the more common insertion-related complications, it is rare today because standard practice includes the use of ultrasound to guide all CVAD insertions (INS, 2011a; Pittiruti, Hamilton, Biffi, MacFie, & Pertkiewicz, 2009; Schulmeister, 2010). In fact, very low complication rates by nurse-led CVAD placement services has been demonstrated (Alexandrou et al., 2012).

Signs and Symptoms

Signs and symptoms of *pneumothorax* include:
- Sudden onset of chest pain or shortness of breath during the procedure
- On auscultation, a crunching sound heard with heartbeat (caused by mediastinal air accumulation)
- Dyspnea, persistent cough
- Tachycardia

Signs and symptoms of *hemothorax* include:
- Sudden onset of chest pain with mild to severe dyspnea
- Bleeding into the pleural cavity

- Tachycardia
- Hypotension
- Delayed symptoms of dusky skin color, diaphoresis, hemoptysis
- Dullness of affected side of chest disclosed by percussion
- Decreased or absent breath sounds detected by auscultation

Signs and symptoms of *chylothorax* are similar to those of hemothorax and include:

- Milk-like substance withdrawn during insertion into the needle or catheter

Prevention

1. Use of ultrasound to guide CVAD insertion
2. Radiography or other technology to verify CVAD tip placement before infusion of medication or solutions
3. Use of highly skilled professional to insert CVAD
4. Careful assessment of patient for signs and symptoms during insertion

Treatment

1. Oxygen is usually administered and a chest tube may be inserted for pneumothorax, hemothorax, or chylothorax.
2. Monitor vital signs.
3. Apply pressure over the vein entry site.
4. Remove the catheter.
5. Consider chest tube placement.

Documentation

Document the insertion site, signs and symptoms, and all interventions. Document verification of the catheter tip location.

Central Vascular Access Device Malposition

Description and Etiology

Malposition of the CVAD can occur during the insertion process—"primary CVAD malposition"—or any time during the dwell period—"secondary CVAD malposition" (INS, 2011a, p. S72). Malposition is simply defined as the catheter tip being in a suboptimal or aberrant location, with the optimal position of the CVAD tip being in the SVC near its junction with the right atrium (INS, 2011a, p. S45). Aberrant locations include contralateral innominate and subclavian veins, internal jugular veins, azygos veins, thoracic veins, right atrium, and right ventricle.

Primary malposition results when the catheter passes into an aberrant location during the catheter insertion procedure. The main contributing factors for primary malposition include failure to use visualization technology (e.g., ultrasound), multiple attempts and needle passes, and lack of skill by the CVAD inserter (Alexander, Corrigan, Gorski, & Phillips, 2014). During the insertion procedure, anatomic abnormalities (e.g., persistent left SVC) or vessel stenosis may also contribute to malposition. The guidewire can puncture the vasculature, and extravascular CVAD tip malposition can cause cardiac tamponade and intrathoracic infiltration/ extravasation (Bullock-Corkhill, 2010; INS, 2011a, p. S73).

Secondary malposition of the catheter tip, also called "tip migration," can occur at any time. Causes include changes in intrathoracic pressure associated with coughing or sneezing, presence of heart failure, neck and arm movement, or forceful flushing of the catheter as occurs with power injection (INS, 2011a). In some instances, CVAD migration has been noted as a result of a disease process (Gorski et al., 2010). For example, in patients with heart failure, catheter tip migration has been thought to result from reduced blood flow and the dilated vessels associated with the disease. Migration has resulted from displacement by invading tissue (tumor) or venous thrombosis. Migration can occur with improper care, for example, when the catheter is repositioned during routine care by accidentally dislodging the catheter or advancing the catheter into the body. Tip migration may also result from external catheter movement of the CVAD out of the insertion site, which could result from excessive arm movement in patients with PICCs or inadequate CVAD stabilization.

Signs and Symptoms

Signs and symptoms of CVAD malposition include the following:
- Patient experiences symptoms associated with pneumothorax/ hemothorax if the pleural covering of the lung has been punctured.
- If fluid is infused through the catheter, then the patient experiences hydrothorax as fluid is infused into the chest.
- Arm or neck swelling
- Change in catheter function is noted. Inability to flush, infuse, or aspirate blood can mean the catheter tip is no longer at the desired position.
- Tip migration into the right atrium may result in dysrhythmias, and the patient may experience palpitations.
- Catheter tip migration to the internal jugular vein has been associated with the "ear gurgling sign"; the patient complains of the sound of a running stream rushing past the ear.
- Patient complains of headache or pain, swelling, redness, or discomfort in the shoulder, arm, or neck, which may indicate catheter migration.
- Changes in the length of the external catheter segment may mean the catheter tip has migrated.

Prevention

1. Extreme care should be taken when using a break-away needle to remove the break-away introducer before threading the catheter. Catheter tip position of *all* CVADs must be verified before device use.
2. Well-qualified, highly skilled professionals should place CVADs.
3. Positioning of the patient: For PICCs inserted through the basilic vein, turn the patient's head toward the side of insertion. For placement of a catheter into the subclavian vein, place the patient in a slight Trendelenburg position with a rolled towel.
4. Right-sided CVAD insertion is suggested.
5. Care must be taken during CVAD site care and stabilization procedures to not inadvertently pull the catheter out of the exit site.

Treatment

1. Medical interventions include removing the catheter and treating any associated complications. Because visualization technologies are used during catheter insertion, quick identification of problems is possible. Catheters can be repositioned using techniques such as rapid flushing and appropriate body positioning.
2. Oxygen and chest tube may be necessary.
3. Monitor vital signs.
4. Catheters that loop back into the axillary or peripheral veins have a lower rate of successful repositioning. Radiographic or direct fluoroscopic observation can be used to reposition catheters.
5. Catheters with simple looping into the subclavian, innominate, or internal jugular veins can often be repositioned by placing the patient in an ipsilateral position with the head of the bed slightly elevated.
6. Guidewire exchange has been used with success for placing a new catheter without repeated percutaneous cannulation.
7. Catheters placed in the right atrium or ventricle can be partially withdrawn.
8. When tip migration is suspected at any time during catheter dwell, notify the LIP and obtain order to hold infusions until correct catheter placement is confirmed. It is important to recognize that catheter tip migration increases the risk for central vein thrombosis, thrombophlebitis, pericardial effusion, cardiac tamponade, and cerebrovascular accident (INS, 2011a).
9. Never reinsert a catheter that has been inadvertently pulled out from the exit site. Stabilize it in place and report to the LIP. Follow-up chest x-ray film may be necessary to ensure correct tip placement.

Documentation

Document the insertion site and positioning of patient, signs and symptoms, type of catheter used, and all interventions. Document radiography or other technology used to verify CVAD tip placement.

 NURSING FAST FACT!

Appropriate CVAD tip placement in the SVC is always verified prior to catheter use.

Catheter Occlusion

Description and Etiology

Catheter occlusion is the most common complication encountered with CVADs. Catheter occlusion is characterized by:

- Inability to aspirate blood
- Inability to flush/infuse
- Sluggish flow

Based on a literature review, Baskin et al. (2009) found that 14% to 36% of patients with CVADs had an occlusion occur within the first 2 years of catheter placement.

Occlusion is a significant complication because it may delay or cause interruptions in infusion therapy. Also, untreated catheter occlusion may result in secondary complications such as loss of venous access, cost/risks of catheter replacement, and risk for BSI. Catheter occlusion may result from mechanical, precipitate, or thrombotic causes.

Mechanical occlusions may result in partial or complete obstruction of the VAD. Causes may be attributed to either external (outside of the body) or internal problems. Causes of internal mechanical problems include pinch-off syndrome and **catheter malposition** as addressed in subsequent sections of this chapter. It is possible that the catheter tip abuts against the blood vessel wall, blocking the ability to aspirate blood on occasion. For example, having the patient cough or change positions may result in ability to aspirate blood. Persistent problems should result in reevaluation of catheter placement. Causes of external mechanical obstruction include:

- Clamped catheter
- Kinked I.V. tubing
- Obstructed I.V. filter
- Constriction of catheter by a suture

The second possible cause of occlusion is precipitate formation. Factors contributing to drug precipitation include:

- Inadequate flushing between incompatible medications
- Simultaneous infusion of incompatible medications

- Infusion of medications with a low or high pH (usually <5 and >9), such as phenytoin or aminophylline
- Lipid emulsions causing occlusion by leaving a waxy buildup on the catheter wall. This is more likely to occur with three-in-one parenteral nutrition (PN) solutions, which include the amino acids, dextrose, lipids, and additives in a single container.

Some common drug combinations that lead to precipitate formation within the catheter have been identified (Hadaway, 2009):

- Phenytoin and most other solutions
- Vancomycin and heparin
- Tobramycin and heparin
- Fluorouracil and droperidol
- Dobutamine and furosemide
- Dobutamine and heparin

The third and most common cause of occlusion is thrombotic catheter occlusion. This type of occlusion occurs when fibrin or blood within and around the CVAD or within the reservoir of implanted ports slows down or disrupts catheter flow. Accumulation of deposits leads to obstruction of the infusion. It is important to recognize that any artificial device placed in the body, including a CVAD, is coated with plasma proteins, blood cells, and fibrin as the coagulation cascade is initiated by the body. The device is covered by a fibrin sheath as a result of a natural protective bodily response (Nakazawa, 2010). This fibrin growth may cause catheter occlusion and require intervention. The presence of a thrombotic occlusion may contribute to CLABSI because the presence of a blood clot in or around the catheter serves as a rich culture medium for microbial growth. Therefore, it is clinically important to recognize and treat thrombotic occlusion. Four categories of thrombotic occlusion are commonly described in the literature:

1. *Fibrin tail*: A layer of fibrin resides on the tip of the CVAD. The tail can grow as more cells and blood components are deposited. With fibrin tails, it is possible to flush the catheter and administer infusions. However, when aspiration of blood is attempted, the tail acts as a one-way valve as it is pulled over the catheter tip. The ability to flush but not aspirate blood is considered a partial occlusion and sometimes is referred to as "withdrawal occlusion."
2. *Fibrin sheath or sleeve*: A layer of fibrin forms around the external surface of the catheter, potentially coating the entire exterior wall and tip of the catheter (Fig. 9-6). When a significant fibrin sheath develops and encases the catheter tip, any medication/solution that is administered can travel retrograde ("back track") along the sheath to the catheter insertion site, resulting in an infiltration/extravasation. Infusate may be observed on the skin (nontunneled catheters), in the subcutaneous tunnel (tunneled catheters), or in the subcutaneous pocket of implanted ports.

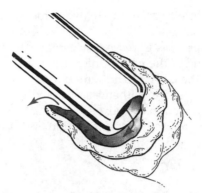

Figure 9-6 ■ Fibrin sleeve.

3. *Intraluminal occlusion*: Fibrin or blood clot accumulates within the internal catheter lumen. Flow through the catheter becomes sluggish and may progress to a complete occlusion, in which it is not possible to flush or aspirate blood from the catheter.
   ■ Frequently, the cause is blood remaining in the catheter after inadequate irrigation or retrograde flow (Figs. 9-7 and 9-8). Also, poor flushing technique after blood sampling may allow

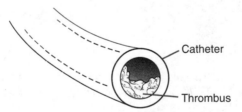

Figure 9-7 ■ Intraluminal occlusion.

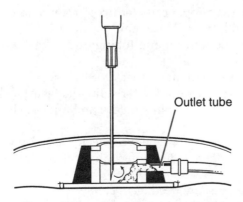

Figure 9-8 ■ Portal reservoir occlusion.

layers of fibrin to accumulate over time, narrowing or obstructing the lumen.

4. *Mural thrombus*: This is caused by catheter tip irritation against the inner lining of the vein (tunica intima). An accumulation of fibrin causes the CVAD to adhere to the vessel wall. A mural thrombus may lead to catheter-associated venous thrombosis, which is addressed in the next section. Contributing factors include frequent attempts at cannulation and use of rigid catheters.

 NURSING FAST FACT!

The presence of a blood clot in or around the catheter increases the risk for BSI because a blood clot is a nidus for microbial growth.

Signs and Symptoms

- Inability to aspirate blood
- Resistance to flushing
- Sluggish infusion
- Complete inability to flush or infuse
- Frequent infusion pump alarms
- Leaking of fluid from the insertion site as fluid tracks back along a fibrin sheath

 NURSING FAST FACT!

A properly functioning catheter is patent, should be easy to flush, and should yield a free-flowing blood return on aspiration.

Prevention

1. Ensure/verify proper catheter tip placement in the SVC near its junction with the right satrium.
2. Make sure the catheter and tubing do not have kinks or closed clamps.
3. Assess suture placement; check for tightness.
4. Use SASH (saline-administer-saline-heparin) technique, flushing the CVAD with saline before and after each medication administration.
5. Know the type of needleless connector used by your organization and use a proper clamping technique after CVAD flushing or access:
   - Positive-pressure needleless connectors: Do not clamp CVAD until after flush syringe is disconnected.

- Negative-pressure needleless connectors: Apply pressure to syringe barrel, close catheter clamp, then remove syringe.
- Neutral-pressure needleless connectors: Clamping sequence does not matter.

6. Meticulous technique in blood sampling using an adequate saline flush after any blood withdrawal.
7. Use 1.2-micron filter for administration with three-in-one parenteral nutrition solutions.
8. Consult with infusion pharmacist to help identify causative agents and solutions and avoid potential drug or solution incompatibilities.

Treatment

1. Rule out/resolve any mechanical causes, such as a clamped CVAD, kinked I.V. tubing, or an obstructed filter.
2. If unable to flush an implanted port, attempt re-access and flushing.
3. Instruct patient to cough or change position. It is possible that the catheter tip is abutted against the blood vessel and a position change may result in aspiration of blood. If this is a persistent problem, radiographic evaluation of catheter placement is indicated.
4. If mechanical causes are ruled out, intervention is based on the suspected cause of occlusion.
5. Catheter salvage is always preferred over catheter replacement.
6. For suspected precipitate formation, collaborate with the LIP for an order to treat and follow organizational procedures. The following solutions can be instilled into the CVAD in a volume that approximates the CVAD internal priming volume and is left in the catheter for at least 60 minutes before withdrawing the solution (INS, 2011a; Gorski et al., 2010):
   - Instill 0.1 N hydrochloric acid to dissolve low pH drug precipitates (e.g., vancomycin).
   - Instill sodium bicarbonate to dissolve high pH drug precipitates (e.g., phenytoin).
   - Instill ethanol, ethyl alcohol, and sodium hydroxide to restore patency to catheters with suspected buildup of lipids.
   - Be aware that use of alcohol solutions such as ethanol or ethyl alcohol may damage catheters made of some types of polyurethane and that manufacturer's instructions should be reviewed and followed.
7. For suspected thrombotic occlusion, collaborate with the LIP for an order to treat and follow organizational procedures.
   - Obtain an order for alteplase.
   - Perform hand hygiene and maintain aseptic technique throughout procedure.

- Prepare alteplase in 10-mL syringe; reconstitute per manufacturer's directions or use as pharmacy prepared.
- Disinfect the needleless connector with antiseptic solution.
- Attach alteplase syringe.
- For inability to withdraw blood or sluggish flow, unclamp catheter and gently instill medication into CVAD.
- For complete occlusion, never push medication into occluded CVAD; a "negative-pressure" method must be used.
  - Unclamp CVAD and, while holding syringe vertical, gently aspirate until plunger reaches approximately 8-mL mark, then slowly release plunger. This step may be repeated several times. The idea is to create a vacuum by aspirating air or catheter dead-space to allow alteplase into the CVAD.
- Clamp catheter, and secure device to patient and label "DO NOT USE."
- Allow the agent to dwell in catheter.
  - Recommendations for alteplase: Allow to dwell for 30 minutes and then assess for blood return. If successful, discard aspirated blood, flush CVAD with 0.9% sodium chloride solution, and resume infusion as ordered.
  - If not successful, allow alteplase to dwell for another 90 minutes and re-assess for blood return. If not successful, a second dose may be used.

NOTE > Agents used to restore CVAD patency (e.g., alteplase) should not be used with peripheral-short or midline catheters (INS, 2011a).

THROMBOLYTIC ADMINISTRATION

It is important to understand the process of fibrinolysis or dissolving of the fibrin clot. In the presence of a blood clot, tissue plasminogen activator (t-PA) is released. The t-PA converts plasminogen to plasmin, which is the activated enzyme that breaks down the blood clot. The drug alteplase, commonly referred to as t-PA, is a recombinant form of the naturally occurring tissue plasminogen activator (tPA). Cathflo Activase® (alteplase) is currently the only approved thrombolytic for catheter clearance; it is safe for use in all health-care settings, including the home (Gorski et al., 2010). The dosage is 2 mg/mL and is instilled into the occluded CVAD. There is a dosage adjustment for pediatric patients weighing 10 to 29 kg; the dosage is adjusted to 110% of the internal lumen volume of the occluded catheter, not to exceed 2 mg/2 mL (Genentech, 2005).

Precautions Related to Thrombolytic Therapy for Central Vascular Access Device Occlusion. Patients who have active internal bleeding, intracranial neoplasm, hypersensitivity to thrombolytic agents, hepatic disease, subacute bacterial endocarditis, or visceral malignancy, who have had a cerebrovascular accident within the past 2 months, or who underwent intracranial or intraspinal surgery should not receive a thrombolytic agent. Alteplase should be used with caution in the presence of suspected or known catheter-related infection because breakdown of a blood clot may release bacteria into the circulation.

Catheter-Associated Venous Thrombosis

Description and Etiology

Venous thrombosis, or formation of a blood clot in a vein, may occur in the veins of the upper extremities or chest, most often associated with presence of a CVAD or a diagnosis of cancer. In fact, the incidence of venous thrombosis is increasing, very likely because of increasing use of CVADs (Grant et al., 2012). The consequences of catheter-associated venous thrombosis include symptomatic pulmonary **embolism** (one in 10 cases), recurrent deep vein thrombosis (2% annual rate), and postthrombotic syndrome (about one-fifth of cases) (Grant et al., 2012). Postthrombotic syndrome is a late complication of venous thrombosis with symptoms of chronic pain, edema, and mobility issues in the affected extremity.

Virchow's triad remains the time-honored pathophysiological explanation for the formation of venous thrombosis (Gorski et al., 2010). Three factors are implicated in the development of a thrombus:

1. Vessel wall damage or injury. Causes include surgery or trauma, the presence of a central venous catheter, and administration of irritating solutions. Injury to the vessel wall at the catheter entry site can be related to catheter infection or exposure of the vessel wall to TPN solutions and chemotherapeutic agents.
2. Alterations in the flow of blood. Causes include venous stasis often associated with immobility, obstruction of the veins, heart failure, and varicosities.
3. Hypercoagulability of the blood. Contributing conditions include a decrease in coagulation inhibitors (e.g., antithrombin III), pregnancy, malignancy, and/or postoperative states.

There are a number of patient factors that increase the risk for central vein thrombosis as summarized based on a review of the literature (INS, 2011a), including:

- Chronic diseases associated with a hypercoagulable state including cancer, diabetes, irritable bowel syndrome, and end-stage renal failure
- Genetic coagulation abnormalities (e.g., factor V Leiden, prothrombin mutation)

- Pregnancy or use of oral contraceptives, surgery, and immobility
- History of multiple CVADs, especially with difficult or traumatic insertion and the presence of other intravascular devices
- Age extremes (young children, older adults)

There are also CVAD-related factors that increase risk, such as:

- PICC insertion sites in the antecubital fossa versus placement in the mid-upper arm
- Suboptimal CVAD tip location in the mid to upper portion of the SVC associated with greater rates of CAVD
- CVADs with larger outer diameters
- Use of anatomic landmark techniques to place CVADs rather than ultrasound; use of ultrasound decreases trauma to the vein during catheter insertion (Grant et al., 2012; INS, 2011a; Pittiiruti, Hamilton, Biffi, et al., 2009)

Signs and Symptoms

- Pain in extremity, shoulder, neck, chest
- Edema, erythema in extremity, shoulder, neck, chest
- Dilated superficial veins
- Dyspnea
- Low-grade fever
- Possible progression to SVC syndrome (addressed in next section)
- Difficulty with neck or extremity motion
- Evidence of catheter occlusion as previously discussed (i.e., inability to withdraw blood, sluggish infusion)

Prevention

1. Place CVADs in patients only when they are definitively indicated.
2. Select the smallest-diameter catheter appropriate for infusion needs.
3. Ensure/verify proper catheter tip placement in the SVC near its junction with the right atrium.
4. Promptly remove CVADs when they are no longer needed

EBP In a prospective study of PICC placements by a specially trained team, the rate of catheter-associated venous thrombosis significantly decreased with an increase in placement of single-lumen 5 Fr and smaller-gauge 5 Fr triple-lumen PICCs over a 3-year period; previously 6 Fr catheters were used. The PICC venous thrombosis rate improved to 1.9% from 3.0% (P <.04) (Evans, Sharp, Linford, et al., 2013).

Treatment

Report signs and symptoms of catheter-associated venous thrombosis to the LIP promptly. Ultrasound is most often used to diagnose the presence of thrombosis. Treatment includes:

1. Anticoagulation, usually with a parenteral anticoagulant (e.g., low molecular weight heparin) bridged to an oral anticoagulant (e.g., warfarin). The purpose is to prevent any extension of the thrombus and pulmonary embolism.
2. Anticoagulation duration usually at least 3 months but may be extended based on patient characteristics (e.g., active cancer)

Superior Vena Cava Syndrome

Description and Etiology

SVC syndrome is a rare but very serious condition caused by an obstruction of blood flow through the SVC. Obstruction occurs by extensive vein thrombosis, tumor compression, or enlarged lymph nodes that compress the SVC. More than 80% of cases are the result of malignant tumors and lymphoma; however, the increased use of CVADs has accounted for an increased incidence of SVC syndrome as a result of catheter-associated venous thrombosis (Shaheen & Alraies, 2012).

Signs and Symptoms

Signs and symptoms of SVC syndrome include:
- Progressive shortness of breath, dyspnea, cough
- Anxiety and fear as a result of feeling of suffocation
- Sensation of skin/chest tightness
- Periorbital edema
- Unilateral edema
- Cyanosis of the face, neck, shoulders, arms
- Extensive edema of the upper body without edema in lower body parts
- Engorged and distended jugular, temporal, and arm veins
- Prominent venous pattern usually present over the chest from dilated thoracic vessels
- Headache, visual disturbances
- Potential for bronchial obstruction, cerebral anoxia (result of increased intracranial pressure), death

Prevention

1. Ensure/verify proper catheter tip placement in the SVC near its junction with the right atrium; this reduces the risk for catheter-associated venous thrombosis.

2. Well-trained, experienced professionals should place the catheter; skillful insertion technique decreases risk of vein wall trauma and risk for subsequent thrombosis.
3. Assess patients for risk factors for venous thrombosis

NOTE > Hypercoagulability increases the risk of clot or thrombus formation in either the arterial or venous circulation.

Treatment

1. Notify the LIP of signs and symptoms immediately.
2. Confirm diagnosis by radiographic studies.
3. Base treatment on cause:
   - If tumor related, treatment may include radiation, chemotherapy, and stent placement.
   - If related to CVAD, treatment is catheter removal and/or thrombolytic therapy.
4. Place head of bed in semi-Fowler position.
5. Provide oxygen to facilitate breathing if needed.
6. Provide emotional support if patient has feeling of suffocating.
7. Monitor fluid volume status to minimize further edema.

Documentation

Document all signs and symptoms, radiographic studies, and interventions.

Table 9-8 provides a summary of the complications related to central venous access.

Pinch-off Syndrome

Description and Etiology

Catheter pinch-off syndrome is a rare but significant and often unrecognized complication. It occurs when the CVAD enters the costoclavicular space medial to the subclavian vein and is positioned outside the lumen of the subclavian vein in the narrow area bounded by the clavicle, first rib, and costoclavicular ligament. Catheter compression causes intermittent or permanent catheter obstruction and, because of the "scissoring" effect of catheter compression between the bones, can result in catheter tearing, transection, and catheter embolism, most often to the right heart or pulmonary artery (Mirza, Vanek, & Kupensky, 2004).

> Table 9-8   SUMMARY OF COMPLICATIONS OF CENTRAL VENOUS ACCESS

Complication and Cause	Signs and Symptoms	Treatment	Prevention
Pneumothorax: Collection of air in the pleural space between the lung and chest wall; caused by puncture of the pleural covering of the lung	Shortness of breath during procedure, crunching sound on auscultation, dyspnea, cyanosis, subcutaneous emphysema Sudden chest pain	Administer oxygen. Chest tube may be inserted. May resolve slowly without evacuation of air. Monitor vital signs. Apply pressure over the site.	Use of ultrasound-guided CVAD placement Radiographic verification of placement Highly skilled professional inserters Careful assessment during insertion
Hemothorax: Blood enters the pleural cavity as a result of trauma or transection of a vein	Sudden onset of chest pain, tachycardia, hypotension, dusky color, diaphoresis, hemoptysis	Usually noted during insertion of catheter (subclavian artery during infraclavicular placement). Remove catheter and apply pressure to the site. Monitor vital signs. Administer oxygen.	Same as for pneumothorax
Chylothorax: Lymph (chyle) fluid enters the pleural cavity as a result of transection of the thoracic duct on the left side where it enters the subclavian vein	Sudden onset of chest pain, dyspnea, withdrawal of a milk-like substance (chyle) into the needle Large amounts of serous drainage from insertion site	Remove the catheter. Monitor vital signs. Administer oxygen. Chest tube may be necessary.	Same as for pneumothorax
Catheter Malposition	Symptoms associated with pneumothorax, hemothorax as above Difficulty with aspiration Complaints of discomfort, swelling, or shoulder pain Edema of neck or shoulder "Ear gurgling sign" Palpitations	Notify LIP of signs/symptoms Catheter may not require removal; interventional radiologist may be able to reposition Rapid flush may sometimes correct malposition with single-lumen reposition.	Ultrasound-guided CVAD placement Radiographic confirmation of tip before use Well-qualified inserter Careful care and maintenance to avoid catheter dislodgement

Continued

> Table 9-8   SUMMARY OF COMPLICATIONS OF CENTRAL VENOUS ACCESS—cont'd

Complication and Cause	Signs and Symptoms	Treatment	Prevention
Pinch-off Syndrome: Central vascular access device (CVAD) inserted via the percutaneous subclavian site is compressed by the clavicle and the first rib; results in mechanical occlusion; can result in complete or partial catheter transection and embolization	Intermittent and positional occlusion Difficulty flushing infusing or aspirating CVAD Occlusion relieved by specific postural changes (often relieved by rolling the shoulder or raising the arm) Infraclavicular pain or swelling	Remove the catheter. Retrieve the embolized segment if necessary.	Ultrasound-guided CVAD placement Radiographic confirmation of tip before use Well-qualified inserter
SVC Syndrome: Condition caused by obstruction of flow through the superior vena cava (SVC)	Progressive shortness of breath; cough; sensation of skin tightness; unilateral edema; cyanosis of face, neck, shoulder, and arms; jugular, temporal, and arm veins engorged and distended; prominent venous pattern present over chest	Notify the LIP immediately. Place the patient in semi-Fowler position. Administer oxygen. Monitor fluid volume status. Monitor cardiac and neurological status. Provide emotional support. Administer anticoagulant therapy for long-term catheters. Catheter may or may not be removed.	Well-trained inserter Awareness of high-risk patients
Nonthrombolytic Occlusion: Precipitation of total parenteral nutrition (TPN) admixtures and drug-to-drug or drug-to-solution incompatibilities	Sluggish flow rates, total occlusion, inability to flush or obtain blood withdrawal	Attempt to restore patency using appropriate solution (HCl or sodium bicarbonate, or ethanol).	Saline flush before and after each I.V. drug administration Use of 1.2-micron filter for three-in-one TPN solutions Consultation with pharmacist to identify possible sources/avoid potential drug or solution incompatibilities
Thrombotic Occlusions: Deposits of fibrin and blood components within and around the CVAD; intraluminal blood clot, fibrin sheath totally or partially	Sluggish flow rates, inability to flush or obtain blood withdrawal	Rule out other causes of occlusion. Obtain order for thrombolytic drug to dissolve clot.	Adequate flushing of catheter

Signs and Symptoms

Pinch-off syndrome may occur with implanted ports or nontunneled or subcutaneously tunneled CVADs inserted via the subclavian vein. Signs and symptoms include:

- Intermittent and positional occlusion
- Difficulty with flushing, infusing, aspirating
- Frequent occlusion alarms
- Occlusion relieved by specific postural changes (e.g., rolling the shoulder back or raising the arm), which open the angle of the costoclavicular space (Gorski et al., 2010)
- In patients in whom catheter partially or completely transect internally, some patients may have no symptoms, whereas others may experience chest pain, palpitations, swelling in the area of the CVAD, or pain with catheter flushing.

NOTE > Radiographic confirmation of the catheter with proper position of the patient during radiography are crucial. It is important to note that because raising the arms or shrugging opens the costoclavicular angle, the films should be taken with the patient upright and with arms by the side (Mirza et al., 2004).

Prevention

1. Use ultrasound guidance for catheter placement. The use of ultrasound was associated with prevention of pinch-off syndrome in implanted port placement (Osawa et al., 2013).
2. Insert the catheter lateral to the midclavicular line to decrease the risk (Mirza et al., 2004).

Treatment

1. Catheter removal is generally recommended.

Documentation

Document any intermittent positional flushing and infusion difficulties, signs and symptoms, radiographic confirmation, and interventions.

NURSING POINTS OF CARE

COMPLICATIONS ASSOCIATED WITH CENTRAL VASCULAR ACCESS

Nursing Assessment
- Confirm tip placement in the SVC.
- Inspect the site for signs of infection and outward catheter migration.
- Assess CVAD patency (ability to flush, ability to aspirate blood).
- Obtain baseline vital signs and monitor for changes.
- Examine PICC and tunneled catheters for line integrity.
- Review patient cardiovascular and neurological history.

Key Nursing Interventions
1. Assist with insertion where appropriate, including correct positioning of patient and adherence to central line bundle interventions.
2. Maintain competency if performing PICC insertion.
3. Follow standard precautions.
4. Perform hand hygiene protocol with all CVAD-related procedures.
5. Use best practice for care and maintenance of catheters.
6. Maintain the integrity of the CVAD dressing.
7. Adhere to aseptic technique with all CVAD-related procedures.
8. Use no smaller than a 10-mL syringe to flush all CVADs.
9. Perform interventions as indicated (e.g., positioning, oxygen).
10. Provide emotional support.

AGE-RELATED CONSIDERATIONS

The Pediatric Client

It is important to assess the infant or child early during the hospital stay and to determine the most appropriate VAD for meeting ongoing infusion needs. All complications discussed for the adult client can occur with the pediatric client. The following focus on the pediatric patient.
- Infiltration/extravasation are common complications in pediatric infusion therapy. Use of the INS Infiltration Scale (see Table 9-4) was found to underestimate the extent of injury as a result of edema measurement in inches. The INS Scale was modified to assess edema based on percentage of swelling in relation to the size of the extremity (Pop, 2012).
- Restricted joint movement is considered an important sign of infiltration in infants (Talbot & Rogers, 2011).
- Be aware that catheters inserted into the cephalic vein most commonly are malpositioned into the axillary and basilic veins.
- Saphenous vein insertions may increase the risk for phlebitis.

The Older Adult

- Hematomas and ecchymoses are frequently seen in elderly persons. Fragile veins are easily injured.
- Older adults, particularly those older than 85 years with multiple comorbidities, multiple medications, and functional or cognitive impairment, are at higher risk for adverse outcomes, including responses to medical or surgical events (Zwicker, 2003).
- The risk of fluid overload and subsequent pulmonary edema is especially increased in older patients with cardiac disease.
- Be alert to the potential presence of infection when even low-grade temperature elevations appear for short periods.

Home Care Issues

Home care nurses must be aware of the risks associated with infusion therapy and peripheral and central vascular access devices (CVADs). The risk of catheter-related infections among home care patients is low, whereas catheter occlusion problems are not uncommon. Many home care patients have VADs in place for long periods because of extended infusion therapy needs. Because nurses are in the patient's home only intermittently, it is critically important that patients understand the signs and symptoms of potential complications. Although home care nurses assess catheter sites and function at each home visit, patient education is critical and must address the importance of regular site assessment and what to report. The patient should be provided with information about the VAD, potential risks, and instruction to promptly report signs or symptoms such as pain, swelling, or redness. Potential problems and complications encountered in home infusion therapy include:

- Mechanical problems
- Occlusion problems
- Catheter-associated venous thrombosis
- Malfunction of electronic infusion devices (EIDs)

Patient Education

- Instruct the patient to report any signs or symptoms of common local complications (e.g., redness, swelling, pain at site).
- Instruct the patient to report any interruption in flow rate.
- Instruct the patient on the purpose of the electronic infusion device (EID).
- Teach the client and family the symptoms of infection that should be promptly reported to the medical caregiver.

◼ Nursing Process

The nursing process is a six-step process for problem-solving to guide nursing action (see Chapter 1 for details on the steps of the nursing process). The following table focuses on nursing diagnoses, nursing outcomes classification (NOC), and nursing interventions classification (NIC) for patients with local and systemic complications of infusion therapy. Nursing diagnoses should be patient specific and outcomes and interventions individualized. The NOC and NIC presented here are suggested directions for development of specific outcomes and interventions.

Nursing Diagnoses Related to Complications	Nursing Outcomes Classification (NOC)	Nursing Interventions Classification (NIC)
Anxiety (mild, moderate, or severe) related to: Threat to change in health status or situational crisis	Anxiety level	Anxiety reduction techniques such as use of a calm reassuring approach, explaining all procedures
Fluid volume deficit related to: Vasodilation of peripheral vessels, leaking capillaries secondary to septicemia	Fluid balance, hydration	Fluid management, hypovolemia management, shock management such as monitoring hydration status and administration of intravenous fluids
Gas exchange impaired related to: Alveolar-capillary membrane changes secondary to pneumothorax	Respiratory status, ventilation	Airway management, monitor blood gases and hemoglobin levels
Pain, acute, related to: Peripheral vascular inflammation, edema, central malposition or occlusion, medication	Injuring agents: Physical or chemical	Comfort level, pain control strategies
Infection risk of related to: Environmental exposure to pathogens; immunosuppression, invasive procedures	Infection control, risk control and detection	Infection control practices, patient and health-care worker education
Protection ineffective related to: Abnormal blood profiles, drug therapies (thrombolytics)	Blood coagulation, immune status	Bleeding precautions, infection prevention, infection protection
Skin integrity, impaired, external related to mechanical factors: Vascular access device (VAD); irritation from I.V. solution, and internal: inflammation, infection	Tissue integrity: Skin	Skin surveillance, wound care, risk identification

Nursing Diagnoses Related to Complications	Nursing Outcomes Classification (NOC)	Nursing Interventions Classification (NIC)
Perfusion ineffective (peripheral) related to: Aggravating factors: Trauma such as infiltration or extravasation of fluid or medication	Circulation status, fluid balance, hydration Tissue perfusion: Peripheral	Circulatory care: Peripheral, such as evaluate peripheral edema and pulses, inspect skin
Perfusion risk for, altered cardiopulmonary, related to: Arterial or venous blood flow exchange problems, hypovolemia, decreased systemic vascular resistance related to sepsis	Circulatory status, fluid balance, hydration Tissue perfusion: Cellular	Cardiac care, cardiac precautions, embolus precautions, vital signs monitoring and shock management: cardiac

Sources: Ackley & Ladwig (2011); Bulechek, Butcher, Dochterman, & Wagner (2013); Moorhead, Johnson, Maas, & Swanson (2013).

Chapter Highlights

- Complications may be local or systemic.
- Some local complications (e.g., exit site infection) can progress to systemic complications.
- Use of evidence-based preventative interventions is critical. Today, the attitude and expectation is that there should be *no* complications.
- Key tips for preventing local complications:
  - Follow aseptic technique for all infusion-related procedures.
  - Perform hand hygiene prior to all infusion-related procedures, and teach patients and caregivers to expect this from all health-care providers.
  - Maintain an appropriate dressing over the insertion site.
  - Stabilize catheters to reduce micromovement at the insertion site.
  - Administer solutions at the prescribed rate.
  - Assess the I.V. site at least every 4 hours in alert and oriented adults and every hour in infants and children.
- Phlebitis (bacterial, chemical, or mechanical) is a frequently encountered problem associated with infusion therapy and can lead to cellulitis, thromboembolic complications, or BSI.
- Infiltration is also frequently encountered and may be a minor or a major complication associated with tissue and/or nerve damage. Infiltration of a vesicant medication is called extravasation.
- Key tips for preventing systemic complications:
  - Follow aseptic technique for all infusion-related procedures.
  - Perform hand hygiene prior to all infusion-related procedures.
  - Inspect solutions and equipment for breaks in integrity.
  - Use luer-lock connectors.
  - Limit the use of add-on devices.
  - Maintain flow rates at the prescribed rate.

- Use a 0.22-micron filter when appropriate.
- Use EIDs as appropriate for fluid/medication administration.
- Use central line bundle interventions with CVAD placement.

Central Venous Catheter Complications
- Insertion-related complications are highly preventable and include:
  - Venous air embolism
  - Pneumothorax/hemothorax/chylothorax
  - Nerve injury
  - Primary CVAD malposition
- Complications that can occur during catheter dwell time include:
  - Secondary malposition
  - Catheter occlusion as a result of mechanical, precipitation, and/or thrombotic causes
  - Catheter-associated venous thrombosis
  - SVC syndrome
  - Pinch-off syndrome

▦ Thinking Critically: Case Study

A 40-year-old woman with insulin-dependent diabetes mellitus is familiar with her disease but does not take care of herself. She is currently admitted with an infected plantar ulcer and had a transmetatarsal amputation. She was discharged home on a regimen of I.V. antibiotics via a PICC, with home care follow-up.

Case Study Questions
1. What potential complications should the home care nurse be alert for?
2. What documentation needs to be addressed at every visit?
3. What patient education needs to be reinforced at home?

 Media Link: Answers to the case study and more critical thinking activities are provided on DavisPlus.

Post-Test

1. Which of the following are local complications associated with infusion therapy?
   a. Speed shock, septicemia, and venous spasm
   b. Phlebitis, venous spasm, and hematoma
   c. Septicemia, thrombophlebitis, and hematoma
   d. Phlebitis, pulmonary edema, and speed shock

2. Which of following will reduce the risk for infiltration?
   a. Use of pumps or controllers to manage the I.V. rate
   b. Avoiding placing the cannula in areas of flexion
   c. Use of needleless systems
   d. Use of larger-bore catheters

3. A patient states that his I.V. site is sore. You assess the site and note redness and swelling but no signs of palpable cord or streak. Using the criteria for infusion phlebitis, what is the severity of this phlebitis?
   a. 3+
   b. 2+
   c. 1+
   d. 0

4. While a solution is infusing, which of the following is a treatment for venous spasm?
   a. Apply a cold pack to the site.
   b. Increase the flow rate of the solution.
   c. Apply a warm compress to the site.
   d. Administer pain medication.

5. You check an infusion site on a patient and find swelling and cool skin temperature. Also, the patient's skin appears blanched and feels rigid, and the infusion rate has slowed. These are signs of:
   a. Phlebitis
   b. Catheter embolus
   c. Hematoma
   d. Infiltration

6. You are performing a venipuncture and an ecchymosis forms over and around the insertion area, which has become raised and hardened. You are unable to advance the cannula into the vein. These are signs of:
   a. Phlebitis
   b. Infiltration
   c. Hematoma
   d. Occlusion

7. Strategies for VAD-related infection prevention include:
   a. Changing the needleless connector daily
   b. Hand hygiene
   c. Wearing a mask during I.V. administration
   d. Daily bathing with Betadine solution

8. Signs and symptoms of circulatory overload include:
   a. Low blood pressure
   b. Weight loss of 2 pounds over 1 day
   c. Bounding pulse
   d. Fever

9. To prevent air embolism during CVAD removal, the nurse should:
   a. Instruct patient to deep breathe during the procedure
   b. Have patient in the supine position during removal
   c. Apply an occlusive dressing after removal
   d. Have patient lie in bed for 1 hour after removal

10. Signs and symptoms of catheter tip migration during the dwell time include:
    a. Loss of hearing
    b. Palpitations
    c. Increased respiratory rate
    d. Fever

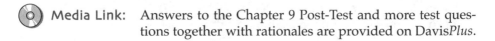 Media Link: Answers to the Chapter 9 Post-Test and more test questions together with rationales are provided on Davis*Plus*.

■ References

Ackley, B. J., & Ladwig, G. B. (2011). *Nursing diagnosis handbook: An evidence-based guide to planning care* (9th ed.). St. Louis, MO: Mosby Elsevier.

Alexander, M., Corrigan, A., Gorski, L., & Phillips, L. (2014). *Core curriculum for infusion nursing* (4th ed). Philadelphia: Lippincott, Williams & Wilkins.

Alexandrou, E., Murgo, M., Calabria, E., Spencer, T. R., Carpen, H., Brennan, K., ... Hillman, K. M. (2012). Nurse-led central venous catheter insertion: Procedural characteristics and outcomes of three intensive care based catheter placement services. *International Journal of Nursing Studies, 49*(2), 162-168.

Baskin, J. I., Pui, C. H., Reiss, U., Wilimas, J. A., Metzger, M. L., Ribeiro, R. C., & Howard, S. C. (2009). Management of occlusion and thrombosis associated with long-term indwelling central venous catheters. *The Lancet, 374*(9684), 159-169.

Bhananker, S. M., Liau, D. W., Kooner, P. K., Posner, K. L., Caplan, R. A., & Domino, K. B. (2009). Liability related to peripheral venous and arterial catheterization: A closed claims analysis. *Anesthesia Analgesia, 109*, 124-129.

Bulechek, G. M., Butcher, H. K., Dochterman, J. M., & Wagner, C. M. (2013). *Nursing interventions classification (NIC)* (6th ed.). St. Louis MO: Mosby Elsevier.

Bullock-Corkhill, M. (2010). Central venous access devices: Access and insertion. In M. Alexander, A. Corrigan, L. Gorski, J. Hankins, & R. Perucca (Eds.), *Infusion nursing: An evidence-based practice* (3rd ed.) (pp. 480-494). St. Louis, MO: Saunders/Elsevier.

Carter, A., Gelchion, K., Saitta, P., & Clark, D. (2011). Dyeing to identify IV medication errors: A clinical nurse specialist group identifies factors contributing
to IV push medication errors, and the resulting housewide education initiative. *Clinical Nurse Specialist, 25*(3), 144.

Clark, E., Giambre, B. K., Hingl, J., Doellman, D., Tofani, B., & Johnson, N. (2013).
Reducing risk of harm from extravasation. *Journal of Infusion Nursing, 36*(1),
37-44.

Clark, D. K., & Plaizier, E. (2011). Devastating cerebral air embolism after central
line removal. *Journal of Neuroscience Nursing, 43*(4), 193-196.

Climo, M. W., Yokoe, D. S., Warren, D. K., Perl, M. M., Bolon, M., Herwaldt, L.
A., ... Wong, E. S. (2013). Effect of daily chlorhexidine bathing on hospital-
acquired infection. *New England Journal of Medicine, 368*, 533-542.

Cook, L. S. (2013). Infusion-related air embolism. *Journal of Infusion Nursing,
36*(1), 26-36.

Doellman, D., Hadaway, L., Bowe-Geddes, L. A., Franklin, M., LeDonner, J.,
Papke-O'Donnell, L., ... Stranz, M. (2009). Infiltration and extravasation:
Update on prevention and management. *Journal of Infusion Nursing, 32*(4),
203-211.

Dychter, S. S., Gold, D. A., Carson, D., & Haller, M. (2012). Intravenous therapy:
A review of complications and economic considerations of peripheral
access. *Journal of Infusion Nursing, 35*(2), 84-91.

Evans, R. S., Sharp, J. H., Linford, L. H., Lloyd, J. F., Woller, S. C., Stevens, S. M., ...
Weaver L. K. (2013). Reduction of peripherally inserted central catheter-
associated DVT. *Chest, 143*(3), 627-633.

Faraj, W., Zaghal, A., El-Beyrouthy, O., & Kutoubi, A. (2010). Complete catheter
disconnection and migration of an implantable venous access device: The
disconnected cap sign. *Annals of Vascular Surgery, 24*, 692.e11-692.e15.

Genentech Inc. (2005). CathFlo Activase package insert January 2005. South San
Francisco, Author. Retrieved from http://www.gene.com/gene/products/
information/pdf/cathflo-prescribing.pdf (Accessed December 4, 2012).

Gorski, L., Hallock, D., Kuehn, S. C. Morris, P., Russell, J., & Skala, L. (2012). INS
position paper: Recommendations for frequency of assessment of the short
peripheral catheter site. *Journal of Infusion Nursing, 35*(5), 290-292.

Gorski, L., Perucca, R., & Hunter, M. (2010). Central venous access devices: Care,
maintenance, and potential complications. In M. Alexander, A. Corrigan, L.
Gorski, J. Hankins, & R. Perucca (Eds.), *Infusion nursing: An evidence-based
practice* (3rd ed.) (pp. 495-515). St. Louis, MO: Saunders/Elsevier.

Grant, J. D., Stevens, S. M., Woller, S. C., Lee, E. W., Kee, S. T., Liu, D. M., ...Elliott,
C. G. (2012). Diagnosis and management of upper extremity deep vein
thrombosis in adults. *Thrombosis and Haemostasis, 108*(6), 1097-1108.

Hadaway, L. (2009). Managing vascular device occlusions, part I. *Nursing, 39*(3),
13-14.

Hadaway, L. (2012). Short peripheral intravenous catheters and infections.
Journal of Infusion Nursing, 35(4), 230-240.

Harnage, S. (2012). Seven years of zero central-line-associated bloodstream
infections. *British Journal of Nursing, 21*(21), S6-S12.

Infusion Nurses Society (INS). (2011a). Infusion nursing standards of practice.
Journal of Infusion Nursing, 34(1S):S1-S110.

INS. (2011b). *Policies and procedures for infusion nursing.* Norwood, MA: Author.

Jurgensonn, S. V. (2010). Prevention and management of air in an IV infusion. *British Journal of Nursing, 10*(10), S28, S30.

Macklin, D. (2010). Catheter management. *Seminars in Oncology Nursing, 26*(2), 113-120.

Maki, D. G., & Mermel, L. A. (2007). Infections due to infusion therapy. In W. Jarvis (Ed.), *Hospital infections* (5th ed.). Philadelphia: Lippincott Williams & Wilkins.

Marschall, J., Mermel, L. A, Classen, D., Arias, K. M., Podgorny, K., Anderson, D. J., ... Yokoe, D. S. (2008). Strategies to prevent central line-associated bloodstream infections in acute care hospitals. *Infection Control and Hospital Epidemiology, 29*(Suppl 1), S22-30.

Masoorli, S. (2007). Nerve injuries related to vascular access insertion and assessment. *Journal of Infusion Nursing, 30*(6), 346-350.

McGoldrick, M. (2010). Infection prevention and control. In M. Alexander, A. Corrigan, L. Gorski, J. Hankins, & R. Perucca (Eds.), *Infusion nursing: An evidence-based practice* (3rd ed.) (pp. 204-228). St. Louis, MO: Saunders/Elsevier.

Mirza, B., Vanek, V. W., & Kupensky, D. T. (2004). Pinch-off syndrome: Case report and collective review of the literature. *Annals of Surgery, 70*, 635-644.

Moorhead, S., Johnson, M., Maas, M., & Swanson, E. (2004). *Nursing outcomes classification (NOC)* (5th ed.). St. Louis, MO: Mosby Elsevier.

Nakazawa, N. (2010). Infectious and thrombotic complications of central venous catheters. *Seminars in Oncology Nursing, 26*(2), 121-131.

Natal, B. L., Doty, C. I., Dire, D. J., Talvera, F., Eitel, D., Halamka, J. D., & Brown, D. F. M. (2012). Venous air embolism. Retrieved from www.emedicine.com/emerg/topic787.htm (Accessed October 31, 2012).

National Institute of Neurological Disorders and Stroke. (2011). Complex regional pain syndrome fact sheet. Retrieved from http://www.ninds.nih.gov/disorders/reflex_sympathetic_dystrophy/detail_reflex_sympathetic_dystrophy.htm (Accessed November 5, 2012).

Nightingale, F. (1859). *Notes on nursing: What it is, and what it is not.* London: Harrison, 59, Pall Mall, 59.

O'Grady, N. P., Alexander, M., Burns, L. A., Dellinger, E. P., Garland, J., Heard, S. O., ...Healthcare Infection Control Practices Advisory Committee (HICPAC). (2011). Guidelines for the prevention of intravascular catheter related infections, 2011. *American Journal of Infection Control, 39*(4 Suppl), S1-S34. Also available at http://www.cdc.gov/hicpac/pdf/guidelines/bsi-guidelines-2011.pdf (Accessed September 15, 2012).

O'Grady, N. P., & Chertow, D. S. (2011). Managing bloodstream infections in patients who have short-term central venous catheters. *Cleveland Clinic Journal of Medicine, 78*(1), 10-17.

Osawa, H., Hasegawa, J., Yamakawa, K., Matsunami, N., Mikata, S., Shimizu, J., ... Nezu, R. (2013). Ultrasound-guided infraclavicular axillary vein puncture is effective to avoid pinch-off syndrome: A long-term follow-up study. *Surgery Today, 43*(7), 745-750.

Perucca, R. (2010). Peripheral venous access devices. In M. Alexander, A. Corrigan, L. Gorski, J. Hankins, & R. Perucca (Eds.), *Infusion nursing: An evidence based approach* (3rd ed.).(pp. 456-479). St. Louis, MO: Saunders Elsevier.

Phillips, L. (2010). Parenteral fluids. In M. Alexander, A. Corrigan, L. Gorski, J. Hankins, & R. Perucca (Eds.), *Infusion nursing: An evidence-based practice* (3rd ed.) (pp. 229-241). St. Louis, MO: Saunders/Elsevier.

Pittiruti, M., Hamilton, H., Biffi, R., MacFie, J., & Pertkiewicz, M. (2009). ESPEN Guidelines on Parenteral Nutrition: central venous catheters (access, care, diagnosis and therapy of complications). *Clinical Nutrition, 28*(4), 365-377.

Polovich, M., Whitford, J. M., & Olsen, M. (2009). *Chemotherapy and biotherapy guidelines and recommendations for practice* (3rd ed.). Pittsburgh, PA: Oncology Nursing Society.

Pop, R. S. (2012). A pediatric peripheral intravenous infiltration tool. *Journal of Infusion Nursing, 35*(4), 243-248.

Rasul, A. T. (2011). Acute compartment syndrome. Retrieved from http://emedicine.medscape.com/article/307668-clinicaleMedicine (Accessed November 5, 2012).

Schulmeister, L. (2010). Management of non-infectious central venous access device complications. *Seminars in Oncology Nursing, 26(2)*, 132-141.

Schulmeister, L. (2011). Extravasation management: Clinical update. *Seminars in Oncology Nursing, 27*(1), 82-90.

Shaheen, K., & Alraies, M. C. (2012). The clinical picture: Superior vena cava syndrome. *Cleveland Clinic Journal of Medicine, 79*(6), 410-412.

Shreve, J., Van Den Bos, J., Gray, T., Halford, M., Rustagi, K., & Ziemkiewicz, E. (2010). *The economic measurement of medical errors.* Schaumburg, IL: Society of Actuaries/Milliman.

Talbot, S. G. & Rogers, G. F. (2011). Pediatric compartment syndrome caused by intravenous infiltration. *Annals of Plastic Surgery, 67*(5), 531-533.

The Joint Commission (TJC). (2012a). Preventing central line–associated bloodstream infections: A global challenge, a global perspective. Retrieved from http://www.jointcommission.org/assets/1/18/CLABSI_Monograph.pdf (Accessed December 3, 2012).

TJC. (2012b). National patient safety goals. Retrieved from http://www.jointcommission.org/standards_information/npsgs.aspx (Accessed October 29, 2012).

Timset, J. F., Schwebel, C., Bouadma, L. Geffroy, A., Garrouste-Orgeas, M., Pease, S., ...Dressing Study Group. (2009). Chlorhexidine-impregnated sponges and less frequent dressing changes for prevention of catheter-related infections in critically ill adults: A randomized controlled trial. *JAMA, 301*(12), 1231-1241.

Traynor, K. (2012). Trauma experts urge cautious use of I.V. fluids. *American Journal of Health-System Pharmacy, 69*, 1846-1847.

Wilkins, R. G., & Unverdorben, M. (2012). Accidental intravenous infusion of air: A concise review. *Journal of Infusion Nursing, 35*(6), 404-408.

Zingg, W., & Pittet, D. (2009). Peripheral venous catheters: An under-evaluated problem. *International Journal of Antimicrobial Agents, 34S*(4), S38-S42.

Zwicker, D. (2003). The elderly patient at risk. *Journal Infusion Nursing, 26*(3), 137-143.

Chapter **10**

Infusion Medication Safety, Methods, and Routes

In the future, which I shall not see, for I am old, may a better way be opened! May the methods by which every infant, every human being will have the best chance of health, the methods by which every sick person will have the best chance of recovery, be learned and practiced! Hospitals are only an intermediate state of civilization never intended, at all events, to take in the whole sick population.
—*Florence Nightingale, 1860*

Procedures Displays
10-1 Administration of
Medication by the Direct
(I.V.) Push: Peripheral
Catheter

10-2 Administration of
Continuous Subcutaneous
Medication Infusion

🔖 LEARNING OBJECTIVES

On completion of this chapter, the reader will be able to:

1. Define terminology related to medication infusion methods and routes.
2. Discuss advantages and risks associated with I.V. medication administration.
3. Describe safe injection practices.
4. Describe interventions aimed at reducing risk of tubing and catheter misconnections.
5. Identify three types of drug incompatibility.
6. Describe potential consequences of drug adsorption.
7. Identify and describe the four categories of I.V. drug delivery.
8. Discuss safety issues related to the use of patient-controlled analgesia.
9. Describe the advantages of a subcutaneous infusion.
10. List potential subcutaneous infusion sites.
11. Identify indications for the administration of chemotherapy via the intraperitoneal route.
12. Describe the intraosseous space.
13. Identify the most common site used in intraosseous access.
14. Differentiate between the epidural and the intrathecal space.
15. List medications that may be given via an intraspinal route.
16. Identify signs and symptoms for medication-associated complications of the intraspinal infusion route.

GLOSSARY

Admixture Combination of two or more infusion medications/solutions

Adsorption Adhesion by a liquid or gas to the surface of a solid

Bolus Concentrated medication or solution given rapidly over a short period of time

Chemical incompatibility Degradation of a drug as a result of change in the molecular structure or pharmacological properties of a substance, which may or may not be visually observed

Compatibility Capable of being mixed and administered without undergoing undesirable chemical or physical changes or loss of therapeutic action

Delivery system A product that allows for the administration of medication

Distribution Process of delivering a drug to the various tissues of the body

Drug interaction An interaction between two drugs; also, a drug that causes an increase or decrease in another drug's pharmacological effects

Epidural A potential space located outside the dura mater, which is the most external protective membrane surrounding the spinal cord

High alert medications Medications associated with increased risk of causing patient harm when used in error

Hypodermoclysis Administration of hydration fluids into the subcutaneous tissues

Incompatibility Chemical, physical, or therapeutic reaction that occurs among two or more drugs or between a drug and the delivery device

Intermittent infusion I.V. therapy administered at prescribed intervals

Intraosseous (IO) Route by which fluids and medications are delivered to the vascular system by percutaneous insertion of a needle into the marrow cavity of a bone

Intraperitoneal (IP) Route by which medication is administered directly into the peritoneal cavity

Intraspinal Spaces surrounding the spinal cord, including the epidural and intrathecal spaces

Intrathecal Space between the arachnoid mater and the pia mater, which contains the cerebrospinal fluid; also called the subarachnoid space

Intravenous push Administration of medication over a short period of time (minutes) in a syringe directly into the vascular access device or through the injection port of an administration set

Metered volume chamber A small container (i.e., chamber) incorporated into the I.V. administration set to which medication can be added to the primary I.V. solution; the chamber may contain from 10 to 150 mL of fluid

Patient-controlled analgesia (PCA)   A drug delivery system that dispenses a preset intravascular dose of a narcotic analgesic when the patient pushes a switch on an electric cord

Physical incompatibility   A reaction between two or more medications resulting in changes in color, haziness, turbidity, precipitate, or gas formation; usually a visible reaction

Single-dose vial   Medication bottle that is hermetically sealed with a rubber stopper and is intended for one-time use; usually does not contain a preservative

Therapeutic incompatibility   Undesirable effect occurring within a patient as a result of two or more drugs being given concurrently

▪ Safe Delivery of Infusion Therapy

Infusion medications may be administered by several routes that are described in this chapter. The intravenous route is by far the most common. Medications and solutions may also be administered via the subcutaneous tissue. Subcutaneous administration is a common way to administer opioid analgesics in the palliative care or hospice patient, and there are many more medications that may be delivered by this route. The **intraosseous (IO)** route is a quick means to vascular access in emergent care for delivery of critical care medications and fluids. The **intraspinal** route may be used to deliver a variety of anesthetic, analgesic, and other medications for patients in acute care and for those with longer-term needs beyond the hospital setting. Chemotherapy drugs may be administered via I.V. and also into the peritoneal cavity. Other less common and very specialized routes are used to administer chemotherapy, including the intravesicular route for bladder cancer and the intra-arterial route for chemotherapy administration directly into an organ (e.g., brain, liver, head, neck, pelvis) (Polovich, Whitford, & Olsen, 2009). Because they are so specialized, they are not addressed in this text.

Standards of Practice

The Infusion Nurses Society (2011, pp. S15, S86) identifies some general criteria for the safe administration of infusion medication administration, including:
   ▪ The nurse should review orders for appropriateness, access device, and rate and route of administration and follow the rights of medication administration.
   ▪ *All* medications (including over-the-counter drugs, via any and all routes) are reconciled at time of admission, transfer within or between health-care systems, and discharge.

- Organizational policies and procedures should include a list of approved parenteral medications and solutions for each type of administration method and route.
- The nurse should verify the patient's identity by using at least two identifiers prior to administration.

Orders

Infusion administration begins with obtaining and verifying the orders from the licensed independent practitioner (LIP) (e.g., physician, nurse practitioner, physician assistant). There is a great potential for patient harm and death from errors related to infusion medications. This is because the effects of an infusion, particularly an I.V. infusion, are immediate, and it is difficult, if not impossible, to reverse the pharmacological effects once administered. Errors are known to occur at various times, such as during prescribing, storage, preparation, dispensing, administration, and monitoring. The following key safety recommendations are reiterated from Chapter 1:

- Verify the completeness of the order. Orders should include:
  - I.V. medication dosage, route, frequency or time of administration, special considerations
    Example: 1000 mg vancomycin I.V. every 12 hours; obtain serum creatinine and vancomycin trough levels twice per week.
  - Standardized dosing protocols should be used for emergency drugs and **high alert medications**.
- Use verbal orders only when medically necessary.
- Use a standardized "read-back" of the order when accepting a verbal or telephone order. Note that telephone orders are regularly taken in alternate sites (e.g., home care and long-term care facilities) by necessity because physicians are generally not available on site.
- Accept only abbreviations approved by the organization.
- Review the order for appropriateness of the prescribed therapy in relation to the patient's age, condition, type of vascular access device (VAD), dose, rate, and route of administration.
- Inspect the infusate to ensure that it is properly labeled, that there is no evidence of leakage/discoloration, that it is the right drug or solution, that the dose is correct, that the expiration or beyond-use date has not passed, and that the drug or solution has been properly stored.
- Verify the patient's identity using two independent identifiers before initiating the infusion.

Compounding of Medications

In general, infusion drugs and admixtures are prepared in a central pharmacy where accuracy and sterility is best assured. The INS Standards (2011, p. S27) state that the nurse should administer pharmacy-prepared or commercially available infusion products whenever possible. The USP (ASHP, 2008) details procedures and requirements for compounding sterile preparations and sets standards applicable to all practice settings in which sterile preparations are compounded. These standards have been widely adopted, are enforced by many state boards of pharmacy, and may be used by accreditation organizations (e.g., The Joint Commission [TJC]) in surveys.

In some cases, and often in alternate sites, certain medications may need to be reconstituted by the nurse. For example, the drug used for declotting a central venous access device (CVAD), alteplase, must be reconstituted just before use. In a hospital setting, the pharmacy may mix the drug and transport it to the nursing unit; however, this is not possible in the home care setting. This is referred to as an "immediate-use" compounded sterile preparation (CSP) by the USP (ASHP, 2008). Once mixed, an immediate-use medication must be started within 1 hour of preparation or else it must be discarded (INS, 2011, p. S27; ASHP, 2008).

Attention to aseptic technique is critical when preparing immediate-use medications and should include the following safe injection practices as defined by the Centers for Disease Control and Prevention (CDC) (Siegel, Rhinehart, Jackson, & Chiarello, 2007) and INS (2011):

- Perform hand hygiene before preparing the medication.
- Always use a sterile syringe and cannula when entering a vial. Never enter a vial with a syringe or cannula that has been used on a patient.
- Never administer medications from the same syringe to more than one patient.
- Discard **single-dose vials** after use. Never use them again for another patient.
- Disinfect the tops of vials and the necks of ampules using friction with 70% alcohol and allow to dry prior to inserting a needle or breaking the ampule.
- Use a 5-micron filter needle or filter straw when withdrawing medications from a glass ampule.

Tubing and Catheter Misconnections

The issue of tubing and catheter misconnections, that is, the accidental or intentional connection of two devices that are not compatible, has received much attention over the years. In 2006, TJC issued a Sentinel Event

Alert addressing misconnection errors as an important, under-reported problem resulting in deaths and disabilities (TJC, 2006). Some examples of misconnections include I.V. solutions connected to **epidural** catheters and vice versa, enteral feeding sets connected to a CVAD, and oxygen tubing connected to an I.V. port.

The major problem is that many administration sets have luer connections that allow the linkage of tubing that should not be connected. The risk is especially great in hospitalized patients who have multiple catheters, tubes, and drains, which all appear similar. Industry changes are occurring as manufacturing companies implement designed incompatibility between tubing. Meanwhile, interventions aimed at reducing risk for misconnections are summarized as follows (Pennsylvania Safety Authority, 2010):

- Trace all lines back to their point of origin to verify that correct connections are made (also addressed in INS Standards, 2011, p. S86).
- Recheck connections and trace all lines to their point of origin after the patient's arrival to a new care area or as part of a handoff process.
- Never force connections; when effort is needed to make a connection, there is a good chance that the connection should not be made.
- Only use adapters that are clearly indicated for a specific application. Additionally, the need for an adapter may mean that the connection should not be made.
- Label high-risk catheters (e.g., epidural, **intrathecal**, arterial).
- Route lines (e.g., tubes, catheters) with different purposes in unique and standardized directions (e.g., route I.V. lines toward the patient's head, route enteral feeding lines toward the patient's feet).
- Identify and manage conditions that may contribute to worker fatigue, which could result in inattentiveness when making tubing connections, and take appropriate action.
- Tell nonclinical staff to get help from the nurse if there is a real or perceived need to connect or disconnect infusions or devices.
- Never use a standard Luer syringe for oral medications or enteral feedings.

▪ Principles of Intravenous Medication Administration

Advantages

The advantages of administration of fluids and medications via the intravenous (I.V.) route include (1) direct access to the circulatory system, (2) a route for administration of fluids and drugs to patients who cannot tolerate oral medications, (3) a method of instant drug action, and (4) a method of instant drug administration termination. This route offers advantages over the subcutaneous (SQ), intramuscular (IM), and oral routes in certain clinical situations (Table 10-1).

Drugs that cannot be absorbed by other routes because of the large molecular size of the drug or destruction of the drug by gastric juices can be administered directly to the site of **distribution**, the circulatory system, with I.V. infusion. Drugs with irritating properties that cause pain and trauma when given via the intramuscular or subcutaneous route can be given intravenously. When a drug is administered intravenously, there is instant drug action, which is an advantage in emergency situations. The I.V. route also provides instant drug termination if sensitivity or adverse reactions occur. This route provides for control over the rate at which drugs are administered. Prolonged action can be controlled by administering a dilute medication infusion intermittently over a prolonged time period.

Intravenous medications are administered to obtain rapid therapeutic or diagnostic responses or as delivery routes for solutions or medications that cannot be delivered by any other route. Nurses administering the solution or medication are accountable for achieving effective delivery of prescribed therapy and for evaluating and documenting deviations from an expected outcome, including the implementation of corrective action.

INS Standard The nurse administering parenteral medications and solutions should have knowledge of indications for therapy, side effects, potential adverse reactions, and appropriate interventions (INS, 2011, p. S86).

> Table 10-1	ADVANTAGES AND DISADVANTAGES OF INTRAVENOUS MEDICATION ADMINISTRATION

Advantages
1. Provides a direct access to the circulatory system.
2. Provides a route for drugs that irritate the gastric mucosa.
3. Provides a route for instant drug action.
4. Provides a route for delivering high drug concentrations.
5. Provides for instant drug termination if sensitivity or adverse reaction occurs.
6. Provides for better control over the rate of drug administration.
7. Provides a route of administration in patients in whom use of the gastrointestinal tract is limited.

Disadvantages/Risks
1. Drug interaction because of incompatibilities
2. Potential for drug adsorption and subsequent loss of drug activity.
3. Errors in compounding (mixing) of medication
4. Speed shock
5. Extravasation of a vesicant drug
6. Chemical phlebitis

Risks

Despite the advantages of I.V. medication, there are also risks not found with other medication administration routes (see Table 10-1). The advantage (as discussed earlier) of immediate, systemic effects with I.V. infusion is also a risk in the event of a drug administration error. As stated earlier, it is difficult, or impossible, to reverse the pharmacological effects after I.V. administration. Other risks specific to the administration of I.V. drugs include potential **drug interactions**; drug loss via **adsorption** of I.V. containers and administration sets; potential errors in compounding techniques; and the potential complications of speed shock, extravasation of vesicant drugs, and phlebitis (see Chapter 9).

▪ Drug Stability and Compatibility

Drug Stability

Stability refers to the length of time that a drug retains its original properties and characteristics (Turner & Hankins, 2010). Factors that affect stability include pH, number of additives in the solution (e.g., parenteral nutrition solutions contain many additives), dilution, time (e.g., some drugs once mixed are only stable for a few hours), light exposure, temperature, order in which additives are put into the solutions, and type of container (e.g., insulin adsorption in polyvinyl chloride [PVC] containers). The pH is one of the most important factors (Turner & Hankins, 2010) because most drugs are stable in a very narrow pH range.

Drug Incompatibility

Incompatibility is an undesirable reaction that occurs between the drug and the solution, the container, or another drug (Turner & Hankins, 2010). There are three types of drug incompatibility: physical, chemical, and therapeutic. Incompatibility may occur when:

- Several drugs are added to a large volume of fluid to produce an **admixture**
- Drugs in separate solutions are administered concurrently or in close succession via the same I.V. line
- A single drug is reconstituted or diluted with the wrong solutions
- One drug reacts with another drug's preservative

Physical Incompatibility

A **physical incompatibility** refers to a visible reaction that occurs, such as changes in color, haziness, turbidity, precipitate formation, and gas formation. The most common type of physical incompatibility is precipitate formation.

Some precipitation may be microcrystalline (i.e., smaller than 50 microns) and not apparent to the eye. Use of a 0.22-micron inline filter reduces the amount of microcrystalline precipitates. Such particulate matter can result in occlusion of pulmonary capillaries. As discussed in Chapter 5, filter use in critically ill patients has been found to be efficacious in preventing complications such as systemic inflammatory response syndrome and others (Jack et al., 2012).

The presence of calcium in a drug or solution increases the risk for precipitation if it is mixed with another drug. Ringer's solution preparations contain calcium, so check carefully for compatibility before adding any drug to this solution. Other physical incompatibilities caused by insolubility include the increased degradation of drugs added to sodium bicarbonate and the formation of an insoluble precipitate when sodium bicarbonate is combined with other medications in emergency situations.

The following are important recommendations regarding physical drug incompatibilities:

- Do not mix drugs prepared in special diluents with other drugs.
- When administering a series of medications, prepare each drug in a separate syringe. This will lessen the possibility of precipitation. Insolubility may also result from the use of an incorrect solution to reconstitute a drug.
- Follow the manufacturer's directions for reconstituting drugs and remember that pharmacy-prepared medications are preferred to reduce the risk of contamination and instability.

 NURSING FAST FACT!

To prevent physical I.V. drug incompatibility during administration, best practice is to always flush the infusion device with 0.9% sodium chloride before and after each medication infusion. However, some drugs, such as amphotericin B, are not compatible with sodium chloride. In such cases, use 5% dextrose in water for flushing before and after administration. The dextrose should always be flushed from the catheter with 0.9% sodium chloride because it can provide nutrients supporting microbial growth if allowed to dwell in the catheter lumen (INS, 2011, p. S60).

Chemical Incompatibility

A **chemical incompatibility** involves the degradation of the drug, which may occur for a variety of reasons, for example, drug decomposition (Turner & Hankins, 2010). It is differentiated from physical incompatibility in that the reaction may not be visible. The most common cause of chemical incompatibility is the reaction between acidic and alkaline drugs or solutions, which results in a pH level that is unstable for one of the drugs. A specific pH or a narrow range of pH values is required for the solubility of a drug and for the maintenance of its stability after it has been mixed.

Therapeutic Incompatibility

A **therapeutic incompatibility** is an undesirable effect that occurs in the patient as a result of two or more drugs being given concurrently. An increased therapeutic or a decreased therapeutic response is produced. This incompatibility often occurs when therapy dictates the use of two antibiotics. For example, with the use of chloramphenicol and penicillin, chloramphenicol has been reported to antagonize the bacterial activity of penicillin (Gahart & Nazareno, 2012). If prescribed, penicillin should be administered at least 1 hour before chloramphenicol to prevent therapeutic incompatibility.

Therapeutic incompatibility may go unnoticed until the patient fails to show the expected clinical response to the drug or until peak and trough levels of the drug show a lack of therapeutic levels. If an incompatibility is not suspected, the patient may be given increasingly higher doses of the drug in an attempt to obtain the therapeutic effect. When more than one antibiotic is prescribed for **intermittent infusion**, it is generally best to stagger the time schedule so that each antibiotic can be infused individually.

Adsorption

Adsorption is the attachment of a liquid or gas to a solid surface. In infusion therapy, some infusion drugs and solutions adsorb to glass or plastic. With adsorption, the patient receives a smaller amount of the drug than was intended. The amount of adsorption is difficult to predict and is affected by the drug concentration, solution of the drug, amount of surface contacted by the drug, and temperature changes.

An example of adsorption is the binding of insulin to plastic and glass containers. The insulin rapidly adsorbs to I.V. containers and tubing until all potential adsorption sites are saturated. The potency of insulin may be reduced by at least 20% and possibly up to 80% before it reaches the vein (Gahart & Nazareno, 2012). Methods for reducing adsorption include use of additives such as albumin, electrolytes, vitamins, or other medications or use of a syringe pump where there is less surface area for adsorption (Gahart & Nazareno, 2012). Another example of a medication that is readily adsorbed into PVC bags or administration sets is nitroglycerin. Non-PVC tubing and non-PVC or glass bottles should be used.

As discussed in Chapter 5, di(2-ethylhexyl)phthalate (DEHP), a known toxin, is a plasticizer used in making PVC bags soft and pliable. DEHP is lipophilic and can leach into lipid-based solutions. In the package inserts, many drug manufacturers recommend nonphthalate **delivery systems**. The INS Standards (2011, p. S56) recommend DEHP-free administration sets for administration of lipid-based infusates. Many companies are manufacturing nonphthalate I.V. bags and tubing to prevent this problem.

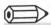

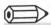 NURSING FAST FACT!

> When mixing medications into glass or plastic systems, refer to the manufacturer's guidelines to prevent/minimize adsorption.

 CULTURAL AND ETHNIC CONSIDERATIONS: DRUG ADMINISTRATION

Data have been collected regarding differences in the effect of some medications on persons of diverse ethnic or cultural origins. Genetic predispositions to different rates of metabolism cause some patients to be prone to overdose reactions to the "normal dose" of medication, whereas other patients are likely to experience a greatly reduced benefit from the standard dose of the medication.

In ethnic and cultural groups (e.g., African Americans and Asian Americans) with a high incidence of glucose-6-phosphate dehydrogenase (G6PD) deficiency, some drugs may impair red blood cell metabolism, leading to anemia. Caffeine, a component of many drugs, is excreted more slowly by Asian Americans. Asian Americans may require smaller doses of certain drugs (Giger & Davidhizar, 2004).

 NURSING FAST FACT!

> ■ Be knowledgeable of the pharmacological implications relative to patient clinical status and diagnosis.
> ■ Verify that all solution containers are free of cracks, leaks, and punctures.

Intravenous Medication Administration

Intravenous medications may be infused via four administration methods: continuous infusion, intermittent infusion, direct injection or I.V. push, and **patient-controlled analgesia (PCA)** (Turner & Hankins, 2010). Factors in the choice of administration method include the type of medication or I.V. solution, the patient's condition, and the desired drug effects.

Continuous I.V. Infusions

A continuous infusion is given over several hours to several days or longer. Some examples of solutions or medications administered as a continuous infusion include parenteral nutrition, hydration fluids, and medications requiring constant plasma concentrations such as nitroprusside and dobutamine. Electronic infusion devices are used to ensure an accurate flow rate.

ADVANTAGES

■ Constant serum levels of medications are maintained.

DISADVANTAGES

■ Potential for fluid overload
■ Potential for incompatibilities between the infusion and any other I.V. medications administered through the same VAD or through a port of the administration set
■ Accidental **bolus** infusion can occur if the medication is not adequately mixed with the solution.

Intermittent I.V. Infusions

Intermittent infusions are used with medications that are mixed in a smaller volume of fluid (e.g., 50 mL) and infused over a short period of time (e.g., 30–60 minutes) at regular intervals. For example, antibiotics are most often administered as intermittent infusions. Methods of delivering intermittent infusions include piggyback infusions, simultaneous infusions, **metered volume chambers**, and primary administration sets (Turner & Hankins, 2010).

The "piggyback" infusion is a very commonly used method. An I.V. solution is attached to a primary administration set, which is the main tubing carrying the infusion from the container to the patient. A secondary administration set is attached to the primary set, entering the tubing at a port with a back check valve. When the drug infusion is completed, the primary I.V. solution then resumes. Although the primary infusion is interrupted during the secondary infusion, the drug from the intermittent infusion container comes in contact with the primary solution below the injection port; therefore, the drug and the primary solution must be compatible (Fig. 10-1A).

In a simultaneous infusion, the main I.V. solution and the drug I.V. solution are infused at the same time through a port near the I.V. catheter. A risk associated with this method is blood reflux back into the VAD when the secondary infusion of the medication is completed because no back check valve is used, as with a piggyback infusion set (Fig. 10-1B).

The metered volume chamber is used less often today and is most often used in pediatric settings. The primary solution is added to the chamber (may hold 100–150 mL; neonatal chambers 10–50 mL), and the medication is added to the chamber via a syringe (Fig. 10-2).

Finally, a small solution container of medication may be attached to a primary administration set and infused directly into the patient's I.V. catheter; there is no secondary set. This method is often used in home care settings and other alternate sites. Use of an elastomeric infusion pump (see Chapter 5) is another way to deliver an intermittent

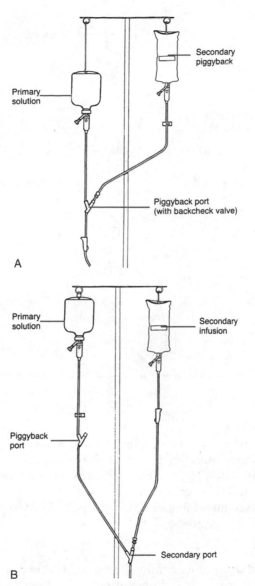

Figure 10-1 ■ Methods of delivery of secondary infusions. *A,* Secondary piggyback infusion. *B,* Simultaneous infusion.

medication through a primary set. The balloon of the reservoir holds the medication, and the pre-attached I.V. tubing is primed. When the clamp is opened, the medication is infused at a rate based on an integrated flow restrictor. This method is also most commonly used in alternate sites for intermittent medication administration.

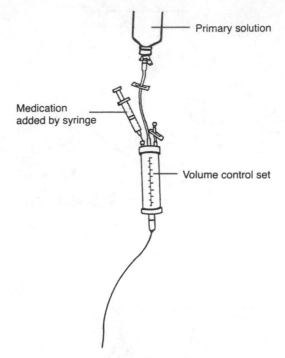

Figure 10-2 ◼ Administration of medication via a volume-controlled chamber.

Advantages

- A larger drug dose can be administered at a lower concentration per milliliter than with the I.V. push method.
- Peak flow concentrations occur at periodic intervals.
- The risk of fluid overload is decreased.
- Metered volume chamber: The volume of fluid in which the drug is diluted can be adjusted.

Disadvantages

- Increased drug concentration in the intermittent solution can cause vein irritation and phlebitis.
- The administration rate may not be accurate unless it is electronically monitored; too rapid a rate can potentially lead to speed shock and/or fluid overload.
- Primary administration set method: I.V. set changes can result in wasting a portion of the drug that remains in the I.V. tubing.
- Risk for incompatibility can occur if the administration set is not adequately flushed between medication administrations.
- Metered volume chamber:
  - A portion of the medication can be left in the tubing after the chamber empties.

- Incompatibilities may develop when the chamber, which is usually within the primary line, is used for multiple drug deliveries.
- Labeling of the chamber must coincide with the drug being delivered. If multiple drugs are delivered, this could present a problem.

 NURSING FAST FACT!

Consider the volume of fluid delivered with an intermittent infusion as part of the patient's overall intake when calculating intake.

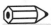 **NURSING FAST FACT!**

Drug incompatibility is a greater risk with the simultaneous infusion method.

NURSING POINTS OF CARE
INTERMITTENT I.V. INFUSION DELIVERY

- Ensure the **compatibility** of the I.V. solution and medication, both the solution in the primary system and the diluent in the secondary system.
- Assess the I.V. site and the patency of the catheter.
- Calculate the amount of medication to add to the solution.
- Use the correct amount and type of diluent solution.
- Use the correct rate of administration.
- Determine the correct primary line port in which to infuse the medication.
- Affix the correct label to the secondary bag, with start date and hour, discard date and hour, and your initials.
- Calculate the amount of medication to be added to the volume-controlled set.
- High alert medications: Consider using a double-check drug process. Follow the organization's procedures.

Intravenous Push

Direct injection, or "**intravenous push**," is the administration of I.V. medication in a syringe directly into the patient's VAD or through the injection port of a continuous infusion. This method is used with drugs that require rapid serum concentrations. In the home care setting, I.V. push is often used for selected antimicrobials, including some in the cephalosporin group (e.g., ceftriaxone) and daptomycin.

It is important to recognize risks associated with I.V. push medications. Speed shock is a systemic reaction that occurs when a substance is rapidly introduced into the circulation (discussed further in Chapter 9). Symptoms include dizziness, facial flushing, headache, and medication-specific symptoms and can progress to chest tightness, hypotension, irregular pulse, and anaphylaxis. It is critical to administer I.V. push medications over the appropriate time frame. Usually the label on the medication syringe will indicate the time (e.g., administer over 3–5 minutes); if not labeled, the nurse should consult with the pharmacist. Refer to Procedures Display 10-1 at the end of this chapter.

 NURSING FAST FACT!

> Studies have shown frequent lapses in correct I.V. push administration, including the fact that nurses often administer I.V. push medications too rapidly (Carter, Gelchion, Saitta, & Clark, 2011).

ADVANTAGES

- Barriers of drug absorption are bypassed.
- The drug response is rapid and usually predictable.
- The patient is closely monitored during the full administration of the medication.

DISADVANTAGES

- Adverse effects occur at the same time and rate as therapeutic effects.
- The I.V. push method has the greatest risk of adverse effects and toxicity because serum drug concentrations are sharply elevated.
- Speed shock is possible from too rapid administration of medication.

NURSING POINTS OF CARE
DIRECT I.V. PUSH MEDICATIONS

- Only use single-use vials for mixing and diluting medication and prepare them aseptically and in accordance with manufacturer's instructions for preparation and organizational procedures. In most cases, the medication should be prepared by the pharmacy.
- Determine the amount of time needed to administer the medication.

- Flush the VAD with 0.9% sodium chloride (USP) before administration of medication.
- Maintain aseptic technique.
- High alert medications: Consider using double-check process with another registered nurse (RN) according to organizational procedures.
- Most medications are delivered slowly, between 1 and 10 minutes. (Example: Morphine I.V. push delivery of 15 mg or a fraction thereof is recommended over 4–5 minutes; Gahart & Nazareno, 2012).

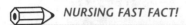 NURSING FAST FACT!

If adverse effects occur, supportive care is the basis for treatment of most symptoms because specific antidotes are available only for certain drugs.

Patient-Controlled Analgesia

PCA is a method of pain management that allows the patient to deliver his or her own analgesic dose when needed. It is a common method of pain management, particularly in postoperative patient care. It is also used in palliative care and hospice care settings to achieve pain control. The goal of PCA is to provide the patient with good pain management with minimal sedation. Putting patients in control of their own pain management makes sense because only they know how much they are suffering. It is more desirable to use small doses of narcotics frequently than large doses of narcotics infrequently.

PCA infusion is delivered with a specific type of electronic infusion pump that is programmed to administer a prescribed amount of analgesic to the patient when activated by the patient pressing a button. PCA pumps may be programmed for only a dose on demand but may also be used in conjunction with a continuous basal infusion of drug, primarily in hospice and palliative care. There are ambulatory PCA pumps available for the home care patient (Fig. 10-3).

It is important to recognize that opioids are considered high alert medications in both acute and community settings by the Institute for Safe Medication Practices (ISMP, 2011, 2012). The INS (2011, p. S90) and ISMP (2008) recommend that a double-check procedure be in place; a second clinician should independently verify the drug, dosage, rate, and route prior to initiation of PCA, when the solution container is changed, and when the drug or dosage is changed. The INS (2011, p. S90) further states that "special attention should be given to drug, concentration, dose, and rate of infusion according to the order and as programmed into the electronic infusion device, in order to reduce the risk of adverse outcomes and medication errors."

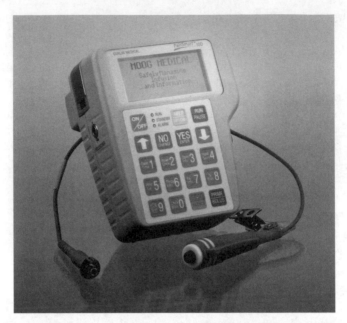

Figure 10-3 ◼ Ambulatory PCA pump: PainSmart IOD (information on demand). (Courtesy of Moog Medical Devices Group, Salt Lake City, UT.)

It is also important to recognize that not all patients are good candidates for PCA. The patient must be able to cognitively understand the relationship between pain, activating the dose button, and achieving a goal of good pain control. Candidates for PCA include those patients who (Simpson, 2010):

- Are anticipating pain that is severe and intermittent
- Have constant pain that worsens with activity
- Can comprehend the technique
- Have the functional ability to press the button
- Are motivated
- Are not sedated from other medications

INS Standard The nurse should assess the patient for the appropriateness of PCA therapy and the patient's comprehension of, and ability to participate in, the intended therapy (INS, 2011, p. S90).

With PCA, in general, no other person should be activating the drug dose. As PCA use grew, the process of identifying appropriate candidates was not always adhered to, and well-meaning nurses and family members would deliver the medication. The problem of "PCA by proxy" was identified (Wuhrman et al., 2007). It is important to recognize that a basic safeguard of PCA is that the excessively sedated patient will be too sleepy to activate the dose; therefore, the risk for opioid-induced respiratory depression is minimized. This safeguard is lost if others are activating the PCA dose.

However, when the patient cannot actively participate in PCA, the patient may be assessed for the appropriateness of "authorized agent-controlled analgesia" (AACA) (INS, 2011, p. S90). As identified by the American Society for Pain Management Nursing (ASPMN) (Wuhrman et al., 2007), with AACA, a consistent, available, and competent person is authorized by the prescriber and educated to activate the dose button when the patient is unable to do so. The ASPMN further identifies the concepts of nurse-controlled analgesia (NCA), where the nurse administers the dose, and caregiver-controlled analgesia (CCA), where a nonprofessional caregiver such as a parent or family member administers the dose.

Patients should be carefully monitored to prevent respiratory depression and other adverse events due to PCA. Patient risk factors for oversedation and respiratory depression associated with opioid use are listed in Table 10-2. The ASPMN (Jarzyna et al., 2011) has published evidence-based guidelines aimed at monitoring opioid-induced sedation and respiratory depression. Key recommendations include:

- Development of an individualized plan for monitoring based on risk factors, iatrogenic risks, and pharmacological regimen
- Outlining of monitoring practices in organizational policies and procedures
- Use of serial sedation and respiratory assessments
    - Perform during wakefulness and during sleep.
    - Use sedation scales that have acceptable validity and reliability.
    - Count respirations for a full minute and qualify according to rhythm and depth of chest excursion while patient is in restful/sleep state.

> Table 10-2	PATIENT RISK FACTORS FOR OVERSEDATION AND RESPIRATORY DEPRESSION WITH PATIENT-CONTROLLED ANALGESIA

- Older adults (>60 years old, risk increases with increasing age)
- Morbid obesity
- Snoring
- No recent opioid use
- Postoperative patients who have had upper abdominal or thoracic surgery
- Long duration of anesthesia
- Taking other sedative medications
- Pre-existing cardiopulmonary disease or major organ failure
- Obstructive sleep apnea or other sleeping disorder

The Joint Commission, 2012.

- Do not transfer patients between levels of care during peak effect of medication.
- If respiratory depression (e.g., rate <8–10 per minute), evidence of advancing sedation, poor respiratory effort, snoring or other noisy respiration, or oxygen desaturation is present, the patient should be aroused immediately and instructed to take deep breaths. Additional interventions may be required (e.g., opioid reversal with naloxone).
- Technology-supported monitoring should be considered.
  - Continuous pulse oximetry
  - Capnography monitoring (measurement of end-tidal CO_2), a more sensitive measure and early indicator of respiratory compromise

Monitoring should be more vigilant when patients are at greater risk, such as during peak medication effects, first 24 hours postoperatively, with dosage increases, with changes in opioid medication, and with changes in route of administration (Jarzyna et al., 2011).

 NURSING FAST FACT!

When opioids are administered, the potential for opioid-induced respiratory depression should always be considered.

Adverse Events and Patient-Controlled Analgesia

Infusion pump PCA programming errors are a significant problem (Simpson, 2010). The ISMP (2008) has received a small but concerning number of reports of overdoses with PCA because of pump programming errors. Errors related to programming the opioid concentration are of particular concern. When higher concentrations are erroneously programmed, a lower dose will be delivered, compromising pain management. On the other hand, erroneously entering a lower concentration will increase the dose, which has led to adverse drug events, including fatalities. Recommendations from the ISMP (2008) include:

- Limiting the concentrations available in the organization
- Distinguishing custom drug concentrations by the pharmacy, such as different-colored pharmacy labels and specific instructions
- Matching the medication administration record to the PCA label so that there is less confusion when comparing the product label to the medication order
- Use of barcode technology
- Use of smart pumps
- Use of independent double-checking

In 2012, TJC issued a Sentinel Event Alert related to the use of opioids and adverse events, including deaths, which occurred in hospitals and were reported to TJC's Sentinel Event database (2004–2011) (TJC, 2012). Errors occurred as follows:

- 47% wrong dose errors
- 29% improper monitoring
- 11% others, such as excessive dosing, drug interactions, and adverse drug reactions

TJC emphasizes the critical need for judicious and safe prescribing and administration of opioids, and appropriate monitoring of patients.

EBP A follow-up survey to evaluate the effectiveness, perceived benefits, and shortcomings of existing monitoring practices was performed by the ASPMN. Overall, a lack of a standard of care for monitoring patients for opioid-induced respiratory depression was identified. The national survey included 147 responses from 90 health-care institutions across the United States. Some findings in relation to PCA included the following: only one-third of patients received increased frequency and timing of monitoring; continuous pulse oximetry was used only about one-third of the time; only about 2% of respondents had access to capnography monitoring; and variations in definition of respiratory depression, with most respondents not considering quality of breaths during assessment. A lack of a standard of care is a factor contributing to adverse events. Since the guidelines were published (Jarzyna et al., 2011), the ASPMN has focused on educational presentations, and a follow-up survey is planned to evaluate effectiveness of their efforts (Willens, Jungquist, Cohen, & Polomano, 2013).

PCA Advantages

- When patients are in control and know they can get more immediate pain relief by pushing a button, they are more relaxed.
- Analgesia is most effective when a therapeutic serum level is consistently maintained.
- Patients whose postoperative pain is controlled are better able to ambulate, cough, and deep breathe.

PCA Disadvantages/Risks

- Opioid administration is associated with excessive sedation and potential respiratory depression. Patients at increased risk must be identified, and all patients should be carefully monitored.
- Not all patients are appropriate candidates, including those whose level of consciousness, psychological condition, or limited intellectual capacity cannot safely manage PCA.
- Misprogramming PCA concentration has been identified as a significant source of error, but errors in initiating PCA infusion can occur at any point in the programming process.

■ There is a risk of someone other than the patient pushing the button on a PCA pump. Place warning labels "For patient use only" on the button. Remind patients and visitors that PCA is for patient use only unless there is a plan in place for AACA.

 NURSING FAST FACT!

> Only the patient should push the PCA button unless there is a clear plan in place for AACA.

NURSING POINTS OF CARE
PCA ADMINISTRATION

■ PCA is a philosophy of treatment rather than a single method of drug administration.
■ Assess the patient's baseline vital signs, cognitive status, and pain level.
■ Insert the pump device containing the medication accurately.
■ Set the pump for the loading dose (if ordered), basal rate (not used with opioid-naïve and postoperative patients, often used with palliative care patients), demand dose, lockout interval, and 1-hour or 4-hour lockout dose limit.
■ Validation by a second clinician or caregiver should be used before initiation and administration of PCA, and when the syringe, solution container, or rate/dose is changed.
■ Put the button that controls dosing within reach of the patient.
■ Monitor for potential adverse events, including excessive sedation and respiratory depression.
■ Consider use of continuous pulse oximetry to maintain pulse oxygen above 90% and/or capnography.
■ Use a sedation scale to monitor patients with I.V. PCA.

TEN SAFE PRACTICE RECOMMENDATIONS TO PREVENT ERRORS ASSOCIATED WITH PCA THERAPY

1. Limit the variety of medications used for PCA.
2. Improve access to information.
   a. Develop a quick reference sheet on PCA that includes programming tips as well as maximum dose warnings.
3. Improve label readability.
   a. Match the sequence of information that appears on PCA medication labels and order sets with the sequence of information that must be entered into the PCA pump.

4. Highlight the drug concentration on the label.
5. Program default settings.
6. Ensure staff competence with PCA infusion pump use.
   a. Involve nurses in selection and evaluation of PCA pumps to ensure patient safety.
7. Consider the possibility of error.
   a. If the patient is not responding to the PCA doses, consider the possibility of an error, especially before administering a bolus dose. Reverify the drug, concentration, pump settings, and line attachment.
8. Use double-checks.
   a. Clearly define a manual, independent double-check process for clinicians to follow when verifying PCA medications, pump settings via a confirmation screen, the patient, and line attachments.
   b. Use barcode technology; use smart PCA pumps that alert clinicians to potential programming errors.
9. Assess the proximity of the PCA pump to the general infusion pump
   a. To decrease the potential for I.V. line mix-ups and possible medication errors.
10. Educate the patient.

INS Standard Patient and caregiver education should be appropriate to duration of therapy and care setting and should include the purpose of PCA therapy, operating instructions for the infusion pump, expected outcomes, precautions, potential side effects, and contact information for support services (INS, 2011, p. S90).

NURSING POINTS OF CARE
DELIVERY OF INTRAVENOUS MEDICATION

Nursing Assessments
- Review the present illness.
- Perform medication reconciliation.
- Review medication history or adverse/side effects.
- Review allergies before starting the medication.
- Assess current medications for potential drug interactions/incompatibility issues.
- Assess vital signs.
- Weigh the patient.
- Identify patient-related factors that may alter the patient's response to the drug, such as age or renal, hepatic, and cardiovascular function.

Continued

■ Assess need for and appropriateness of I.V. medication infusion beyond the acute care setting (e.g., home care, long-term care setting).

Key Nursing Interventions
1. Follow the rights of medication administration.
2. Verify order before administering the drug.
3. Check expiration date on medication container.
4. Determine the correct dilution, amount, and length of administration time as appropriate.
5. Administer medications using the appropriate infusion method.
6. Maintain aseptic technique at all times.
7. Monitor for:
   a. Signs/symptoms of VAD site complications (e.g., phlebitis, infiltration)
   b. Laboratory values as appropriate (e.g., drug levels, renal function)
   c. Therapeutic response
   d. Adverse reactions/side effects
   e. Intake and output
8. Maintain I.V. access.
9. Dispose of unused or expired drugs according to organizational policy.
10. For I.V. PCA:
    a. Monitor sedation level.
    b. Monitor respiratory rate, rhythm and chest excursion; count respirations for full minute.
    c. Monitor oxygen saturation via pulse oximetry and monitor end-tidal CO_2 using capnography if available.
    d. Intervene promptly if excessive sedation.
    e. Intervene promptly if respiratory depression present.
11. Document medication administration and patient responsiveness.

◾ Other Infusion Medication Routes

Subcutaneous

The subcutaneous administration of medications or fluids is an alternative option to I.V. infusion and has become a more commonly used route. As a brief review of anatomy, the subcutaneous tissue is located beneath the dermal layer of the skin. It contains blood vessels, nerves, and adipose tissue. Fluids or medications administered subcutaneously are absorbed into the blood vessels located in the subcutaneous space.

There are two main categories of subcutaneous infusion therapy: medication administration and isotonic fluid administration. Continuous subcutaneous infusion (CSI) of opioid drugs (e.g., morphine, hydromorphone) for pain management is a common practice in palliative care and hospice settings. In general, the subcutaneous dose for opioids is considered equianalgesic to the I.V. dose, that is, 1 mg of morphine I.V. is equal to 1 mg of morphine subcutaneous (Weisman, 2009). Other medications administered via CSI include insulin, terbutaline (preterm labor), deferoxamine (iron chelation for iron overload), some antiemetics, steroids, and immunoglobulin therapy (Parker & Henderson, 2010; Younger et al., 2013). The optimal infusion rate for CSI of medications is not known, but infusion rates of 2 to 3 mL/hr are commonly reported (INS, 2011, p. S84). With subcutaneous immunoglobulin infusions, it is important to follow the manufacturer's specific recommendations for subcutaneous rates; depending on the manufacturer, rates of 15 to 25 mL/hr are not uncommon.

Subcutaneous infusion of isotonic fluids is called **hypodermoclysis**. This was a widely used mode of infusion until the 1950s, when complications from improper care related to poor patient selection, incorrect rates of administration, and poor choices of fluids led to the severe decline of this infusion modality. Today, hypodermoclysis is recognized as a relatively easy, low-risk, and cost-effective method for delivery of hydration fluids in patients with mild to moderate dehydration (Humphrey, 2011; Scales, 2011). The isotonic fluids most commonly administered include 0.9% sodium chloride and 5% dextrose in water.

Hypodermoclysis is used often in long-term care facilities to manage mild dehydration in the older patient and is increasingly being used in the home care setting. Pediatric patients with limited or difficult venous access are also candidates for hypodermoclysis, although there is scarce evidence for use in this population (Rouhani, Meloney, Ahn, Nelson, & Burke, 2011). Up to 1500 mL over 24 hours (approximately 60 mL/hr) can be delivered to a single subcutaneous site, and up to 3 L may be given using two different sites. A simple Y tubing connected to the I.V. administration set can deliver fluids via two different sites simultaneously (INS, 2011; Parker & Henderson, 2010). There are also specially designed subcutaneous infusion sets that allow for simultaneous infusion via two or more sites (Fig. 10-4).

There are three options for devices used to access the subcutaneous tissue: (1) stainless steel winged needles; (2) over-the-needle catheters (i.e., small-gauge [24-gauge] catheters used for peripheral I.V. insertion); and (3) specially designed subcutaneous needles (Figs. 10-5, 10-6). Key issues related to device placement include the following:

- Site selection: Any area where there is adequate subcutaneous tissue and the skin is intact (no evidence of bruising, irritation) can be used. The most common sites include the abdomen (avoid area around navel because of blood vessel proximity), anterior

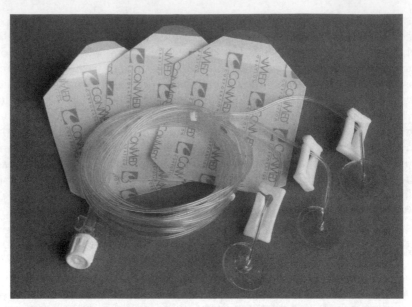

Figure 10-4 ■ ClearView™ MS: multiple site subcutaneous delivery set. (Courtesy of Norfolk Medical, Skokie, IL.)

thighs, subclavicular chest wall, upper back, and upper arm (INS, 2011, p. S84).

■ Site preparation: As with placement of any VAD, skin antisepsis is an important step. Attention to proper hand hygiene and washing of visibly dirty skin with soap and water followed by skin antisepsis are critical steps. Antiseptic agents are the same as those used for I.V. preparation, including chlorhexidine-alcohol solutions and 70% alcohol (Scales, 2011).

■ Device insertion: It is important to review and follow the manufacturer's directions for use with any device. When using an over-the-needle catheter, enter the subcutaneous tissue at a 30- to 45-degree angle, depending on the thickness of the tissue. Specially designed subcutaneous sets are inserted at a 90-degree angle. Once placed, the device should be aspirated to ensure that there is no blood return, which confirms that the device is in the tissue and not in a small blood vessel (INS, 2011, p. S84).

■ Device securement and dressing: Generally a transparent semipermeable dressing is placed over the site, which allows for continuous site observation and assessment.

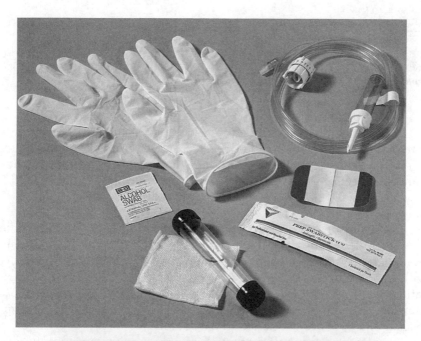

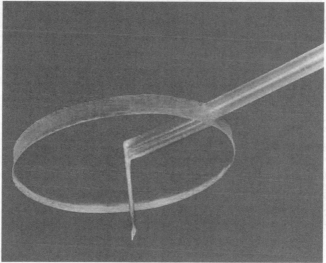

Figure 10-5 ■ Aqua-C™ hydration set for hypodermoclysis and ClearView™ Sub-Q. A clear disk allows for ongoing subcutaneous site assessment. (Courtesy of Norfolk Medical, Skokie, IL.)

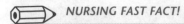 *NURSING FAST FACT!*

Based on a review of the literature, the use of nonmetal subcutaneous devices was found to be more comfortable for patients. They also lasted longer and required less frequent site changes (Parker & Henderson, 2010).

The infusion is set up the same as an I.V. A standard I.V. administration set is used for hypodermoclysis, and gravity administration is recommended (Scales, 2011). When administering CSI of medications, an electronic infusion device is used. Syringe pumps are often used, especially with immunoglobulin administration (INS, 2011, p. S84).

Complications related to subcutaneous infusions are generally minor. They include itching or burning at the site, erythema, induration, pain, leaking, bleeding, infection, and tissue slough. Some edema is expected with hypodermoclysis but will subside as the fluid is absorbed. Complications are managed by ongoing site assessment and site rotation. The infusion rate may need to be reduced, and use of a plastic-type device instead of a steel needle should be considered.

Site rotation is an important aspect related to subcutaneous infusions. For hypodermoclysis, the site should be changed after 1500 mL of fluid has been administered in a single site. Depending on tolerance and site assessment, the site may need to be rotated earlier. When administering medications via CSI, the recommendation is every 2 to 7 days and as clinically indicated, based on the integrity of the access site (INS, 2011, p. S84). The nurse's assessment of individual patient tolerance is an important aspect when considering frequency of site rotation.

Candidates for CSI:
- Patients unable to take medications by mouth
- Patients with evidence of mild to moderate dehydration
- Patients with limited or difficult venous access
- Patients requiring continuous medication delivery

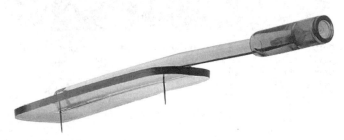

Figure 10-6 ▪ Aqua-C subcutaneous device with two needles; used for hypodermoclysis. (Courtesy of Norfolk Medical, Skokie, IL.)

INS Standard The responsibility of the nurse caring for a patient with CSI therapy includes, but is not limited to, knowledge of anatomy and physiology, care and maintenance practices, potential complications, and patient and caregiver education (INS, 2011, p. S84).

> *EBP Walsh (2005) conducted a study of 30 long-term care residents from 24 to 90 years of age who received subcutaneous infusions from 1 to 2 days. All treatments were for dehydration, and all infusions were completed without adverse effects except for one incidence of local edema at the site.*

ADVANTAGES

- Ease of initiation and maintenance by RN or licensed vocational nurse (LVN)/licensed practical nurse (LPN)
- Reduction in transfers to acute care facilities from long-term care for intravenous access
- Fewer complications, less pain reported by patients, decreased cost

DISADVANTAGES

- Not appropriate for patients with severe dehydration who require a larger volume of fluid replacement
- Local irritation at the infusion site
- Edema

NURSING POINTS OF CARE
CONTINUOUS SUBCUTANEOUS INFUSIONS

- A number of medications can be administered subcutaneously; use of subcutaneous opioids is common in palliative care.
- Isotonic fluids are acceptable for hypodermoclysis.
- Suitable sites for subcutaneous infusion include posterior upper arms, subclavicular chest, anterior thighs, upper back, and upper arms.
- Rotate the site every 2 to 7 days for continuous medication infusions or after 1500 mL of fluid has been administered in a single site (hypodermoclysis).
- Change the dressing with each site rotation.
- Monitor the access site:
  - Observe site for bleeding, bruising, inflammation, drainage, edema, and cellulitis.
  - Monitor the patient for complaints of burning or itching at the site.

Intraperitoneal

Infusions via the **intraperitoneal (IP)** route involve the administration of chemotherapy agents directly into the peritoneal cavity. The delivery of chemotherapeutic agents directly into the peritoneum has been practiced since the 1950s, and although it has lost and gained popularity over the years, it is a standard of care for certain types of cancers within the peritoneal space, most often with advanced ovarian cancer (Anastasia, 2012; Drake, 2009). Other diagnoses with the potential for IP chemotherapy include malignant peritoneal mesothelioma, malignancy of the appendix, and peritoneal dissemination from pancreatic cancer (Polovich, Whitford, & Olsen, 2009). The IP route is limited to select patients who have minimal residual tumors. The administration of IP as well as I.V. chemotherapy requires specialized knowledge and competency (Anastasia, 2012; INS, 2011, p. S87).

The semipermeable membrane of the peritoneal cavity acts as a barrier. When chemotherapy drugs are administered via the IP route, the malignant cells are directly exposed to the chemotherapy agent, and the exposure is prolonged. There is limited passage of the drug back into the systemic circulation, and most of the drug is absorbed by the portal vein to the liver where the drug is metabolized.

The average infusion time for IP drug instillation is between 30 minutes and 2 hours. For patients who experience abdominal pain and discomfort, infusion time may be extended. The chemotherapy infusion is generally warmed to body temperature using an inline fluid warmer or water bath (never microwaved). The IP chemotherapy is generally reconstituted in 2 L of normal saline, which facilitates distribution within the peritoneal cavity (Potter & Held-Warmkessel, 2008). After the infusion is completed, patients are asked to turn at intervals to facilitate drug distribution. Side effects include abdominal pain, cramping, nausea and vomiting, and difficulty breathing from pressure on the diaphragm. Other adverse reactions to the chemotherapy include neutropenia, ototoxicity, and neuromuscular toxicity. Patient education and preparation are critical. Comfort may be promoted by eating a small meal, voiding, and moving bowels before the procedure; antianxiety and pain medications are often helpful (Drake, 2009).

Types of IP devices include external peritoneal catheters with cuffs to hold them in place and implanted ports that are accessed using a noncoring needle (Fig. 10-7). There are also specially designed IP catheters that have multiple holes along the lumen; however, they have been linked to fibrin sheaths, plugging, higher infection rates, perforation, and bowel adhesions (Drake, 2009; Potter & Held-Warmkessel, 2008). Many surgeons use the same vascular ports for IP chemotherapy as those used for I.V. chemotherapy. Ports are generally placed below the bra line to avoid irritation. This port is restricted only to IP chemotherapy, and

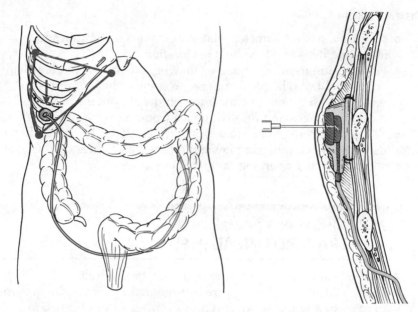

Figure 10-7 ■ Intraperitoneal port placement. (Courtesy of Ron Boisvert, RGB Medical Imagery, Inc., with permission.)

the catheter is never used for I.V. administration of drugs or blood products. As with I.V. ports and catheters, strict attention to aseptic technique with access is critical in infection prevention. Once therapy has concluded, the port should be removed to prevent bowel and infectious complications.

 NURSING FAST FACT!

■ *IP catheter care and infusion is only performed by nurses with specialized knowledge and competency.*
■ *The nurse and family must be familiar with the therapeutic effects of antineoplastic agents.*

Advantages

■ Increased dose goes directly to malignant cells.
■ IP chemotherapy diffuses into the peritoneal surface where it is absorbed systemically, prolonging exposure to the tumor via capillary flow.
■ Lower drug doses can be used, which may decrease adverse drug reactions.

DISADVANTAGES

- There is a risk for catheter-related infections or complications, including ileus and intestinal perforation.
- Postinfusion rotation schedules may be difficult for patients with arthritis, those who have undergone spine or hip surgeries, or patients who cannot tolerate lying on the abdomen.

List of advantages and disadvantages from Polovich, Whitford, and Olsen, 2009 and Potter and Held-Warmkessel, 2008. IP chemotherapy can cause greater fatigue; pain; hematological, gastrointestinal (GI), and metabolic events; and neurological toxicities.

NURSING POINTS OF CARE
INTRAPERITONEAL INFUSIONS

- Premedication for nausea and pain may be ordered.
- Comfort during the procedure is promoted by instructing patients to eat a small meal, void, and move bowels prior to infusion.
- Average infusion time is between 30 minutes and 2 hours.
- Infusion is via gravity and never by infusion pumps.
- Because a small amount of systemic absorption is desirable, fluid infused is not drained from the abdominal cavity.
- Patients are turned at intervals after the infusion is complete to facilitate distribution of drug.
- Heparinization of the IP port or catheter after the infusion currently is not standardized and varies among institutions. IP ports are not placed in the vascular system; therefore, there is no blood return.
- Monitor for:
  - Presence of asymmetry around the port or leaking around the Huber needle
  - Pain level
  - Respiratory rate or difficulty breathing due to fluid pressure on diaphragm (repositioning may be helpful)
  - Vital signs before and after the infusion

Intraosseous

The timely delivery of fluids and medications is critical for a patient in need of emergency treatment for injuries or underlying disease. A relatively easy and rapidly accessed vascular route is via the matrix of the bone, which is called the IO route. The primary indication for the IO route is emergent use in patients with limited or no vascular access. The IO route is recommended as the first alternative to I.V. access during cardiac arrest in advanced cardiac life support (ACLS) and pediatric advanced life support (PALS) (Kleinman et al., 2010; Neumar et al., 2010). A position statement endorsed by multiple nursing organizations supports consideration of IO access when I.V. access cannot be obtained and concern exists for morbidity and mortality if treatment cannot be delivered (Phillips et al., 2010). Vizcarra and Clum (2010) also discuss the expanding use of the IO route for nonemergent clinical situations in hospitals, such as immediate and short-term vascular access needs in patients with difficult venous access. Technology has evolved to make access to the IO route easy and cost effective for use in all age groups.

The long bones of the body have two ends, the diaphysis and the epiphysis. The epiphysis is sponge-like bone, whereas the diaphysis contains hard bone with a hollow interior space called the medullary cavity. The IO space is the spongy cancellous bone of the epiphysis and the medullary cavity of the diaphysis. The IO space is like a noncollapsible vein (Fig. 10-8). Within this space are thousands of noncollapsible intertwined blood vessels, which absorb any fluid, like a sponge, and which is rapidly transported to the central circulation (Vizcarra & Clum, 2010). A series of longitudinal canals contain tiny intertwined blood vessels, which connect to the central circulation. Bone marrow, which consists of blood, blood-producing cells, and connective tissue, fills the space. Within

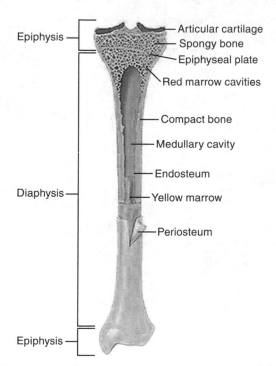

Figure 10-8 ■ Anatomy of a long bone. (Courtesy of MCV & Associates Healthcare, Inc., Indianapolis, IN.)

the IO space, blood flow is steady even during states of shock. Any medication that can be given as an I.V. can be given via the IO route because both are vascular access routes. The blood pressure in the IO space is about 35/25 mm Hg, or approximately one-third the systemic arterial pressure (Parker & Henderson, 2010). A bolus of approximately 10 mL of 0.9% sodium chloride must be rapidly given before starting an infusion to open the pathway and establish a good IO flow rate. Infusion rates are similar to that of a 21-gauge I.V. needle; infusion pumps or a pressure pump around the I.V. bag can deliver fluids at a rate of 20 to 25 mL/min (Vizcarra & Clum, 2010).

The site most often used for IO access in both adults and children is the proximal tibia. Other sites for adults include the proximal humerus, sternum, distal femur, humeral head, radius, ulna, pelvis, and clavicle. In children, the distal tibia and distal femur are also used (Fig. 10-9).

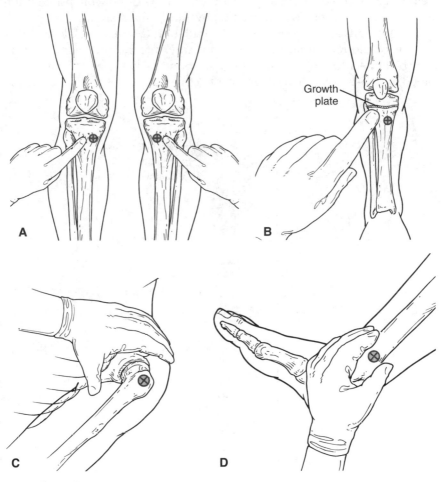

Figure 10-9 ■ Sites for intraosseous infusions. *A*, Tibia; *B*, pediatric tibia; *C*, proximal humerus; *D*, distal tibia.

There are a variety of IO devices that are easy to use and very fast, providing access within seconds. Pain management during insertion and infusion should always be considered, especially in the conscious patient. The use of lidocaine is widely recommended, both subcutaneously at the intended site and into the IO space prior to starting an infusion. There are three categories of IO devices (Phillips et al., 2010; Vizcarra & Clum, 2010). It is important to emphasize that any nurse who inserts such a device must be properly educated and trained in IO access and device use.

1. **Manual:** A hollow, steel needle with a removable trocar. It is inserted by applying pressure and twisting the device. The manual method is dependent on the preparation and insertion time, patient's condition, and skill of the inserter. The steel needles are difficult to insert in adult bones because of the density and hardness of the bone.
2. **Impact driven:** A spring-loaded device with a hollow needle and removable trocar. The device triggers penetration into the sternum or the tibia via direct force.
3. **Powered drill:** A battery-operated drill with a hollow needle and removable stylet. The device drills the needle to the appropriate depth into IO space. This type of device can be used for IO access into the proximal and distal tibia and the humeral head. The manufacturer of this device had reported insertion success rates of 100% when access steps are followed (Figs. 10-10 and 10-11).

It is important to recognize that the IO route is a temporary route, and the device should not be allowed to dwell more than 24 hours (INS, 2011, p. S83). Complications are rare with IO access but include extravasation from dislodgement, iatrogenic fracture, growth plate injury, infection, fat emboli, compartment syndrome, and osteomyelitis. The risk of infectious complications is increased with prolonged infusion or if bacteremia is present during the time of insertion (INS, 2011).

Indications for IO access:

1. Pediatric and adult patient resuscitation
2. To provide access in patients in whom peripheral I.V. access is difficult or impossible (e.g., those with trauma, obesity, diabetes)
3. Prehospital emergency access by paramedic staff

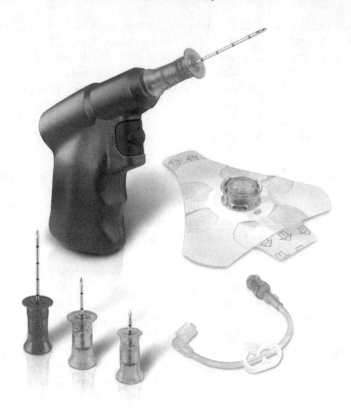

Figure 10-10 ■ EZ-IO® drill and products. (Courtesy of Vidacare, San Antonio, TX.)

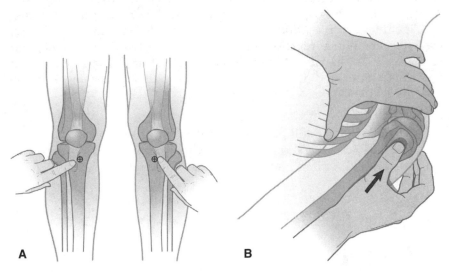

A **B**

Figure 10-11 ■ EZ-IO steps. *A,* Proximal tibia; *B,* humerus in shoulder;

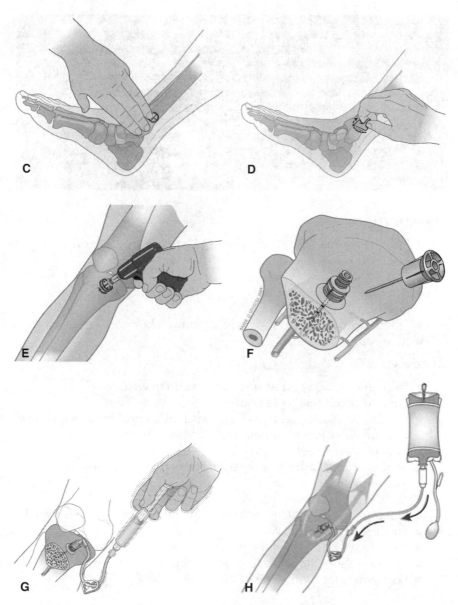

Figure 10-11—cont'd ■ *C,* distal tibia; *D,* site preparation; *E,* insertion of drill; *F,* hub removal; *G,* flush; *H,* infusion. (Courtesy of Vidacare, San Antonio, TX.)

EBP Success rates of first attempts and procedure times for IO access were compared to CVAD placement in a prospective, observational study. The population included 40 adults undergoing resuscitation, each receiving simultaneous IO and CVAD access. Success rates on first attempt were significantly higher for IO cannulation than for CVAD catheterization (85% vs 60%, p = 0.024), and procedure times were significantly lower for IO access compared to CVC (2.0 vs 8.0 minutes, p <0.001). Complications included failure to gain IO access (n = 6) and need for two or more CVAD placement attempts (n=16). There were no other complications reported. The researchers conclude that IO access is more efficacious with a higher success rate on first attempt and a lower procedure time compared to CVAD placement (Leidel et al., 2012).

Advantages

- Provides immediate alternative to I.V. access; average time for insertion is less than a minute
- Easy to stabilize device
- Any fluid that can be given I.V. (colloid, crystalloid, or blood product) can be infused via IO.
- Blood samples drawn IO can be used for laboratory studies.
- Rare complications

Disadvantages

- Pain on insertion and during infusion (manageable)
- Limited dwell time (<24 hours)
- Possibility of complications (rare), such as compartment syndrome, osteomyelitis, extravasation, and microfat emboli

Contraindicated for patients with:

- Bone diseases such as osteogenesis imperfecta and severe osteoporosis

Areas to avoid include:

- Previously used IO sites or areas where IO access was attempted
- Fractures at or above sites of previous bone surgery
- Presence of infection at the insertion site
- Recent orthopedic procedures in the area of insertion
- Local vascular compromise (INS, 2011, p. S83).

NURSING POINTS OF CARE
INTRAOSSEOUS INFUSIONS

- Premedication with lidocaine subcutaneously at the site and into the IO space is recommended.
- Allows for rapid intravascular access within 1 minute

- Mechanically easier to perform than I.V. access
- Any drug that is administered via the I.V. route may be administered via the IO route, without dosage adjustments.
- Dwell time should not exceed 24 hours.

Intraspinal

Analgesic, anesthetic, and adjuvant medications may be administered via an intraspinal route. Intraspinal access devices are defined as those placed in the epidural or intrathecal spaces in the spinal cord. An access device placed into the intraventricular space in the brain is also often categorized as an intraspinal device (INS, 2011, p. S81). Access to the intraventricular space is gained via a device called an Ommaya reservoir, which is implanted surgically under the scalp, providing access to the cerebrospinal fluid (CSF). It is a dome-shaped device with a self-sealing silicone reservoir attached to a catheter (Fig. 10-12). Like an implanted venous access port, the reservoir is accessed with a needle. This is a highly

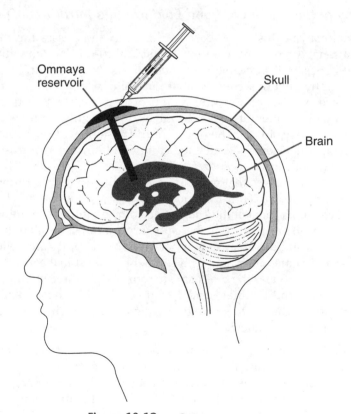

Figure 10-12 ■ Ommaya reservoir.

specialized infusion route and is only briefly addressed. In most cases, an LIP administers medications via the intraventricular route. Because many chemotherapy drugs do not cross the blood–brain barrier, this route is sometimes used to treat head, neck, or spine cancers. Other medications such as antibiotics or antifungals may also be given via the intraventricular route. Additionally, samples of CSF may be extracted for laboratory analysis, and CSF pressure can be measured (Stearns & Brant, 2010).

Intraspinal infusions via the epidural or intrathecal route may be used to control pain with surgical procedures and for patients in labor. Intraspinal infusions may also be indicated for long-term pain management, as occurs in patients who have not achieved pain relief despite escalating analgesic doses or those who are experiencing excessive systemic side effects. In addition, chemotherapy may be given via an intraspinal catheter for neurological cancers or neoplastic meningitis (Camp-Sorrell, 2011).

For pain management, drugs are administered directly to opiate receptor sites located in the spinal cord. Pain impulses are intercepted before they are transmitted to the brain. There is less central nervous system (CNS) depression associated with intraspinal analgesic administration.

Anatomy of the Spinal Cord and Epidural and Intrathecal Spaces

The spinal cord begins at the base of the skull and passes through the vertebral canal of the spinal column. The spinal cord is located within the vertebral bones and protective connective tissue. In the adult, the spinal cord ends at the first or second lumbar vertebra.

The cord consists of a central region of gray matter surrounded by bundles of white matter (Stearns & Brant, 2010). The gray matter is shaped like a butterfly (Fig. 10-13). The dorsal horn (posterior) of the spinal cord is rich in opioid receptors, and medications administered intraspinally directly bind with these receptors to block pain transmission. There are 31 pairs of spinal nerves that are named according to their position with respect to associated vertebra: 8 cervical, 12 thoracic, 5 lumbar, and 5 sacral, and 1 coccygeal. The area of the body affected by an intraspinal infusion is dependent on where the tip of the catheter is located in relation to the sensory nerves and the areas they innervate. Dermatomes are delineated areas of skin that are innervated by a segment of the spinal cord.

The spinal cord and the brain are surrounded by three meninges that protect and suspend the brain and spinal cord within the cranial cavity and the vertebral canal (Drake, Vogl, & Mitchell, 2010). The meninges are as follows (Figs. 10-13 and 10-14):

1. The dura mater is the outermost layer. It is a tough membrane consisting of dense fibrous connective tissue.
2. The arachnoid mater is the middle layer that is located against, but not adherent to, the internal surface of the dura mater. It is a thin and delicate membrane.

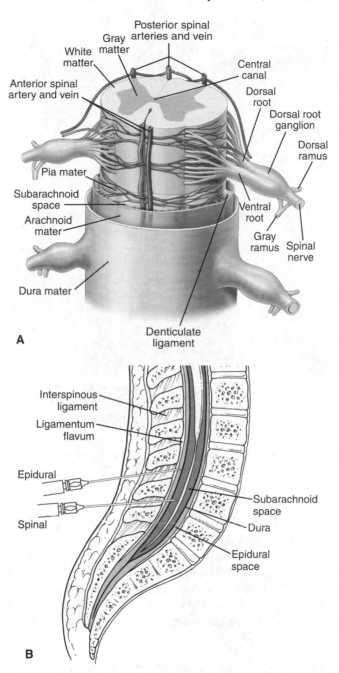

Figure 10-13 ■ *A.* Cross sectional view of the spinal cord. *B.* Intraspinal anatomy. Note epidural and spinal (intrathecal) spaces.

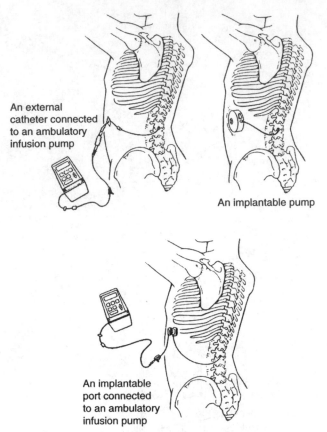

An external
catheter connected
to an ambulatory
infusion pump

An implantable pump

An implantable
port connected
to an ambulatory
infusion pump

Figure 10-14 ■ Methods of epidural administration. (Courtesy of Smith Medical, Inc., St. Paul, MN.)

3. The pia mater is a vascular membrane that firmly adheres to the surface of the spinal cord.

In between the arachnoid and the pia mater is the subarachnoid space, which contains CSF. The subarachnoid space is also called the intrathecal space. Medications in the CSF flow in two directions: primarily to the brain (rostral flow) and passively toward the base of the spine. Rostral spread of drugs can increase drug effects away from the targeted area (Stearns & Brant, 2010).

Epidural versus Intrathecal Medication Administration

The epidural space is the space surrounding the spinal cord and its meninges. This space contains fatty tissue, veins, spinal arteries, and nerves. It is considered a potential space that is not created until medication or air is injected. Medications administered via the epidural route must pass through the dura mater. Medications administered via the epidural route are about one-tenth of an I.V. dose and about 10 times greater than an intrathecal dose (Stearns & Brant, 2010) (see Fig. 10-13b).

Intrathecal medications are administered directly into the subarachnoid, or intrathecal, space where the CSF circulates; therefore, they do not have to pass through any membranes. For this reason, medication doses are very low, about one-tenth of an epidural dose. The intrathecal route is often used for long-term drug administration through long-term catheter systems. In addition to the low doses of medication required, potential advantages of intrathecal access compared to epidural access include ease of catheter placement; superior analgesia in the presence of epidural pathology (e.g., metastatic disease), and a lower incidence of catheter problems, such as catheter migration or tip occlusion (Reisfield & Wilson, 2009). Specific indications for intrathecal access include widespread pain, multiple pain locations, pain more distant from the catheter site, or pain poorly responsive to epidural therapy.

Intraspinal devices are aspirated prior to medication administration as part of an assessment of placement. With an epidural catheter, aspiration should ascertain the *absence* of fluid or blood; with an intrathecal catheter, aspiration should ascertain the *presence* of spinal fluid and absence of blood (INS, 2011, p. S81; Stearns & Brant, 2010).

Types of Catheters and Administration Systems

Catheters may be temporary or long term. Temporary catheters are typically used for no longer than a week. They may be used for postoperative analgesia or during labor, or they may be placed as part of a trial in a patient who might benefit from long-term intraspinal pain management. Short-term catheters may also be placed in patients with limited life expectancy in palliative care (Reisfield & Wilson, 2009). Long-term or permanent catheters include:

- Subcutaneously tunneled catheters: Surgically placed catheter with a synthetic cuff to hold it in place. It is generally tunneled around the flank area to an exit site in the abdominal area. Advantages include ease of activities of daily living and decreased risk of catheter dislodgement.
- Implanted ports: Surgically placed device that is also tunneled through the skin so that the port exits in the abdominal area (see Fig. 10-14). The port, like an implanted venous port, is accessed using a noncoring needle. Advantages include ease of activities of daily living, decreased risk for catheter dislodgement, and low risk for infection.
- Completely implanted systems that include a catheter and an implanted infusion pump: This is an expensive and complex system (Fig. 10-15). Access to the implanted infusion pump is via a noncoring needle. The pump is typically refilled with medication every 1 to 3 months. The pump can be programmed via a computer externally (Camp-Sorrell, 2011; Stearns & Brant, 2010).

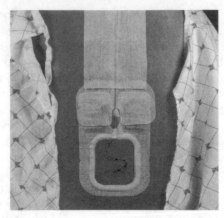

Figure 10-15 ■ Epidural site covered with SorbaView® Shield transparent dressing. (Courtesy of Centurion Medical Products, Williamston, MI.)

Intraspinal Medication Administration

Medications administered via an intraspinal catheter include opioids, local anesthetic agents, clonidine, baclofen, and sometimes chemotherapy agents. Medications must be preservative-free because preservatives are potentially neurotoxic. Morphine is the most commonly administered intraspinal opioid. It is a hydrophilic agent and has a high affinity for the opiate receptors in the dorsal horn of the spinal cord. Hydrophilic opioids decline more slowly in the CSF, which results in more rostral, or upward, spread. Because of this, delayed respiratory depression can occur. Hydromorphone may also be used, and although it is also hydrophilic, there is less rostral spread. Fentanyl and sufentanil are lipophilic, which results in faster analgesia and less rostral spread. Fentanyl clears rapidly but may be less available to the opiate receptors.

Local anesthetics may be used in conjunction with opioids. Bupivacaine is the most frequently used. Clonidine, an antihypertensive medication, may be used to treat neuropathic pain when given intraspinally. Table 10-3 provides a summary of intraspinal medications.

There are various approaches to the administration of narcotics and anesthetics via the intraspinal route: a single-bolus injection of opioid or local anesthetic, a continuous infusion of opioid with or without local anesthetics, or a continuous infusion of opioid with a patient-activated bolus.

A single injection of an opioid may be used for procedures that produce a short course of postoperative pain. This method may be appropriate for a patient having a cesarean section or vaginal hysterectomy, or for a patient after a same-day surgical procedure. Care must be taken to avoid the inadvertent administration of additional opioids by another route, which may oversedate the patient and cause respiratory depression.

> Table 10-3   **EPIDURAL AND INTRATHECAL MEDICATIONS**

Type of Medication	Actions and Issues

Opioids
  Fentanyl
  Hydromorphone
   hydrochloride
  Morphine sulfate
  Sufentanil
	Bind with opiate receptors.
	Morphine is hydrophilic; slower movement through cerebrospinal fluid results in longer duration of action and slower clearance; more rostral spread; risk for respiratory depression.
	Hydromorphone is hydrophilic with less rostral spread.
	Fentanyl and sufentanil are lipophilic with more rapid onset and less rostral spread.

Anesthetic agents Most often bupivacaine and ropivacaine	Given in low doses to block nerve fibers with minimal sensory and motor effect. May be used in conjunction with opioids and reduce opioid dose. Have long duration of action. Toxicity signs and symptoms include tinnitus, metallic taste, slow speech, irritability, twitching, seizures, circumoral tingling, numbness. Side effects include motor blockade, hypotension, diarrhea, urinary retention.
Baclofen	Used primarily for spasticity but may be combined with other medications for pain control. Side effects include hypotonia, sedation, constipation, erectile dysfunction, loss of sphincter control, respiratory depression.
Clonidine	Centrally acting alpha2-adrenergic agonist used to treat chronic neuropathic pain. Side effects include hypotension, sedation, dry mouth, bradycardia.
Ziconotide	Nonopioid analgesic administered intrathecally. Used with refractory pain in patients with cancer, chronic pain. Side effects include dizziness, nausea, asthenia, sedation, diarrhea, confusion, ataxia.

INS (2011, p. S81); Stearns & Brant (2010).

Continuous infusion is administered for short or long periods of time. Patients with pain from surgery, trauma, and acute medical disorders creating severe pain may benefit from short-term continuous infusions. Long-term patients include those with chronic intractable cancer or those with back or pelvic pain. Patients with chronic spasticity may be treated with the drug baclofen given intraspinally.

Most commonly intraspinal medication is administered by a certified RN anesthetist or an anesthesiologist, and the catheter is managed by the staff nurse. Administration of medication by a nurse through an intraspinal catheter must be based on an order from an LIP and in accordance with rules and regulations with each state's Board of Nursing and organizational policies, procedures, and/or practice guidelines (INS, 2011, p. S81). Nursing responsibilities also include (1) patient and family education, (2) site and dressing assessment and management, and (3) evaluation of pain relief.

 NURSING FAST FACT!

> ■ *Patients should be frequently monitored for the first 24 hours after starting an intraspinal infusion. Recommendations include every hour for the first 24 hours followed by assessment every 4 hours (INS, 2011, p. S82).*

ADVANTAGES OF INTRASPINAL MEDICATION ADMINISTRATION

- Permits control or alleviation of severe pain without the sedative effects
- Permits delivery of smaller doses of a narcotic to achieve the desired level of analgesia
- Allows for continuous infusion, if needed
- Can be used for short-term or long-term therapy
- Does not produce motor paralysis

DISADVANTAGES/RISKS OF INTRASPINAL MEDICATION ADMINISTRATION

- Only preservative-free opioids can be used.
- Medication-related complications include pruritus, paresthesia, urinary retention, and respiratory depression.
- Catheter-related risks include infection, dislodgement, and leaking.
- Intraspinal catheters and medications must be clearly labeled as a specialized infusion system as a safety precaution to prevent inadvertent intravenous infusion.

INS Standard Medications administered via an intraspinal route shall be preservative-free (INS, 2011, p. S81).

 NURSING FAST FACT!

> *Ineffective pain control should be reported to the LIP or anesthesiologist who is managing care of the epidural catheter.*

MONITORING THE PATIENT WITH AN INTRASPINAL CATHETER

Careful monitoring is critical for patients with an intraspinal catheter. For the first 24 hours after placing and initiating an intraspinal infusion, the patient is monitored for response to the therapy and for any adverse reactions as outlined in Table 10-4. Frequency of monitoring should be hourly for the first 24 hours and then every 4 hours thereafter. For home care or

> Table 10-4 | **MONITORING PARAMETERS FOR THE PATIENT RECEIVING AN INTRASPINAL INFUSION**

Pain rating, at rest and with activity
Vital signs
Level of sedation
Infusion pump: Number of bolus doses, if patient-controlled epidural analgesia; correctness of administration parameters
Fetal status, response of patient in labor
Presence of adverse reactions: Pruritus, nausea, urinary retention, orthostatic hypotension
Changes in sensory or motor function
Status of dressing (e.g., intact)
Measurement of external catheter length (changes may indicate potential migration)
Signs of infection/epidural abscess: Back pain, tenderness, erythema, drainage, fever, malaise, neck stiffness, progressive numbness
Oxygen saturation levels, CO_2 levels per organizational policy

INS, 2011, p. S82.

outpatients, a thorough assessment should be done with every patient encounter (INS, 2011, p. S82).

CARE AND MANAGEMENT OF INTRASPINAL CATHETERS

Temporary epidural catheters should be handled carefully during site care because they are easily dislodged. In acute-care, short-term catheterization, often only the anesthesiologist will change the dressing, if needed (see Fig. 10-15). Chlorhexidine-impregnated foam dressings are recommended for use because research has demonstrated a reduction in exit site colonization and decreased risk for CNS-related infection (INS, 2011, p. S82).

Patients who have long-term external intraspinal catheters in place require regular site care and dressing changes. Permanent catheters have a synthetic cuff that acts as a protective barrier against bacterial migration and secures the catheter. Key steps in the dressing procedure include:

1. Gather needed supplies and establish a sterile field with antiseptic solution and dressings.
2. Perform hand hygiene. Don gloves and mask.
3. Remove the old dressing and discard.
4. Perform hand hygiene and don sterile gloves. Apply antimicrobial solution without alcohol (usually povidone-iodine) in a circular motion, starting at the exit site and working outward. Allow the solution to air dry.
5. Apply a new dressing, gauze or transparent, and make sure that the catheter is well secured to reduce the risk for inadvertent dislodgement. Use a chlorhexidine dressing per organizational

policy. Transparent dressings are most often used and are changed at least every 7 days in conjunction with site care.
6. Check that the catheter is coiled near the insertion site, which will prevent accidental dislodgement.
7. Document the dressing change, assessment of the exit site, and how the patient tolerated the procedure.

INS Standard The potential for catheter tip migration should be routinely assessed by checking for changes in external catheter length (INS, 2011, p. S82).

 NURSING FAST FACT!

Do not use alcohol on skin or at the dressing site because of the risk of migration of alcohol into the intraspinal space and the possibility of neural damage.

COMPLICATIONS ASSOCIATED WITH INTRASPINAL PAIN MANAGEMENT

Medication-related side effects of intraspinal medication administration include pruritus, nausea and vomiting, respiratory depression, urinary retention, hypotension, and constipation. Pruritus is a common side effect that may be an allergic-type reaction or may be caused by stimulation of histamine in response to opioid administration (Stearns & Brant, 2010). Tolerance tends to develop to this side effect with long-term administration. Cool clothing and diversion may help. Also, low doses of the opioid antagonist naloxone can be administered to relieve pruritus without reversal of analgesia. Nausea and vomiting is less common with intraspinally administered opioids. Urinary retention is a common side effect that is theorized to be a result of inhibition of the parasympathetic nervous system on the bladder. This may require intermittent catheterization.

Conditions requiring immediate LIP notification include:
■ Inadequate pain relief. This can occur for three reasons: catheter migration, insufficient dosages of opioid and local anesthetics, and undetermined surgical complication.
■ Respiratory depression from epidural or intrathecal narcotic administration. Vital signs, including assessment of respiratory rate for a full minute, should be regularly assessed. Naloxone should be available to reverse the depressant effects of a narcotic.
■ Extreme dizziness as a result of orthostatic hypotension or excessive opioid effect
■ New onset of paresthesia or paresis
■ Pain at the insertion site
■ Displacement or migration of the epidural catheter. Catheter migration may occur as follows: (1) an epidural catheter can migrate through the dura mater into the intrathecal space, leading to an

opioid overdose; or (2) the catheter may migrate into an epidural vein or subcutaneous space, creating inadequate pain relief.

■ Infections. These are rare from epidural catheters, but precautions should be instituted to keep the catheter insertion process and exit site sterile. If an infection develops elsewhere in the body, the patient should be evaluated for removal of the epidural catheter.

■ Excessive drowsiness or confusion occurring when too much narcotic is being administered. This is usually improved by decreasing the amount of epidural narcotic infusion. Titrating an opioid antagonist, such as naloxone (Narcan) or an agonist/antagonist subcutaneously, may reverse side effects without eliminating the analgesia.

Other complications that may not warrant immediate notification but need to be reported at the earliest convenience include the inability to urinate and pruritus, which may be treated with parenterally administered medication while the infusion continues.

 NURSING FAST FACT!

If catheter migration is suspected, the LIP should be notified and the placement check verified by an anesthesiologist.

NURSING POINTS OF CARE

ADMINISTRATION OF INTRASPINAL PAIN CONTROL

■ Nurses caring for intraspinal catheters must demonstrate competency in maintenance, assessment of placement, and function of the access device and have an understanding of anatomy and physiology, neuropharmacology, and potential complications.

■ Only preservative-free medications are administered via the intraspinal route to prevent nerve damage.

■ Preservative-free morphine, which is water soluble and has a slower onset of action and longer duration of action, is generally the first choice of opioid analgesic. Lipid-soluble fentanyl and sufentanil penetrate the dura mater faster than water-soluble opioids, providing a faster onset of action but a shorter duration of action.

■ Aseptic technique, including donning of mask and gloves, is used when accessing, caring for, and maintaining an intraspinal access device.

■ Alcohol, disinfectants containing alcohol, or acetone **are never** to be used for site preparation or for cleansing the catheter hub because of the potential for neurotoxic effects of the alcohol.

Continued

- For intraspinal infusions, a 0.2-micron filter that is surfactant-free, particulate retentive, and air eliminating must be in place.
- Epidural devices should be aspirated to ascertain the *absence* of spinal fluid and blood before medication administration (INS, 2011, p. S81).
- Intrathecal and ventricular devices should be aspirated to *ascertain the presence* of spinal fluid and the absence of blood prior to medication administration (INS, 2011, p. S81).
- Inspect the catheter–skin junction visually and palpate for tenderness daily through the intact dressing.
- The potential for catheter migration should be monitored by assessing for changes in external catheter length, changes in pain control. or increase in side effects.
- After insertion of the external catheter, lay the exposed catheter length cephalad along the spine and over the shoulder. Tape the entire length of the exposed catheter in place to provide stability and protection.
- Evaluate the effects of the drug on the patient's alertness. Caregivers should also be taught to observe for levels of sedation.
- Clearly label the epidural catheter after placement to prevent accidental infusion of fluids or medications. Use yellow striped tubing for epidural infusions only. DO NOT USE EPIDURAL TUBING FOR I.V. SOLUTIONS.

■ Infusion Medication Delivery

General Guidelines

Nursing responsibilities related to infusion drug administration are summarized as follows:

1. Identify whether a prescribed route or method of administration (i.e., continuous, intermittent, or push) is appropriate.
2. Administer solutions and medications prepared and dispensed from the pharmacy or as commercially prepared solutions and medications whenever feasible (INS, 2011, p. S86).
3. Medications admixed outside of the pharmacy, pharmacy-labeled solutions, and medications labeled for emergent use should be administered within 1 hour of preparation (INS, 2011, p. S86).
4. Check all labels (drugs, diluents, and solutions) to confirm appropriateness for infusion use.
5. Use a filter needle or straw when withdrawing I.V. medications from ampules to eliminate possible pieces of glass (INS, 2011, p. S86).

6. Ensure adequate mixing of all drugs added to a solution.
7. Examine solutions for clarity and any possible leakage.
8. Double-check with another RN prepackaged medication syringes for use in specific pumps.
9. Use only single-dose vials for parenteral additives or medications.
10. Monitor the patient for therapeutic response to the medication.

The eight rights of safe medication administration are summarized in Table 10-5.

> Table 10-5	EIGHT RIGHTS OF MEDICATION ADMINISTRATION

1. Right patient
   - Verify identity using two patient identifiers.
   - Ask patient to identify himself/herself.
   - Technology: Barcode
2. Right medication
   - Review medication order against the medication label.
3. Right dose
   - Review medication dose against medication label.
   - Confirm appropriateness of the dose using a current drug reference.
   - Technology: Smart pump use; do not bypass drug library.
   - Independent double-checking of high-risk medications
   - Calculate the dose and have another nurse independently calculate the dose as well.
4. Right route
   - Review order for the appropriateness of the ordered route.
   - Make sure patient can take or receive the medication by the ordered route.
   - Make sure infusion drug is appropriate for the type of vascular access device (INS, 2011, p. S86).
5. Right time
   - Review order for frequency of medication.
   - Double-check that you are giving the ordered dose at the correct time.
   - Confirm when the last dose was given.
6. Right documentation
   - Document administration AFTER giving the ordered medication.
   - Document other specific information as necessary, such as laboratory values reviewed prior to administration (e.g., vancomycin trough level, serum creatinine).
7. Right reason
   - Confirm the rationale for the ordered medication.

INS Standard Review the order for appropriateness of prescribed therapy for the patient's age and condition (INS, 2011, p. S86).

8. Right response
   - Make sure that the drug led to the desired effect.

INS Standard The nurse should be accountable for evaluating and monitoring the effectiveness of prescribed therapy; documenting patient response, adverse events, and interventions; and communicating the results of laboratory tests (INS, 2011, p. S86).

INS (2011); Nursing 2012 Drug Handbook.

AGE-RELATED CONSIDERATIONS

Older adults and pediatric patients require special consideration when infusion medications are to be delivered. Each poses special problems that must be carefully addressed to ensure safe infusion therapy. Medications may have many greater side effects and adverse consequences in these populations.

Pediatric Patients

Medication errors occur more frequently in the pediatric inpatient population. There are a number of reasons for this:

• Availability of different dosage forms of same medication
• Few standardized dosing regimens for children compared to adults
• Variance among children in body weight, body surface area (BSA), and organ maturity (e.g., renal and hepatic function)
• Children are often unable to communicate adverse reactions.
• Limited physiological capacity to buffer medication errors (Gonzalez, 2010).

Based on a systematic review of the literature, Gonzales (2010) found that antibiotics, sedative medications, and opioids were most often involved in medication errors. Medication errors occurred because of distractions, interruptions, miscommunication, incorrect dose calculation, and lack of knowledge, and such errors tended to be underreported.

INS Standard The nurse should exercise particular care when administering solutions and medications to pediatric and neonatal patients because the incidence of medication errors is significantly higher for these patients. The use of standardized drug concentrations is strongly recommended for this population (INS, 2011, p. S86).

Calculations for Delivery of I.V. Medications in Pediatric Patients

Most medications for children are dosed based on body weight or BSA.

Body Weight

Many drugs are ordered in milligrams per kilogram of body weight.

Formula	Case example: Child weighs 35 pounds. Requires ampicillin for treatment of septicemia. The pediatric dose ordered is 100 mg/kg/24 hours in equally divided doses every 4 hours (Gahart & Nazareno, 2012).
Convert pounds to kilograms (1 kg = 2.2 pounds)	35 pounds divided by 2.2 pounds/kg = 15.9 kg
Calculate 24 dose in milligrams	15.9 kg × 100 mg/day = 1590 mg
Calculate dose based on frequency	1590 mg/day divided by six doses per day = 265 mg every 4 hours

BODY SURFACE AREA

As with adults, many chemotherapy drugs are dosed according to BSA. BSA requires measurement of height and weight and is reflected in meters squared (M^2). A nomogram is used to calculate the BSA. There are many online sources for calculation of BSA (see table below).

Formula	Case example: Child weighs 35 pounds and is 95 cm tall. Requires cytarabine 200 mg/M^2/24 hours for treatment of leukemia (Gahart & Nazareno, 2012).
Measure height	95 cm
Convert pounds to kilograms (1 kg = 2.2 pounds)	35 pounds divided by 2.2 pounds/kg = 15.9 kg
Calculate BSA*	0.63 M^2
Calculate dose in milligrams	200 mg/ M^2 × 0.63 M^2 = 126 mg

*Cornell University Medical School Web site (http://www-users.med.cornell.edu/~spon/picu/calc/bsacalc.htm) used for body surface area (BSA) calculation.

The Older Adult

The older is adult is more susceptible to adverse drug reactions. Physiological changes associated with aging may have an impact on or alter drug metabolism. There is a decrease in total body water and a relative increase in body fat that may affect water- and fat-soluble medication bioavailability. Changes on all levels of bodily function—cellular, organic, and systemic—occur as a result of the normal aging process. Because many older adults have multiple diseases, they are more likely to be taking multiple medications, which increases the risk of drug interactions. Because of the decline in organ function with aging, older adults are more likely to experience drug toxicity. It is important to realize that drug side effects in older adults, such as an increase in confusion, may be mistaken for signs of aging. Age-related changes are most pronounced in those older than 85 years; however, there is great variability among individuals (Smith & Cotter, 2012). Physiological changes particularly pertinent to infusion nursing include the following:
- Cardiovascular
  - Decreased cardiac reserve
  - Increased risk for dysrhythmias
  - Increased risk for postural and diuretic-induced hypotension
- Pulmonary
  - Decreased respiratory muscle strength
  - Decreased cough reflex
  - Decreased response to hypoxia, hypercapnia
- Renal
  - Decrease in kidney mass
  - Decreased drug clearance

Continued

- Increased risk for fluid volume overload
- Increased risk for dehydration
- Immune system
- Increased susceptibility to infection (Smith & Cotter, 2012)

INS Standard The nurse providing infusion therapy to the older adult should have knowledge and demonstrated skill competency in physiological changes related to older adults and their effect on drug dosage and volume limitations, pharmacological actions, interactions, side effects, monitoring parameters, and response to infusion therapy (INS, 2011, p. S7).

Home Care Issues

Many infusion medications and solutions are safely administered in the home care setting. These include antimicrobial drugs, parenteral nutrition, chemotherapy, analgesics for pain management, some cardiovascular medications, chelation therapy (e.g., iron unloading), factor replacement for bleeding disorders, biological drugs, enzyme replacement therapy (e.g., Prolastin), and both I.V. and subcutaneous immunoglobulin therapies. Most often, infusion medications are delivered via an infusion pump. Exceptions include some antibiotics that may be administered via I.V. push or gravity infusions.

Other than the I.V. route, medications may also be administered in the home via the subcutaneous and intraspinal (epidural/intrathecal) routes. Subcutaneous infusions include both hydration fluids (i.e., hypodermoclysis) or medications. Opioid drugs for pain management (e.g., morphine, hydromorphone) are the most common subcutaneously administered drugs in the home setting.

Intravenous antimicrobial medications are the most common medication class administered in the home. Administration methods include intermittent and continuous infusions, and I.V. push. The type of method selected is based on the characteristics of the medication (e.g., only a few antimicrobials can be given as I.V. push), the frequency of the infusion, and patient factors. In most cases, the patient or a caregiver is expected to learn how to administer the antimicrobial medications after the home care nurse teaches the techniques and validates competency and home safety with the plan. Elastomeric pumps (see Chapter 5) are commonly used for intermittent infusions. It is very easy to teach patients how to use these pumps and they are safe for the home environment. Programmable infusion pumps may be used for antibiotics that must be given every 4 to 6 hours, for example. In these cases, a full day's supply of antibiotic is prepared in a container, the infusion pump is programmed to administer the dose as ordered, and the pump delivers a keep vein open rate between infusions. Syringe and bedside infusion pumps may also be used.

Monitoring for potential adverse reactions to the home infusion is an important role of the home care nurse. Depending on the medication or infusion solution ordered, regular laboratory studies may be part of the monitoring process, for example, drug levels and serum creatinine levels for the patient receiving nephrotoxic medications (e.g., vancomycin, gentamicin). The nursing role includes timely review of laboratory work, ensuring results are received by the LIP, and communicating any changes in the plan of care to the patient. Before administering each dose, pertinent laboratory studies should be reviewed.

INS Standard The nurse administering parenteral medications should have knowledge of indications for therapy, side effects, potential adverse reactions, and appropriate interventions (INS, 2011, p. S86).

Special attention must be paid to administration of the first doses of an infusion medication in the home and/or when there is an ongoing risk for severe antibody/anaphylactic reactions (e.g., some biological drugs, immunoglobulin therapy). Emergency drugs (e.g., epinephrine, diphenhydramine) must be available in the home with orders and protocols established for their use. Additional criteria for first-dose administration include:

- The patient should have no history of severe drug reactions and minimal medication allergies.
- All nurses should be certified in basic life support.
- The nurse should remain in the home for the entire duration of the first-dose administration.
- Telephone access must be available (Gorski et al., 2010).

Patient education is crucial to safe home infusion of medications. Home care situations vary in terms of the patient's ability to manage the infusion. Based on the type of infusion and the patient's or caregiver's ability, the level of independence in home infusion therapy will vary. For example, drugs/fluids with a high risk for adverse reactions with every infusion, such as I.V. immunoglobulin therapy and other biological drugs, are administered by the nurse, whereas in most cases, self-administration of antimicrobial drugs is typically taught to the patient or caregiver.

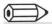 *NURSING FAST FACT!*

When programmable infusion pumps are used, in general the pharmacist programs and locks the program into the pump. Double-check systems should be in place in the pharmacy prior to dispensing the infusion pump and medications to the home. The nurse must also review and verify the infusion pump program against the drug label and against the medication order. When infusion pump parameters are changed in the home (e.g., increasing a PCA dose), the home care agency should have systems in place for a double-check, for example, calling the pharmacy on the telephone and reading the infusion pump parameters to the pharmacist.

Patient Education

- Patient education related to I.V. medication administration is vital for all health-care settings. When infusion medication will continue beyond the acute care setting, patient education should begin before hospital discharge to facilitate a smooth transition to home care.
- The education should include VAD placement, care and management, and signs and symptoms to report (INS, 2011 S16).
- Medication administration should address infection prevention (i.e., hand hygiene and aseptic technique), infusion delivery method, frequency of administration, and proper catheter flushing.
- Include troubleshooting instructions and telephone numbers to call for 24-hour assistance.
- Expected actions and adverse effects of medication must be addressed and reinforced throughout care.
- Use of a checklist is helpful and provides a method for documenting the completion of self-drug administration.

Patient Education Related to PCA
- Make sure the postoperative patient is alert enough to understand the directions for use of PCA. Make sure hearing aids or glasses are in place before instruction.
- Instruct on how to use PCA.
- Instruct on when to push the bolus button.
- Instruct on when to communicate with the nurse (e.g., pain not controlled with PCA, feeling of sedation).
- Discuss fears (of addiction to medication, receiving too much medication).
- Discuss expected outcomes for the patient: Pain scale use, prevention of breakthrough pain, and early ambulation.

◾ Nursing Process

The nursing process is a six-step process for problem-solving to guide nursing action (see Chapter 1 for details on the steps of the nursing process). The following table focuses on nursing diagnoses, nursing outcomes classification (NOC), and nursing interventions classification (NIC) for patients with medication administration via intravenous and alternate modalities. Nursing diagnoses should be patient specific and outcomes and interventions individualized. The NOC and NIC presented here are suggested directions for development of specific outcomes and interventions.

Nursing Diagnoses Related to Central Venous Access	Nursing Outcomes Classification (NOC)	Nursing Interventions Classification (NIC)
Anxiety (mild, moderate, and severe) related to: Threat to or change in health status; misconceptions regarding therapy	Coping; anxiety level	Anxiety reduction strategies
Comfort impaired, related to illness related symptoms: Pruritus	Comfort level; symptom control; coping	Pruritus management; distraction
Health maintenance ineffective, related to: Limited skills of family members in delivering intravenous medications and fluids; deficient communication skills	Health beliefs, perceived resources, health-promoting behaviors	Health education, health systems guidance, support system enhancements
Injury, risk for related to: Internal: Toxic or effects of medications	Knowledge of medication, medication response	Health education Medication management Surveillance: Safety
Knowledge deficit, related to: Lack of motivation to learn and/or decreased energy available for learning	Knowledge of treatment regimen Participation in health-care decisions	Decision-making support Health system guidance Mutual goal setting Teaching: Procedure/ treatment
Mobility impaired (physical), related to: Pain and discomfort resulting from placement and maintenance of I.V. catheters	Activities of daily living	Exercise therapy, ambulation, joint mobility, positioning assistance
Tissue integrity impaired, related to: Adverse reaction to medication	Wound healing	Skin care, skin surveillance, wound care management

Ackerley & Ladwig (2011); Bulechek, Butcher, Dochterman, & Wagner (2013); Moorhead, Johnson, Maas, & Swanson (2013).

Chapter Highlights

- Advantages of I.V. medications include the fact that they provide a direct access to the circulatory system, a route for instant drug action, a route for delivering high drug concentrations, instant drug termination if sensitivity or an adverse reaction occurs, and a route of administration in patients in whom use of the GI tract is limited.
- Disadvantages and risks of I.V. medications include the potential for drug interaction because of incompatibilities, drug adsorption, errors in compounding of medication, speed shock, extravasation of a vesicant drug, and chemical phlebitis.
- Drug incompatibilities fall into three broad categories: physical, chemical, and therapeutic.
- The four main methods of I.V. medication administration are continuous infusion, intermittent infusion, I.V. push, and patient-controlled analgesia.

- The subcutaneous route may be used to administer certain medications (e.g., opioids) and fluids (hypodermoclysis).
- The IP route is used for administration of chemotherapy in patients with certain cancers in the peritoneal space, most often for ovarian cancer.
- IO access for medication infusion is used in adults and children in emergency care, severely dehydrated patients, adults in whom peripheral I.V. access is impossible, and for rapid and reliable prehospital emergency access.
- Disadvantages of IO include pain on insertion, compartment syndrome, osteomyelitis, or cellulitis.
- There are two types of intraspinal catheters: epidural and intrathecal.
- Epidural and intrathecal administrations provide good pain control, require small doses, and produce longer periods of relief between doses while preventing many systemic side effects.
- Alcohol must NEVER be used for site preparation or for accessing an intraspinal catheter. Only preservative-free medications can be delivered by the intraspinal routes.

■■ Thinking Critically: Case Study

Mrs. Robertson is 1 day postoperative from an abdominal hysterectomy. She has an epidural catheter in place. Her baseline vital signs are blood pressure 110/80; respiration 18 breaths/min, and pulse 72 bpm. Your assessment finds she is difficult to arouse, but she does respond to simple commands. She is able to move her legs and can squeeze your fingers. Her blood pressure is 90/60, pulse 100 bpm, and respirations 14 breaths/min. She is moaning in pain but is unable to rate her pain on the pain scale.

Case Study Questions
1. What further assessments need to be done?
2. What further actions should the nurse initiate?
3. What could be the reason for her change in status?

Media Link: Answers to the case study and more critical thinking activities are provided on Davis*Plus*.

Post-Test

1. An I.V. medication reconstituted by the nurse:
   a. Must be initiated within 1 hour of preparation
   b. Must be initiated within 2 hours of preparation
   c. Must be used within 8 hours of reconstitution
   d. Nurses should not reconstitute I.V. medications

2. The risk for a misconnection between an I.V. administration set and an epidural tubing is best prevented when:

   a. The nurse identifies that the administration sets appear different
   b. The nurse traces the administration set to the I.V. catheter before initiating the infusion
   c. The nurse assesses that it is easy to connect the administration to the epidural catheter
   d. The nurse asks the patient to help in a double-check of the infusion set

3. The risk for physical drug incompatibilities is reduced when:

   a. All I.V. medications are filtered with a 0.2-micron filter
   b. The nurse reconstitutes the drug
   c. The I.V. catheter is routinely flushed with 0.9% sodium chloride between drug infusions
   d. The I.V. catheter is routinely flushed with 5% dextrose in water between drug infusions

4. Risks associated with I.V. push medication administration include:

   a. Increased risk for infection
   b. Increased risk for infiltration
   c. Increased risk for speed shock
   d. A slow drug response

5. The risk for oversedation and respiratory depression associated with PCA is associated with the following patient population:

   a. Patients who have been taking hydromorphone regularly
   b. Patients who have had orthopedic surgery
   c. Patients who are in their 50s
   d. Patients who have heart failure

6. Safety precautions to prevent errors associated with PCA therapy include which of the following? (*Select all that apply.*)

   a. Use double-checks.
   b. Highlight the drug concentration on the label.
   c. Limit the variety of medications used for PCA.
   d. Develop a reference sheet on PCA that includes programming tips and maximum dose warnings.

7. The subcutaneous infusion site should be rotated:

   a. Every 24 hours when administering medications
   b. Every 24 hours when administering hypodermoclysis
   c. Every 48 hours when administering hypodermoclysis
   d. After 1500 mL has been administered with hypodermoclysis

8. The most common site used for intraosseous access is:
   a. Sternum
   b. Distal femur
   c. Humeral head
   d. Proximal tibia

9. Which of the following is a known adverse reaction associated with an intraspinal infusion?
   a. Hypertension
   b. Tachypnea
   c. Urinary retention
   d. Elevated oxygen saturation levels

10. Clear fluid in the syringe after aspiration of an epidural catheter is an indication of catheter:
   a. Patency
   b. Kinking
   c. Migration
   d. Damage

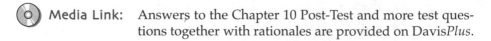 **Media Link:** Answers to the Chapter 10 Post-Test and more test questions together with rationales are provided on Davis*Plus*.

■ References

Ackerly, B. J., & Ladwig, G. B. (2011). *Nursing diagnosis handbook: An evidence-based guide to planning care* (9th ed.). St. Louis, MO: Mosby Elsevier.

ASHP. (2008). *The ASHP Discussion Guide on USP Chapter <797>*. Retrieved from www.ashp.org/s_ashp/docs/files/discguide797-2008.pdf (Accessed October 30, 2012).

Anastasia, P. (2012). Intraperitoneal chemotherapy for ovarian cancer. *Oncology Nursing Forum, 39*(4), 346-349.

Bulechek, G. M., Butcher, H. K., Dochterman, J. M., & Wagner, C. M. (2013). *Nursing interventions classification (NIC)* (6th ed.). St. Louis: MO: Mosby Elsevier.

Camp-Sorrell, D. (2011). *Access device guidelines: Recommendations for nursing practice and education* (3rd ed.). Pittsburgh, PA: Oncology Nursing Society.

Carter, A., Gelchion, K., Saitta, P., & Clark, D. (2011). Dying to identify IV medication errors: A clinical nurse specialist group identifies factors contributing to IV push medication errors, and the resulting housewife education initiative. *Clinical Nurse Specialist, 25*(3), 144.

Drake, B. (2009). Intraperitoneal chemotherapy: A reemerging approach in the treatment of ovarian cancer. *Journal of Infusion Nursing, 32*(6), 314-322.

Drake, R. L., Vogl, W., & Mitchell, A. W. (2010). *Gray's anatomy for students* (2nd ed.). St. Louis, MO: Elsevier.

Gahart, B. L., & Nazareno, A. R. (2012). *Intravenous medications* (28th ed.). St. Louis, MO: Elsevier Mosby.

Giger, J. N., & Davidhizar, R. E. (2004). *Transcultural nursing: Assessment & intervention* (2nd ed.). St. Louis, MO: C. V. Mosby.

Gonzales, K. (2010). Medication Administration Errors and the Pediatric Population: A Systematic Search of the Literature. *Journal of Pediatric Nursing, 25*(6), 555-565.

Gorski, L. A., Miller, C., & Mortlock, N. (2010). Infusion therapy across the continuum. In M. Alexander, A. Corrigan, L. Gorski, J. Hankins, & R. Perucca (Eds.), *Infusion nursing: An evidence-based approach*. St. Louis, MO: Saunders Elsevier.

Humphrey, P. (2011). Hypodermoclysis: An alternative to IV infusion therapy. *Nursing, 41*(11), 16-17.

Infusion Nurses Society (INS). (2011). Infusion Nursing Standards of Practice. *Journal of Intravenous Nursing, 34*(1S), S1-S110.

Institute of Safe Medication Practices (ISMP). (2008). Misprogramming PCA concentration leads to dosing errors. Retrieved from http://www.ismp.org/newsletters/acutecare/articles/20080828.asp (Accessed April 22, 2013).

ISMP. (2011). ISMP list of high-alert medications in community/ambulatory healthcare. Retrieved from http://www.ismp.org/communityRx/tools/ambulatoryhighalert.asp (Accessed April 22, 2013).

ISMP. (2012). ISMPs list of high alert medications. Retrieved from http://www.ismp.org/Tools/institutionalhighAlert.asp (Accessed April 22, 2013).

Jack, T., Boehne, M., Brent, B. E., Hoy, L., Köditz, H., Wessel, A., & Sasse, M. (2012). In-line filtration reduces severe complications and length of stay on pediatric intensive care unit: A prospective, randomized, controlled trial. *Intensive Care Medicine, 38*, 1008-1016.

Jarzyna, D., Jungquist, C. R., Pasero, C., Willens, J. S., Nisbet, A., Oakes, L., ... Polomano, R. C. (2011). American Society for Pain Management Nursing guidelines on monitoring for opioid-induced sedation and respiratory depression. *Pain Management Nursing, 12*(3), 118-145.

Kleinman, M. E., de Caen, A. R., Chameides, L., Atkins, D. L., Berg, R. A., Berg, M. D., ... Zideman, D. (2010). Pediatric basic and advanced life support: 2010 international consensus on cardiopulmonary resuscitation and emergency cardiovascular care science with treatment recommendations. *Circulation, 122*(18 Suppl 3), S466-S515.

Leidel, B. A., Kirchhoff, C., Bogner, V., Braunstein, V., Biberthaler, P., & Kanz, K.-G. (2012). Comparison of intraosseous versus central venous vascular access in adults under resuscitation in the emergency department with inaccessible peripheral veins. *Resuscitation, 83*(1), 40-45.

Moorhead, S., Johnson, M., Maas, M., & Swanson, E. (2013). *Nursing outcomes classification (NOC)* (5th ed.). St. Louis, MO: Mosby Elsevier.

Neumar, R. W., Otto, C. W., Link, M. S., Kronick, S. L., Shuster, M., Callaway, C. W., ... Morrison, L. J. (2010). Part 8: Adult advanced cardiovascular life support: 2010 American Heart Associate guidelines for cardiopulmonary resuscitation and emergency cardiovascular care. *Circulation, 122*(18 Suppl 3), S729-S767.

Nightingale, F. (1860). *Notes on nursing*. New York: Appleton & Co.

Nursing 2012 Drug Handbook. (2012). Philadelphia: Lippincott, Williams and Wilkins.

O'Grady, N. P., Alexander, M., Burns, L. A., Patchen Dellinger, E., Garland, J., Heard, S. O., ... the Healthcare Infection Control Practices Advisory Committee (HICPAC). (2011). Healthcare Practices Advisory Committee (HICPAC). Guidelines for the prevention of intravascular catheter-related infections, 2011. *American Journal of Infection Control, 39*(4 Suppl), S1-S34. Also available at http://www.cdc.gov/hicpac/pdf/guidelines/bsi-guidelines-2011.pdf (Accessed September 15, 2012).

Parker, M., & Henderson, K. (2010). Alternative infusion access devices. In M. Alexander, A. Corrigan, L. Gorski, J. Hankins, & R. Perucca (Eds.), *Infusion nursing: An evidence-based practice* (3rd ed.) (pp. 516-524). St. Louis: Saunders/Elsevier.

Pennsylvania Safety Authority. (2010). Tubing misconnections: Making the connection to patient safety. Retrieved from http://patientsafetyauthority.org/ADVISORIES/AdvisoryLibrary/2010/Jun7(2)/Pages/41.aspx (Accessed April 25, 2013).

Phillips, L., Brown, L., Campbell, T., Miller, J., Proehl, J., & Youngberg, B., & Consortium on Intraosseous Vascular Access in Healthcare Practice. (2010). Recommendations for the use of intraosseous vascular access for emergent and nonemergent situations in various healthcare settings: A consensus paper. *Journal of Emergency Nursing, 36*(6), 551-556.

Polovich, M., Whitford, J. M., & Olsen, M. (2009). *Chemotherapy and biotherapy guidelines and recommendations for practice* (3rd ed.). Pittsburgh, PA: Oncology Nursing Society.

Potter, K. L., & Held-Warmkessel, J. (2008). Intraperitoneal chemotherapy for women with ovarian cancer: Nursing care and considerations. *Clinical Journal of Oncology Nursing, 12*(2), 265-271.

Reisfield, G. M. & Wilson, G. R. (2009). Fast facts and concepts #098. End of Life/Palliative Education Research Center (EPERC). Retrieved from http://www.mcw.edu/FileLibrary/User/jrehm/fastfactpdfs/Concept098.pdf (Accessed October 10, 2013).

Rouhani, S., Meloney, L., Ahn, R., Nelson, B. D., & Burke, T. F. (2011). Alternative rehydration methods: A systematic review and lessons for resource-limited care. *Pediatrics, 127*, e748-e757.

Scales, K. (2011). Use of hypodermoclysis to manage dehydration. *Nursing Older People, 23*(5), 16-22.

Siegel, J. D., Rhinehart, E., Jackson, M., & Chiarello, L. (2007). Guideline for isolation precautions: Preventing transmission of infectious agents in healthcare settings 2007. Retrieved from www.cdc.gov/ncidod/dhqp/hai.html (Accessed December 11, 2012).

Simpson, M. H. (2010). Alternative infusion access devices. In M. Alexander, A. Corrigan, L. Gorski, J. Hankins, & R. Perucca (Eds.), *Infusion nursing: An evidence-based practice* (3rd ed.) (pp. 372-390). St. Louis: Saunders/Elsevier.

Smith, C. M., & Cotter, V. T. (2012). Nursing standard of practice protocol: Age-related changes in health. Retrieved from http://consultgerirn.org/topics/normal_aging_changes/want_to_know_more (Accessed May 5, 2013).

Stearns, C. K., & Brant, J. M. (2010). Intraspinal access and medication adminis-
    tration. In M. Alexander, A. Corrigan, L. Gorski, J. Hankins, & R. Perucca
    (Eds.), *Infusion nursing: An evidence-based practice* (3rd ed.) (pp. 525-539).
    St. Louis: Saunders/Elsevier.
The Joint Commission (TJC). (2006). Sentinel event: Issue 36. Tubing
    misconnections—A persistent and potentially deadly occurrence.
    Retrieved from http://www.jointcommission.org/assets/1/18/SEA_36.
    PDF (Accessed April 20, 2013).
TJC. (2012). Sentinel event: Issue 49. Safe use of opioids in hospitals. Retrieved
    from http://www.jointcommission.org/assets/1/18/SEA_49_opioids_
    8_2_12_final.pdf (Accessed April 20, 2013).
Turner, M. S., & Hankins, J. (2010). Alternative infusion access devices. In M.
    Alexander, A. Corrigan, L. Gorski, J. Hankins, & R. Perucca (Eds.), *Infusion
    nursing: An evidence-based practice* (3rd ed.) (pp. 263-298). St. Louis: Saunders/
    Elsevier.
Vizcarra, C., & Clum, S. (2010). Intraosseous route as alternative access for
    infusion therapy. *Journal of Infusion Nursing, 33*(3), 162-174.
Walsh, G. (2005). Hypodermoclysis: An alternate method for rehydration in
    long-term care. *Journal of Infusion Nursing, 28*(2), 123-129.
Weisman, D. E. (2009). Fast facts and concepts #028 subcutaneous opioid infu-
    sion. End of Life/Palliative Education Research Center (EPERC). Retrieved
    from http://www.eperc.mcw.edu/EPERC/FastFactsIndex/ff_028.htm
    (Accessed October 10, 2013)
Willens, J. S., Jungquist, C. R., Cohen, A., & Polomano, R. (2013). ASPMN survey—
    Nurses' practice patterns related to monitoring and preventing respiratory
    depression. *Pain Management Nursing, 14*(1), 60-65.
Wuhrman, E., Cooney, M. F., Dunwoody, C. J., Eksterowicz, N., Merkel, S.,
    Oakes, L. L., & American Society for Pain Management Nursing. (2007).
    Authorized and unauthorized ("PCA by proxy") dosing of analgesic infu-
    sion pumps: Position statement with clinical practice recommendations.
    Pain Management Nursing, 8(1), 4-11.
Younger, M. E. M., Aro, L., Bouin, W., Duff, C., Epland, K. B., Murphy, E., ...
    Nurse Advisory Committee Immune Deficiency Foundation. (2013). Nurs-
    ing guidelines for administration of immunoglobulin replacement therapy.
    Journal of Infusion Nursing, 36(1), 58-68.

PROCEDURES DISPLAY 10-1

Administration of Medication by the Direct (I.V.) Push: Peripheral Catheter

Equipment Needed
Alcohol wipes
Two prefilled syringes of 0.9% sodium chloride
Labeled medication prepared by pharmacy in syringe

Delegation
This procedure **cannot** be delegated.

Procedure	Rationale
1. Verify the authorized prescriber's order.	1. A written order is a legal requirement.
2. Verify the allergy status of the patient.	2. Patient safety
3. Introduce yourself to the patient.	3. Establishes nurse–patient relationship.
4. Verify patient identity using two patient identifiers.	4. Patient safety
5. Perform hand hygiene.	5. The single most important means of infection prevention.
6. Explain procedure to patient and its expected outcome, potential adverse reactions, and signs/symptoms to report.	6. Prepares patient for procedure.
7. Disinfect the needleless connector with 70% isopropyl alcohol for at least 15 seconds using a twisting motion.	7. Reduces risk for intraluminal introduction of microbes.
8. Attach syringe of sodium chloride and aspirate to assess for blood return. Slowly flush the solution; disconnect and discard.	8. Assess patency of catheter and clears the line of any medication. Never forcibly flush catheter.
9. Disinfect the needleless connector with 70% isopropyl alcohol for at least 15 seconds using a twisting motion.	9. Reduces risk for intraluminal introduction of microbes.

PROCEDURES DISPLAY 10-1

Administration of Medication by the Direct (I.V.) Push: Peripheral Catheter—*cont'd*

Procedure	Rationale
10. Attach medication syringe and inject slowly over the time indicated on the syringe label or according to pharmacist; disconnect and discard.	**10.** Slow injection reduces the risk for speed shock and provides time for the nurse to observe the patient for adverse effects. Studies have indicated nurses often administer I.V. push medications too rapidly.

Note: If administering medication with a running I.V. solution, the medication MUST be compatible with the I.V. solution, or the administration set needs to be clamped before the first flush.

Procedure	Rationale
11. Disinfect the needleless connector with 70% isopropyl alcohol for at least 15 seconds using a twisting motion.	**11.** Reduces risk for intraluminal introduction of microbes.
12. Attach syringe of sodium chloride and slowly inject the sodium chloride after the medication administration to decrease the chance of a "bolus" of medication.	**12.** Positive pressure must be maintained within the lumen of the catheter during and after administration of a flush solution to prevent reflux of blood into the luer-activated systems. Follow guidelines below.

Note: There are different types of needleless connector devices, so be sure you know which devices are used in your facility.

Procedure	Rationale
13. a. For negative-displacement devices: Flush all solution into the catheter lumen, maintain force on the syringe plunger as a clamp on the catheter or extension set is closed, then disconnect the syringe.	**13.** Manufacturer requires "positive pressure" flushing technique to prevent reflux of blood.

Continued

PROCEDURES DISPLAY 10-1

Administration of Medication by the Direct (I.V.) Push: Peripheral Catheter—*cont'd*

Procedure	Rationale
b. **For positive-displacement device:** Flush all solution into the catheter lumen, disconnect the syringe, then close the catheter clamp.	Catheter is clamped *after* disconnection of the syringe.
c. **For neutral-displacement device:** Flush all solution into the catheter lumen; it does not matter if the catheter clamp is closed before or after the flush procedure	
14. Assess patient response and any side effects/adverse reactions; ensure plan in place for ongoing monitoring.	14. Patient safety
15. Discard all used supplies per organizational policy.	
16. Perform hygiene.	
17. Document the procedure.	17. Maintains a legal record and communication with the health-care team.

PROCEDURES DISPLAY 10-2

Administration of Continuous Subcutaneous Medication Infusion

Equipment Needed
Transparent semipermeable membrane (TSM) dressing
Prepackaged dedicated subcutaneous set from manufacturer (if using instead of butterfly needles)
Antiseptic solution (chlorhexidine gluconate)
Sterile 10 mL syringe
Prescribed fluids or prefilled medication container or cassette
Infusion pump (medication infusion)

Delegation
This procedure can be delegated to LPN/LVN in some states that allow by nurse practice act to administer subcutaneous infusions for hypodermoclysis.

Procedure	Rationale
1. Verify authorized prescriber's order.	1. A written order is a legal requirement for infusion therapy.
2. Verify the allergy status of the patient.	2. Patient safety.
3. Gather all equipment.	3. Having all equipment at hand will save time and lessen patient anxiety.
4. Introduce yourself to the patient.	4. Establishes nurse–patient relationship.
5. Verify the patient's identity using two patient identifiers	5. Patient safety
6. Perform hand hygiene.	6. The single most important means of infection prevention.
7. Explain procedure to patient and its expected outcomes, potential adverse reactions, and signs/symptoms to report.	7. Prepares patient for procedure.
8. Assess skin and select insertion site with adequate subcutaneous tissue: a fat fold of at least 1 inch (2.5 cm) when thumb and forefinger are pinched together. Site	8. Reduces risk of infusion outside of subcutaneous tissue.

Continued

PROCEDURES DISPLAY 10-2

Administration of Continuous Subcutaneous Medication Infusion—*cont'd*

Procedure	Rationale
selection is also based on the patient's anticipated mobility and comfort. *Note:* Avoid areas that are scarred, infected, irritated, edematous, bony, or highly vascularized.	
9. Don gloves.	9. Standard precautions
10. Prime the administration set and into pump per manufacturer's directions.	
11. Perform skin antisepsis with chlorhexidine gluconate and let dry. (*Note:* If skin is visibly dirty, wash with soap and water prior to skin antisepsis.)	11. Reduces risk for infection.
12. Follow the manufacturer's labeled use and direction for access device placement; prime set with 0.9% sodium chloride.	
13. Lift the skin up into a small mound between the thumb and index finger.	
14. Insert the primed subcutaneous infusion device into the skin.	14. Ensures secure entry of the needle into the subcutaneous tissue and not into muscle.
15. Aspirate subcutaneous device using sterile syringe.	15. Presence of blood may be indicative of entry into blood vessel. Remove and replace device in new site if positive blood aspirate.

PROCEDURES DISPLAY 10-2

Administration of Continuous Subcutaneous Medication Infusion—*cont'd*

Procedure	Rationale
16. Stabilize the device, secure connection junctions, and apply TSM dressing over the site.	16. Protects the site and stabilizes the catheter or needle to prevent dislocation.
17. Initiate therapy and adjust the rate per order and medication label.	17. Accurate medication administration
18. Discard used equipment and supplies in the appropriate receptacle.	18. Occupational Safety and Health Administration (OSHA) standard
19. Remove gloves and perform hand hygiene.	
20. Document in the patient's permanent medical record.	20. Maintains a legal record and communication with the health-care team.

Note: Rotate the access site every 2–7 days. Monitor the access site and equipment; observe the site for bleeding, bruising, inflammation, drainage, edema, and cellulitis. Monitor the patient for complaints of burning or itching.

Sources: INS (2011), Parker & Henderson (2010).

Chapter **11**

Transfusion Therapy

*Let whoever is in charge keep this simple question in her head (not, how can
I always do this right thing myself, but) how can I provide for this right thing
to be always done?*
—*Florence Nightingale, 1860*

Chapter Contents

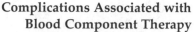

 **LEARNING
OBJECTIVES**

On completion of this chapter, the reader will be able to:

1. Define terminology related to transfusion therapy.
2. Identify the antigens and antibodies in the blood system.
3. Identify the universal red blood cell donor type.
4. Identify the Rh antigens located on the red blood cells.
5. Identify the preservatives used in donor blood storage.
6. Summarize the tests used to screen donor blood.
7. Distinguish among homologous, autologous, and designated blood.
8. Describe each of the blood components, their indications, and key points in administration.
9. Describe the procedure for administration of blood components.
10. Establish a plan of action for a patient exhibiting symptoms of hemolytic transfusion, febrile transfusion, and mild allergic transfusion reactions.

GLOSSARY

ABO system Blood group of antigens that reside on structurally related carbohydrate molecules

ADSOL Additive solution of 100 mL containing saline, dextrose, and adenine that is added to packed red blood cells

Agglutinin An antibody present in the blood that attaches to an antigen that causes clumping, or agglutination; agglutinins cause transfusion reactions when blood from a different group is transfused

Agglutinogen An antigen that stimulates production of an agglutinin

Allergic reaction Reaction from exposure to an antigen to which the person has become sensitized

Allogeneic Blood transfused to someone other than the donor

Allogeneic/homologous donation Blood donation by someone other than the recipient

Alloimmunization Development of an immune response to alloantigens; occurs during pregnancy, blood transfusions, and organ transplantation

Antibody A protective substance that resides in plasma produced by B lymphocytes in response to an antigen; antibodies identify and neutralize or destroy antigens

Antigen A substance that induces an immune system response.

Autologous/Autotransfusion donation Originating within an individual, especially a factor present in tissues or fluids; donation of a unit of blood to be reinfused, if needed, back to the original donor

Blood component Product made from a unit of whole blood such as platelet concentrate, red blood cells, fresh frozen plasma, or cryoprecipitate

Crossmatch The process of mixing a sample of the donor's red blood cells with the recipient's serum (major crossmatching) and mixing a sample of the recipient's blood with the donor's serum (minor crossmatching) to determine compatibility

Cryoprecipitate A plasma component rich in fibrinogen and other clotting factors

Delayed transfusion reaction Adverse effect occurring after 48 hours and up to 180 days after transfusion

Directed/designated donation Use of blood or components from a specific donor for a specific patient

Febrile reaction Nonhemolytic reaction to antibodies formed against leukocytes

Fresh frozen plasma Collection of the fluid portion of the circulating blood by separation and freezing the plasma within 8 hours of collection

Hemoglobin Respiratory pigment of red blood cells having the reversible property of taking up oxygen or releasing oxygen

Hemolysis Rupture of red blood cells, with the release of hemoglobin

Hemolytic transfusion reaction Blood transfusion reaction in which an antigen–antibody reaction in the recipient is caused by an incompatibility between red blood cell antigens and antibodies

Human leukocyte antigen (HLA) Used for tissue typing and relevant for transplant histocompatibility; essential to immunity

Hypothermia Abnormally low body temperature

Immunohematology   Study of blood and blood reactions as it relates to immune systems and its response

Microaggregate   Microscopic collection of particles such as platelets, leukocytes, and fibrin that occurs in stored blood

Packed red blood cells   A blood product consisting of concentrated cells, most of the plasma having been removed

Pheresis   Derived from the Greek word *aphairesis*, meaning "to take away"; used to denote the removal of blood, the separation into component parts, the retention of only the parts needed, and the return of the rest to the donor (e.g., removal of plasma is plasmapheresis)

Plasma   Fluid portion of the blood, composed of a mixture of proteins in solution

Platelets   An irregularly shaped, disc-like cell that functions in clotting

Refractory   Not responsive or readily yielding to treatment

Rh system   Second most important system determining compatibility; Rh antigens are inherited and located on the surface of red blood cells; classified as positive or negative based on whether D antigen is present

Serum   Term used to describe plasma after fibrinogen has been removed

Thrombocytopenia   Abnormally small number of platelets in the blood

To ensure the delivery of safe transfusion therapy, nurses must possess a knowledge and understanding of the blood system as well as basic immunohematology. Nurses must also be knowledgeable about the theory and practical management of **blood component** therapy. Today, "blood management" is the standard of care aimed at reducing, eliminating, or optimizing blood transfusions to ensure the best possible patient outcome.

The manufacture and distribution of blood products is overseen by the Food and Drug Administration (FDA), although the FDA does not directly inspect transfusion services. Rather, the FDA accepts inspections sanctioned by the Centers for Medicare & Medicaid Services (CMS), which is most often based on certificates of accreditation from an approved organization (Clark, 2011). The AABB (formerly the American Association of Blood Banks) is a major accreditation organization for hospital transfusion services. Safe transfusion practices are critical. Transfusion errors are likely to occur in three areas: labeling of the pretransfusion sample, patient identification at the bedside (a major nursing responsibility), and the initial decision to transfuse (i.e., appropriateness for transfusion).

The first part of this chapter presents the fundamental concepts of immunohematology, blood grouping, and the criteria for donor blood, including designated, **autologous**, and donation. Blood components, administration equipment, administration techniques for each blood component, and management of transfusion reactions are presented in the second part of the chapter.

INS Standard The registered nurse (RN) administering transfusion therapy should have knowledge and understanding of immunohematology; blood grouping; blood and its components; administration equipment, including vascular access devices and filters; techniques appropriate for each component; transfusion reactions and nursing interventions; and associated risks of transfusion therapy (Infusion Nurses Society [INS], 2011, p. S93).

■ Basic Immunohematology

Immunohematology is the science that deals with antigens of the blood and their **antibodies**. The antigens and antibodies are genetically inherited and determine each person's blood group. An **antigen** is a substance capable of stimulating the production of an antibody and then reacting with that antibody in a specific way. Antigens of the blood are also called **agglutinogens**. Any substance that can elicit an immunological response is an antigen and is located on the blood cell membrane. The three antigens on the red blood cells (RBCs) that cause problems and are routinely tested for are A, B, and Rh D. The **human leukocyte antigen (HLA)** is located on most cells in the body except mature erythrocytes. Antibodies are found in the **plasma** or **serum**.

Antigens (Agglutinogens)

ABO System

The **ABO system** was developed in 1901 by Dr. Karl Landsteiner. The most significant antigens in the blood are the surface antigens A and B, which are located on the RBC membranes in the ABO system (Table 11-1). The name of the blood type is determined by the name of the antigen on the RBC. Individuals who have A antigen on the RBC membrane are classified as group A; B antigens, group B; A and B surface antigens, group AB; and neither A nor B antigens, group O. Table 11-2 provides an ABO compatibility chart.

Unique to the ABO system is the presence of antibody in the serum of persons who lack the corresponding antigen; that is, the antibody is present even when the body is not stimulated with the foreign antigen. These naturally occurring antibodies are responsible for the rapidity and severity of reactions that occur when ABO-incompatible blood is administered. This phenomenon occurs occasionally in other blood systems but appears to be ubiquitous within the ABO system. As a result, if antigen A is present on the RBC, then antibody to B (anti-B) is present in the serum. If antigens A and B are present, no antibody exists in serum; conversely, if no antigen is present, then both anti-A and anti-B are present in the serum. Table 11-3 provides ABO compatibility for plasma.

> Table 11-1	ABO BLOOD GROUPING CHART	
Blood Groupings	Recipient Antigens on Red Blood Cells	Antibodies Present in Plasma
A	A	Anti-B
B	B	Anti-A
AB	A and B	None
O	None	Anti-A and Anti-B

> Table 11-2	ABO COMPATIBILITIES FOR RED BLOOD CELL COMPONENTS							
	→ Can Receive							
Recipient ↓	O NEG	O POS	A NEG	A POS	B NEG	B POS	AB NEG	AB POS
O NEG	√							
O POS	√	√						
A NEG	√		√					
A POS	√	√	√	√				
B NEG	√				√			
B POS	√	√			√	√		
AB NEG	√		√		√		√	
AB POS	√	√	√	√	√	√	√	√

Note: *The universal red blood cell donor is O-negative; the universal recipient is AB-positive.*

> Table 11-3	ABO COMPATIBILITY FOR FRESH FROZEN PLASMA	
Recipient	Donor Unit	
A	A or AB	
B	B or AB	
AB	AB	
O	O, A, B, or AB	

CULTURAL AND ETHNIC CONSIDERATIONS: BLOOD TYPES AND RH FACTOR

Blood groups differentiate people in certain racial groups. A prevalence for type O blood has been found among Native Americans, with some incidence of type A blood and virtually no incidence of type B blood. Almost equal incidences of types A, B, and O blood occur in Japanese and Chinese people, whereas AB blood type occurs in only about 10% of this population.

African Americans and European Americans have been found to have equal incidences of A, B, and O blood types, with predominant blood types of A and O (Giger & Davidhizar, 2004).

Persons with type O blood are at a greater risk for duodenal ulcers, and those with type A blood are more likely to develop cancer of the stomach. The Rh-negative factor is most common in European Americans, is much rarer in other racial groups, and is absent in Eskimos (Giger & Davidhizar, 2004).

Rh System

After A and B, the most significant RBC antigen is the D antigen, which was discovered in 1940 by Drs. Landsteiner and Wiener. The **Rh system** is so called because of its relationship to the substance in the RBCs of the Rhesus monkey. There are approximately 50 Rh-related antigens; the five principal antigens are D, C, E, c, and e. A person who has D antigen is classified as Rh-positive; one lacking the D antigen is Rh-negative. The majority of the population is classified as D–Rh-positive (Chou & Westhoff, 2011). The prevalence of D–Rh-negative is approximately 15% to 17% among Caucasians, 3% to 5% in African Americans, and rare in persons of Asian descent. There are no naturally occurring anti-D antibodies; however, D antibodies build up easily in D-negative recipients when stimulated with D-positive blood. Therefore, typing is done to ensure that D-negative recipients receive D-negative blood. Because the Rh-antigen resides on the red cell, an Rh-negative recipient should receive Rh-negative blood if the components might contain RBCs. Rh-negative blood can be administered to Rh-positive persons. Table 11-4 lists the most common blood types.

HLA System

The HLA antigen was originally identified on leukocytes, but it has been established that HLA is present on most cells in the body. The HLA system

> Table 11-4	BLOOD TYPES BY POPULATION			
Type	**% Population/Ethnic Groups**			
	Caucasian	*African American*	*Hispanic*	*Asian*
O Rh-positive	37	47	53	39
O Rh-negative	8	4	4	1
A Rh-positive	33	24	29	27
A Rh-negative	7	2	2	0.5
B Rh-positive	9	18	9	25
B Rh-negative	2	1	1	0.4
AB Rh-positive	3	4	2	7
AB Rh-negative	1	0.3	0.2	0.1

Source: American Red Cross (n.d.).

includes a complex array of genes and their protein products. It is located on the surface of white blood cells (WBCs), platelets, and most tissue cells. HLA typing, or tissue typing, is important in patients with transplants or multiple transfusions and is used for identification in paternity testing. The HLA system is very complex and is essential to immune regulation and cellular differentiation.

The HLA system is important in transfusion therapy because HLA antigens and antibodies play a role in complications of transfusion therapy, such as platelet refractoriness, febrile nonhemolytic transfusion reaction (FNHTRs), transfusion-related acute lung injury (TRALI), and posttransplant and posttransfusion graft-versus-host disease (GVHD). The HLA antigen of the donor unit can induce **alloimmunization** in the recipient. Methods used to decrease HLA alloimmunization include HLA matching and leukocyte depletion of the donor unit (Gebel, Pollack, & Bray, 2011).

The incidence of HLA alloimmunization and platelet refractoriness among patients receiving repeated transfusion ranges from 20% to 71% (Gebel et al., 2011). In the refractory state, platelet transfusions fail to increase the recipient's platelet count. HLA alloimmunization can be lessened with leukocyte-reduced blood components. Blood may be depleted of leukocytes during three periods: (1) immediately after collection, (2) 6 to 24 hours after collection, and (3) at the time of infusion. The trend today is for prestorage leukocyte depletion of packed red blood cells (PRBCs) and platelets. Early removal of leukocytes reduces the development of cytokines that appear to be implicated in many transfusion reactions.

 NURSING FAST FACT!

Patients receiving multiple transfusions are at particular risk for developing complications related to leukocytes, such as sensitization to leukocyte antigens, nonhemolytic febrile reactions, transmission of leukocyte-mediated viruses, and GVHD (Gebel et al., 2011).

Antibodies (Agglutinins)

An antibody is a protein that reacts with a specific antigen. Each blood antibody has the same name as the antigen with which it reacts. For example, anti-A reacts with antigen A. The antibodies anti-A and anti-B are produced spontaneously in the plasma after birth and usually mature in the first 3 months of life.

Antibodies of the blood system are **agglutinins**; that is, when stimulated by a specific antigen, they bind to the antigen to cause clumping. In the case of a red cell incompatibility, the interaction of the antibody with the like antigen (e.g., anti-B with antigen B) causes the red cells to clump together.

Antibodies, also known as immunoglobulins (Igs) or immune antibodies, are a group of glycoproteins (i.e., complex molecules containing protein and sugar molecules) in the serum and tissues of mammals that have the ability to interact with foreign objects, such as bacteria or viruses, and neutralize them. There are five categories of Ig molecules in human blood: IgA, IgD, IgE, IgG, and IgM. These antibodies are classified as either complete or incomplete. The naturally occurring antibody in the blood, which occurs within the inherited blood group (ABO), is from the class of antibodies called immunoglobulin M (IgM). These antibodies have the ability to cause agglutination of blood cells even when suspended in saline. In vivo, these antibodies cause total cellular destruction and lead to intravascular **hemolysis** when stimulated by foreign antigen.

The other four antibody groups and some IgM antibodies are incomplete antibodies, meaning they are not capable of causing agglutination in saline. These Igs are produced by the immune system in response to previous exposure to an antigen via previous transfusion, pregnancy, and from immunizations; they are not genetically inherited. When these antibodies contact the corresponding antigen, the cells are affected but not destroyed in the intravascular system. The sensitized cells are removed intact by the reticuloendothelial system, primarily the spleen and liver (Porth & Matfin, 2010).

Other Blood Group Systems

The International Society of Blood Transfusion (ISBT) recognizes 30 blood group systems. The ABO and Rh systems are best known and clinically most significant. The antigens of the H, Lewis, I, P, and globoside systems are carbohydrate structures that are biochemically closely related to ABO antigens. The most important aspect of blood groups in transfusion medicine is whether the antibodies are hemolytic and have potential to cause **hemolytic transfusion reactions** (HTRs) and hemolytic disease of the fetus and newborn (Daniels, 2011).

Pretransfusion Testing

At the time of donation, every unit of blood intended for **homologous (allogeneic)** and **directed (designated) donation** must undergo the following tests by the blood bank:

1. The ABO group must be determined by testing the RBCs with anti-A and anti-B sera and by testing the serum or plasma with A and B cells.
2. The Rh type must be determined with anti-D serum. Units that are D-positive must be labeled as Rh-positive.
3. Most blood banks test all donor blood for clinically significant antibodies. If all donors are not tested, then at least blood from

donors with a history of previous transfusion or pregnancy should be tested for unexpected antibodies before the **crossmatch**.
4. All donor blood must be tested to detect transmissible disease. The blood component must not be used for transfusion unless the test results are nonreactive, negative, or within the normal range.
5. Each unit must be appropriately labeled. The label must include the following information: name of the component, type and amount of anticoagulant, volume of unit, required storage temperature, name and address of collecting facility, a reference to the circular of information, type of donor (i.e., volunteer, autologous), expiration date, and donor number (Fig. 11-1).
6. The facility performing the compatibility testing must do ABO and Rh grouping confirmation tests on a sample obtained from the originally attached segment of all units of whole blood or RBCs.

 NURSING FAST FACT!

Since 2006, the FDA has required that blood and blood components contain specific labeled barcoded information about (1) the unique facility identifier (registration number), (2) the lot number relating to the donor, (3) the product code, and (4) the ABO group and Rh type of the donor. These four pieces of information must also be present in eye-readable format (FDA, 2009).

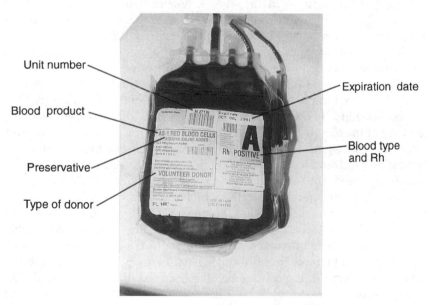

Figure 11-1 ■ Correct labeling of a unit of blood.

After blood is drawn from a donor, it is tested for ABO group (blood type) and Rh type (positive or negative), as well as for any unexpected RBC antibodies that may cause problems in the recipient. Screening tests are also performed for evidence of donor infection including the following:

Viruses
- Hepatitis B virus (HBV)
- Hepatitis C virus (HCV)
- Human immunodeficiency virus (HIV) types 1 and 2
- West Nile virus (WNV)
- Human T cell lymphotropic virus

Bacteria
- Syphilis
- *Trypanosoma cruzi*, a protozoan parasite transmitted by insects (Galel, 2011).

Blood Preservatives

There are several available RBC preservatives. Understanding of the RBC preservative is necessary because adverse reactions may occur in some patients as a result of the preservative. The solutions in the blood collection bag have a dual function: anticoagulation and RBC preservation. Citrate is used as an anticoagulant in all blood preservatives. Citrate binds with free calcium in the donor's plasma. Blood will not clot in the absence of free or ionized calcium. Citrate prevents coagulation by inhibiting the calcium-dependent steps of the coagulation cascade. Preservatives provide proper nutrients to maintain RBC viability, function, and metabolism. In addition, refrigeration at 1° to 6°C preserves RBCs and minimizes the proliferation of bacteria (Lockwood, Leonard & Liles, 2008).

In 1971, citrate-phosphate-dextrose (CPD) became a common preservative for blood. Phosphate is added to buffer the decrease in pH. The compound in the RBC that facilitates the transport of oxygen is 2,3-diphosphoglycerate (2,3-DPG). When the pH of the blood drops, there is a decrease in 2,3-DPG and therefore a lowering of the oxygen-carrying capacity of the blood. The 2,3-DPG levels remain higher in blood stored in CPD than in that stored with adenine-citrate-dextrose preservative. The expiration of RBCs preserved in CPD is 21 days stored at 1° to 6°C. Additional approved anticoagulant preservatives include citrate-phosphate-dextrose-dextrose solution (CP2D), which also has a shelf-life of 21 days, and citrate-phosphate-dextrose-adenine (CPDA-1), which has a shelf-life of 35 days (Lockwood et al., 2011). CPDA-1 contains adenine, which helps the RBCs synthesize adenosine triphosphate (ATP) during storage. Cells have improved viability in this anticoagulant preservative because the energy requirements of the cell are better preserved than with plain CPD.

There are three forms of additive solution (AS) approved by the FDA: AS-1, AS-3, and AS-5. The additive solution for red cell preservative

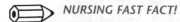

system AS contains sodium chloride, dextrose, adenine, and other substances that support red cell survival and function up to 42 days (Lockwood et al., 2011).

> ### NURSING FAST FACT!
>
> RBCs prepared with AS-1, AS-3, and AS-5 have better flow rates and do not require dilution with saline. Hypocalcemia is an adverse reaction that can occur when large amounts of citrated blood are infused in a person with impaired hepatic function.

■ Blood Donor Collection Methods

Allogeneic/Homologous

The term **allogeneic,** or homologous, donation describes transfusion of any blood component that was donated by someone other than the recipient. Most transfusions are provided by volunteer donors.

Guidelines for Allogeneic Donation

Donor selection for homologous collection is based on a limited physical examination and a medical history to determine the safety of the donated unit. Strict criteria have been established for selection of prospective donors:

1. Donor history questionnaire (DHQ). In October 2006, the FDA (2006) recognized the DHQ in a final guidance document that is currently used by the majority of blood centers in the United States (Eder, 2011). The AABB recommends the use of specific donor screening materials, which can be found on the following Web site. An abbreviated donor history questionnaire is available for frequent donors.

 Website

FDA: www.fda.gov/BiologicsBloodVaccines/BloodBloodProducts/ApprovedProducts/LicensedProductsBLAs/BloodDonorScreening/ucm164185.htm

2. Age: 17 years old without parental permission; some states allow 16-year-olds with parental permission
3. Provisions must be made for donors not fluent in English or who are illiterate
4. Provisions for donors who are hearing or vision impaired

---

5. **Hemoglobin** (Hgb) and hematocrit (Hct) of at least 12.5 g/dL
   and 38%, respectively, in males and females
6. Temperature: Less than or equal to 37.5°C (99.5°F) measured orally
7. No evidence of skin lesions at site of venipuncture for blood
   collection
8. Has not donated blood or plasma within the last 8 weeks
9. Medications: The DHQ medication deferral list contains the
   required deferrals (Fig. 11-2.)

Designated or Directed Donors

Directed (designated) donation refers to the donation of blood from selected friends or relatives of the patient. Most blood centers and hospitals
provide this service. Designated donations have been requested more frequently because of the concern over the risk of transfusion-transmitted diseases. However, there is no evidence that directed donations are safer than
blood provided by transfusion services (Eder, 2011). Relatives or friends
who may be members of a risk group may feel forced into donating and
hesitate to identify themselves as a risk group member. Fig. 11-3 identifies
the unit as designated or directed to a specific recipient.

Guidelines for Designated Donation

The selection and screening of directed donors are the same as for other
homologous (allogeneic) donors, except that the units collected are
labeled for a specific recipient. The designated donor must pass all the
history and screening tests required, and the unit must be compatible
with the intended recipient (Eder, 2011).

Autologous Donors

Autologous donation is the collection, storage, and reinfusion of a recipient's own blood. This is also called autotransfusion. In 2008, U.S. autologous collections comprised less than half a million units, or 1.5% of total
blood collections (Eder, 2011). Decreased interest in autologous donations
reflects the decline in viral risk associated with allogeneic blood transfusion and consequently the minimal medical benefit and increased cost of
autologous blood. The use of autologous blood avoids the possibility of

MEDICATION DEFERRAL LIST

Please tell us if you are now taking or if you have _EVER_ taken any of these medications:

❏ **Proscar® (finasteride)** – usually given for prostate gland enlargement

❏ **Avodart® (dutasteride)** – usually given for prostate enlargement

❏ **Propecia® (finasteride)** – usually given for baldness

❏ **Accutane® (Amnesteem, Claravis, Sotret, isotretinoin)** – usually given for severe acne

❏ **Soriatane® (acitretin)** – usually given for severe psoriasis

❏ **Tegison® (etretinate)** – usually given for severe psoriasis

❏ **Growth Hormone from Human Pituitary Glands** – used usually for children with delayed or impaired growth

❏ **Insulin from Cows (Bovine, or Beef, Insulin)** – used to treat diabetes

❏ **Hepatitis B Immune Globulin** – given following an exposure to hepatitis B.
NOTE: This is different from the hepatitis B vaccine which is a series of 3 injections given over a 6 month period to prevent future infection from exposures to hepatitis B.

❏ **Plavix (clopidogrel) and Ticlid (ticlopidine)** – inhibits platelet function; used to reduce the chance for heart attack and stroke.

❏ **Feldene** – given for mild to moderate arthritis pain

❏ **Experimental Medication or Unlicensed (Experimental) Vaccine** – usually associated with a research protocol

---

IF YOU WOULD LIKE TO KNOW WHY THESE MEDICINES AFFECT YOU AS A BLOOD DONOR, PLEASE KEEP READING:

• If you have taken or are taking **Proscar, Avodart, Propecia, Accutane, Soriatane, or Tegison,** these medications can cause birth defects. Your donated blood could contain high enough levels to damage the unborn baby if transfused to a pregnant woman. Once the medication has been cleared from your blood, you may donate again. Following the last dose, the deferral period is one month for Proscar, Propecia and Accutane, six months for Avodart and three years for Soriatane. Tegison is a permanent deferral.

• **Growth hormone from human pituitary glands** was prescribed for children with delayed or impaired growth. The hormone was obtained from human pituitary glands, which are found in the brain. Some people who took this hormone developed a rare nervous system condition called Creutzfeldt-Jakob Disease (CJD, for short). The deferral is permanent.

• **Insulin from cows (bovine, or beef, insulin)** is an injected material used to treat diabetes. If this insulin was imported into the US from countries in which "Mad Cow Disease" has been found, it could contain material from infected cattle. There is concern that mad cow disease is transmitted by transfusion. The deferral is indefinite.

• **Hepatitis B Immune Globulin (HBIG)** is an injected material used to prevent infection following an exposure to hepatitis B. HBIG does not prevent hepatitis B infection in every case; therefore persons who have received HBIG must wait 12 months to donate blood to be sure they were not infected since hepatitis B can be transmitted through transfusion to a patient.

• **Feldene** is a non-steroidal anti-inflammatory drug that can affect platelet function. A donor taking Feldene will not be able to donate platelets for 2 days; however, its use will not affect whole blood donations.

• **Plavix and Ticlid** are medications that can decrease the chance of a heart attack or stroke in individuals at risk for these conditions. Since these medications can affect platelets, anyone taking Plavix or Ticlid will not be able to donate platelets for 14 days after the last dose. Use of either medication will not prohibit whole blood donations.

• **Experimental Medication or Unlicensed (Experimental) Vaccine** is usually associated with a research protocol and the effect on blood donation is unknown. Deferral is one year unless otherwise indicated by Medical Director.

Figure 11-2 ■ Medication deferral list. (Source: http://www.fda.gov/)

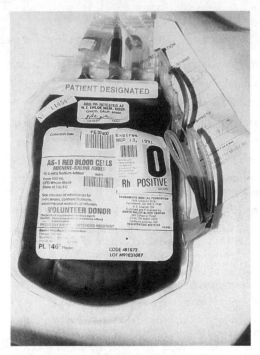

Figure 11-3 ■ Designated donor unit.

alloimmunization because it does not contain foreign RBCs, platelets, and leukocyte antigens. The risk of exposure and disease transmission is also eliminated. Because of this, the use of autologous blood is regarded as safer than homologous transfusion. However, risks associated with labeling and documentation remain. The same precautions used for preparing and administering a homologous blood component must be observed.

Donor Requirements

1. Age is the same as for allogeneic donor selection.
2. All blood collection shall be completed more than 72 hours before the time of surgery or transfusion.
3. Vital signs are the same as for allogeneic donor selection.
4. There is a deferral for conditions presenting risk of bacteremia.
5. Hgb is greater than or equal to 11 g/dL or Hct is greater than or equal to 33%.
6. There must be a prescription or order from the patient's LIP.
7. Candidates must be evaluated by the blood bank (Eder, 2011).

Advantages

■ Eliminates the risk of alloimmunization (sensitization to RBCs, platelets, and leukocyte antigens).

- Eliminates the risk of exposure to bloodborne infectious agents.
- Expands the blood resources.
- Reduces the need for allogeneic blood (decreases dependence on the volunteer donor supply).
- Provides an option for patients who find homologous transfusion unacceptable on religious grounds.
- Allows perioperative isovolemic hemodilution.

DISADVANTAGES

- Cost of predeposited autologous blood and increased paperwork because of special handling required
- Used only for the donor-patient.

Types

There are four categories of autologous transfusion: (1) preoperative autologous blood transfusion, (2) perioperative isovolemic hemodilution, (3) intraoperative autologous transfusion, and (4) postoperative blood salvage (Richardson, 2014).

PREOPERATIVE AUTOLOGOUS DONATION

Predeposit or preoperative autologous blood donation is the collection and storage of the recipient's own blood several weeks before scheduled surgery for reinfusion during or after surgery. Patients may be able to donate their own blood up to 72 hours before surgery. Approximately half of preoperatively donated units are discarded, which is a waste of resources (Waters, 2011).

Indication
- Elective surgical procedure with realistic possibility of transfusion

Typical Uses
- Total joint replacement (most common)
- Other major orthopedic surgeries
- Vascular surgery
- Cardiothoracic surgery (Eder, 2011)

Disadvantages
- Relatively costly
- Risk of clerical error

PERIOPERATIVE ISOVOLEMIC HEMODILUTION

Blood is collected in the operating room after anesthesia induction, removing whole blood just before surgery so that blood lost during surgery has a lower concentration of RBCs (Waters, 2011). Up to 2 L of blood is collected and replaced with crystalloid or colloid solutions for fluid replacement. The collected blood can be stored at room temperature in the operating room but should be transfused within 8 hours (Richardson, 2014). If the operating room procedure is expected to last more than

8 hours, then the blood should be refrigerated and must be transfused within 24 hours (Richardson, 2014).

INTRAOPERATIVE AUTOLOGOUS TRANSFUSION (BLOOD RECOVERY)

Intraoperative blood salvage is the collection and use of shed blood during surgery. Typically, 2 units of blood are collected early in the surgery from the surgical site. Shed blood can be readministered after concentrating and washing (washed recovered blood) with a blood recovery device, or it can be filtered and readministered (unwashed recovered blood). Unwashed recovered blood is usually reserved for the postoperative environment where small quantities of blood are collected and reinfused (Waters, 2011). This blood must be reinfused within 8 hours (Richardson, 2014).

Indications
- Surgical procedure with anticipated major blood loss
- Patient unable to donate preoperatively

Surgical Procedures Associated With Large Blood Loss
- Cardiac: Valve replacement, coronary artery bypass graft surgery
- Orthopedic: Knee replacement, hip replacement; major spine surgery, hemipelvectomy
- Urology: Radical prostatectomy, cystectomy, nephrectomy
- Liver transplant
- Neurosurgery: Arteriovenous malfunction resection
- Pregnancy: Ectopic pregnancy, cesarean section with placenta accreta/percreta/increta (Waters, 2011)

Contraindications
- Malignancy at operative site
- Bacterial contamination at operative site
- Use of microfibrillar collagen materials

Advantages
- May be acceptable to patients opposed to transfusions for religious reasons
- May eliminate need for allogeneic transfusion

Disadvantage
- Risk of air embolism and cell salvage syndrome

POSTOPERATIVE BLOOD SALVAGE

Postoperative salvage involves the salvage of blood from the surgical field in a single-use, self-contained reservoir for immediate return and reinfusion to the patient. This technique is used most often after cardiac surgeries and, recently, with orthopedic surgeries.

Indication
- Substantial bleeding in postoperative period

Typical Uses
- Cardiac surgery
- Orthopedic surgery

Contraindication
- Same as for intraoperative blood collection

Advantage
- May decrease allogeneic transfusion in some clinical settings

Disadvantages
- **Febrile reaction** to washed blood
- Cost increases if shed blood is washed
- Air embolism and cell salvage syndrome

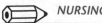 *NURSING FAST FACT!*

> Any autologous blood must be filtered during reinfusion to eliminate the possibility of microclot or debris infusion into the patient.

Blood Management

Blood management is an evidence-based, multidisciplinary process that is designed to reduce, eliminate, or optimize blood transfusions to improve patient outcomes (Seeber & Shander, 2013). The goal of blood management is to ensure the safe and efficient use of the many resources involved in the complex process of blood component therapy. Blood management includes nursing time, technician time, medical supplies, medical devices, laboratory tests, pharmaceuticals, hospital patients, and financial resources. In terms of nursing time, it takes more than 75 minutes of nursing time from prescription through completion of transfusion (Tolich, Blackmur, Stahorsky, & Wabeke, 2013).

Transfusion of blood products is a commonly performed procedure in the hospital setting (Tolich et al., 2013). The fact is that many blood components are not administered according to evidence-based practices, thereby consuming precious resources without benefit to patients (Tolich et al., 2013). The following facts should be considered before transfusions:
- Transfusions are not risk free.
  Transfusions today are the safest in history; however, they can cause some degree of harm. The leading causes of transfusion-related morbidity and mortality are unrelated to viral transmission and include bacterial contamination of platelets, transfusion errors from patient misidentification, and TRALI. Blood transfusions can improve outcomes but only when used in the right patient for the right indication and in the right dose (Boucher & Hannon, 2007).
- Blood is a human tissue transplant (Tolich et al., 2013).
  Infusing blood is not different from solid organ transplant. Blood transfusions can cause changes in the immune system

function of patients, which present a new set of immune challenges.

> EBP Based on controlled studies, the best evidence for transfusion therapy indicates that a more conservative approach to blood transfusion not only saves blood but also improves patient outcomes (Corwin, 2006).

- Transfusions can increase health-care–associated infections.
- Transfusion education is necessary to address the gaps in education of physicians and nurses in appropriate ordering and administration of blood products.
- Financial penalties for poor clinical outcomes related to inappropriate transfusion practices are increasing. The CMS and many commercial health insurance carriers will not pay for the cost of treating transfusion errors, bleeding complications in cardiac surgery, and a growing number of hospital-acquired infections that are increased two- to fivefold by blood transfusions.

Strategic Approach to Blood Management

Blood should only be administered based on appropriate indications. For example, transfusions should be restricted to an Hgb level of 7 to 8 g/dL in stable, hospitalized patients and to 8 g/dL or less in the presence of clinical symptoms for patients with cardiovascular disease (Carson et al., 2012). Decisions regarding transfusion should be based on the patient's clinical condition in conjunction with laboratory values.

The role of nurses in transfusion-related practices is critical. Some implications include:

- Reduce the risk of iatrogenic anemia from excessive laboratory testing and loss of blood. Repeated phlebotomy is implicated as a contributing factor to blood loss and need for transfusion (Welden, 2010). Nurse-driven blood conservation strategies can reduce the need for transfusion (Table 11-5).
- Check Hgb levels on admission to the hospital. Patients admitted with an Hgb less than 10 g/dL are at risk for transfusion, so an in-depth assessment of contributing factors and physical assessment should be performed.
- Recognize that iron deficiency is a major contributor to anemia and that iron studies are warranted.
- Follow all organizational procedures related to blood and blood product verification.
- Transfuse 1 unit of RBCs at a time, then reassess the patient (Tolich et al., 2013).

> Table 11-5	BLOOD CONSERVATION METHODS

Minimize laboratory draws; consolidate all daily draws.

Evaluate laboratory orders for redundancy and make sure there are stop times on serial orders for testing.

Use low-volume or pediatric collection tubes.

Record the amount of blood obtained for laboratory tests and document the output.

Use point-of-care testing methods (e.g., international normalized ratio [INR] meters, glucometers).

Consider the mixing method for blood sampling from central venous access devices (CVADs) (avoids blood discard before laboratory sampling).

Sources: INS (2011, p. S79); Tolich et al. (2013); Welden (2010).

 NURSING FAST FACT!

> *It has been reported that patients lose approximately 41.1 mL of blood from blood draws within a 24-hour period (Zaccheo & Bucher, 2010).*

 ## Websites

Strategic Blood Management: www.bloodmanagement.com
Society for Advancement of Blood Management: www.sabm.org/
  professionals

INS Standard Only the volume of blood needed for accurate testing should be obtained. Phlebotomy contributes to iron deficiency and blood loss in critically ill patients and neonates, so efforts to conserve blood should be considered (INS, 2011, p. S79).

■ Blood Component Therapy

Blood is a "liquid organ" with extraordinary and unique functions. Blood carries oxygen to cells, carries waste away from cells, contains disease-fighting cells, and helps in regulation of body pH and temperature. Fifty-five percent of blood is composed of plasma (fluid); the remaining cellular portion (45%) is made up of solids (RBCs, WBCs, and platelets).

Whole Blood

Whole blood is composed of RBCs, plasma, WBCs, and platelets. The volume of each unit is approximately 500 mL and consists of 200 mL of RBCs and 300 mL of plasma, with a minimum of 33% Hct. Whole blood is rarely used for allogeneic transfusion; RBCs and crystalloid solutions have become the standard for most cases of active bleeding in trauma and surgery with supplementation of hemostatic elements as needed.

Uses

Most whole blood units are now used to prepare separate RBC and plasma components to meet specific clinical needs. A whole blood unit can be centrifuged and separated into three components: RBCs, plasma, and platelet concentrate. By transfusing the patient with the specific component needed rather than with whole blood, the patient is not exposed to unnecessary portions of the blood product, and valuable blood resources are conserved (Fig. 11-4).

Few conditions require transfusion of whole blood. Indications include acute, massive blood loss with signs and symptoms such as hypotension, dyspnea, tachycardia, and pallor (Richardson, 2014). A unit of whole blood increases RBC mass, which provides oxygen-carrying capacity and plasma for blood volume expansion.

Administration

- Amount: Volume of 500 mL
- Catheter size: 22 to 14 gauge, with 20 to 18 gauge appropriate for general populations. With use of smaller gauge catheters (22 gauge), blood dilution and a pump are helpful to administer the unit (Sink, 2011).
- Usual rate: 2 to 4 hours
- Administration set: Straight or Y type with 170- to 260-micron filter

Compatibility

Whole blood requires type and crossmatching. Must be ABO compatible.

Red Blood Cells

RBC units are prepared by removing 200 to 250 mL of plasma from a whole blood unit. The remaining **packed red blood cells** concentrate has a volume of approximately 250 to 350 mL. Each unit contains the same RBC mass as whole blood, as well as 20% to 30% of the original plasma, leukocytes, and some platelets. The advantages of RBCs over whole blood are decreased plasma volume and decreased risk of circulatory overload. Another advantage is that because most of the plasma has been removed, less citrate, potassium, ammonia, and other metabolic byproducts are transfused.

 NURSING FAST FACT!

In a normal adult patient, 1 unit of RBCs should raise the Hgb level approximately 1 g/dL and the Hct level 3%, the same as with a unit of whole blood (Nester & AuBuchon, 2011).

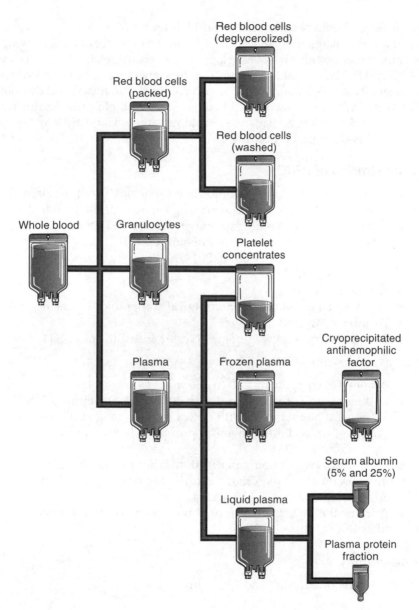

Figure 11-4 ■ Derivation of transfusible blood products.

Uses

RBCs are used to improve the oxygen-carrying capacity in patients with symptomatic anemia. The administration of RBCs should be considered only if improvement of the RBC count cannot be achieved through nutrition, drug therapy, or treatment of the underlying disease. As stated earlier, transfusions should be restricted to an Hgb level of 7 to 8 g/dL in stable, hospitalized patients and to 8 g/dL or less in the presence of clinical symptoms for patients with cardiovascular disease (Carson et al., 2012). Per the AABB (2009), RBCs should not be used to treat anemia that can be corrected with hematinic medications (e.g., iron, vitamin B_{12}, folic acid, erythropoietin). Criteria for transfusion should be based on multiple variables, including Hgb and Hct levels, patient symptoms, amount and time frame of blood loss, and surgical procedures.

Administration of PRBC

- Increase red cell mass when volume expansion is not required
- Restore or maintain oxygen-carrying capacity of the blood
- Symptomatic anemia unresponsive to other treatments
- Acute or chronic blood loss with symptoms (i.e., tachycardia, dyspnea, pallor) (Richardson, 2014)

Do not transfuse RBCs:
- For volume expansion
- In place of a hematinic (nonbiological compound for raising Hgb)
- To enhance wound healing
- To improve general well-being (Nester & AuBuchon, 2011)

ADMINISTRATION SUMMARY

- Amount of component: 250 to 350 mL
- Catheter size: 22 to 14 gauge, with 20 to 18 gauge appropriate for general populations. With use of smaller gauge catheters (22 gauge), blood dilution and a pump are helpful to administer the unit (Sink, 2011).
- Usual rate: 1½ to 2 hours per unit, maximum 4 hours. (If longer infusion times are required, the unit may be split and aliquots administered over 1.5–2 hours.)
- Administration set: Straight or Y type with 170- to 260-micron filter (Fig. 11-5).

Compatibility

Crossmatch required. ABO and Rh compatible.

Leukocyte-Reduced Red Blood Cells

Leukocyte-poor RBCs are grouped in a category referred to as modified blood products. A unit of whole blood contains more than 1 to 10×10^9 WBCs. Leukocyte-reduced PRBCs result from removal of the number of leukocytes in whole blood to 5×10^6. In the United States, leukocyte reduction by filtration of RBCs must not result in a red cell loss greater than 15%; in addition, 40 g of Hgb must be present in each unit after leukocyte reduction (AABB, 2009). Leukocyte reduction is achieved either by using

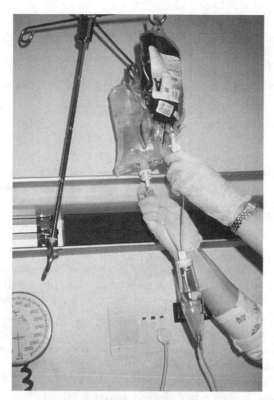

Figure 11-5 ■ Hanging PRBCs with Y administration set. Always wear gloves when handling blood products.

filtration before transfusion or by using a special filter at the bedside during transfusion. Leukocyte-reduced RBCs require ABO compatibility.

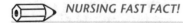 *NURSING FAST FACT!*

> *The leukocyte-reduced component will have therapeutic efficacy equal to at least 85% that of the original component (Kakaiya, Aronson, & Julleis, 2011).*

Uses

Leukocyte-reduced components are indicated as follows:
- In patients with a known history of febrile non-HTRs caused by donor WBC antigens
- To reduce the incidence of urticarial and anaphylactic reactions
- To prevent transmission of cytomegalovirus (CMV)
- In immunosuppressed patients (Richardson, 2014)

Safety Concern: On rare occasions, patients may develop severe hypotension when leukocyte reduction is performed at the bedside. This happens more often in patients who take angiotensin-converting enzyme (ACE) inhibitors (Sink, 2011). In general, leukocyte reduction at the time of collection is preferred over filtration at the bedside.

Deglycerolized Red Blood Cells (Freezing Red Blood Cells)

Deglycerolized RBCs are prepared to allow for freezing of cells for long-term storage; this increases the storage rate for rare units of RBCs (such as B-negative) and autologous donor units. The RBCs are frozen after the plasma is removed and glycerol (a cryoprotective agent) is added. The RBCs are stored at –65°C or colder. Glycerol enters the cell and protects the cell from damage caused by cellular dehydration and mechanical injury from ice formation. RBC units are usually placed in canisters to protect the polyolefin plastic bag during freezing, storage, and thawing.

To thaw the deglycerolized RBCs, the canister is placed in a 37°C dry heater or, after overwrapping, is placed in a 37°C water bath. If the red cells have been frozen in the primary blood container, then the container should be thawed at 42°C. Thawing should be complete within 40 minutes (Kakaiya et al., 2011). The glycerol cryopreservative must be removed before the component is transfused. The removal is accomplished in a slow "deglycerolization" process to minimize hemolysis; it is performed using washing techniques. The manufacturer's instructions must be followed to ensure maximum red cell recovery and minimal hemolysis.

The shelf-life for thawed deglycerolized RBCs depends on the type of system used. Closed system devices allow storage for up to 14 days, but components prepared using open systems expire within 24 hours of thawing.

Use: Special needs for rare donor antigen-negative units and autologous units. ABO compatibility is required.

Washed Red Blood Cells

RBCs can be "washed" with sterile normal saline to remove cellular debris, plasma, platelets, and leukocytes (Richardson, 2014). Limited clinical indications for washed RBCs may include recurrent or severe allergic reactions to one or more plasma proteins, and neonatal and intrauterine transfusions. A disadvantage is that up to 20% of the RBC yield is lost during the washing procedure (Lockwood et al., 2011). Anticoagulant-preservative solutions are removed during the washing procedure; therefore, washed RBC units expire 24 hours after washing.

Irradiated Blood Products

Cellular blood components can be irradiated for certain patient populations to prevent transfusion-associated GVHD. Irradiation is accomplished with the use of gamma irradiators, linear accelerators, ultraviolet-A irradiation, and other nonradioisotope equipment.

Uses

- Prevention of GVHD
- Patients with acute leukemia and lymphoma (Hodgkin's disease and non-Hodgkin's disease)
- Bone marrow or stem cell transplant recipients
- Patients with immunodeficiency disorders
- Neonates and low-birth-weight infants

 NURSING FAST FACT!

A label marked "irradiated" must be placed on the bag containing the product. Whole blood, RBCs, platelets, or granulocytes can be irradiated.

Safety Concern: The shelf-life of irradiated RBCs is limited to 28 days because irradiation damages the cells and reduces their viability (Kakaiya et al., 2011). Platelets and granulocytes are not damaged, so their shelf-life is not affected.

Granulocytes

Granulocyte concentrations are prepared by leukapheresis from a single donor of whole blood. Each unit contains granulocytes and variable amounts of lymphocytes, platelets, and RBCs suspended in 200 to 300 mL of plasma. They are obtained for transfusion by granulocytapheresis.

Granulocyte infusions should be administered as soon after collection as possible because of the well-documented possibility of deterioration of granulocyte function during short-term storage. If stored, units should be maintained at 20° to 24°C without agitation and will expire in 24 hours (AABB, 2009). In general, the administration of granulocytes is controversial and their use has declined (AABB, 2009; Kakaiya et al., 2011). Transfusion may not significantly increase the granulocyte count.

Uses

- Neutropenia
- Patients with chronic granulomatous disease (CGD), a hereditary neutrophil function defect; myeloid hypoplasia; hematopoietic stem cell transplantation; aplastic anemia; neonatal sepsis

Administration of granulocytes is accompanied by a high frequency of nonhemolytic febrile reactions. These side effects can be managed with the use of diphenhydramine, steroids, and nonaspirin antipyretics and by slowing the transfusion rate (AABB, 2009).

Safety Concern: Granulocytes must be transfused before testing for infectious diseases can be completed. Authorization to permit the transfusion is obtained from the patient's LIP before testing of the current donation is completed (Kakaiya et al., 2011).

Administration

There is no set standard for the amount or duration of granulocyte therapy, but generally transfusion therapy is delivered for at least 4 consecutive days.

- Amount: 300 to 400 mL suspended in 200 to 300 mL of plasma
- Catheter size: 22 to 14 gauge
- Usual rate: 1 to 2 hours; slower if reaction occurs
- Administration set: Straight or Y type with 170-micron filter; *microaggregate or leukocyte-reduction filter contraindicated*
- Storage of unit is for the least time possible at room temperature without agitation

Compatibility

Crossmatch required. ABO/Rh compatibility required.

Platelets

Platelets are normally suspended in plasma and are responsible for hemostasis. **Platelets** live up to 12 days in the blood, do not have nuclei, and are unable to reproduce. They contain no Hgb. Normal platelet counts are 150,000 to 300,000/μL. Platelets can be supplied either as random-donor concentrates or from single-donor apheresis. Random-donor concentrates are prepared from individual units of whole blood by centrifuging the unit to separate the platelets. The platelets are stored at approximately room temperature, between 20° and 24°C, for up to 7 days. To prevent agglutination of the cells, platelets must be continuously agitated during storage. The expiration date is 24 hours without agitation (Kakaiya et al., 2011). Single-donor platelet apheresis products are collected from a single donor. During **pheresis**, the platelets are harvested, and all unneeded portions of the blood are returned back to the donor. A single pheresis unit is equivalent to 6 to 8 units of random-donor platelets (Fig. 11-6).

Use of a single-donor unit has the obvious advantage of exposing the recipient to fewer donors and is ideal for treating patients who have developed HLA antibodies from previous transfusions and have become **refractory** (unresponsive) to random-donor platelets. HLA typing may be indicated when patients become refractory to platelets after multiple transfusions. Platelet crossmatch procedures are also being evaluated for their usefulness with refractory patients.

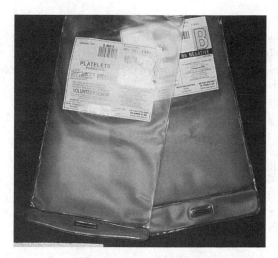

Figure 11-6 ■ Platelets.

 NURSING FAST FACT!

One platelet concentrate should raise the recipient's platelet count 5000 to 10,000/mL. The usual dose is 6 to 10 units of random or 1 unit of pheresis (AABB, 2009).

Uses

Platelets are administered in the presence of **thrombocytopenia** to control or prevent bleeding from platelet deficiencies or to replace functionally abnormal platelets. Current prophylactic platelet transfusion triggers:

- Patients with acute thrombocytopenia: Platelet count less than 10,000/μL **OR**
- Stable patients with chronic thrombocytopenia: 5000/μL
- Patients with fever or recent hemorrhage (with bleeding controlled): 10,000/μL
- Patients with coagulopathy, on heparin, or with anatomic lesion likely to bleed: 20,000/μL (Nester & AuBuchon, 2011)

Platelet transfusions at higher platelet counts may be required for patients with systemic bleeding and for those at high risk for bleeding because of additional coagulation defects, sepsis, or platelet dysfunction related to medication or disease. Significant spontaneous bleeding with platelet counts greater than 20,000/μL is rare. Platelet transfusions usually are not effective in patients with conditions in which rapid platelet destruction occurs, such as idiopathic autoimmune thrombocytopenic purpura (ITP) and untreated disseminated intravascular coagulation (DIC). In patients with these conditions, platelet transfusions should be used only in the presence of active bleeding.

Do not transfuse platelets:

- To patients with ITP (unless there is life-threatening bleeding)
- Prophylactically with massive blood transfusions
- Prophylactically after cardiopulmonary bypass (Nester & AuBuchon, 2011)
- Transfusion in DIC remains controversial.

Administration

Single-donor platelets are normally suspended in 40 to 70 mL of plasma; the volume of aphered units is 350 to 500 mL total (plasma plus platelets). Platelets may be infused rapidly as the patient tolerates, with infusion rates ranging from 1 to 2 mL/min up to 5 minutes per single-donor bag. Platelets should be delivered to infants by means of a syringe-type device and can be transfused at a rate of 1 mL/min.

The effectiveness of platelet transfusions may be altered if fever, infection, or active bleeding is present. To determine the effectiveness of a transfusion, platelet counts may be checked 1 hour and 24 hours after transfusion. Poor platelet count recovery may also indicate that the patient may be refractory to random-donor platelets.

ADMINISTRATION SUMMARY

- Amount: 40 to 70 mL/unit; usual dose 4 to 8 units (pediatric patients: 1 unit per 7 to 10 kg of body weight)
- Catheter size: 22 to 14 gauge
- Usual rate: Generally over 1 hour
- Filter: 170 to 260 microns; leukocyte-reduction filter, if indicated
- Administration set: Component syringe or Y drip set; tubing should be rubber free to prevent platelets from sticking; use 0.9% sodium chloride as primer

Platelet concentrates may be pooled before administration or infused individually; after they are pooled, platelets should be transfused within 4 hours.

Safety Concern: HLA alloimmunization: Although patients receiving multiple platelet transfusions usually are immunosuppressed, they are still able to mount an immune response against antigens on platelets; antibodies to HLA antigens can occur (Nester & AuBuchon, 2011).

Compatibility

ABO match is not required for the administration of platelets but is preferred (Sink, 2011). The amount of red cells and platelets harvested with the platelets is generally minimal but occasionally is sufficient to elicit an antigen–antibody response.

Plasma Derivatives

Plasma and Fresh Frozen Plasma

Plasma is the liquid portion of the blood in which nutrients are carried to body tissues and wastes are transported to areas of excretion. It is a colorless, thin, aqueous solution (91% water) that contains chemicals (bile pigments, bilirubin, electrolytes, enzymes, fats, and hormones), protein (7%), carbohydrates (2%), and clotting factors. When the clotting factors are removed, plasma is referred to as serum. Plasma does not contain any cellular portion of blood.

Fresh frozen plasma (FFP) is prepared from whole blood by separating and freezing the plasma within 8 hours of collection (Kakaiya et al., 2011). FFP may be stored for up to 1 year at 18°C or lower. FFP stored at 65°C may be stored for up to 7 years. The volume of a typical unit is 200 to 250 mL. FFP does not provide platelets, and loss of factors V and VIII (i.e., the labile clotting factors) is minimal (Fig. 11-7).

Uses

- Active bleeding with multiple coagulation factor deficiencies
- Warfarin reversal
- DIC
- Massive transfusions in trauma

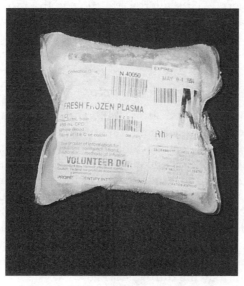

Figure 11-7 ■ Fresh frozen plasma.

Administration

Plasma must be frozen or administered within 8 hours of harvest to preserve labile coagulation factors. Plasma is administered as rapidly as tolerated after the first 5 minutes, at a rate of 300 mL/hr, unless there is a potential for fluid volume overload (Sink, 2011). Medications and diluents are never to be added to plasma.

FFP must be thawed in a 30° to 37°C water bath with gentle agitation or kneading. The thawing process takes up to 30 minutes, and the FFP should be transfused immediately after thawing or refrigerated once thawed and used within 24 hours. FFP must be delivered through a standard blood filter.

Do not transfuse FFP:

- For volume expansion
- When coagulopathy can be more effectively corrected with a specific therapy (e.g., vitamin K for warfarin overdose)

Administration Summary

- Amount: 200 to 300 mL (pediatric patient: 10–15 mL per kilogram of body weight and transfused at 1-2 mL/min)
- Catheter size: 22 to 18 gauge
- Usual rate: 1 to 2 hours
- Administration set: Straight or Y type with a 170-micron filter, primed with 0.9% sodium chloride

Compatibility

Crossmatch not required. Must be ABO compatible.

Safety Concern: Acute allergic reaction is the most common reaction after plasma administration. Most reactions are mild with primarily local symptoms such as hives. Rarely anaphylactic reactions can occur (DomBourian & Holland, 2012).

Cryoprecipitated Antihemophilic Factor

Cryoprecipitate is prepared from FFP and is the insoluble portion of plasma that remains as a white precipitate after FFP is thawed at 4°C under special conditions. The cold-insoluble precipitate is refrozen. Cryoprecipitate has a shelf-life of 1 year. AABB standards require that cryoprecipate contain at least 80 units of factor VIII, 150 mg of fibrinogen per unit; von Willebrand factor (vWF); and factor XIII (about 60 units per bag) (Kakaiya et al., 2011). It is the only concentrated source of fibrinogen and in today's practice is used for its fibrinogen content. The frozen component is thawed in a protective plastic overwrap in a water bath at 30° to 37°C for up to 15 minutes. It should not be used if there is evidence of container breakage or thawing during storage.

The development of cryoprecipitated antihemophilic factor (AHF) in the 1970s represented the first effective treatment of hemophilia, allowing patients to receive a short infusion at home versus long transfusions in the hospital (Nester & AuBuchon, 2011; Hitch, 2013). In the 1980s, the discovery of HIV and other disease contamination of the blood supply changed the picture as many persons with hemophilia contracted HIV and HCV. Today, the uses of cryoprecipitate have declined. The development of factor products without human plasma, through recombinant technology, is used for hemophilia treatment. Cryoprecipitate may be used in conditions with systemic fibrinolysis, such as those resulting from certain types of chemotherapy or DIC; however, virus-inactivated fibrinogen concentrates have largely replaced the use of cryoprecipitate.

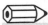 *NURSING FAST FACT!*

- *Do not refreeze after thawing.*
- *Good patient management requires that the cryoprecipitate AHF treatment responses of factor VIII–deficient recipients be monitored with periodic plasma factor VIII:C assays.*

USES

- Main use today: As a source of fibrinogen in acquired coagulopathies: DIC, massive hemorrhage
- May be used in the treatment of hemophilia A (factor VIII deficiency) and vWF disease if factor concentrate is not available (factor concentrate is preferred)

ADMINISTRATION

Cryoprecipitate is thawed before it is transfused and should be transfused as soon as possible after thawing (Sink, 2011). It is usually supplied as a single-donor pack or as a pack of six or more single-donor units that have been pooled. The inside of the bag should be rinsed with a small amount of saline to maximize recovery. Cryoprecipitate should be administered through a standard blood filter, and, as with platelet administration sets, small priming volumes are recommended to decrease loss of the product in the set. Cryoprecipitate should be transfused as rapidly as the patient can tolerate. The cryoprecipitate units are usually pooled to simplify administration, but pooling of cryoprecipitate is not universally done.

Administration Summary
- Amount: 10 to 15 mL of diluent added to precipitate (3–5 mL) unit; usual dose 6 to 10 units
- Catheter size: 22 to 18 gauge
- Usual rate: 1 to 2 mL/min for both adult and pediatric patients
- Administration set: Component syringe or standard blood component set, with 170-micron filter primed with 0.9% sodium chloride

Compatibility

Crossmatch and ABO compatibility is not required (Sink, 2011).

Recombinant Factor Replacement Products

Today, most of the factor replacement products used in managing hemophilia are derived from recombinant DNA rather than processed from donated plasma.

Administration

- Usually administered by slow I.V. bolus infusion in the acute or home care environment. Infusion time varies by product, so it is important to follow the manufacturer's directions.
- Packaged in kits that include a vial of factor (powder), a diluent, and a mixing device; most with a built-in filter. Sometimes, a steel needle I.V. device is included in the kit.
- Generally supplied by the blood center. Stored in refrigerator or at room temperature (as directed by the manufacturer); shelf-life up to 2 years.
- Dosage varies and is based on units per kilogram.

Factor VIII

Hemophilia A is a deficiency of coagulation factor VIII that occurs in about 1:10,000 males (Hitch, 2013). Factor VIII replacement either is used routinely for patients with severe hemophilia or may be used situationally in moderate to mild cases, such as patients undergoing prophylactic therapy with planned surgery or with a traumatic event.

Factor IX

Hemophilia B is a deficiency of coagulation factor IX that occurs in about 1:50,000 males (Hitch, 2013).

Safety Concern: Patients can develop antibodies to replacement factor, making it more difficult to control bleeding. This may require higher doses or a bypassing agent that allows clotting to occur without factor VIII or IX (Hitch, 2013).

Albumin

Albumin is a natural plasma protein that is commercially extracted from plasma. It supplies 80% of the osmotic activity of plasma and is the principal product of fractionation (dividing plasma into its component parts). It is administered as plasma protein fraction (PPF) and as purified albumin. Both products (albumin and PPF) are derived from donor plasma, prepared by the cold alcohol fractionation process, and then subsequently heated. Both products do not transmit viral diseases because of the extended heating process. Normal serum albumin is composed of 96% albumin and 4% globulin and other proteins. It is available as a 5% (isotonic) or 25% (hypertonic) solution.

NOTE > Additional information on albumin as a plasma expander is provided in Chapter 4.

Plasma Protein Fraction

PPF is a similar product to albumin except that it is subjected to fewer purification steps in the fractionation process and contains about 83% albumin and 17% globulin. PPF is available only in a 5% solution.

USES

PPF and 5% albumin are isotonic solutions and therefore are osmotically equivalent to an equal volume of plasma. They cause a plasma volume increase, are used interchangeably, and share the same clinical uses. Both are used primarily to increase plasma volume resulting from sudden loss of intravascular volume as seen in patients with hypovolemic shock from trauma or surgery. Their use may also be indicated in individual cases to support blood pressure during hypotensive episodes or to induce diuresis in those with fluid overload by assisting in fluid mobilization. The plasma derivatives lack clotting factors and other plasma proteins and therefore should not be considered plasma substitutes. Neither component (albumin or PPF) will correct nutritional deficits or chronic hypoalbuminemia.

Twenty-five percent albumin is hypertonic and is five times more concentrated than 5% albumin. This hyperosmotic product is used to draw fluids out of tissues and body cavities into intravascular spaces. This solution must be given with caution. Principal uses for 25% albumin include plasma volume expansion, hypovolemic shock, burns, and prevention or treatment of cerebral edema.

 NURSING FAST FACT!

> *Albumin 25% must not be used in dehydrated patients without supplemental fluids or in those at risk for circulatory overload.*

ADMINISTRATION

Albumin and PPF are supplied in glass bottles. Depending on the brand, albumin in 5% concentrations is available in units of 50-, 250-, 500-, and 1000-mL vials, and 25% concentrations are supplied in units of 20-, 50-, and 100-mL vials (Richardson, 2014). Manufacturers recommend that the solution be used within 4 hours of opening. Depending on the manufacturer, the solutions are sometimes supplied with an infusion set. If no administration set is provided, a standard administration set without a filter is used. Blood transfusion sets and filters are not required for infusion of albumin.

Albumin 5% and 25% may be given as rapidly as the patient tolerates for reduced blood volumes. When the blood volume is normal or only slightly reduced, rates of 2 to 4 mL/min have been suggested for 5% albumin and 1 mL/min for 25% albumin. More caution is used when infusing PPF because hypotension may occur with a rate greater than 10 mL/min (AABB, 2008).

Administration Summary
- Amount: 5% solution = 250 mL; 25% solution = 50 to 100 mL
- Catheter size: 22 to 18 gauge
- Usual rate: 5% solution: 2 to 4 mL/min; 25% solution: 1 mL/min
- Administration set: May come with administration set in package

COMPATIBILITY

ABO or Rh matching and compatibility testing are not necessary for these components because antigens and antibodies are not present in these products.

Table 11-6 provides a summary of blood components.

Immunoglobulins

Immune Globulin

Concentrates of plasma Igs were developed in the early 1980s to treat congenital immunodeficiencies and certain viral exposures by the intravenous route. Ig products are made from carefully screened and tested donors. Ig production includes dedicated steps to remove and inactivate bloodborne pathogens. Ig replacement therapy is indicated for patients who have primary immune deficiencies characterized by hypogamma-globulinemia and/or the inability to make protective levels of antibody in response to antigen exposure (Younger, Aro, Blouin et al., 2013). Ig therapy is also used for immunomodulation in some autoimmune diseases as well. Ig infusions may be administered intravenously or subcutaneously and may be administered to patients in outpatient settings, in the home, and in the hospital. Subcutaneous infusion of Ig is used in patients who have primary immune deficiency, and its use has been increasing. It is well tolerated with fewer systemic effects, and patients can become completely independent in self-infusing and monitoring.

USES

- Reduce infections in patients with primary immune deficiencies
- Secondary (acquired) immune deficiencies (e.g., chronic lymphocytic leukemia, multiple myeloma, reduction of bacterial infection in pediatric acquired immune deficiency syndome [AIDS])

> Table 11-6   SUMMARY OF COMMON BLOOD COMPONENTS

Blood Component	Volume	Action and Use	Infusion Guide	Special Considerations
Red Blood Cells (RBCs)	250–350 mL	Symptomatic anemia Hemoglobin level of 7–8 g/dL in stable, hospitalized patients Hemoglobin ≤8 g/dL in the presence of clinical symptoms for patients with cardiovascular disease	Filter 170–260 microns Y administration set, primed with 0.9% sodium chloride Transfuse each unit in ≤4 hours or less	Crossmatch required ABO and Rh compatible Each unit raises the hemoglobin 1 g and hematocrit 3% Smaller aliquots of RBC volume can be made for use with neonatal, pediatric, or adult patients with special needs
Irradiated RBCs	Same as above.	Prevention of graft-versus-host disease (GVHD) Acute leukemia and lymphoma Bone marrow or stem cell transplant recipients Immunodeficiency disorders Neonates and low-birth-weight infants	Same as above	Same as above
Deglycerolized RBCs (frozen)	Same as above.	Prolonged storage of blood for rare blood types and autologous donations For special needs antigen-negative donors	Same as above	Must be used within 24 hours of being thawed

Continued

> Table 11-6   SUMMARY OF COMMON BLOOD COMPONENTS—cont'd

Blood Component	Volume	Action and Use	Infusion Guide	Special Considerations
Granulocytes	200–300 mL	Chronic granulomatous disease Neutropenia Aplastic anemia	Filter 170–260 microns Y administration set, primed with 0.9% sodium chloride No leukocyte-reduction filter or depth-type microaggregate filters Administer slowly over 2 hours, slower if reactions occur	Crossmatch required ABO and Rh compatible May be human leukocyte antigen (HLA) matched Transfusion of granulocytes controversial *Note:* High frequency of febrile nonhemolytic reactions Premedication used (e.g., diphenhydramine, steroids, nonaspirin antipyretics
Platelets, Random Donor	40–70 mL/unit Usual dose: 4–10 units	Acute thrombocytopenia: Platelet count <10,000/μL Stable patients with chronic thrombocytopenia: 5000/μL Fever or recent hemorrhage (with bleeding controlled): 10,000/μL Patients with coagulopathy, on heparin, or with anatomic lesion likely to bleed: 20,000/μL	Filter 170–260 microns Y administration set, primed with 0.9% sodium chloride Administer as rapidly as patient can tolerate; generally transfused over 1 hour Leukocyte reduction if indicated	Crossmatch not required ABO/Rh preferred but not necessary May be HLA matched Prophylactic medication with antihistamines, antipyretics may be needed
Fresh Frozen Plasma (FFP)	Prepared from whole blood 200–250 mL	Replacement of clotting factors in patients with a demonstrated deficiency or for single-factor deficiency when concentrate not available Correct coagulation deficiencies Before an invasive procedure	Standard blood filter May be infused rapidly: 20 mL over 3 minutes or more slowly within 4 hours	Crossmatch not required ABO compatible with recipient red cells Does not provide platelets 1 unit (200 mL) raises the level of clotting factor 2%–3% Requires 20 minutes thawing time by blood bank Must be ABO compatible

Component		Uses	Administration	Notes
Cryoprecipitate	Each unit contains factor VIII, von Willbrand factor (vWF), factor XIII, fibrinogen 15 mL plasma (5–10 mL/unit) Usual order is for 6–10 units	Main use today as a source of fibrinogen in acquired coagulopathies: disseminated intravascular coagulation (DIC), massive hemorrhage Alternative to factor VIII	Standard blood filter or component syringe Administer as fast as patient tolerates 10–15 mL of diluent added to each unit Rate 1–2 mL/min	Crossmatch and ABO compatibility not required Infuse as soon as possible after thawing
Albumin (5% = 12.5 g/250 mL; 25% = 12.5 g/ 50 mL)	5% solution is in concentration of 250 or 500 mL; 25% solution is in concentration of 50–100 mL	Plasma volume expander For hypovolemic shock Supports blood pressure during hypotensive episodes; induces diuresis in fluid overload	May be administered as rapidly as tolerated for reduced blood volume Normal rates: 2–4 mL/min for 5% solution; 1 mL/min for 25% solution Supplied in glass bottles with tubing for administration	25% albumin is hypertonic and is five times more concentrated than 5% solutions. Give with extreme caution; can cause circulatory overload No type and crossmatching necessary Store at room temperature
Plasma Protein Fraction (PPF) (5% solution)	Glass: 250-mL bottle with tubing (83% albumin, 17% globulin)	Same as for albumin Osmotically equal to plasma	Equivalent to 5% albumin	Has fewer purification steps than albumin No type and crossmatching necessary Has high sodium content

- Autoimmune thrombocytopenia (ITP)
- Presumed autoimmune disorders (Kawasaki's disease, Guillain-Barré syndrome, multiple sclerosis, myasthenia gravis, dermatomyositis, systemic vasculitides, factor VIII inhibitors)
- Prevention/treatment of infections
- Other immunological conditions (GVHD, asthma, myocarditis, inflammatory bowel disease, Stevens–Johnson syndrome)
- Other conditions: Alzheimer's disease, atherosclerosis, autism, chronic fatigue syndrome, multifocal motor neuropathy (Nester & AuBuchon, 2011)

ADMINISTRATION

- Intravenous Ig usually is administered via a peripheral I.V. catheter.
- Subcutaneous Ig is administered using 24- to 27-gauge catheter with varying lengths based on amount of subcutaneous tissue.
- Administer at room temperature.
- Do not mix with other medications or piggyback into other infusions.
- Reconstitute medication only after I.V. access is established.
- Use I.V. administration set provided with product if included. Some formulations will also require filtration.
- Premedications are sometimes ordered to minimize infusion-related symptoms.
- Use a large vein because of the relative concentration of the product.
- Most infusions are given over 2 to 4 hours. Follow the manufacturer's recommendations for maximum rates.
- Monitor vital signs throughout the infusion.

NOTE > Not all Ig formulations are the same, and each product must follow the manufacturer's recommendations for administration.

Safety Concern: Infusion-associated allergic reactions (e.g., fever, chills, facial flushing, tachycardia, dyspnea, wheezing) may occur. Other associations are renal dysfunction, venous thromboembolism, and aseptic meningitis.

■ Alternatives to Blood Transfusions

Alternatives to blood transfusion focus on management of anemia and blood loss prevention. Many new strategies are now being used in blood management because of the shortages in the U.S. blood supply, risks associated with blood transfusions, and lack of evidence in efficacy of blood transfusions under certain conditions, along with blood product ordering practice inconsistencies. The following are some of the alternatives to blood transfusions or transfusion augmentations.

1. Augmentation of volume with colloid solutions
2. Autologous cell salvage
3. RBC substitutes
4. Modified Hgb or hemoglobin-based oxygen carriers (HBOCs) made from human, animal, or genetically engineered (recombinant) Hgb
5. Perfluorocarbons (PFCs)
6. Erythropoietic-stimulating agents (ESAs)
7. White cell growth factors
8. Hematinics

Augmentation of Volume with Colloid Solutions

Using allogeneic blood to maintain blood volume is not appropriate; plasma expanders can be used for this purpose. Crystalloid and colloid volume expanders are discussed in Chapter 4.

Intraoperative Autologous Transfusion (Blood Recovery)

As discussed earlier, intraoperative autologous transfusion is the collection of blood that would otherwise be lost during a surgical procedure. Collection systems remove debris and return the blood to the patient.

Red Blood Cell Substitutes

A variety of means have been explored to provide the oxygen-carrying capacity of Hgb without using red cells. The goal of creating an Hgb substitute that is safe as donor cells continues to be "elusive" (Nester & AuBuchon, 2011, p. 579).

Erythropoietic-Stimulating Agents

Erythropoietin is an endogenous hormone secreted by the kidneys that stimulates RBC production in the bone marrow. Recombinant human erythropoietin is successfully used for dialysis patients who experience anemia as a result of kidney disease. It can increase a patient's Hgb level before a surgical procedure where major blood loss is anticipated and is used for patients receiving chemotherapy for malignancy. It should be used with caution because of its thromboembolic risks. Furthermore, the majority of preoperative anemia is related to iron deficiency, and simple iron replacement is indicated (Waters, 2011). It is administered subcutaneously or by I.V. push.

White Cell Growth Factors

Recombinant granulocyte colony-stimulating factor (G-CSF) is used to stimulate the production of granulocytes. Patients receiving chemotherapy have seen the greatest benefit of these medications. A dangerously decreased white cell count that puts the patient at risk for infection is a dose-limiting side effect of many cancer chemotherapy drugs. G-CSF products help maintain levels at near-normal levels, allowing patients to continue to receive scheduled doses of chemotherapy. It is administered subcutaneously or by I.V. push.

Hematinics

Hematinics are medications that are not biological products or substitutes but are able to increase cell efficiency by pharmacological means, such as intravenously administered iron preparations. Some of these medications can raise a patient's Hgb level 2 g/dL over 3 weeks, reducing the need for transfusion in some cases.

 ### Websites

Synthetic Blood International, Inc.: www.sybd.com
Network for Advancement of Transfusion Alternatives: www.nataonline.com

■ Administration of Blood Components

The procedure for obtaining a blood component from a hospital blood bank varies from institution to institution. Regardless of the specific institutional procedure, certain essential guidelines must be followed (Table 11-7).

Step 1: Recipient Consent

Recipient consent for transfusion must be obtained from patients who are competent to make such decisions. Documents of informed consent must contain indications, risks/benefits, possible side effects, and alternatives to transfusion with allogeneic blood components (Sink, 2011).

Step 2: Verifying the Authorized Prescriber's Order

There are two steps in orders. The authorized prescriber's order for the clinical laboratory must specify the type of component to be prepared for the patient (e.g., an order for crossmatching for RBCs). The second order for the nurse should specify:
- The patient's name and other identifiers
- The component to transfuse

> Table 11-7	STEPS IN THE ADMINISTRATION OF A BLOOD COMPONENT

Step 1: Recipient consent
Step 2: Verifying the authorized prescriber's order
Step 3: Pretransfusion
Step 4: Venous access; selecting and preparing the equipment
Step 5: Preparing the patient
Step 6: Dispensing and transportation of the component
Step 7: Initiating the transfusion
Step 8: Monitoring the transfusion
Step 9: Completing the transfusion

- Any special processing required for the component (e.g., washing, irradiation, or filtration)
- The number of units or volume to be administered
- Date and time of infusion
- Flow rate or duration of the transfusion (up to 4 hours) (Sink, 2011)

NOTE > When multiple types of components are transfused, the order should specify the sequence in which they are to be transfused. Orders must specify any premedications that are to be given before transfusion.

INS Standard The administration of transfusion therapy shall be initiated on the order of a licensed independent practitioner (LIP) in accordance with the rules and regulations promulgated by the state Board of Nursing, state regulations, AABB standards, and organizational policies, procedures, and/or practice guidelines (INS, 2011, p. S93).

Step 3: Pretransfusion

Laboratory Testing

Once the order has been obtained, the transfusion service initiates a series of steps to ensure the provision of compatible components. The laboratory must have a sample of the patient's blood, which generally must be drawn within 3 days of the individual being transfused; the draw date is considered day 0 (Sink, 2011).

Identification Wristband

Most transfusion agencies require patients to be identified with an armband that matches the recipient to the intended product. Barcode-based ID systems are available for safety in transfusion.

Testing of Transfusion Recipient's Blood Specimen

ABO group and Rh type must be determined in order to transfuse ABO- and Rh-compatible components. The serum or plasma of the recipient must be tested for expected and unexpected antibodies before components containing red cells are issued for transfusion (AABB, 2009). ABO "forward typing" is the process in which the recipient's RBCs are mixed with anti-A or anti-B. This process identifies the antigens present in the RBCs by visually apparent agglutination of the cells when the antibody combines with its corresponding antigen. ABO "reverse typing" is the testing of the recipient's serum for the presence of predicted ABO antibodies by adding RBCs of a known ABO type to it.

Rh typing of both recipient and donor blood is accomplished by testing the RBCs against anti-D serum. If agglutination occurs, the RBCs possess the D antigen and the blood is Rh-positive. If no agglutination is apparent, the RBCs must be tested further to rule out the presence of the weakly expressed D antigen, called weak D (formerly referred to as D). This antigen can be identified most reliably by indirect antiglobulin testing (IAT) after incubating the RBCs with anti-D sera. RBCs that possess the weak D are given to Rh-positive recipients (Downes & Shulman, 2011).

Compatibility testing is performed between the recipient's plasma and the donor's RBCs to ensure that the specific unit intended for transfusion to the recipient is not incompatible. Blood samples from the donor and recipient are mixed and incubated under a variety of conditions and suspending medium. If the recipient's blood does not agglutinate the donor cells, compatibility is indicated. Blood bank personnel are responsible for providing serologically compatible blood for transfusion.

When testing is complete, transfusion therapy can begin. The blood bank has two objectives: (1) to prevent antigen–antibody reactions in the body and (2) to identify an antibody that the recipient may have and supply blood from a donor who lacks the corresponding antigen. The testing of donor blood and recipient blood is intended to prevent adverse effects of transfusion therapy.

Labeling of Blood and Blood Components with the Recipient's Information

At the time of issue, the following must be in place:
- A tag or label indicating the recipient's two independent identifiers, the donor unit number, and the compatibility test interpretation, if performed, must be attached securely to the blood container.
- A final check of records maintained in the blood bank for each unit of blood or component must be made:
  - Two independent identifiers, one of which is usually the patient's name

- The recipient's ABO group and Rh type
- The donor unit or pool identification number
- Donor's ABO group and, if required, Rh type
- Interpretation of the crossmatch tests (if performed)
- Date and time of issue
- Special transfusion requirements (e.g., CMV reduced risk, irradiated, antigen-negative)
- A process must exist to confirm that the identifying information, the request, the records, and the blood or component are all in agreement, and that any and all discrepancies have been resolved before issue (Downes & Shulman, 2011).

Step 4: Vascular Access; Selecting and Preparing the Equipment

It is important for the transfusionist to determine whether a central or peripheral intravenous line is in place and if it is acceptable for infusion of blood components. Selecting the proper equipment includes catheter and solution selection, and obtaining administration sets, special filters, blood warmers, and electronic monitoring devices.

Vascular Access

The recommendation for catheter size is dependent on how quickly the blood needs to be administered. A 20- to 18-gauge catheter is the catheter of choice for peripheral infusions in most situations. A 22- to 24-gauge catheter can be considered for pediatric patients or those patients with small veins. The use of a central vascular access device for administration of blood is dependent on the catheter gauge and the manufacturer's recommendations for use of infusion device. When smaller catheters are used, blood dilution and use of an infusion pump are helpful. Of note, units that have the preservative solution **ADSOL** do not require additional dilution (Sink, 2011).

NOTE > It is important that vascular access be obtained before the component is received at the patient's bedside.

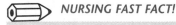 *NURSING FAST FACT!*

Forcing blood through a tiny or damaged catheter may cause lysis of the cells. If the patient requires medication or solution administration while the blood component is being administered, a second I.V. site should be initiated.

Equipment

SOLUTION

No medication or solution other than 0.9% sodium chloride should be administered simultaneously with blood components through the same tubing (AABB, 2009). The use of dextrose in water or hypotonic solutions can cause RBC hemolysis as a result of cell swelling. Lactated Ringer's solution is not recommended because it contains enough ionized calcium to overcome the anticoagulant effect of CPDA-1 and allows small clots to develop.

> **INS Standard** Blood or blood components should be administered only with 0.9% sodium chloride. No other solutions or medications should be added to blood and blood products (INS, 2011, p. S93).

NOTE > The AABB (2009) allows exceptions to the restrictions mentioned earlier when:
1. The drug or solution has been approved by the FDA for use with blood administration
2. There is documentation in the literature showing that the addition is safe and does not adversely affect the blood components

---

ADMINISTRATION SETS

Blood administration sets are available as a Y-type tubing or as single-lead tubing. Y-type administration sets allow for infusion of 0.9% sodium chloride before and after each blood component. A Y-type set also allows for dilution of RBCs that are too viscous to be transfused at an appropriate rate by allowing for sterile transfer of saline into the unit. Platelets and cryoprecipitate should be infused through a filter similar to the standard blood filter but with a smaller drip chamber and shorter tubing so that less priming volume is needed. A syringe device designed specifically for platelets and cryoprecipitate may also be used to administer these products.

Blood administration sets come with an inline filter. Most routine blood filters have a pore size of 170 to 260 microns designed to remove the debris that accumulates in stored blood. It is necessary to fill the filter chamber completely to use all the surface area. Red cell filters are designed to filter 1 unit of whole blood or PRBCs. Filters used for platelets and cryoprecipitate may be used to administer multiple units. Filters are changed for two reasons: debris in the blood clogs the filter pores, slowing the rate; and the risk of bacterial contamination increases when filter-trapped blood particles are maintained at room temperature.

> **INS Standard** The transfusion administration set and filter should be changed after the completion of each unit or every 4 hours. If

more than 1 unit can be infused in 4 hours, the transfusion set can be used for a 4-hour period (INS, 2011, p. S93).

SPECIAL FILTERS

Microaggregate filters are not used routinely. These second-generation filters were developed to remove leukocytes and to complement or replace the standard clot screen. They have been replaced by third-generation leukocyte-reduction filters. Today, microaggregate filters are used for reinfusion of shed autologous blood collected during or after surgery (Sink, 2011).

Leukocyte-reduction filters are third-generation filters used for the delivery of RBCs and platelets. Filtration may occur immediately after blood collection in the blood bank or at the time of administration.

These filters are capable of removing more than 99.9% of the leukocytes present in the unit, which decreases the risk of febrile transfusion reactions, the risk HLA alloimmunization, and the risk for transmission of CMV (Sink, 2011). There are different leukocyte reduction filters for red cells and platelets, and it is important to use the correct filter based on the blood component. It is preferred that leukocyte reduction occur prestorage shortly after unit collection as compared to bedside filtration. This is because bedside filtration is associated with dramatic hypotension in some patients (Sink, 2011). These filters are more expensive than standard blood filters and require a LIP order before use.

BLOOD WARMERS

Blood warmers are rarely needed but may be indicated when rapid transfusion is required. The transfusion of cold components may cause **hypothermia** and cardiac complications (Sink, 2011). The risk of clinically significant hypothermia is heightened when transfusing via a central vascular access device. They are also useful for transfusions to neonates or patients with cold agglutinin syndrome.

NOTE > The AABB Standards (Carson, 2011, p.6) state that "warming devices shall be equipped with a temperature sensing device and a warning system to detect malfunctions and prevent hemolysis or other damage to blood and blood components."

Blood is warmed only by using a specifically designed blood/fluid warmer (Richardson, 2014). Adhere to the manufacturer's guidelines when using any of the many types of blood and fluid warmers. The temperature control should not warm the blood or fluid above 42°C because this will cause hemolysis (AABB, 2008).

INS Standard Blood and fluid warmers should be used when warranted by patient history, clinical condition, and prescribed therapy, including, but not limited to, avoiding or treating hypothermia, during cardiopulmonary bypass, when the patient is known to have cold agglutins, or during replacement of large blood volumes (INS, 2011, p. S35).

 NURSING FAST FACT!

> Blood components should NEVER be placed in microwave ovens or hot water baths because of damage to RBCs and the lack of temperature control, which may cause fatal complications for the patient.

Electronic Infusion Device

Some transfusions may require an electronic infusion device (EID) to control the blood flow. Only pumps designed for the infusion of whole blood and RBCs may be used because other types of infusion pumps may cause hemolysis. Pumps require the use of pump-compatible tubing. Little if any increased hemolysis occurs secondary to the use of most infusion pumps. A pump's manufacturer should be consulted for detailed information on the pump's suitability for transfusing blood components.

INS Standard EIDs can be used to deliver blood or blood components without significant risk of hemolysis of RBCs. However, the EID should be analyzed to evaluate the safety and rate of hemolysis. The nurse should follow the manufacturer's directions for use of EIDs for blood and blood component administration (INS, 2011, p. S93).

Pressure Devices

The use of an externally applied pneumatic pressure device may achieve flow rates of 70 to 300 mL/min depending on the pressure applied. The use of pressure devices has been reported to provide only a small increment in component flow rates. This is considered a safe practice in the majority of red cell transfusions. Before use, verify that the I.V. access device is functioning appropriately. Forcing cells through a damaged catheter may increase the risk of cell hemolysis.

INS Standard External compression devices, if used, should be equipped with a pressure gauge and should exert uniform pressure against all parts of the blood container. A blood pressure cuff should not be used because it is unable to apply uniform pressure (INS, 2011, p. S93).

NOTE > When rapid infusion is desired, an increase in cannula size typically provides better results.

Step 5: Preparing the Patient

Patient preparation begins when the transfusion of a blood component is anticipated. Urgency factors related to the transfusion may affect the amount of time available to prepare the patient for the transfusion. The steps of the nursing process are activated, including assessment and the establishment of new goals and interventions related to the transfusion.

Patient/Family Education

The patient's and the patient's family's understanding of the need for blood, the procedure, and related concerns need to be assessed. Concerns are typically expressed regarding the risks of disease transmission and need to be addressed.

The patient should be instructed regarding the length of time for the procedure and the need for monitoring his or her vital signs and physical condition. Signs and symptoms that may be associated with a complication of the component to be given should be explained to the patient and family members. It is not necessary to offer graphic explanations regarding symptoms; rather, a brief description of possible symptoms should be provided and the patient should be asked to report any different sensations after the transfusion has been started. Because transfusions typically take several hours, preparation includes making the patient physically comfortable.

Assessment

A baseline assessment of the patient should include the following:
- Vital signs
- Presence of any signs or symptoms that might be confused with a transfusion reaction, such as dyspnea, rashes, pruritus, chills, wheezing
- Presence of diseases that increase risk for fluid volume overload (e.g., heart failure) and may require a slower infusion rate (Sink, 2011)

If the vital signs are abnormal, consult with the LIP before initiating the transfusion. An elevated temperature may destroy cellular components at an increased rate and mask symptoms of a transfusion reaction (Sink, 2011). Premedication with diuretics, antihistamines, or antipyretics may be necessary to help keep the vital signs at acceptable levels.

Assessment of the lungs and renal function should be documented before transfusion. The nurse should review the laboratory data (Hgb, Hct, platelets, clotting times) and anticipate how the component to be administered will affect these values over the next 24 hours. The patient should also be questioned regarding any symptoms he or she may be experiencing that could be confused with a transfusion reaction.

NURSING FAST FACT!

Patient education, assessment including vital signs, and current symptoms are documented in the medical record.

Step 6: Dispensing and Transportation of the Component

As a rule, except in emergency situations, if blood is obtained from an on-site blood bank, only one product will be issued at a time and must be initiated within 30 minutes (usually) or returned to the blood bank for proper storage (Sink, 2011). The blood component should not be obtained until the patient is ready to receive the component. If blood is obtained from an offsite blood bank, multiple units may be issued at one time. These units will be packaged to provide optimum storage conditions, and time limits for safe initiation will be detailed by the blood bank.

Placing a unit of blood in the nursing unit refrigerator is not acceptable practice. Most refrigerators cannot ensure the rigid temperature controls required. Accidental freezing can destroy the unit. If the transfusion will be initiated within 30 minutes, the blood should be left at room temperature. If a longer period of time will pass (for alternate sites), the blood should be stored in the container in which it was sent.

 NURSING FAST FACT!

Refrigerators on the nursing units are never used to store blood products.

Proper identification is essential to ensure that the blood component is going to the intended recipient. Several items must always be verified and recorded before the transfusion is initiated.

- The order should always be verified before the component is picked up.
- When the blood is issued, the intended recipient's two independent identifiers should be verified (name, date of birth, or patient identification number and/or unique identifier given at the time the crossmatch sample is drawn).
- The donor unit or pool identification number, donor ABO group, and, if required, the Rh type should be verified.
- The notation of ABO group and Rh type must be the same on the primary blood bag label as on the transfusion form. This information is to be recorded on the attached compatibility tag or label.
- The donor number must be identically recorded on the label of the blood bag, the transfusion form, and the attached compatibility tag.
- The color, appearance, and expiration date of the component must be checked.

■ The name of the person issuing the blood, the name of the person to whom the blood is issued, and the date and time of issue must be recorded. Often this is in a book in the laboratory.

Step 7: Initiating the Transfusion

The identification of the unit and the recipient must be verified by the nurse and another health-care provider qualified in performing identification verification (often a second nurse).

> **INS Standard** Validation of correct patient and blood product shall be simultaneously performed at the bedside by two qualified clinicians prior to administration (INS, 2011, p. S93).

The transfusion check includes:
■ *Prescriber's order*: Check the blood or component against the prescriber's written order to verify that the correct component and amount are being given. If leukocyte reduction or irradiation was ordered, check that this was performed.
■ *Transfusion consent form*: Check that the form is completed per organizational policy.
■ *Recipient identification*: The name and identification number on the patient's identification band must be identical with the name and number attached to the unit.
■ *Unit identification*: The unit identification number on the blood container, the transfusion form, and the tag attached to the unit must agree.
■ *Blood type*: The patient's blood type should be compatible with the unit.
■ *Expiration*: The expiration date and time of the donor unit should be verified as acceptable.
■ *Compatibility*: The interpretation of compatibility testing must be recorded on the transfusion form and on the tag attached to the unit.
■ *Appearance*: The unit should be returned if there is any discoloration, foaming, presence of bubbles, cloudiness, presence of clots or clumps, or loss of integrity of the container (Sink, 2011).

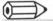 *NURSING FAST FACT!*

■ *It is helpful if one nurse reads the information for verification to the other nurse; errors can be made if both nurses look at the tags together.*
■ *Unless the exact time is given, the component expires at midnight on the expiration date.*
■ *Watch for any discrepancies during any part of the identification process. The transfusion should not be initiated until the blood bank is notified and any discrepancies are resolved.*

Use proper hand hygiene and follow standard precautions when administering blood components. Wear gloves! When using a Y-type blood set, spike one port with 0.9% sodium chloride and prime the tubing, being sure to saturate the filter. To administer whole blood or RBCs, spike the blood container on the second port and hang it up. Turn off the 0.9% sodium chloride and turn on the blood component. It is recommended that transfusions of RBCs be started at 1 to 2 mL/min for the first 15 minutes of the transfusion (Sink, 2011).

This small amount is large enough to alert the nurse to a possible severe reaction but small enough that the reaction probably can be successfully treated. If the patient shows signs or symptoms of an adverse reaction, the transfusion must be stopped immediately; only a small amount of blood product will have been infused. After the first 15 minutes has safely passed, the rate of flow can be increased to complete the transfusion within the amount of time indicated by the LIP or by policy. The rate of infusion should be based on the patient's blood volume, hemodynamic condition, and cardiac status.

Red cell products should be infused within a 4-hour period. When a longer transfusion time is clinically indicated, the unit may be divided by the blood bank, and the portion not being transfused can be properly refrigerated.

Step 8: Monitoring the Transfusion

The patient's vital signs should be taken within 5 to 15 minutes of initiating the transfusion and then according to organizational policy. There is little evidence requiring routine assessment of vital signs other than before initiation, shortly after starting the transfusion, and after the transfusion (Sink, 2011).

Step 9: Completing the Transfusion

At the completion of the transfusion, the patient's vital signs should be obtained. The bag and tubing are discarded in a biohazard container. At this point, another unit may be infused, the unit and line may be discontinued, the vascular access device may be locked, or a new administration set and solution container may be added.

▷ *NURSING FAST FACT!*

Do not save previous solutions and tubing that were interrupted to give the blood component; they are considered contaminated. Restart with a fresh set and solution.

Documentation is an important part of the nursing intervention. The documentation should be made in the patient's medical record. At a minimum, the AABB Standards (Carson, 2011) require the following:

1. Medical order for transfusion
2. Documentation of recipient consent
3. Name or type of component
4. Donor unit or pool identification number
5. Date and time of transfusion
6. Pre- and post-transfusion vital signs
7. Volume transfused
8. Identification of the transfusionist
9. Any adverse events possibly related to the transfusion

Some transfusion service departments require that a copy of the completed transfusion form be returned to them. Returning the blood component after an uncomplicated transfusion is not required in all facilities. If disposal is allowed on the unit, use hospital standards in disposing the blood bag in contaminated trash.

NOTE > If an additional unit needs to be transfused, the institution's guidelines should be followed. A new blood administration set is to be used with each component. Blood unit administration must be completed within 4 hours.

NURSING POINTS OF CARE
DELIVERY OF BLOOD COMPONENT THERAPY

Nursing Assessments
- Interview the patient regarding his or her understanding of the need for the blood component.
- Determine the patient's understanding of options as appropriate: autologous, allogeneic, and directed donations.
- Assess vital signs.
- Assess renal and cardiovascular function.
- Assess and evaluate the I.V. site before requesting blood component from the blood bank.
- Assess the patient's level of consciousness.
- Review laboratory test results.
- Assess current intake and output ratios.

Key Nursing Interventions

1. Verify that the patient's written informed consent has been obtained.
2. Verify with another health-care provider that the blood product matches the patient's blood type.
3. Validate patient identification with two identifiers.
4. Administer blood products properly and according to organizational procedure.
5. Prime the administration system with 0.9% sodium chloride.
6. Use an EID, if indicated.
7. Do not administer I.V. medications into blood or blood product lines.
8. Monitor:
   a. The I.V. site for signs and symptoms of complications
   b. Vital signs: Baseline (prior to transfusion), within 5 to 15 minutes of initiating transfusion, on completion of transfusion
   c. Fluid status
   d. Flow rate of the transfusion
9. Change the blood administration set after every unit of red cells transfused or every 4 hours, whichever comes first.
10. Document the time frame of the transfusion and volume infused.
11. Document patient tolerance to first 15 minutes of transfusion.
12. Document nursing interventions and response to interventions.
13. Document all patient teaching.
14. Stop the transfusion immediately if a reaction is suspected and follow policy and procedure for interventions related to the reaction.
15. Notify the laboratory and the LIP in the event of a blood reaction.
16. Maintain aseptic technique and standard precautions with all transfusion/infusion procedures.
17. Evaluate the effect of transfusion on laboratory test results at 24 hours.

■ Complications Associated With Blood Component Therapy

Significant, and sometimes life-threatening, complications are associated with transfusion therapy (Table 11-8). Adverse reactions are often classified into immunological and nonimmunological categories. Table 11-9 lists the complications in a quick-guide format.

INS Standard In the event of an adverse reaction, the transfusion should be stopped, the LIP and the blood bank notified, and interventions implemented (INS, 2011, p. S94).

> Table 11-8 **RISKS OF TRANSFUSION THERAPY**

Viral Infection	Estimated Risks per Unit
Human immunodeficiency virus (HIV)-1 and HIV-2	1:1,467,000
Hepatitis B virus (HBV)	1:280,000
Hepatitis C virus (HCV)	1:1,149,000
Acute Transfusion Reactions <24 hours	
Hemolytic transfusion reactions	ABO/Rh mismatch: 1:40,000
	Acute hemolytic transfusion reaction (AHTR): 1:76,000
	Fatal HTRs 1:1.8 million
Febrile nonhemolytic transfusion reaction	0.1%–1% with universal leukocyte reduction
Minor allergic reaction	1%–3%
Anaphylaxis	1:20,000 to 1:50,000
Transfusion-related acute lung injury (TRALI)	1:1200 to 1:190,000
Circulatory overload	<1%
Delayed Reactions	
Alloimmunization, human leukocyte antigen (HLA) antigens	1:100 (1%)
Delayed hemolytic	1:2500 to 11,000

Sources: Galel (2011); Mazzei et al. (2011).

Summary: Patient-Focused Interventions

1. Stop the transfusion immediately but keep the line open with saline. Because the blood setup contains a significant amount of blood, in some cases it is necessary to replace the saline primed administration set (e.g., acute hemolytic transfusion reaction).
2. Reconfirm that the unit of blood is being administered to the intended recipient; document this recheck of identification. The labels on the component, patient records, and patient identification should be examined to detect any identification errors. Transfusion facilities may require repeat ABO and Rh typing of the patient on a new sample.
3. Contact the treating LIP immediately for instructions for patient care.

Summary: Component-Focused Interventions

1. Contact the transfusion service for directions for investigation.
2. Follow organizational policy for return of the remaining component and complete I.V. setup (fluid and tubing) (Sink, 2011).

Text continued on page 741

> Table 11-9 　SUMMARY OF TRANSFUSION REACTIONS

Transfusion Reaction	Etiology	Signs and Symptoms	Key Interventions	Prevention
Acute Immediate (<24 hours)				
Acute hemolytic transfusion reaction (AHTR)	Hemolysis occurs when antibodies in plasma attach to antigens on the donor's red blood cells (RBCs). Caused by infusion of ABO-incompatible RBCs.	Fever with/without chills Tachycardia Abdominal, chest, flank, back pain Hypotension Shortness of breath Red/dark urine Shock	*STOP TRANSFUSION!* Get help immediately. Change administration set and infuse 0.9% sodium chloride Treat shock. Maintain blood pressure (BP)/renal perfusion. Administer diuretics to maintain blood flow.	Exercise extreme care during the entire identification process. Start transfusion slowly and monitor for first 15 minutes.
Febrile nonhemolytic reaction	Occurs as a result of antibodies directed against leukocytes or platelets. Febrile reactions occur immediately or 1–2 hours after transfusion is completed.	Fever rise of 1° C (2°F) in association with transfusion Chills Headache Vomiting	Stop the transfusion. Change administration set and infuse 0.9% sodium chloride. Notify the LIP. Monitor vital signs. Anticipate order for antipyretic agents. If ordered, restart transfusion slowly.	Use leukocyte-reduced blood component.
Allergic reactions (mild)	Caused by recipient sensitivity to allergens in the blood component.	Itching Hives (local) Urticaria Facial flushing Runny eyes Anxiety Angioedema	Stop the transfusion. Keep vein open with normal saline. Notify the LIP. Monitor vital signs. Anticipate antihistamine order. If ordered, restart transfusion slowly. Mild reactions can precede severe allergic reactions.	If known mild allergic reaction occurs with blood transfusion, may premedicate with diphenhydramine 30 minutes before the transfusion.

Reaction	Cause	Signs and Symptoms	Nursing Interventions	Prevention
Severe allergic reactions: Anaphylaxis	Antibodies to donor blood plasma (e.g., immunoglobulin A [IgA] proteins are transfused into an IgA-deficient recipient who has developed IgA antibody)	Hypotension Urticaria Bronchospasm Anxiety Shock	Stop the transfusion. Keep the vein open with normal saline. Administer cardiopulmonary resuscitation (CPR) if necessary. Anticipate order for steroids. Maintain BP.	Use autologous blood. Use blood from donors who are IgA deficient or administer only well-washed RBCs in which all plasma has been extracted.
Transfusion-related acute lung injury (TRALI)	Infrequent Related to antibodies to leukocyte antigens and the infusion sequence of events damage basement membrane **Leading cause of transfusion-related deaths**	Fever Chills Dyspnea Cyanosis Hypoxemia Hypotension Bilateral pulmonary edema	Stop transfusion. Provide respiratory support. Administer oxygen. May require mechanical ventilation. Administer vasopressor agents.	Monitor patient frequently. Reduce flow rate in high-risk patients. Monitor intake and output.
Transfusion-related circulatory overload (TACO)	Administration of blood faster than the recipient's cardiac output	Dyspnea Orthopnea Cyanosis Tachycardia Jugular venous distention Increased BP Cough	Stop the transfusion. Place patient in sitting position. Notify the LIP. Administer diuretics. Administer oxygen.	Monitor patient frequently. Reduce flow rate in high-risk patients. Monitor intake and output.

Continued

> Table 11-9   SUMMARY OF TRANSFUSION REACTIONS—cont'd

Transfusion Reaction	Etiology	Signs and Symptoms	Key Interventions	Prevention
Complications of Massive Transfusions				
Citrate toxicity	Infrequent High-rate infusions, liver unable to keep up with the rapid administration and cannot metabolize the citrate (which chelates calcium), reducing the ionized calcium concentration in the recipient's blood.	Hypocalcemia-induced cardiac dysrhythmias Tingling of fingers Muscular cramps Confusions Hypotension Cardiac arrest	Slow rate of infusion. Administer calcium chloride or calcium gluconate. Do not add calcium to infusing blood!	Administer fresh blood. Monitor calcium levels. Monitor patients with hepatic impairment more closely for hypocalcemia.
Hyperkalemia/ hypokalemia	Rare Administration of blood that has been stored. Related to release of potassium from the RBCs as they go through lysis. Occurs most frequently in multiple transfusions.	Elevated/low potassium levels Slow, irregular heart rate Nausea Muscle weakness Electrocardiographic (ECG) changes Diarrhea Renal failure	Stop or slow the transfusion. Monitor the ECG. Notify the LIP. Remove excess potassium: Concurrently administer hypertonic dextrose and insulin or administer polystyrene sulfonate orally or by enema.	In patients receiving multiple transfusions, use only the freshest blood.
Hemostatic abnormalities in massive transfusions	Coagulopathy related to massive transfusions. Caused by dilution of platelets and clotting factors.	Occurs after replacement of 2–3 blood volumes Clinical evidence of bleeding Platelet count <50,000 Shock and disseminated intravascular coagulation (DIC)	Intraoperative laboratory testing	No specific guidelines

Delayed Transfusion Reactions

Delayed Transfusion Reactions	Result of RBC antigen incompatibility other than the ABO group. Occur due to destruction of transfused RBCs by alloantibodies not discovered during the crossmatch procedures	Fever (continual, low grade) Malaise Jaundice (mild) Malaise Decreased hematocrit and hemoglobin Increased bilirubin levels	No acute treatment required Monitor hematocrit level Renal function Coagulation profile Notify LIP and transfusion services	Exercise extreme care during identification processes.
Transfusion-associated graft-versus-host disease (TA-GVHD)	Rare and fatal Viable t-lymphocytes in transfusion component engraft in recipient and react against recipient tissue antigens Highest risk in the immunocompromised patient	Fever Maculopapular rash Increase levels on hepatic function tests Watery diarrhea Pancytopenia	No effective therapy Treatment of symptoms	Administer irradiated blood products in immunocompromised patients.
Iron overload	Multiple units of RBC chronically transfused. Excretion of iron from 1 unit slow.	Development of organ failure Signs and symptoms associated with heart failure, cirrhosis, diabetes	Iron chelation	Iron chelation

Continued

> Table 11-9   SUMMARY OF TRANSFUSION REACTIONS—cont'd

Transfusion Reaction	Etiology	Signs and Symptoms	Key Interventions	Prevention
Infection-Related Complications				
Bacterial contamination	Occurs at the time of donation or in preparing the component for infusion. Highest risk in platelets	High fever Flushing of skin Shock Hemoglobinuria Renal failure DIC	Stop transfusion. Aggressively treat shock and anticipate order of steroids and antibiotics. Culture patient's blood, component, and all I.V. solutions.	Preventable Exercise proper care of blood product from procurement through administration. Pay attention to skin antisepsis prior to venipuncture during blood donation process. Inspect unit before administration and do not administer if clots, bubbles, leaks in bag, or discoloration of the blood or plasma is present. Complete transfusion within 4 hours.

Acute or Immediate Transfusion Reactions

Acute or immediate adverse reactions to blood or blood products are those that occur within 24 hours of transfusion and may occur during the transfusion. The clinical significance of an acute reaction often cannot be determined by clinical history or signs and symptoms alone but requires laboratory evaluation.

Acute Hemolytic Transfusion Reactions

The most serious and potentially life-threatening reaction is acute **hemolytic transfusion reaction** (AHTR), which occurs when the donor's red cells are incompatible with the patient's plasma as a result of identification errors during the transfusion process. As few as 10 mL of the wrong blood can produce AHTR symptoms. Death from AHTR is estimated to occur in 1:1.8 million transfusions (Mazzei, Popovsky, & Kopko, 2011).

Signs and Symptoms

- Typically begin with fever and tachycardia
- Mild: Abdominal, chest, flank/back pain
- Severe: Fever, chills, hypotension, dyspnea, flank pain, shock, oliguria or anuria, abnormal bleeding
- Red/dark urine may be first sign in an anesthetized patient
- If infusion is allowed to continue, symptoms progress to shock and DIC.

Interventions

Prompt recognition of AHTR is critical to successful outcome.
- Stop the transfusion immediately.
- Disconnect the tubing from the I.V. catheter and prepare/infuse fresh administration set primed with fresh 0.9% sodium chloride.

 NURSING FAST FACT!

   If AHTR is suspected, you must not give the recipient another drop of donor blood.

- Notify the LIP and blood bank or transfusion service *immediately.*
- Monitor vital signs.
- Anticipate the following interventions:
   - Intravascular volume may be maintained with fluids to improve hypotension and promote renal circulation.
   - The patient's respiratory status may have to be supported.
   - Low-dose dopamine may be administered to increase renal function (controversial).

- Furosemide may be ordered to maintain urine output greater than 100 mL/hr to decrease the risk of renal damage.
- Therapies, such as heparin to prevent DIC or mannitol to produce an osmotic diuresis, are controversial but are sometimes used cautiously (Mazzei et al., 2011).

Extreme care during the entire identification process is the first step in prevention. Clerical and human errors involving proper patient, sample, and blood unit identification are the most common causes of AHTR. The transfusion must be started slowly, and evaluation of the patient for reactions during the first 15 minutes is needed to monitor for initial AHTR.

Febrile Nonhemolytic Febrile Reactions

The nonhemolytic febrile reaction is manifested by a rise in temperature of 1°C (2 F°) or more occurring in association with transfusion and not having any other explanation (AABB, 2009). It usually occurs as a result of reactions to antibodies directed against leukocytes or platelets. Febrile reactions occur in only 1% of transfusions; repeat reactions are uncommon. Such reactions can occur immediately or within 1 to 2 hours after transfusion is completed.

SIGNS AND SYMPTOMS

- Fever, increase greater than 1°C (2 F°)
- Chills
- Headache
- Vomiting

INTERVENTIONS

- Stop transfusion and initiate transfusion reaction workup.
- Change administration set and administer 0.9% sodium chloride to keep the vein open.
- Notify LIP and blood bank, and institute transfusion reaction protocol.
- Monitor vital signs.
- Administer antipyretic agents as ordered.
- Another transfusion unit may be safely infused once symptoms subside.

NOTE > The remainder of the implicated component should not be transfused.

PREVENTION

Patients who experience repeated, severe febrile reactions may benefit from leukocyte-reduced components.

Allergic Reactions

In its mild form, **allergic reactions** are a common type of reaction. They are probably caused by allergens in the component or less often by antibodies from an allergic donor (Mazzei et al., 2011). The patient may experience mild localized urticaria, pruritus, and flushing. Allergic reactions usually occur within seconds to minutes of starting the transfusion. Most reactions respond to antihistamines. Severe anaphylactic reactions include symptoms of urticaria and angioedema but progress to severe hypotension, shock, and loss of consciousness.

SIGNS AND SYMPTOMS

- Mild: Itching, hives, urticaria, angioedema (deep swelling around eyes/lips)
- Severe: Anxiety, bronchospasm, wheezing, hypotension, shock, loss of consciousness

INTERVENTIONS

- Stop the transfusion.
- Keep the vein open with normal saline.
- Notify the LIP.
- Monitor vital signs.
- For a mild reaction, administer antihistamines per LIP order and resume transfusion after symptoms have resolved.
- Anaphylactic reaction: Give fluids, place patient in Trendelenberg position, administer epinephrine, antihistamines, steroids

 NURSING FAST FACT!

> *Mild allergic reactions characterized by urticaria is the only transfusion reaction in which administration of the component may be resumed after treatment (Mazzei et al., 2011).*

PREVENTION

For mild reactions, premedicate with diphenhydramine 30 minutes before the transfusion. For patients whose reactions are severe, washing red cells or platelets may be considered. Administration of deglycerolized rejuvenated RBCs has met with some success (Mazzei et al., 2011). For patients with anaphylactic reactions, IgA-deficient components are required.

Transfusion-Related Acute Lung Injury

TRALI is a severe and life-threatening reaction characterized by symptoms associated with acute respiratory distress syndrome, such as fever, chills, dyspnea, cyanosis, and hypotension. Pulmonary edema occurs secondary to leakage of protein-rich fluid into the alveolar space (Mazzei et al., 2011).

TRALI is the leading cause of transfusion-associated mortality (5%–15%) (Richardson, 2014). It most often begins within 1 to 2 hours after transfusion but can occur up to 6 hours after transfusion. TRALI is a clinical diagnosis without specific diagnostic tests; rather, it is a diagnosis of exclusion (Kopko, 2010). Three main conditions need to be differentiated from TRALI:

1. *Anaphylactic transfusion reactions*: They usually do not include symptoms of fever and pulmonary edema.
2. *Transfusion-associated circulatory overload (TACO)*: This is a cardiac syndrome whereas TRALI is not.
3. *Transfusion-related sepsis*: Does not usually include symptoms of respiratory distress (Mazzei et al., 2011).

Although the exact mechanism for TRALI is not known, it is associated with antibodies to leukocyte antigens and the infusion of biological response modifiers (Mazzei et al., 2011). Infusion of either is thought to initiate a sequence of events that results in cellular activation and damage of the basement membrane. TRALI has been associated with transfusion of blood components from female donors with HLA and human neutrophil antigen (HNA) antibodies (Mazzei et al., 2011; Richardson, 2014). Studies have found an increased prevalence of HLA antibodies in female blood donors (with history of pregnancy) with each additional pregnancy, up to four (Mazzei et al., 2011).

Signs and Symptoms

- Acute respiratory distress
- Hypoxemia
- Hypotension
- Fever/chills
- Cough
- Bilateral pulmonary edema

NOTE > TRALI is a life-threatening complication.

Interventions

Respiratory and Volume Support
- Oxygen therapy with or without mechanical ventilation
- Pressor agents to support blood pressure
- Notify LIP and blood bank

Prevention

Strategies to reduce the risk of TRALI are complicated. Because it is the main cause of transfusion-related deaths, great attention is being paid to reducing the risk. A number of measures have been put in place by blood centers, including deferring a donor if a blood component from that donor resulted in TRALI and reducing the amount of plasma from female donors (Kopko, 2010).

Transfusion-Associated Circulatory Overload

The rapid administration of any blood product can lead to TACO. RBC products, plasma products, and 25% albumin are the blood components most commonly associated with circulatory overload. Patients at greatest risk are infants and adults older than 70 years (Mazzei et al., 2011). Individuals with compromised cardiac or pulmonary function are also at risk. Signs and symptoms generally occur within 1 to 2 hours of transfusion.

SIGNS AND SYMPTOMS

- Dyspnea
- Orthopnea
- Cyanosis
- Tachycardia
- Jugular venous distention
- Increased blood pressure
- Severe headache
- Cough

INTERVENTIONS

- Stop transfusion if symptoms are suggestive of TACO.
- Maintain patent vascular access device.
- Place the patient in a sitting position.
- Administer oxygen therapy.
- Administer diuretics.

PREVENTION

Patients identified as being at risk for TACO should have blood infused at a reduced rate. Recommendations are to administer blood at a rate of 1 mL/kg body weight/hr, which is about 4 hours per unit to prevent overload (Richardson, 2014). Consider administration of a diuretic when beginning the transfusion in at-risk recipients. Monitor vital signs and intake and output throughout the transfusion (Mazzei et al., 2011).

Less Common Complications

Complications of Massive Transfusions

Citrate Toxicity

A reaction to toxic proportions of citrate, which is used as a preservative in blood, can cause hypocalcemia. The citrate ion can combine with the recipient's serum calcium, causing a calcium deficiency; normal citrate metabolism is hindered by the presence of hepatic disease. Patients at risk for development of citrate toxicity or a calcium deficit are those who receive large volume transfusions or in patients who have hepatic disease. The liver, unable to keep up with the rapid administration, cannot metabolize the citrate, which chelates calcium, reducing the ionized calcium concentration. Hypocalcemia may induce cardiac dysrhythmias. Slow the infusion rate and, based on symptoms and blood values of calcium, administer calcium chloride or calcium gluconate solution. Do not administer calcium via the administration set infusing the blood.

SIGNS AND SYMPTOMS

- Paresthesias
- Tetany
- Dysrhythmias
- Hypotension
- Nausea and vomiting

INTERVENTIONS

- Slow the transfusion.
- Monitor serum calcium and potassium levels.
- Replace calcium.

PREVENTION

Massively transfused patients may benefit from calcium replacement. Slowing the transfusion rate may prevent the occurrence of hypocalcemia unless the patient has a predisposing condition that hinders citrate metabolism.

Hyperkalemia and Hypokalemia

Potassium toxicity is a rare complication. As the blood ages during storage, potassium is released from the cells into the plasma during RBC lysis. When RBCs have been stored at 1° to 6°C, there is leakage of intracellular potassium into the plasma. Because there is rapid dilution during transfusion, redistribution of potassium into cells, and excretion, hyperkalemia is a rare problem. It may be a problem in patients with renal failure, in premature infants, and in newborns who have large transfusions. Hypokalemia is generally of greater concerns because potassium-depleted donor red cells reaccumulate this ion intracellularly, and citrate metabolism causes further movement of potassium into the cells (Mazzei et al., 2011). Single-unit transfusion is generally not a problem, but individuals who receive multiple units of aged blood may experience this reaction. Patients with renal failure, premature infants, and newborns receiving large transfusions are at risk.

SIGNS AND SYMPTOMS

- Slow, irregular heartbeat
- Nausea

- Muscle weakness
- Electrocardiographic changes

INTERVENTIONS

- No interventions are usually needed.
- Monitor serum potassium levels and notify LIP.

PREVENTION

- Ascertain history of renal disease and chronic transfusions.

Hemostatic Abnormalities in Massive Transfusions

Coagulopathy can be observed when massive transfusion is required for severe blood loss, especially when the lost blood is initially replaced with red cells. It is caused by the dilution of platelets and clotting factors, which occurs as the patient loses hemostatically active blood, and by reduction of enzymatic activity (Mazzei et al., 2011).

SIGNS AND SYMPTOMS

- Occurs after replacement of two to three blood volumes
- Clinical evidence of bleeding
- Platelet counts below $50,000/\mu L$ with alteration in other coagulation factors
- Shock and DIC

TREATMENT AND PREVENTION

There are no specific guidelines for treatment and prevention. Frequently monitor prothrombin time (PT) and activated partial thromboplastin time (aPTT) when using platelets and plasma products to avoid overuse (Mazzei et al., 2011).

Delayed Transfusion Reactions

Delayed Hemolytic Transfusion Reaction

Delayed **hemolytic transfusion reactions** are a result of RBC antigen incompatibility other than with the ABO group. Rapid production of RBC antibody occurs shortly after transfusion of the corresponding antigen as a result of sensitization during previous transfusions or pregnancies. Destruction of the transfused RBCs gradually occurs over 2 or more days or up to several weeks after the transfusion. Reactions are common but often go unnoticed.

SIGNS AND SYMPTOMS

- Occur days to weeks after transfusion of red cell component
- Decreased Hgb and Hct levels
- Persistent low-grade fever, malaise

- Increased bilirubin levels
- Jaundice

INTERVENTIONS

- Usually no acute treatment is required.
- Monitor Hct level, renal function, and coagulation profile routinely for all patients receiving transfusions.
- Notify the LIP and transfusion services if delayed reaction is suspected.

PREVENTION

Reactions can be prevented by transfusion of antigen-negative red cells. Past transfusion records should be reviewed because alloantibodies may have been identified.

Transfusion-Associated Graft-versus-Host Disease

Transfusion-associated graft-versus-host disease (TA-GVHD) is a rare and fatal complication. It occurs when viable T lymphocytes in the transfused component engraft in the recipient and react against recipient tissue antigens (AABB, 2009). In essence, the T lymphocytes proliferate and begin to attack host tissue cells. Symptoms typically occur 8 to 10 days after the transfusion and include rash, fever, and diarrhea. Patients with risk factors for TA-GVHD include those with severe cellular immunodeficiency including leukemia, lymphoma, use of immunosuppressive drugs administered post-transplant or myeloablative chemotherapy, congenital immunodeficiency disorders, and neonates (Mazzei et al., 2011). Death from bleeding or infection occurs within 3 weeks. There is no cure for TA-GVHD. Gamma irradiation of all cellular components is the only way to prevent TA-GVHD (Mazzei et al., 2011).

 NURSING FAST FACT!

Immunocompromised recipients are at risk for TA-GVHD.

 CULTURAL AND ETHNIC CONSIDERATIONS: RISK FOR TRANSFUSION-ASSOCIATED GRAFT-VERSUS-HOST DISEASE

The degree of genetic diversity in populations affects the risk of developing TA-GVHD. In Japan the range is 1:874, whereas in France the range is 1:16,835. The difference is related to a decreased diversity in HLA antigen expression in the Japanese population (Mazzei et al., 2011).

SIGNS AND SYMPTOMS

- Typically occur within 8 to 10 days after transfusion
- Maculopapular rash
- Fever
- Enterocolitis with watery diarrhea
- Elevated hepatic function tests
- Pancytopenia

INTERVENTIONS

- Use of a variety of immunosuppressive agents
- Almost universally fatal

PREVENTION

Administer irradiated blood components.

Iron Overload

Patients who are chronically transfused for diseases are at risk for iron overload (Mazzei et al., 2011). Diseases associated with frequent transfusion include sickle cell disease, beta-thalassemia major, and myelodysplasia (Eckes, 2011).

A unit of RBCs contains approximately 250 mg of iron. Normally, 1 to 2 mg/day of iron is excreted through sloughing of the intestinal mucosa and the skin; small amounts are excreted in urine and bile (Mir, 2012). As red cells are destroyed, the majority of the released iron cannot be excreted and is stored in the body as hemosiderin. Hemosiderin does not circulate in the blood but is deposited in tissues. The main organs affected by this iron surplus are the liver, heart, lung, and endocrine glands. The damage to organs occurs long before clinical symptoms appear (Richardson, 2014). The consequences of unchelated iron overload include heart failure, cirrhosis, and endocrine diseases (e.g., diabetes).

SIGNS AND SYMPTOMS

- Development of organ failure, tissue damage
- Heart failure
- Diabetes
- Hypothyroidism
- General fatigue and weight loss
- Bronze/gray skin

INTERVENTIONS

- Iron chelation is used to bind iron from end organs and eliminate iron molecules through urine or feces without reducing the circulating Hgb.
- Chelation drugs include parenteral deferoxamine (administered subcutaneously or I.V.), deferiprone, and deferasirox.

Prevention

Identify patients at risk and assess need for iron chelation.

Infection-Related Complications

Transfusion-Transmitted Diseases

Despite all of the advances and attention to safety in blood banking and trans-fusion medicine, there are still risks to blood component therapy. Patients should be informed about alternatives to transfusion as well as the risks to them if transfusion is not undertaken. Furthermore, patients need to know about the blood center's autologous transfusion and patient-designated donor programs.

A uniform donor history is designed to ask questions that protect the health of both the donor and the recipient. Questions asked of the donor help determine whether donating blood might endanger his or her health. If a prospective donor responds positively to any of these questions, he or she will be "deferred" or asked not to donate blood. The health history also is used to identify prospective donors who have been exposed to or who may have disease, such as HIV, hepatitis, or malaria (AABB, 2008). Table 11-8 lists the incidence of transfusion-acquired infections.

Viruses

Transfusion transmission of HIV, HCV, and HBV is "now so rare that the rate of transmission cannot be measured by prospective studies ... only estimated by theoretical modeling" (Galel, 2011, p. 251). The estimated risks given in Table 11-8 are based on calculations.

Cytomegalovirus

CMV is a virus belonging to the herpes group that can be transmitted from a blood transfusion, primarily from white cells present in blood compo-nents. Most adults have been exposed to CMV because the majority of blood donors have CMV antibodies (Galel, 2011). CMV infection usually is mild but may be serious or fatal for those who are immunocompromised, for low-birth-weight infants, and for bone marrow and organ transplant patients. Patients at risk for CMV infection should receive blood components from donors who are CMV-negative or components that are leukocyte reduced.

Bacteria

Bacterial contamination of blood components, mainly platelets, is a major cause of transfusion-related death, after TRALI and hemolytic reactions (Galel, 2011). Bacteria are present in 1:3000 cellular blood components.

Sources of bacteria include the donor's skin and asymptomatic bacteria in the donor's bloodstream. Immediately following blood collection, the level of bacteria is too low to detect or cause recipient symptoms. However, the bacteria proliferate during storage. Because platelets are stored at room temperature, the risk is greatest.

Attention to skin antisepsis during venipuncture preceding blood donation is a critical step. Most often, two-stage procedures involving use of chlorhexidine, alcohol, and iodophors (e.g., Betadine) are used in skin antisepsis. Also, "diversion pouches" are used to discard the first 10 to 40 mL of donor blood away from the blood collection container. This is required for all platelet collections and whole blood collection where platelets are extracted (Galel, 2011). There are additional methods used to detect the presence of bacteria in platelets as part of quality control. Refrigerated storage limits the growth and viability of most bacteria in RBC products.

Prions

Prions are proteinaceous infectious particles that cause fatal infections of the nervous system called transmissible spongiform encephalopathies (TSEs). The best-known TSE disease in humans is Creutzfeldt–Jakob disease (CJD). This is a rare degenerative and fatal nervous system disorder. CJD has been transmitted via infusion or implantation of devices extracted from infected central nervous system tissues but has not been known to be transmissible via blood transfusion (Galel, 2011). Although there is no screening test for the disease, as a precaution the FDA prohibits blood donation by individuals who may be at risk. These include potential donors who have received injections of human-derived pituitary hormone, those with a family history of CJD, and those who have undergone surgeries that involved transplanted dura mater.

Similar to CJD, variant CJD (vCJD), commonly known as the human form of "mad cow" disease, is a rare degenerative and fatal nervous system disorder. There have been four cases of vCJD transmission via blood transfusions; these occurred in the United Kingdom where bovine spongiform encephalopathy (i.e., mad cow disease) is most endemic (Galel, 2011). There are no cases of transmission in the United States. Screening for risk is via questioning, and any patients at risk are excluded.

Infections Transmitted by Insect Vectors

West Nile Virus

WNV is spread by the bite of an infected mosquito. The virus can infect people, horses, and many types of birds. It was first detected in the United States in 1999, and the first documented cases of WNV transmission through organ transplantation and transfusion were noted in 2002. The most common symptoms of transfusion-transmitted WNV are fever and headache. Screening is by blood bank interview for history of fever and headache. Blood screening with nucleic acid amplification testing (NAT) for WNV is now required by both the AABB and the FDA (Galel, 2011).

Parasitic Infections

A variety of parasitic infections may be transmitted through transfusions:

- *Babesia*: These are intraerythrocyte parasites; infections are acquired through tick bites. In many individuals there are no symptoms; however, in immunocompromised, elderly, and asplenic patients, it may present as a fatal flu-like illness (Galel, 2011).There are no FDA-approved tests for blood donor screening at this time.
- *Trypanosoma cruzi*: This is a protozoan parasite that causes Chagas' disease, which is usually a self-limited disease but can be severe in immunocompromised individuals. A blood donor screening test was widely implemented across the United States in 2007 (Galel, 2011).
- *Malaria*: There is no FDA-approved test. Malaria is rare in the United States, and the blood supply has been effectively protected by donor questioning.

AGE-RELATED CONSIDERATIONS

Neonatal and Pediatric Patients

Special guidelines must be applied to neonatal and pediatric patients. The most significant differences between this young group and adults are:

- Smaller blood volume. Blood volumes for pediatric patients vary with body weight. A full-term newborn has a blood volume of approximately 85 mL/kg compared to 100 mL/kg in a preterm newborn. Blood banks and transfusion services must be capable of providing smaller, appropriately sized blood components to meet the needs of this population.
- Because of their smaller volume of blood, neonatal and pediatric patients have a decreased ability to tolerate blood loss.
- Neonatal and pediatric patients have immature organ function (Josephson, 2011).

The most frequently transfused blood component in children is RBCs, and this is often needed because of iatrogenic blood loss from repeated phlebotomy (Josephson, 2011). Attention to blood loss from laboratory testing is critical, as outlined in Table 11-6. Transfusion is based on the presence of symptomatic anemia or target Hct levels. The most frequently published guidelines for RBC transfusion in infants less than 4 months old include:

- Hct less than 20% with low reticulocyte count and symptomatic anemia (e.g., tachycardia, tachypnea, poor feeding)
- Hct less than 30% *and* on 35% oxygen; or on oxygen by nasal cannula; or on continuous positive airway pressure or intermittent mandatory ventilation; or with significant tachycardia or tachypnea; or with significant apnea or

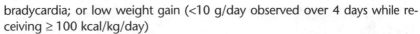

bradycardia; or low weight gain (<10 g/day observed over 4 days while receiving ≥ 100 kcal/kg/day)
• Hct less than 35% and either of the following: on greater than 35% oxygen hood or on continuous positive airway pressure/intermittent ventilation
• Hct less than 45% and either on extracorporeal membrane oxygenation or with congenital cyanotic heart disease (Josephson, 2011)

Transfusion Administration Issues

The most difficult aspect of transfusion in those younger than 4 months is vascular access. The umbilical vein is most frequently used for fluids and transfusions after birth; small-gauge catheters (24G) or needles (25G) can be safely used without causing hemolysis (Josephson, 2011).

Because rate control with small-volume and slow-rate transfusions are important, the use of infusion pumps, such as syringe pumps, is common in the neonatal/pediatric population. As discussed earlier, the manufacturer's infusion pump instructions should be reviewed to ensure the pump is safe to use with blood and blood products. Blood warmers are not routinely used.

Standard filtration using filters between 170 and 260 microns is required, as they are with adults. There are special pediatric transfusion administration sets that have less dead space than a standard set.

Complication Prevention

Leukocyte Reduction

Transfusion reactions are not frequent in those younger than 4 months because of their immature immune system; therefore, routine use of leukocyte reduction is controversial. However, based on studies, benefits of leukocyte reduction include reducing CMV risk, retinopathy of prematurity, and bronchopulmonary dysplasia (Josephson, 2011).

Irradiation

Irradiated blood components are administered to prevent TA-GVHD in the immunocompromised pediatric population. Indications include:
• Premature infants weighing less than 1200 g at birth
• Known or suspected cellular immune deficiency
• Significant immunosuppression related to chemotherapy or radiation treatment
• Patient receiving blood components from blood relatives or HLA-matched or crossmatched platelet components (Josephson, 2011)

Saline Washing

Saline washing of RBCs and platelets reduces the risk of adverse reactions to certain components from plasma, anticoagulant preservatives, and high levels of potassium (Josephson, 2011).

The Older Adult

The older adult receiving transfusion therapy is at increased risk for TACO. Nursing interventions include careful monitoring of intake and output, laboratory test results, and daily weight, and assessment of pulmonary and renal function.

Home Care Issues

In the 1980s, transfusing blood (i.e., red blood cells, platelets) in the home care setting was not uncommon. Such programs required extensive planning, relationships with blood centers, emergency plans and availability of emergency medications, and great attention to nurse education and competency. Today such programs are *not* common. The reality is that with today's focus on blood management and available alternatives to blood transfusion, there is limited need for home-based transfusion programs. Outside of the hospital, outpatient settings such as oncology clinics are more likely and more appropriate settings for transfusing the nonhospitalized patient.

However, there are some blood component infusion therapies that are appropriate for home administration, such as factor replacement for patients with hemophilia and intravenous or subcutaneous Ig infusions. In the case of factor replacement, such infusions are often either administered in the home by a nurse or self-infused by the patient, most often using recombinant, rather than plasma-derived, products.

The role of the home care nurse is also important in providing patient education and identifying and reporting signs and symptoms of delayed transfusion reactions (e.g., delayed hemolytic transfusion reaction) for patients who have received recent transfusions.

Patient Education

- Patients who are aware of the steps involved in a transfusion experience less anxiety.
- The nurse should explain how the transfusion will be given, how long it will take, what the expected outcome is, what symptoms to report, and that vital signs will be taken.
- The LIP has the responsibility to explain the benefits and risks of transfusion therapy as well as the alternatives.
- Informed consent is obtained, addressing the risks and benefits of transfusion.
- Instruct the patient on the need and physiological benefits of blood product.
- Inform the patient of options: autologous, homologous, or directed donation.

■ Nursing Process

The nursing process is a six-step process for problem-solving to guide nursing action (see Chapter 1 for details on the steps of the nursing process related to vascular access). The following table focuses on nursing diagnoses, nursing outcomes classification (NOC), and nursing interventions classification (NIC) for patients receiving transfusion therapy. Nursing diagnoses should be patient specific and outcomes and interventions individualized. The NOC and NIC presented here are suggested directions for development of specific outcomes and interventions.

Nursing Diagnoses Related to Transfusion Therapy	Nursing Outcomes Classification (NOC)	Nursing Interventions Classification (NIC)
Anxiety related to: Situational crisis, stress, lack of knowledge; possibility of harm from transfusion	Anxiety level, anxiety self-control, coping	Anxiety reduction strategies
Fatigue related to: Physiological: Anemia, decreased oxygen supply to the body, increased cardiac workload	Energy conservation, nutritional status	Energy management (conservation and restoration)
Fear related to: Phobic stimulus, hospital procedures, unfamiliarity with environmental experiences, homologous blood transfusion, transmission of disease, fear of needles	Fear control	Anxiety reduction strategies, coping enhancements
Gas exchange impaired related to: Ventilation perfusion imbalance, decreased oxygen-carrying capacity of the blood	Gas exchange, ventilation	Acid–base management
Hypothermia related to: Exposure to cool or cold blood	Thermoregulation	Temperature regulation
Infection risk for related to: Inadequate secondary to leukopenia, suppressed inflammatory response, environmental exposure to pathogens	Immune status, knowledge of infection management, risk control, risk detection	Infection control, infection protection
Knowledge deficit related to: Purpose of blood component therapy; signs and symptoms of complications	Knowledge: Treatment regimen (transfusion)	Teaching: Disease process, transfusion component risk and benefits
Protection ineffective related to: Abnormal blood profiles	Health-promoting behavior, blood coagulation, immune status	Bleeding precautions, infection prevention, infection protection

Sources: Ackley & Ladwig (20011); Bulechek, Butcher, Dochterman, &Wagner (2013); Moorhead, Johnson, Maas, & Swanson (2013).

Chapter Highlights

- Immunohematology is the science that deals with antigens of the blood and their antibodies.
- Blood groups are based on the antigens present on the cell surface of RBCs. The two major antigen groups are the ABO and Rh systems. Every human being has two genotypes that, when paired, determine one of four blood types (A, B, AB, or O).
- The universal RBC donor is O-negative; the universal plasma donor is AB.
- The majority of people (85%) have the Rh antigen D, making them Rh-positive. Those without antigen D are Rh-negative.
- ABO incompatibility is the major cause of fatal transfusion reactions.
- Blood donor collection methods include:
  - Allogeneic: Blood donated by someone other than the intended recipient
  - Autologous: Recipient's own blood; collected in one of four ways: preoperative autologous transfusion, perioperative isovolemic hemodilution, intraoperative autologous transfusion, and postoperative blood salvage.
  - Designated (directed): Blood donated from selected friends or relatives of the recipient
- Blood product transfusions are indicated for:
  - Maintenance of oxygen-carrying capacity of the blood
  - Replacement of clotting factors
  - Replacement of vascular volume
- Governmental agencies (e.g., FDA), accreditation organizations (e.g., AABB), and professional organizations (e.g., INS) provide guidelines and standards for responsibilities of nurses in the safe administration of blood products.
- Biological (immune) reactions include AHTRs, **delayed transfusion reactions**, nonhemolytic febrile reactions, allergic reactions, TRALI, and TA-GVHD reactions.
- Nonimmune complications associated with transfusion therapy include circulatory overload, citrate toxicity, potassium toxicity, hypothermia, hypocalcemia, bacterial contamination, and infectious disease transmission.
- Key steps in the procedure to delivery of blood transfusion are:
  Step 1: Recipient consent
  Step 2: Verifying the authorized prescriber's order
  Step 3: Pretransfusion
  Step 4: Venous access; selecting and preparing the equipment
  Step 5: Preparing the patient
  Step 6: Dispensing and transportation of the component
  Step 7: Initiating the transfusion
  Step 8: Monitoring the transfusion
  Step 9: Completing the transfusion.

▪▪ Thinking Critically: Case Study

At the beginning of your shift, you check on a unit of PRBCs that had been hung just prior to your shift. The unit of RBCs is infusing slowly, with approximately 200 mL left. You agitate the bag slightly and discover a pinhole at the top of the bag.

Case Study Questions
1. What do you do?
2. What legal factors are involved in this scenario?
3. What are the risks to the patient?
4. What assessments should have taken place prior to hanging this blood component?

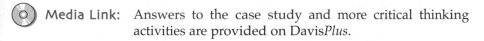

Media Link: Answers to the case study and more critical thinking activities are provided on DavisPlus.

Post-Test

1. Antibodies in the blood system are called:
   a. HLA
   b. Agglutinogens
   c. Agglutinins
   d. Antigens

2. Which of the following diseases is donor blood screened for? (*Select all that apply.*)
   a. Hepatitis B
   b. West Nile virus
   c. Crohn's disease
   d. Epstein–Barr virus (EBV)

3. The initial nursing intervention for an acute hemolytic transfusion reaction would be to:
   a. Slow the transfusion and call the LIP.
   b. Stop the transfusion and turn the saline side of the administration set on at a slow keep open rate.
   c. Stop the transfusion, disconnect the tubing from the I.V. catheter, and initiate new saline and tubing to keep the vein open.
   d. Stop the transfusion and turn the saline side of the administration set on at a rapid rate.

4. The component albumin 25% is hypertonic. Caution should be used by nurses when infusing 25% albumin because this product can:
   a. Cause circulatory overload
   b. Cause clotting disorders

    c. Increase RBC hemoglobin
    d. Lower the blood pressure

5. Which of the following must an RN check with another nurse before initiating a unit of blood? (*Select all that apply.*)

    a. ABO and Rh
    b. Patient name
    c. Unit number
    d. Expiration date
    e. Preservative

6. The universal recipient is a person with blood type:

    a. A-positive
    b. AB-positive
    c. O-negative
    d. AB-negative

7. Which of the following PRBC preparations is considered to prevent TA-GVHD?

    a. Leukocyte-reduced RBCs
    b. Washed RBCs
    c. Irradiated RBCs
    d. Frozen-washed RBCs

8. If a patient receives 2 units of packed red blood cells for an Hct of 24%, what would the anticipated Hct be 24 hours postinfusion?

    a. 26%
    b. 28%
    c. 30%
    d. 32%

9. Which of the following adverse effects of transfusion therapy has the greatest potential for a fatal outcome for the patient?

    a. TACO
    b. Febrile reaction
    c. Citrate toxicity
    d. TA-GVHD

10. A patient with group O blood type may receive which of the following RBCs?

    a. Group A only
    b. Group O only
    c. Group AB and O
    d. Any blood group

Media Link: Answers to the Chapter 11 Post-Test and more test questions together with rationales are provided on Davis*Plus*.

References

American Association of Blood Banks (AABB). (2009). Circular of information for the use of human blood and blood components. Retrieved from https://www.aabb.org/resources/bct/Pages/aabb_coi.aspx (Accessed March 14, 2013).

AABB. (2008). T. H. Price (Ed.), *Standards for blood banks and transfusion services* (25th ed.). Bethesda MD: Author.

Ackley, B. J., & Ladwig, G. B. (2011). *Nursing diagnosis handbook: An evidence-based guide to planning care* (9th ed.). St. Louis, MO: Mosby Elsevier.

American Red Cross. (n.d.). Blood types. Retrieved from http://www.redcrossblood.org/learn-about-blood/blood-types (Accessed March 16, 2013).

Boucher, B. A., & Hannon, T. J. (2007). Blood management: A primer for clinicians. *Pharmacotherapy, 27*, 1394-1411.

Bulechek, G. M., Butcher, G. M., Dochterman, J. M., & Wagner, C. M. (2013). *Nursing interventions classification (NIC)* (6th ed.). St. Louis, MO: Mosby Elsevier.

Carson, T. H. (ed) (2011) Standards for blood banks and transfusion services. (27th ed.). Bethesda, MD: AABB.

Carson, J. L., Grossman, B. J., Kleinman, S., Tinmouth, A. T., Marques, M. B., Fung, M. K., ... Clinical Transfusion Medicine Committee of the AABB. (2012). Red blood cell transfusion: A clinical practice guideline from the AABB. *Annals of Internal Medicine, 157*(1), 49-58.

Chou, S. T., & Westhoff, C. M. (2011). The Rh system. In J. D. Roback, B. J. Grossman, T. Harris, & C. D. Hillyer (Eds.), *AABB technical manual* (17th ed.) (pp. 389-411). Bethesda, MD: AABB Press.

Clark, C. T. (2011). Recent efforts and available technologies for safety in delivery of blood products. *Journal of Infusion Nursing, 34*(1), 23-27.

Corwin, H. K. (2006). Anemia and red blood cell transfusion in the critically ill. *Seminars in Dialysis, 19*, 513-518.

Daniels, G. (2011). Other blood groups. In J. D. Roback, B. J. Grossman, T. Harris, & C. D. Hillyer (Eds.), *AABB technical manual* (17th ed.) (pp. 411-436). Bethesda, MD: AABB Press.

DomBourian, M., & Holland, L. (2012). Optimal use of fresh frozen plasma. *Journal of Infusion Nursing 35*(1), 28-32.

Downes, K. A., & Shulman, I. A. (2008). Pretransfusion testing. In J. D. Roback, B. J. Grossman, T. Harris, & C. D. Hillyer (Eds.), *AABB technical manual* (17th ed.) (pp. 437-462). Bethesda, MD: AABB Press.

Eder, A. F. (2011). Allogeneic and autologous blood donor selection. In J. D. Roback, B. J. Grossman, T. Harris, & C. D. Hillyer (Eds.), *AABB technical manual* (17th ed.) (pp. 137-186). Bethesda, MD: AABB Press.

Food and Drug Administration (FDA). (2006). Guidance for industry: Implementation of acceptable full-length donor history questionnaire and accompanying materials for use in screening donors of blood and blood components. Rockville, MD: CBER Office of Communication, Training and Manufacturer.

FDA. (2009). Vaccines, blood & biologics: Bar code label requirements. Retrieved from http://www.fda.gov/BiologicsBloodVaccines/DevelopmentApprovalProcess/AdvertisingLabelingPromotionalMaterials/BarCodeLabelRequirements/default.htm (Accessed March 9, 2013).

Galel, S. A. (2011). Infectious disease screening. In J. D. Roback, B. J. Grossman, T. Harris, & C. D. Hillyer (Eds.), *AABB technical manual* (17th ed.) (pp. 239-270). Bethesda, MD: AABB Press.

Gebel, H. M., Pollack, M. S., & Bray, R. A. (2011). The HLA system. In J. D. Roback, B. J. Grossman, T. Harris, C. D. Hillyer (Eds.), *AABB technical manual* (17th ed.) (pp. 547-570). Bethesda, MD: AABB Press.

Giger, J. N., & Davidhizar, R. E. (2004). *Transcultural nursing: Assessment and intervention* (2nd ed.) (p. 140). St. Louis, MO: C. V. Mosby.

Hitch, D. (2013). What every nurse should know about hemophilia. *American Nurse Today, 8*(3), 22-26.

Infusion Nurses Society (INS). (2011). Infusion nursing standards of practice. *Journal of Intravenous Nursing, 34*(1S), S1-S110.

Josephson, C. D. (2011). Neonatal and pediatric transfusion practice. In J. D. Roback, B. J. Grossman, T. Harris, & C. D. Hillyer (Eds.), *AABB technical manual* (17th ed.) (pp. 645-670). Bethesda, MD: AABB Press.

Kakaiya, R., Aronson, C. A., & Jullcis, J. (2011). Whole blood collection and component processing at blood collection centers. In J. D. Roback, B. J. Grossman, T. Harris, & C. D. Hillyer (Eds.), *AABB technical manual* (17th ed.) (pp. 187-226). Bethesda, MD: AABB Press.

Kopko, P. M. (2010). Transfusion-related lung injury. *Journal of Infusion Nursing* 33 (1), 32-37.

Lockwood, W. B., Leonard, J., & Liles, S. L. (2011). Storage, monitoring, pretransfusion processing and distribution of blood components. In J. D. Roback, B. J. Grossman, T. Harris, & C. D. Hillyer (Eds.), *AABB technical manual* (17th ed.) (pp. 271-292). Bethesda, MD: AABB Press.

Mazzei, C. A., Popovsky, M. A., & Kopko, P. M. (2011). Noninfectious complications of blood transfusion. In J. D. Roback, B. J. Grossman, T. Harris, & C. D. Hillyer (Eds.), *AABB technical manual* (17th ed.) (pp. 727-762). Bethesda, MD: AABB Press.

Mir, M.A. (2012). Transfusion-induced iron overload. Retrieved from http://emedicine.medscape.com/article/1389732-overview (Accessed October 13, 2013).

Moorhead, S., Johnson, M., Maas, M., & Swanson, E. (2013). *Nursing outcomes classification (NOC)* (5th ed). St. Louis, MO: Mosby Elsevier.

Nester, T., & AuBuchon, J. P. (2011). Hemotherapy decisions and their outcomes. In J. D. Roback, B. J. Grossman, T. Harris, & C. D. Hillyer (Eds.), *AABB technical manual* (17th ed.) (pp. 571-616). Bethesda, MD: AABB Press.

Porth, C. M., & Matfin, G. (2010). *Pathophysiology: Concepts of altered health states* (6th ed.). Philadelphia, PA: Lippincott Williams & Wilkins.

Richardson, D. (2014). Transfusion therapy. In M. Alexander, A. Corrigan, L. Gorski, & L. Phillips (Eds.), *Core curriculum for infusion nursing* (4th ed) (pp. 235-257). Philadelphia: Lippincott, Williams & Wilkins.

Seeber, P., Shander, A. (2013). *Basics of blood management*. Chichester, UK: Wiley-Blackwell.

Sink, B. L. (2011). Administration of blood components. In J. D. Roback, B. J. Grossman, T. Harris, & C. D. Hillyer (Eds.), *AABB technical manual* (17th ed.) (pp. 617-629). Bethesda, MD: AABB Press.

Tolich, D. J., Blackmur, S., Stahorsky, K., & Wabeke, D. (2013). Blood management: Best practice transfusion strategies. *Nursing, 43*, 41-47.

Waters, J. H. (2011). Blood management. In J. D. Roback, B. J. Grossman, T. Harris, & C. D. Hillyer (Eds.), *AABB technical manual* (17th ed.) (pp. 671-686). Bethesda, MD: AABB Press.

Welden, L. (2010). Transfusion confusion. *Nursing Management, 41,* 24-29.

Younger, M. E. M., Aro, L., Blouin, W., Duff, C., Epland, K. B. (2013). Nursing guidelines for the administration of immunoglobulin replacement therapy. *Journal of Infusion Nursing, 36*(1), 58-68.

Zaccheo, M., & Bucher, D. (2010). Establishing evidence-based transfusion education for best practice. *Nursing Critical Care, 5*(5), 41-44.

PROCEDURES DISPLAY 11-1

Initiation of Transfusion

Equipment Needed
0.9% sodium chloride
Blood or blood component
Blood filter
Blood administration set
Needleless infusion administration equipment
Requisition slip
0.9% sodium chloride (USP) flushes or heparin as appropriate
Blood pressure cuff, stethoscope, thermometer, alcohol prep pads

Delegation
This procedure cannot be delegated. An LVN/LPN or NAP can assist by monitoring vital signs. *Note:* In California the LVN can administer blood and blood products through a peripheral line if state I.V. certified and supported by agency policy.

Procedure	**Rationale**
1. Verify the authorized prescriber's order and that informed consent is signed. Order type and crossmatch, and order blood or blood components.	1. A written order is a legal requirement for infusion therapy. Informed consent is required for blood product administration.
2. Confirm blood is available in the blood bank.	
3. Introduce yourself to the patient.	3. Establishes the nurse–patient relationship
4. Verify patient identity using two forms of identification	4. Patient safety

Continued

PROCEDURES DISPLAY 11-1

Initiation of Transfusion—*cont'd*

Procedure	Rationale
5. Use proper hand hygiene throughout procedure.	5. The single most important means of infection prevention
6. Review patient understanding of the procedure and provide the patient with the opportunity to ask questions and express any concerns.	6. The patient who is well informed is better able to cope with the treatment regimen.
7. Verify patency of existing I.V. catheter or place new peripheral I.V. catheter before obtaining blood from transfusion services.	7. The blood component must be started within 30 minutes from removal from blood bank.

8. Obtain and open Y-tubing blood administration set
  a. Close all clamps
  b. Spike 0.9% sodium chloride bag with one extension of Y tubing and prime tubing per manufacturer's directions
  c. Maintain clamp on other Y tubing extension in closed position.
	8. Prime the set and have equipment integrity checked and in place before obtaining the blood component from the transfusion service.

9. Obtain baseline vital signs. Notify the LIP if temperature is elevated 1°F above normal. The transfusion may be held.	9. Fever can conceal the symptoms of an untoward reaction. Vital signs serve as baseline for the identification of changes that may transpire during the transfusion.
10. Obtain the blood component from blood bank. a. Inspect the component and its container for clots, bubbles, leaks in the bag, or discoloration.	10. Most serious reactions are the result of clerical errors. There is shared accountability between the nurse obtaining the component and the transfusion services. The presence of clots, bubbles,

PROCEDURES DISPLAY 11-1

Initiation of Transfusion—*cont'd*

Procedure	Rationale
b. Compare ABO group and Rh type on the blood label to the tag attached to it and ensure that they match.	leaks in the bag, or discoloration may indicate bacterial contamination or inadequate anticoagulation of the unit and should not be used.
c. Check the expiration date.	
11. Return to the unit with one component (only one blood unit is released from the blood bank at a time). NEVER put a blood component in a refrigerator that is not specifically intended to store blood.	**11.** To ensure the safety and integrity of the blood component
12. Reassess the patient's condition and level of consciousness. Check the component at the bedside with another nurse. Verify the following: **a.** Patient identification is correct using at least two patient identifiers **b.** Patient name is correct on all documents **c.** Blood component is what was ordered (e.g., platelets) **d.** The numbers on the patient's ID band correlate with those on the laboratory form and component. **e.** Blood type matches on transfusion records and blood bag **f.** Patient is compatible with donor ABO and Rh type.	**12.** There is less probability of error when two people verify the needed information. One person should read all of the information to the other as the second person verifies it.

Continued

PROCEDURES DISPLAY 11-1

Initiation of Transfusion—*cont'd*

Procedure	Rationale
g. Expiration date has not passed.	
13. Perform hand hygiene and don gloves.	**13.** Infection prevention and standard precautions
14. Using aseptic technique, spike the blood component bag and open the clamp to initiate the transfusion at the rate of approximately 2 mL/min or slower. Turn off the sodium chloride.	**14.** Transfusions are initiated slowly so that minimal blood is transfused in the event of a reaction.
15. Stay with the patient for 15 minutes. Obtain a second set of vital signs and record in the medical record.	**15.** Most transfusion reactions occur within the first 15 minutes.
16. Monitor and document the patient's level of consciousness and vital signs according to organizational policy	**16.** Primary indicators of patient tolerance of transfusion
17. Transfuse within 4 hours.	**17.** There is risk for bacterial growth if the unit is allowed to hang and infuse over >4 hours.
18. On completion of the transfusion, close the clamp to the blood product, open up the clamp to the saline bag, and infuse 0.9% sodium chloride to clear the I.V. catheter at the prescribed rate. If another unit of blood is required, a new administration set must be added. Only one administration set can be used in 4 hours.	**18.** Clears the remaining blood product that is in the tubing and maintains patency of the I.V. catheter

PROCEDURES DISPLAY 11-1

Initiation of Transfusion—*cont'd*

Procedure	Rationale
19. Discard the empty blood container and administration set in biohazard container.	19. Standard precautions
20. Document the time the blood component terminated and the amount infused. During the transfusion, the patient's response should also be documented, along with vital signs. *Transfusion Reaction:* If a transfusion reaction occurs, notify the LIP immediately; do not discard the blood container—return to transfusion services. Complete the transfusion record and place in the patient's permanent medical record. Draw post-transfusion laboratory samples as ordered. Follow agency policy on transfusion reaction. Document signs and symptoms, component administered, amount infused, time LIP notified and response, time of blood bank notification, medication and treatment ordered and administered, patient's response, and patient outcome.	20. To maintain the legal record. Immediate reactions can occur within 2 hours of completion of a transfusion. To maintain proper documentation and communicate that transfusion was administered. The remainder of the blood must be sent to the laboratory blood bank where it can be analyzed to determine the cause of the reaction. Medication and treatment will vary depending on the type of reaction.

Sources: INS (2011); Sink (2011).

Chapter **12**

Parenteral Nutrition

Every careful observer of the sick will agree in this that thousands of patients are annually starved in the midst of plenty, from want of attention to the ways which alone make it possible for them to take food.
—Florence Nightingale, 1859

Chapter Contents

Chapter Highlights   Post-Test
Thinking Critically: Case Study   References

LEARNING   *On completion of this chapter, the reader will be able to:*
OBJECTIVES
1. Define terminology related to nursing care of the patient receiving parenteral nutrition.
2. Describe the three types of malnutrition.
3. Identify the key elements of a nutritional assessment.
4. Identify at least four laboratory tests used in nutritional assessment.
5. Discuss the potential consequences of drug interactions with the parenteral nutrition formula.
6. Describe potential candidates for parenteral nutrition administration.
7. Discuss the advantages and disadvantages of peripheral parenteral nutrition.
8. Define total nutrient admixture.
9. Describe the advantages of cyclic parenteral nutrition.
10. Describe parenteral nutrition administration issues related to administration set changes and use of filters.
11. Discuss potential complications of parenteral nutrition and associated interventions.
12. Discuss physiological differences in the pediatric patient and the older adult patient relative to nutrition.

GLOSSARY

Amino acid   An organic compound that is the building block of protein

Anabolism   The constructive phase of metabolism; the building of body tissues

Anergy   Lack of immune response to an antigen

Anthropometry   Measurement of the size, weight, and proportions of the human body

Basal energy expenditure (BEE)   The amount of energy produced per unit of time under "basal" conditions

Carbohydrate   A group of organic compounds including sugars, starches, and glycogen

Catabolism   The destructive phase of metabolism; the opposite of anabolism

Cyclic parenteral nutrition   Delivery of parenteral nutrition over a reduced time frame, over 8 to 18 hours rather than a 24-hour continuous infusion

Essential fatty acid deficiency (EFAD)   Complication resulting from a lack of adequate intake of fat in the diet; essential fatty acids cannot be synthesized by the body but must be obtained from the diet or by intravenous infusion of lipids

Fat   Biological substances that are insoluble in water but soluble in other solvents; break down into fatty acids and glycerol

Intravenous fat emulsion (IVFE)   A combination of liquid, lipid, and an emulsifying system for intravenous use; the solution has limited ability to be mixed with other solutions

Kwashiorkor   Malnutrition characterized by decreased intake of calories with an adequate protein-calorie ratio

Marasmus   Malnutrition characterized by decreased intake of calories with adequate amounts of protein intake

Parenteral nutrition (PN)   Nutrients that are administered intravenously, including carbohydrates, proteins, fats, electrolytes, vitamins, and trace elements

Peripheral parenteral nutrition (PPN)   Intravenous administration of parenteral nutrition via the peripheral veins

Refeeding syndrome   A rare syndrome associated with the institution of nutritional support in a severely malnourished patient and result-ant metabolic and hormonal changes including hypophosphatemia, which can lead to cardiac failure

Total nutrient admixture (TNA)   A parenteral nutrition solution formula that includes amino acids, fat, dextrose, and all other additives in a single container

■ Nutritional Support

The American Society for Parenteral and Enteral Nutrition (A.S.P.E.N.) is a multidisciplinary professional organization of physicians, nurses, dieti-tians, pharmacists, allied health professionals, and researchers dedicated to patients receiving optimal nutrition care. Nutritional support nursing is a professional nursing specialty that focuses on the care of individuals with potential or known nutritional alterations. The nutrition support nurse encompasses all nursing activities that promote optimal nutritional health, prevention of nutrition-related illness, and advocacy for persons, communities, and populations with known or potential alterations in nutrition (A.S.P.E.N. Board of Directors, 2007). Nursing interventions are based on scientific principles. The scope of practice includes, but is not limited to, direct patient care; consultation with nurses and other health-care professionals in a variety of clinical settings; education of patients, students, colleagues, and the public; participation in research; and administrative functions. Nurses can attain certification as a nutrition support clinician (CNSC) through the National Board of Nutrition Support, an independent credentialing board established by A.S.P.E.N.

All nurses, whether or not specialized in nutrition support, should recognize the importance of adequate nutrition and the adverse effects of malnutrition. Specialized nutritional support, such as parenteral or enteral nutrition, may be indicated in some patients. The focus of this chapter is administration of **parenteral nutrition (PN)**. The goals of PN are:

1. To provide all essential nutrients in adequate amounts to sustain nutritional balance during periods when oral or enteral routes of feedings are not possible or are insufficient to meet the patient's caloric needs
2. To preserve or restore the body's protein metabolism and prevent the development of protein or caloric malnutrition
3. To diminish the rate of weight loss and to maintain or increase body weight
4. To promote wound healing
5. To replace nutritional deficits

 Websites

American Society for Parenteral and Enteral Nutrition:
   www.nutritioncare.org
National Board of Nutrition Support Certification, Inc.:
   https://www.nutritioncare.org/NBNSC/index.aspx

■ Concepts of Nutrition

Nutritional balance occurs when nutrients are provided in sufficient quantities to provide energy, to support the growth of tissues, and to regulate physiological processes within the body (Krzywda & Meyer, 2010). Nutritional balance is based on three factors: (1) intake of nutrients (quantity and quality), (2) relative need for nutrients, and (3) the ability of the body to use nutrients.

Nutritional Deficiency

When nutritional deficiency exists, body stores are used to provide energy for essential metabolic processes. Excess carbohydrates are stored in the muscle and liver as glycogen. Adipose tissue is the body's long-term energy reserve of fat. Body protein is not stored in excess of the body's needs; therefore, use of body protein without replacement adversely affects total body function.

Malnutrition

Malnutrition is defined as an acute, subacute, or chronic state of nutrition, in which a combination of varying degrees of overnutrition or undernutrition with or without inflammatory activity has led to a change in body composition and diminished function (A.S.P.E.N. Board of Directors and Clinical Practice Committee, 2012). A.S.P.E.N. further identifies three nutrition diagnoses based on etiology for adults in clinical practice settings:

- *Starvation-related malnutrition*: Chronic starvation without inflammation (e.g., anorexia nervosa).
- *Chronic disease-related malnutrition*: Inflammation is chronic and of mild to moderate degree (e.g., organ failure, pancreatic cancer, rheumatoid arthritis).
- *Acute disease or injury-related malnutrition*: Inflammation is acute and of a severe degree (e.g., major infection, burns, trauma, closed head injury).

Malnutrition is a result of diminished nutrient intake, abnormal digestion, alterations in absorption of nutrients, and/or increase in nutrient needs. Hospitalized patients who are malnourished have longer hospitalizations, more infectious and noninfectious complications, and greater risk of mortality (Mueller et al., 2011). Clinical guidelines from A.S.P.E.N. recommend the following:

- Nutritional risk screening for all hospitalized patients (there are a number of nutritional risk screening tools available)
- Nutritional assessment for all those patients screened to be at risk
- Nutritional support intervention for those screened and assessed to be at risk (Mueller et al., 2011)

Death from protein energy malnutrition and other nutritional deficiencies occurs within 60 to 70 days of total starvation in normal-weight adults. After total starvation for less than 2 to 3 days in healthy adults, the losses are mainly glycogen and water. Starvation alters the distribution of carbohydrates, fats, and protein substrates. Brief starvation (24–72 hours) rapidly depletes glycogen stores and uses protein to produce glucose (gluconeogenesis) for glucose-dependent tissue. Prolonged starvation (>72 hours) is associated with an increased mobilization of fat as the principal source of energy, reduction in the breakdown of protein, and increased use of ketones for central nervous tissue fuel. Stress in the form of pain, shock, injury, and sepsis intensifies the metabolic change seen in those with brief and prolonged starvation.

 NURSING FAST FACT!

> The prevalence of malnutrition among hospitalized patients is estimated to be as high as 30% to 50%. Malnutrition is associated with increased risk for complications such as poor wound healing, compromised immune status, impaired organ function, and increased mortality (Jensen, Hsiao, & Wheeler, 2012).

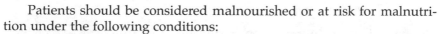

Patients should be considered malnourished or at risk for malnutrition under the following conditions:

- Inadequate nutrient intake for 7 or more days
- Involuntary weight loss of 10% or greater of usual body weight over 6 months
- Involuntary weight loss of 5% or greater of usual body weight in 1 month (Krzywda & Meyer, 2014)

Three types of malnutrition have been defined and classified by an International Classification of Diseases (ICD) diagnostic code: **marasmus**, **kwashiorkor**, and mixed malnutrition.

Marasmus

Marasmus, or simple starvation, is caused by a decrease in the intake of calories with adequate protein–calorie ratio. In this type of malnutrition, a gradual wasting of body fat and skeletal muscle takes place with preservation of visceral proteins. The individual appears emaciated and has decreased anthropometric measurements (e.g., history of weight loss) and **anergy** to common skin test antigens.

 NURSING FAST FACT!

Marasmus may be seen in patients with chronic illness and prolonged starvation as well as in the elderly and patients with anorexia nervosa.

Kwashiorkor

Kwashiorkor is characterized by an adequate intake of calories but with a poor protein intake. This condition causes visceral protein wasting with preservation of fat and somatic muscle. It is seen during a period of decreased protein intake, as seen in patients on liquid diets, fad diets, and long-term use of I.V. fluids containing dextrose. Loss of body protein is caused by depleted circulating proteins in the plasma. Individuals may appear well nourished or obese and have adequate anthropometric measurements but decreased visceral proteins and depressed immune function.

Mixed Malnutrition

Mixed malnutrition is characterized by aspects of both marasmus and kwashiorkor. The person presents with skeletal muscle and visceral protein wasting, depleted fat stores, and immune incompetence. The affected person appears cachectic and usually is in acute catabolic stress. This mixed protein–calorie disorder is associated with the highest risk of morbidity and mortality (Krzywda & Meyer, 2014).

Effects of Malnutrition

The hazards of malnutrition on bodily function are decreased visceral protein stores, albumin depletion, and impaired immune status. Without visceral protein stores in the body, a deficiency of total body protein results first in decreased strength and endurance (loss of muscle mass) and ultimately in decreased cardiac and respiratory muscle function. Skeletal muscle wasting occurs in a ratio of about 30:1 compared with visceral protein loss. The loss of gastrointestinal (GI) function follows skeletal muscle wasting and is associated with hypoalbuminemia. Protein–calorie malnutrition is one of the most common causes of impaired immune function. Both B- and T-cell–mediated immune functions are impaired, causing enhanced susceptibility to infections (Porth & Matfin, 2010).

The effects of malnutrition on the body include:

- Loss of muscle mass
- Impaired wound healing
- Impaired immunological function
- Loss of calcium and phosphate from bone
- Anovulation and amenorrhea in women
- Decreased testicular function in men

■ Nutritional Screening

The purpose of nutritional screening is to identify individuals who are malnourished or who are at risk for malnutrition, thus determining the need for a more detailed nutrition assessment. Practice guidelines for nutrition screening from A.S.P.E.N. include:

- A nutrition screening incorporating objective data such as height, weight, weight change, primary diagnosis, and presence of comorbidities should be a component of the initial evaluation of all patients in an ambulatory, hospital, home, or alternate care setting.
- The health-care organization should determine who will perform the screening and the elements to be included.
- A procedure to rescreen patients who are not immediately identified at nutritional risk should also be in place (Ukleja et al., 2010).

Assessment

Performance of an overall health history provides information for identifying nutrition-related problems. It includes subjective data about the client's dietary history and related factors. The nutritional assessment encompasses anthropometric measurements, diagnostic testing, and a complete physical examination (Jensen et al., 2012) (Table 12-1).

The history includes medical, weight, social, dietary, and medications. The medical history should include a specific history of weight; diseases that

> Table 12-1	COMPONENTS OF A NUTRITIONAL ASSESSMENT

History
■ Medical
■ Social
■ Dietary
Anthropometric measurements
■ Height and weight
■ Mid-arm circumference/skinfold testing (appropriate training required)
Laboratory assessment
■ Serum albumin and transferrin levels
■ Prealbumin and retinol-binding protein
■ Serum electrolytes, serum glucose
■ Liver enzymes
■ Lipid levels
■ Coagulation studies
■ Vitamin/trace element levels
■ Total lymphocyte count
■ Urine assays (creatinine, height index, nitrogen balance)
Energy requirements
■ Indirect calorimetry
Physical examination
Other indices

affect ingestion, digestion, or absorption of oral nutrients such as GI obstructions or fistulas; surgical history; presence of increased losses, such as from draining wounds and fistulas; and factors such as age and drug, alcohol, and tobacco use. The social history affecting nutrient intake includes income, education, ethnic background, and environment during mealtime, along with religious considerations. The dietary history often provides clues to the cause and degree of malnutrition. The components of a dietary history include appetite, GI disturbances, mechanical problems such as ill-fitting dentures, food allergies, medications, and food likes and dislikes (Jensen et al., 2012).

CULTURAL AND ETHNIC CONSIDERATIONS: NUTRITION

Assess for the influence of cultural beliefs, norms, and values on the patient's nutritional knowledge. What the patient considers normal dietary practices may be based on cultural perceptions. Culture can determine the foods a patient eats and how the foods are prepared and served. Culture and religion together often determine if certain foods are prohibited and if certain foods and spices are eaten. When taking a dietary history, the nurse must be sensitive to culture and religious beliefs related to foods (Smeltzer, Bare, Hinkle, & Cheever, 2010).

Anthropometric Measurements

Anthropometry is the physical measurement of subcutaneous fat and of muscle mass (somatic protein) stores, with muscle mass representing the largest concentration of body protein stores (Krzywda & Meyer, 2014). Anthropometry includes accurate measurement of height and weight. A practical measure of body size and an indirect measure of body fat is provided by the body mass index (BMI), which is defined as weight (kg)/[height (m)]^2. Interpretations of BMI are as follows:

BMI <18.5: Underweight, at risk for malnutrition

BMI 18.5–24.9: Desirable

BMI 25–29: Overweight

BMI ≥30: Obese (Centers for Disease Control and Prevention [CDC], 2011)

Serial weight measurements over time provide the most reliable and clinically relevant information for the nutritional assessment (Krzywda & Meyer, 2014). Weight loss is important because it reflects inadequate calorie intake.

Additional anthropometric measurements may include the skinfold test and the mid-arm circumference. To estimate the size of the body fat mass, a skinfold test is done on the triceps of the nondominant arm using a caliper. The mid-arm circumference is an indirect measurement of body protein stores. These measurements are compared to established tables. Limitations to such tests include variability by the clinician performing the tests and the comparative standards; appropriate training to perform such tests is required (Jensen et al., 2012; Krzywda & Meyer, 2010).

NURSING FAST FACT!

Weight loss greater than 10% in any time period may be clinically significant (Krzywda & Meyer, 2014).

In simple starvation, 20% loss of body weight is associated with marked decreases in muscle tissue and subcutaneous fat, giving the patient an emaciated appearance. Gross loss of body fat can be observed not only from appearance but also by palpating a number of skinfolds. When the dermis can be felt between the fingers on pinching the triceps and biceps skinfolds, considerable loss from body stores of fat has occurred. Protein stores can be assessed by inspection and palpation of a number of muscle groups, such as the triceps, biceps, and subscapular and infrascapular muscles. The long muscles in particular are profoundly protein depleted when the tendons are prominent to palpation.

Laboratory Assessment

A number of tests are used to assess a patient's biochemical nutritional status. In the past, anergy testing was recommended for assessing immunological response involving the intradermal injection of antigens. This type of testing is no longer a standard in clinical assessment (Krzywda & Meyer, 2014).

Biochemical assessment reflects both the tissue level of a given nutrient and any abnormality of metabolism. Studies of serum protein, albumin, prealbumin, transferrin, retinol-binding protein, hemoglobin, serum vitamin A, carotene, and vitamin C can reflect the utilization of nutrients.

Serum Albumin and Transferrin Levels

Albumin is a major protein synthesized by the liver. Approximately 40% of protein mass is in the circulation. The serum albumin concentration is normally between 3.5 and 5.0 g/dL (Krzywda & Meyer, 2014). An albumin level of 2.8 to 3.4 g/dL represents mild protein depletion, 2.1 to 2.7 g/dL reflects moderate depletion, and less than 2.1 g/dL indicates severe depletion.

Serum transferrin is a beta globulin that transports iron in the plasma and is synthesized in the liver. Transferrin is present in the serum in concentrations from 250 to 300 mg/dL. The serum levels are affected by nutritional factors and iron metabolism. Levels lower than 100 mg/dL indicate severe depletion (Krzywda & Meyer, 2014).

 NURSING FAST FACT!

The half-life of albumin is about 20 days, meaning that changes in protein synthesis are reflected slowly; acute changes in nutrition are not reflected (Krzywda & Meyer, 2014).

Prealbumin and Retinol-Binding Protein

Prealbumin is required for thyroxine transport and as a carrier for retinol-binding protein. Normal serum concentration is 20 mg/dL. Levels from 10 to 20 mg/dL reflect mild depletion, 5 to 9 mg/dL reflect moderate depletion, and less than 5 mg/dL indicate severe depletion (Krzywda & Meyer, 2014). The half-life of prealbumin is 24 to 48 hours, so it is sensitive to acute changes and is a more accurate indicator of protein malnutrition during refeeding. Retinol-binding protein is another measurement of visceral protein status with normal values from 3 to 5 meq/L. It is a sensitive measure to very short-term changes in nutrition but because it is affected by stress and inflammation, the utility of retinol-binding protein is limited (Jensen et al., 2012).

Nitrogen Balance

A sensitive indicator of the body's gain or loss of protein is its nitrogen balance. A 24-hour urine collection can be analyzed for urine urea nitrogen to determine nitrogen balance. An adult is said to be in nitrogen equilibrium when the nitrogen intake from food equals the nitrogen output in urine, feces, and perspiration. The nitrogen balance is a measure of daily intake of nitrogen minus the excretion. It is used to assess protein turnover. A positive nitrogen balance indicates an anabolic state with an overall gain in body protein for the day. A negative nitrogen balance indicates a catabolic state with a net loss of protein.

 NURSING FAST FACT!

> *One gram of nitrogen is equivalent to 6.25 grams of protein. Nitrogen balance is measured by calculating total protein intake divided by 6.25 to obtain nitrogen grams, subtracting urinary nitrogen as measured by the 24-hour urine collection, and adding in factors for insensible and fecal losses. Accurate urine collection is required for this test.*

Other Laboratory Tests

Serum electrolyte levels provide information about fluid and electrolyte balance and kidney function. The creatinine/height index is an indicator of muscle depletion. It requires a 24-hour urine collection to determine urinary creatinine excretion and is calculated based on ideal urinary creatinine for the patient's sex and height. Serum levels of glucose, vitamins, trace elements, liver enzymes, and lipid levels may be monitored as well as coagulation studies and hemoglobin/hematocrit levels.

Energy Requirements

Energy requirements are dependent on a number of factors, which include the body surface area (derived from height and weight), age, and gender. Total daily energy expenditure has three components: (1) basal metabolic rate (BMR) or resting metabolic rate (RMR); (2) energy expenditure associated with activity; and (3) energy required for digestion (Wooley & Frankenfield, 2012). Determination of energy needs can be determined from the BMR (measured in a fasting state, immediately on awakening before any activity) or resting metabolic expenditure (measured in a fasting state but some activity allowed). The RMR accounts for 60% to 75% of energy expenditure and may be measured (calorimetry) or estimated. Estimates are most commonly used, and there are a number of equations that may be used. A traditional method used to estimate **basal energy expenditure (BEE)** is the Harris–Benedict equation, which takes into consideration the influence of the patient's weight in kilograms, height in centimeters, age, and gender. An easier and widely accepted method to estimate daily caloric requirements for adults is to use 20 to 35 calories/kg/day (Krzywda & Meyer, 2014).

Calorimetry

Calorimetry refers to the measurement of heat or energy metabolism. The BMR/RMR can be measured using indirect or direct calorimetry. Indirect calorimetry measures heat consumption through the measurement of oxygen consumption and carbon dioxide production and is considered the most accurate method for determining energy expenditure in critically ill patients (Wooley & Frankenfield, 2012). Hospitals must have access to a metabolic cart to measure RMR, and this tool remains underutilized because of the expense and clinical expertise required. Direct calorimetry measures heat produced by the body and is not used because of the expense and the cumbersome techniques required.

Physical Examination

A critical component of the nutritional assessment is a complete physical examination. Findings from a physical examination can reflect protein/calorie malnutrition along with vitamin and mineral deficiencies. The physical examination should include evaluation of the patient's hair, nails, skin, thorax and lungs, eyes, oral cavity, glands, heart, muscles, and abdomen, along with a neurological evaluation and evaluation of delayed healing and tissue repair (Table 12-2). The physical examination should also include objective measurements of wound healing, grip strength, skeletal muscle function, and respiratory muscle function.

> Table 12-2 | **PHYSICAL FINDINGS ASSOCIATED WITH DEFICIENCY STATES**

Area Assessed	Physical Findings	Nutrient Deficiencies
Hair	Dull, sparse, thinning	Protein, vitamin B_{12}, folate
	Hair easily pluckable	Protein, biotin, zinc
	Color change	Zinc
	Dry	Vitamins A and E
Nails	Thin, concave, spoon shaped	Iron
Skin	Dry, flaking	Vitamin A, essential fatty acid deficiency (EFAD)
	Follicular hyperkeratosis (like gooseflesh)	Vitamins A, C; essential fatty acids
	Desquamation	
	Petechiae	Riboflavin
	Hyperpigmentation on sun-exposed areas	Niacin
	Subcutaneous fat loss	Calorie
Eyes	Blepharitis	Riboflavin
	Bitot spots (small blemishes on conjunctiva)	Vitamin A
	Night vision difficulty	Vitamin A

Continued

> Table 12-2 | **PHYSICAL FINDINGS ASSOCIATED WITH DEFICIENCY STATES—cont'd**

Area Assessed	Physical Findings	Nutrient Deficiencies
Perioral	Glossitis (scarlet, raw)	Niacin, folate, vitamin B_{12}
	Magenta tongue	Riboflavin
	Swollen, bleeding gums, gingivitis	Vitamin C
	Painful, sensitive, tongue fissuring	B vitamin deficiency
Heart	Enlargement, tachycardia, high output failure	Thiamine ("wet" beriberi)
Abdomen	Hepatomegaly	Protein
Muscles, extremities	Muscle pain	Thiamine, ascorbic acid
	Edema	Protein, thiamine
	Muscle wastage (especially temporal area, dorsum of hand, spine)	Calorie
Bones, joints	Osteoporosis	Vitamin D, calcium, phosphorus
Neurologic	Cognitive decline, paresthesias, unsteadiness, confusion	Vitamin B_{12}, thiamine
Other	Delayed healing and tissue repair (e.g., wound, infarct, abscess)	Ascorbic acid, zinc, protein

NURSING FAST FACT!

Signs of nutritional deficiency are seen most often in skin, hair, eyes, and mouth (Krzywda & Meyer, 2014).

■ Nutritional Requirements/Parenteral Formulations: Adults

PN formulations are based on the patient's nutrient requirements. Basic formulas contain protein and nonprotein calories: carbohydrates and fat, along with electrolytes, vitamins, trace elements, and fluid requirements. Also included are essential macro- and micronutrients for adequate energy production, support of synthesis, replacement, and repair of structural or visceral proteins; cell structure; production of hormones and enzymes; and maintenance of immune function.

Fluid Requirements

Basic fluid requirements for maintenance are 30 to 35 mL/kg/day or 1500 mL for the first 20 kg plus 20 mL/kg for actual weight beyond 20 kg

(Krzywda & Meyer, 2014). Factors that may increase fluid needs are significant fluid losses, as occurs with diarrhea or the presence of an enterocutaneous fistula.

Proteins/Amino Acids

Proteins are required for **anabolism**, that is, for tissue growth and repair and replacement of body cells. Proteins are also components in antibodies, scar tissue, and clots. **Amino acids** are the basic units of protein. There are eight essential amino acids needed by adults that must be supplied in the diet: isoleucine, leucine, lysine, methionine, phenylalanine, threonine, tryptophan, and valine. There are also nonessential amino acids; these amino acids can be synthesized by the body and include alanine, aspartic acid, asparagine, glutamic acid, glycine, proline, and serine. Conditionally essential amino acids required in the diet during certain disease states include histidine, cysteine, tyrosine, arginine, and glutamine.

Protein in PN is provided as synthetic crystalline amino acids. They are available in concentrations of 3% to 20%, with and without electrolytes. There are also specialty amino acid formulations that may be used with certain disease states, such as hepatic encephalopathy and renal failure; however, these products are more expensive and improvement of outcome with their use has not been well demonstrated (Krzywda & Meyer, 2014).

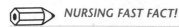 NURSING FAST FACT!

Protein requirement for maintenance of healthy adults is 0.8 to 1 g/kg/day.
Catabolic patients require 1.2 to 2 g/kg/day.
Chronic renal failure patients require 1.5 to 1.8 g/kg/day.
Acute renal failure + catabolic state patients require 1.5 to 1.8 g/kg/day
Critically ill patients require 2.0 g/kg/day (Krzywda & Meyer, 2014).

Carbohydrates

Carbohydrates are the major source for energy and also spare body protein. When glucose is supplied as a nutrient, it is stored temporarily in the liver and muscle as glycogen. When glycogen storage capacity is reached, the excess carbohydrate is stored as fat. Carbohydrate types include dextrose (glucose), fructose, sorbitol and xylitol, and glycerol. There is not a specific requirement for carbohydrates; rather, needs are determined based on estimations of energy requirements. Carbohydrates generally provide about 50% of total calories.

NURSING FAST FACT!

- *Carbohydrates provide 3.4 calories/g.*
- *Excessive dextrose intake can lead to increased production of carbon dioxide, which can cause respiratory failure.*
- *Hepatic dysfunction may occur from excessive dextrose intake as a result of increased synthesis and fat storage in the liver.*

Dextrose is the most commonly used source of carbohydrate in PN solutions and is commercially available in concentrations from 5% to 70%. In addition to caloric need, considerations in the amount and concentration of glucose are based on respiratory, cardiac, renal, and fluid volume status. Table 12-3 provides a list of dextrose solutions, osmolarity, and kcal/L.

Dextrose may be administered with amino acids as the only nonprotein source of calories or administered in conjunction with lipids. When PN is administered peripherally, the final concentration of dextrose must be 10% or less to prevent vein irritation, damage to the vein, and thrombosis. Hypertonic concentrations of 10% and above must be administered through a central vascular access device (CVAD). Of note, glycerol is another carbohydrate that is available for use in **peripheral parenteral nutrition (PPN)** formulas, although it is not well studied.

INS Standard PN solutions containing final concentrations exceeding 10% dextrose should be administered through a CVAD with the tip located in the central vasculature (Infusion Nurses Society [INS], 2011, p. S91).

Fats

Fat is a primary source of heat and energy. Fat provides twice as many energy calories per gram as either protein or carbohydrate. When fat is used to supply a portion of calories, less dextrose is required. In patients with glucose intolerance, this may be beneficial.

> Table 12-3 **DEXTROSE SOLUTIONS FOR PARENTERAL NUTRITION**

Solution (%)	g/L	kcal/L	mOsm/L
5	50	170	252
10	100	340	505
20	200	680	1010
30	300	1020	1515
40	400	1360	2020
50	500	1700	2525
60	600	2040	3030
70	700	2380	3535

Fat is essential for the structural integrity of all cell membranes. Linoleic acid and linolenic acid are the only fatty acids essential to humans and are required to prevent essential fatty acid deficiency (EFAD). These two acids prevent **essential fatty acid deficiency (EFAD)**. Linoleic acid is the primary essential fatty acid and is required for growth. Linolenic acid may not be necessary for adults but may be needed for proper visual and neural development in infants and young children and with certain diseases (Krzywda & Meyer, 2014). Signs and symptoms of EFAD include desquamating dermatitis, alopecia, brittle nails, delayed wound healing, thrombocytopenia, decreased immunity, and increased capillary fragility.

NOTE > EFAD can occur in as few as 5 days without fat supplementation (Krzywda & Meyer, 2014).

Intravenous Fat Emulsion Administration

When fat or lipids are used as a calorie source in PN, there are fewer problems with glucose homeostasis, carbon dioxide (CO_2) production is lower, and hepatic tolerance to I.V. feedings may improve. Primarily, intravenous fats are supplied by safflower or soybean oil, with egg yolk phospholipids and glycerol to provide tonicity. Fat emulsions provide 1.1 kcal/mL (10% solution) or 2.0 kcal/mL (20% solution) (Gahart & Nazareno, 2012). Lipids may be administered as a separate infusion, concurrently with the amino acid/dextrose solution via a Y tubing, or as part of a total nutrient admixture (discussed later). Of note, all fat emulsion products are isotonic, have a pH between 6 and 9, and can be administered via a peripheral vein (Gahart & Nazareno, 2012).

NOTE > A 30% fat emulsion is available but is never given by direct I.V. infusion; rather, it is used by the pharmacy in admixtures (Gahart & Nazareno, 2012).

 NURSING FAST FACT!

- *1 g of fat = 9 kcal*
- *Use of fat for a portion of the calories in the PN solution will allow for a decrease in dextrose and may improve glucose management in stress states.*

In patients with respiratory failure, the use of fat as a part of the total calories allows for a decrease in glucose calories and therefore may decrease carbon dioxide production. The primary purpose of fat emulsions in patients with PN is to prevent or treat EFAD. To prevent EFAD, approximately 250 mL of 20% or 500 mL of 10% lipid emulsions is required twice per week or 500 mL of 20% lipids once per week (Kumpf & Gervasio, 2012).

Lipids are extracted from administration sets that contain di(2-ethylhexyl) phthalate (DEHP) plasticizers; therefore, non-DEHP administration sets that are available with most commercially available products are used. Lipids may be supplied in glass containers or special non–polyvinyl chloride (non-PVC) bags (Fig. 12-1).

 NURSING FAST FACT!

> The initial rate of fat emulsions should be 1 mL/min or 0.1 g of fat/min for the first 15 to 30 minutes of the infusion for a 10% solution; if no untoward effects, the rate can be increased to 2 mL/min. For 20% solution, 0.5 mL/min or 0.1 g of fat/min for the first 15 to 30 minutes; if no untoward effect, the rate can be increased to 1mL/min (Gahart & Nazareno, 2012).

INS Standard Administration sets used to administer lipid-based infusates should be free of DEHP (INS, 2011, p. S56).

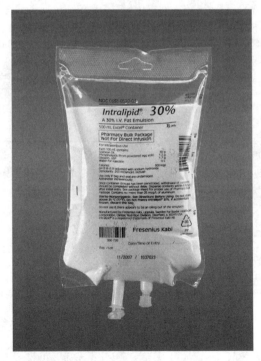

Figure 12-1 ▪ Example of fat emulsion (intralipid 30%). (Courtesy of Baxter Healthcare Corp., Round Lake, IL.)

Electrolytes

Electrolytes may be given either in a premixed PN formula or adjusted based on the patient's status. Standard ranges for parenteral electrolytes assume normal organ function and normal losses. Electrolytes are available in several salt forms and are added or adjusted based on the patient's metabolic status. The electrolytes necessary for long-term PN include sodium, potassium, magnesium, calcium, chloride, and phosphorus. Potassium is needed for the transport of glucose and amino acids across cell membranes. The basic requirement for potassium is approximately 1 to 2 mEq/kg of potassium per day. Potassium may be given as potassium chloride, potassium phosphate, or potassium acetate salt. Serum potassium levels must be closely monitored during PN administration. (See Chapter 3 for a review of the physiological roles of electrolytes.)

 NURSING FAST FACT!

Patients with impaired renal function may need a decreased amount of potassium.

Standard daily requirements for electrolytes included in PN solutions include:

- Sodium: 1–2 mEq /kg
- Potassium: 1–2 mEq /kg
- Phosphorous: 20–40 mmol
- Magnesium: 8–20 mEq
- Calcium: 10–15 mEq
- Chloride/acetate: As needed based on acid–base status (Barber & Sacks, 2012).

Vitamins

Vitamins are necessary for growth and maintenance, as well as for multiple metabolic processes. Vitamins cannot be synthesized by the body and must be provided in the diet. Fat-soluble vitamins are vitamins A, D, E, and K. Water-soluble vitamins include vitamin C and the B complex vitamins: thiamine (B_1), riboflavin (B_2), niacin (B_3), pantothenic acid (B_5), pyridoxine (B_6), biotin (B_7), folic acid (B_9), and cyanocobalamin (B_{12}). Vitamin supplements are added to the PN formulation. There are commercially available multivitamin products. There are daily recommendations for I.V. vitamin requirements established by the American Medical Association (Krzywda & Meyer, 2014).

Trace Elements

Trace elements are micronutrients found in the body in minute amounts. Basic requirements are very small, measured in milligrams. Each trace element is a single chemical and has an associated deficiency state. The functions of trace elements are often synergistic. Trace elements commonly used in PN solutions include:

- Zinc: RNA, DNA, and protein synthesis; important to wound healing
- Copper: Works with iron to form red blood cells
- Chromium: Potentiates insulin reactions
- Manganese: Antioxidant protection; involved in enzyme reactions; carbohydrate synthesis
- Selenium: Catalyst in an important antioxidant pathway (Krzywda & Meyer, 2014).

NOTE > Iron is not included as a component in the PN solution; it is administered as a separate infusion when needed.

Medication Administration with Parenteral Nutrition

PN solutions are complex, and the potential for physicochemical interactions exists with drug–nutrient combinations. Potential interactions between drugs and the nutrients in the solution include physical changes such as precipitation, altered viscosity of the solution, changes in consistency, clumping or curdling of the solution, and loss of drug activity or toxicity (Rollins, 2012). Medications that are generally compatible with and may be added to PN include insulin, heparin, and histamine receptor agonists (e.g., famotidine and ranitidine). Histamine receptor agonists are used to decrease gastric acid secretion and reduce risk for stress ulcers.

Hyperglycemia is a frequent complication of PN. It is caused by the high concentration of glucose in the PN solutions and altered glucose metabolism associated with stress and disease. Insulin aids in adequate metabolism of carbohydrates. It is chemically stable in PN and is often added to the solution. However, insulin can be adsorbed into the plastic solution container, the administration set, and the filter, so doses often need to be increased until blood glucose (BG) control is achieved. (Adsorption is addressed in Chapters 5 and 10.)

Heparin may be added to reduce the risk of thrombotic problems with the I.V. catheter, to reduce the frequency and severity of phlebitis with PPN, and to improve the clearance of fat emulsions from the bloodstream (INS, 2011, p. S92; Krzywda & Meyer, 2014).

Compatibility is always an issue whenever two agents are combined. Stability of the admixed component dictates the appropriate length of time that the solution may be stored before use.

INS Standard Medications added to PN solutions prior to administration of the solution should be assessed for compatibility in compliance with pharmacy rules and regulations (INS, 2011, p. S92).

 NURSING FAST FACT!

- *Always check current information about drug compatibility with PN solutions.*
- *Medications should not be "piggybacked" directly into PN solutions.*
- *Only regular insulin is appropriate for I.V. administration.*

Parenteral Nutrition Compounding

PN solutions must be prepared and stored safety and accurately according to regulations established by the United States Pharmacopeia (USP) <797> entitled "Pharmaceutical Compounding: Sterile Preparations" (Ukleja et al., 2010). It is the responsibility of the dispensing pharmacist to assure that PN is prepared, labeled, controlled, stored, dispensed, and distributed properly. Compounding of an accurate solution that is free of microbial and particulate matter is essential to the process (Barber & Sacks, 2012).

Automated or manual methods of PN compounding are available (Fig. 12-2). Most compounding PN formulations are classified by USP as medium-risk level because of the multiple injections, detachments, and attachments of nutrient source products to be delivered into a final sterile container. They may become high risk when any added component is high risk (e.g., adding compounded l-glutamine to the solution) (Barber & Sacks, 2012). Because of the risk, PN solutions are prepared in compounding rooms that must meet certain conditions, and pharmacy personnel must wear protective equipment such as gloves, masks, and hair/shoe covers during the compounding process.

 NURSING FAST FACT!

The USP Chapter <797> Pharmaceutical Compounding: Sterile Preparations (2008) details the procedures and requirements for compounding sterile preparations and sets standards that are applicable to all practice settings in which sterile preparations are compounded. These standards have been widely adopted, are enforced by many state boards of pharmacy, and may be used by accreditation organizations (e.g., The Joint Commission) in surveys.

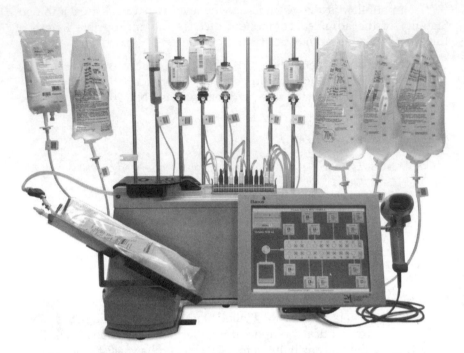

Figure 12-2 ■ Automated method of compounding parenteral nutrition. (Courtesy of Baxter Healthcare Corp., Round Lake, IL.)

■ Delivery of Nutritional Support

Nutritional Support Candidates

Patients who are candidates for nutritional support are those who suffer from a multiplicity of problems. Their clinical course can be complicated by malnutrition and depletion of body protein (Fig. 12-3). Enteral nutrition is the preferred route of nutrition support.

Indications for PN include patients who cannot meet their nutritional needs with enteral nutrition and already are or have the potential for becoming malnourished (Mirtallo & Patel, 2012). PN may be given via a peripheral I.V. catheter for short-term situations up to 2 weeks and when central vascular access is not feasible, or via a CVAD for long-term feeding (over 2 weeks), when peripheral access is limited, and/or when nutrient needs are large (Mirtallo & Patel, 2012). Examples of diagnoses associated with a need for PN include paralytic ileus, mesenteric ischemia, small bowel obstruction, and enterocutaneous fistulas.

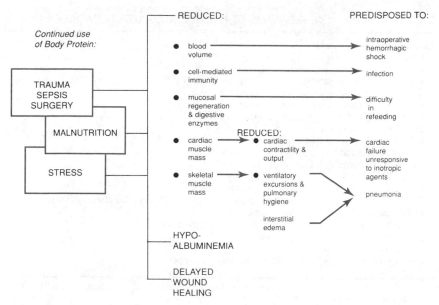

Figure 12-3 ■ Body protein depletion.

Parenteral Nutrition Orders

Life-threatening errors are possible when preparing and delivering PN admixtures to patients. Some factors associated with the PN prescribing errors include:

- Inadequate knowledge of PN therapy
- Lack of knowledge related to patient characteristics pertinent to PN (e.g., age, impaired renal function)
- Calculation of PN dosages
- Specialized PN dosage formulation characteristics and prescribing nomenclature (Mirtallo et al., 2004)

Criteria that must be included in the PN order form are listed in Table 12-4.

Nutritional Support Delivery Methods

Routes for delivery of nutritional support include the enteral and the intravenous routes. The enteral route is the preferred feeding route when the GI tract is functioning. Intravenous nutritional support may be administered via the peripheral or central veins. Fig. 12-4 shows an algorithm for determining the choice of nutritional support.

> Table 12-4	COMPONENTS OF PARENTERAL NUTRITION ORDER FORM

Mandatory Components
  Clarity of the form
  Contact number for person writing the order
  Contact number for assistance with parenteral nutrition (PN) ordering
  Time by which orders need to be received for processing
  Location of venous access device (central or peripheral)
  Height, weight/dosing weight, diagnosis, PN indication
  Hang time guidelines
  Institutional policy for infusion rates
  Information regarding potential incompatibilities
Strongly Recommended Components
  Educational tools
  Guidelines to assist in nutrient/volume calculations
  Recommended PN laboratory tests (baseline, monitoring, special circumstances)
  Guidelines for stopping/interrupting PN
  Contents of multivitamin and trace element preparations
  Brand names of products (e.g., amino acids, IVFE)
  Guidelines for use of insulin
  Guidelines for recognizing additional calorie sources

Source: Mirtallo et al., Journal of Parenteral and Enteral Nutrition 28(6), p. S44. Copyright 2004. Reprinted by permission of SAGE Publications.

Enteral Nutrition

Enteral nutrition (i.e., tube feeding) is indicated for patients with a functional GI tract when oral nutrient intake is insufficient to meet needs. Options for enteral access devices include nasoenteric tubes for short-term use and long-term devices such as gastrostomy, jejunostomy, and gastrojejunostomy tubes. In addition to anticipated duration of need, access device selection is also based on the patient's disease state, GI anatomy and function, and ability to safely access the GI tract via radiological, surgical, or endoscopic techniques (Ukleja et al., 2010).

Advantages of enteral access include the following:

1. Maintenance of the functional integrity of the GI tract
2. Efficient utilization of nutrients
3. Ease and safety of administration
4. Lower cost compared to PN

Disadvantages/risks include:

1. Contraindications, which include severe short gut syndrome, severe GI malabsorption, severe GI bleed, high-output fistulas, intractable vomiting and/or diarrhea, paralytic ileus
2. Gastric feedings that require adequate gastric emptying; gastric residuals are used to monitor the safety and effectiveness of tube feedings
3. Risk for aspiration
4. Tube placement issues

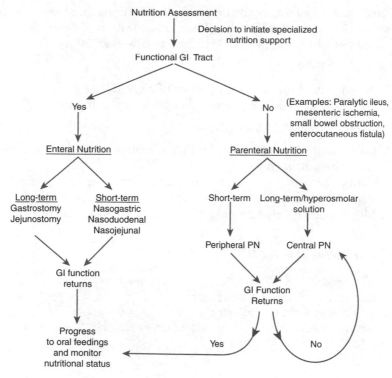

Nutrition Assessment

Decision to initiate specialized
nutrition support

Functional GI Tract

Yes

No

(Examples: Paralytic ileus,
mesenteric ischemia,
small bowel obstruction,
enterocutaneous fistula)

Enteral Nutrition

Parenteral Nutrition

Long-term
Gastrostomy
Jejunostomy

Short-term
Nasogastric
Nasoduodenal
Nasojejunal

Short-term   Long-term/hyperosmolar
solution

Peripheral PN   Central PN

GI function
returns

GI Function
Returns

Progress
to oral feedings
and monitor
nutritional status

Yes

No

Figure 12-4 ■ Routes to deliver nutritional support to adults. This clinical decision algorithm outlines the selection process for choosing the route of nutritional support in adult patients. Major considerations for selecting the feeding route and nutritional support formula include gastrointestinal function, expected duration of nutritional therapy, aspiration risk, and the potential for or actual development of organ dysfunction.

5. GI alterations resulting from the feeding: Diarrhea, constipation, metabolic alterations
6. Feeding tubes, which develop mechanical complications, especially clogging (Brantley & Mills, 2012).

Peripheral Parenteral Nutrition

PPN is used to nourish patients who either already are malnourished or have the potential for developing malnutrition and who are not candidates for enteral nutrition. Patients who are candidates for PPN must meet the criteria of (1) good peripheral I.V. access and (2) able to tolerate large volumes of fluid, up to 3 L/day. PPN is considered a controversial therapy; some believe that the risks of PPN outweigh the benefits because candidates for this therapy have minor nutritional deficits (Mirtallo & Patel, 2012).

Prolonged infusions should be limited to solutions that are lower than 600 mOsm/L. No greater than 10% final concentration of dextrose should be infused peripherally (INS, 2011; Krzywda & Meyer, 2014).

ADVANTAGES OF PPN

1. Avoids insertion and maintenance of a CVAD.
2. Has reduced risk of metabolic complications compared to PN.

DISADVANTAGES/LIMITATIONS OF PPN

1. Contraindications include significant malnutrition, compromised renal/hepatic status.
2. Cannot be used in volume-restricted patients because higher volumes of solution are needed to provide adequate calories.
3. May cause phlebitis because of high solution osmolarity.

 NURSING FAST FACT!

A standardized ordering sheet is used to specify the protein, calories, and electrolyte content of each solution tailored to the client. Standard PPN includes the following basic formula: final concentration of dextrose 5% to 10%; final concentration of amino acids 3% acids; electrolytes, trace elements, and vitamins. Lipids may be included in the formula.

INS Standard PN solutions in final concentrations of 10% dextrose or lower administered via a short peripheral catheter or midline catheter should be reserved for situations in which a CVAD is not currently feasible and delay of feeding would be detrimental to the patient (INS, 2011, p. S92).

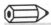 *NURSING FAST FACT!*

Assess for an appropriate peripheral catheter for delivery of PPN. A midline catheter should be considered for PPN anticipated to last longer than 6 days (O'Grady et al., 2011); however, the risk of thrombophlebitis is not eliminated with a midline catheter.

Parenteral Nutrition via a Central Vein

PN via central vein (often called total parenteral nutrition [TPN]) is used to provide nutrients at greater concentrations and fluid volumes than is possible with PPN. Central vascular access can be maintained for prolonged periods (weeks to years) with a variety of catheters (e.g., peripherally inserted central catheter [PICC]) (see Chapter 8). The PN formula may be administered with the lipids mixed together with dextrose/amino acid components (total nutrient admixture; addressed in next section), or the lipids may be administered as a separate intermittent infusion.

PN solutions infused through a central vein are highly concentrated. Final concentrations of standard PN solutions include 4.25% amino acids, 25% dextrose along with electrolytes, trace elements, and vitamins. PN is usually administered at rates of no more than 200 mL/hr.

The delivery of centrally delivered PN involves both advantages and disadvantages.

ADVANTAGES

- Dextrose solution of 20% to 70% can be administered as a calorie source.
- Is beneficial for long-term use (usually longer than 2 weeks).
- Large caloric and nutrient needs can be met.
- Provides calories; restores nitrogen balance; and replaces essential vitamins, electrolytes, and minerals.
- Promotes tissue synthesis, wound healing, and normal metabolic function.
- Improves tolerance to surgery.
- Is nutritionally complete.

DISADVANTAGES

- Requires placement of a CVAD.
- May cause metabolic complications, including glucose intolerance, electrolyte imbalances, and EFAD.
- Fat emulsions may not be used effectively in some severely stressed patients (especially burn patients).
- Potential complications related to CVADs (see Chapter 9).

 NURSING FAST FACT!

> Because of the high dextrose content in PN, it is an ideal medium for microbial growth. Historically, the recommendation has been to use a designated lumen of the CVAD for PN administration as an infection prevention strategy. This is now considered an unresolved issue (insufficient evidence/lack of consensus for efficacy) by the CDC (O'Grady et al., 2011). It is important to review and follow organizational policies regarding TPN administration.

PRACTICE CRITERIA FOR PN

- PN should be delivered through a CVAD as defined by the catheter tip located in the superior vena cava.
- Verification of catheter tip placement must be obtained before use of the catheter.
- The central line bundle interventions are followed during CVAD insertion (see Chapter 2).

Total Nutrient Admixtures (Three-in-One Admixtures)

Total nutrient admixtures (TNAs) are PN solutions containing dextrose, amino acids, and fat emulsions in one large solution container. TNAs are often referred to as "all-in-one solutions" or "three-in-one solutions" (3-in-1 solutions). The solution is compounded in the pharmacy and is usually milky white and opaque, although a faint yellow hue may be evident with the addition of vitamins. "Multichamber bags" are often used in home infusion. This is defined as a container designed to promote extended stability of the PN formulation by separating some components (e.g., intravenous fat emulsion) from the rest of the formulation. It consists of two or more chambers separated by a seal or tubing that is clamped (Fig. 12-5). At the time of administration, the seal or clamp is opened to allow the contents of the chambers to mix and create an admixture (A.S.P.E.N. Board of Directors and Clinical Practice Committee, 2012).

TNA solutions offer some important advantages, including the following:

- All components compounded aseptically in the pharmacy
- Less manipulation during administration and less risk of contamination (compared to administering lipids as a separate infusion)
- Less nursing time required

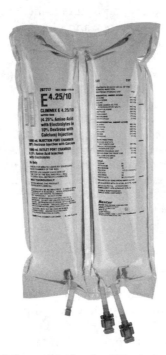

Figure 12-5 ■ Multichamber PN solution container.

- Less supply and equipment expense (e.g., one infusion pump and administration set)
- Dextrose and venous access tolerance in some cases
- May be more cost effective
- Improved fat clearance when administered over more than 12 hours (Barber & Sacks, 2012)

Disadvantages may include less solution stability and risk for separation of lipids, difficulty in visualizing precipitate or particulate matter in the solution, more risk for drug-nutrient incompatibilities, and increased risk for catheter occlusion over time (Barber & Sacks, 2012).

Total nutrient admixtures must be administered through a 1.2-micron filter because of the risk of particulate matter (Fig. 12-6). Although bacterial contaminants such as *Staphylococcus epidermidis* and *Escherichia coli* will not be filtered out, large organisms such as *Candida albicans* will be trapped by the 1.2-micron filter (Barber & Sacks, 2012). The stability of TNA is affected by many factors, including admixture contents, storage time and conditions, addition of non-nutrient drugs, pH of the solution, and variability in temperature.

 NURSING FAST FACT!

Examine the solution for signs of instability before hanging the bag and periodically throughout administration. Monitor the TNA infusion for physical or chemical phenomena, which may occur with TNA solutions before administration and include:

a. Aggregation (stratification): Rare white "streaks," which are an early stage of creaming. It is not harmful to the patient.

b. Creaming: Dense white color at top of solution ("cream") layer. Reverses with gentle agitation and is not harmful. Creaming that reappears in 1 to 2 hours may indicate an unstable emulsion.

c. Chemical phenomena ("oiling" or "cracking" of the solution): Oil globules on the surface of creamed emulsion fuse and form larger oil droplets. This is irreversible; it cannot be dispersed, and the solution should not be administered. If started, it must be immediately stopped.

Cyclic Parenteral Nutrition

For patients requiring long-term PN support, cyclic PN is widely used. This therapy delivers the PN solution over a reduced time frame between 8 and 16 hours, versus a 24-hour continuous infusion. **Cyclic parenteral nutrition** is indicated for patients who have been stable on continuous PN and require long-term PN; for those receiving home PN; for patients who can handle total infusion volume in a shortened time period; and for patients who require PN for only a portion of their nutritional needs (Krzywda & Meyer, 2014).

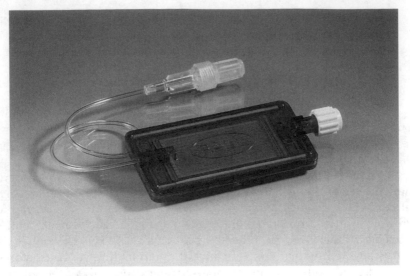

Figure 12-6 ■ Lipopor™ TNA filter set for total nutrient admixture administration with 1.2 micron air- and particle-eliminating filter. (Provided compliments of Pall Corporation. Copyright Pall Corporation, 2013.)

Patients are transitioned to cyclic parenteral nutrition once they are stable on a 24-hour continuous infusion. The hourly rate of PN infusion is increased as the number of infusion hours is decreased. Because of the increased fluid volume and increased glucose delivery over less time, the patient is monitored carefully for signs of fluid volume excess and hyperglycemia. Symptoms of excess fluid administration should be monitored, such as weight gain resulting in edema or infusion-related shortness of breath. If too much fluid is administered during the cyclic period, the time frame should be extended.

Cyclic PN administration requires twice as many central line manipulations as continuous PN because of the initiation of the infusion and the discontinuation of the infusion every 24 hours. This increases the risk of introducing bacteria via the internal catheter lumen and thus the risk for bloodstream infection.

ADVANTAGES

1. Allows for more physiological hormonal response and appetite stimulation because of periods of time without infusion
2. Prevents or treats hepatotoxicity induced by continuous PN; reverses fatty liver and liver enzyme elevations; faster albumin level recovery (Krzywda & Meyer, 2014)
3. For patients on long-term PN, improved quality of life by encouraging normal daytime activities and enhances psychological well-being; patient does not need to carry around an infusion pump

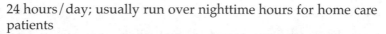

24 hours/day; usually run over nighttime hours for home care patients

DISADVANTAGES

1. Patients must be observed for symptoms of hypoglycemia, hyperglycemia, dehydration, excessive fluid administration, and sepsis associated with central-line manipulation.
2. Patients require monitoring for hyperglycemia, which can develop during the peak flow rate (>250 mg/dL). Inability to control BG levels may require a change back to continuous PN.
3. There is also a risk for hypoglycemia generally during the first hour after cyclic PN discontinuation. BG levels should be checked whenever the patient displays symptoms of nausea, tremors, sweating, anxiety, or lethargy. Tapering the infusion rate for 1 to 2 hours at the end of the infusion may be needed (Winkler, Hagan, & Albina, 2012; Krzywda & Meyer, 2014).

 NURSING FAST FACT!

- *Cyclic PN is indicated for long-term PN.*
- *The patient's cardiovascular status must be able to accommodate large fluid volume during the infusion period.*
- *For patients without complications such as glucose intolerance or a precarious fluid balance, a 12-hour cycling regimen can be used.*

EBP A systematic literature review was conducted to evaluate the metabolic effects of cyclic PN in adults and children. Twenty-five studies were included in the review. When cyclic was compared to continuous infusion, the results included similar nitrogen balance. For patients on continuous PN, converting to a cyclic regimen can stabilize hepatic function tests. Risks include hyper-/hypoglycemia with abrupt initiation/discontinuation of the cyclic infusion; tapering the rate is helpful. The researchers concluded that there is a favorable risk–benefit profile of cyclic PN in most patients (Stout & Cober, 2010).

Specialized Parenteral Formulas

Some parenteral formulas are specifically designed to meet the needs of patients with certain disease states. Although current clinical evidence does not support improved outcomes with specialty formulas, they may be used in limited circumstances (Barber & Sacks, 2012). The following are some special formulas developed for the patient with renal, hepatic, and special metabolic stress needs.

RENAL FORMULAS

Specialty PN formulations used in renal failure are composed mainly of essential amino acids and are based on a theory that nonessential amino acids can be recycled from urea (Barber & Sacks, 2012). It is believed that these formulas do not offer significant advantages and that indications for these special formulations are limited. Examples of commercial preparations include Aminess, Aminosyn-RF, and NephrAmine (Gahart & Nazareno, 2012). Consideration to fluid restriction is also important in patients with renal disease.

HEPATIC FORMULAS

Protein/calorie malnutrition and nutritional deficiencies are common in hepatic diseases. Altered amino acid metabolism is a hallmark of hepatic disease, characterized by low levels of circulating branched-chain amino acid (BCAA) and elevated levels of circulating aromatic amino acids. Solutions high in BCAAs are designed for hepatic disease. Most commonly, these formulas are limited to patients with encephalopathy. The administration formulas high in BCAAs would seem to be beneficial; however, as with formulas for renal failure, controversy exists (Barber & Sacks, 2012). Examples of commercial preparations include HepatAmine and Hepatosol (Gahart & Nazareno, 2012).

Stress Formulas

Patients with severe metabolic stress, as occurs with infection, sepsis, and the trauma of burns, surgery, shock, and blunt or penetrating injuries, have increased breakdown of skeletal muscle (**catabolism**) and may require increased protein to meet increased nutritional needs. High metabolic stress formulas, which are similar to hepatic formulas, are available for this patient population. This group of patients has a predilection to break down BCAAs in muscles. Examples of stress formulas include Aminosyn-HBC, BranchAmine, FreAmine HBC, and Novamine 15% (Barber & Sacks, 2012; Gahart & Nazareno, 2012).

■ Parenteral Nutrition Administration

Vascular Access

As previously discussed, the proper selection of vascular access (central vs. peripheral) depends on the type of PN formula. The hypertonic nature of PN requires the placement of a CVAD for administration. PN may be administered via any type of CVAD: nontunneled, PICC, subcutaneously tunneled, or vascular access port. PPN is administered via a short peripheral catheter or a midline peripheral catheter.

> **NOTE** > Care of peripheral I.V. catheters is addressed in Chapter 6, and care of CVADs is discussed in Chapter 8.

Medical Equipment

Filters

The use of filters is recommended during the administration of PN formulations. Use of a 0.22-micron filter for PN administration can remove microorganisms, but this practice is limited to use with lipid-free formulas. PN formulas with lipids (i.e., TNAs) require the use of a 1.2-micron filter (see also Chapter 5 for a discussion and illustrations of filters).

 NURSING FAST FACT!

PN formulations are considered high-risk admixtures and can become contaminated during compounding or administration setup.

Catheter Locking

The use of ethanol to lock the CVAD rather than heparin (or saline) may be considered because its use is associated with a decreased rate of bloodstream infections (Huang et al., 2011; Maiefski, Rupp, & Hermsen, 2009; Oliveira, Nasr, Brindle, & Wales, 2012). Ethanol is an antiseptic with bactericidal and fungicidal activity against a broad range of microorganisms (Maiefski et al., 2009). Because there are conflicting data about the effect ethanol may have on polyurethane CVADs, recommendations are for use with silicone catheters.

Because patients receiving PN are at increased risk for bloodstream infection, antimicrobial drug locking (e.g., dilute vancomycin heparin solution) may be considered. However, the CDC (O'Grady et al., 2011) recommends its use only in patients who have long-term CVADs and a history of repeated bloodstream infections despite optimal aseptic technique.

Administration Sets and Infusion Pumps

There are specific recommendations to guide the use of PN administration tubing sets. PN administration sets shall be changed using aseptic technique. If any add-on devices (e.g., extension sets) are used, they are changed with each administration set change. INS standards in relation to administration set changes are as follows (INS, 2011, p. S56):

- PN with lipids (i.e., total nutrient admixture): Administration set (and solution container) is changed every 24 hours.

- PN without lipids: Administration set is routinely changed no more often than every 96 hours.
- Intermittent infusions of fat emulsions: Administration set is changed with each new container unless additional units of fat emulsions are administered consecutively; then administration sets can be changed every 24 hours.

Another important issue related to administration sets and containers used with lipid-based infusions is that they should be DEHP free. DEHP is a toxin, is lipophilic, and is extracted into the solution with commonly used PVC administration sets and containers (INS, 2011, p. S56). This issue is also discussed in Chapter 5.

PN is always administered using an electronic infusion device (EID) with free-flow protection (INS, 2011, p. S91). Infusion pumps are addressed in Chapter 5.

Practice Criteria for Administration of Parenteral Nutrition

Establish Goals

Once it is determined that the individual will receive PN, goals for nutritional support should be set with specific markers and outcomes to be measured (Ukleja et al., 2010). Goals should address energy and nutrient requirements and intake goals, route for nutritional support, and short- and long-term measureable goals.

Examples of patient goals include:

1. Normalization of laboratory values
2. Increase, or decrease, in weight (amount specified)
3. Wound healing
4. Improvement in functional status

Monitoring

The monitoring of patients receiving PN consists of assessment of the clinical and therapeutic response to the PN regimen. Assessment focuses on nutritional status, progress toward nutritional goals as discussed earlier, and anticipating and monitoring for potential complications as discussed in the next section. Specific areas for monitoring identified by A.S.P.E.N. (Ukleja et al., 2010) are physical assessment, functional status, vital signs, actual intake (oral, I.V., enteral), weight, medication reviews, and changes in GI function. Monitoring of laboratory data is also important. Laboratory testing is more frequent when PN is initiated and then is decreased in frequency as clinically indicated. Also, regular assessment and meticulous care of the VAD and infusion system are important.

NURSING POINTS OF CARE
ADMINISTRATION OF PARENTERAL NUTRITION

Focus Assessment
- History of weight changes
- Dietary intake
- History of diseases/surgeries
- Identification of allergies
- Medications including over-the-counter and herbal products
- Vital signs
- Neurological status including level of consciousness
- Assessment of skin, hair, nails, oral cavity
- Intake and output
- Before initiation of nutritional support, determination of baseline serum BG levels, serum albumin, total protein, electrolyte, and chemistry profile
- Assessment for most appropriate VAD based on PN formula; hypertonic solutions require a CVAD

Key Nursing Interventions
1. Assist with insertion of central line, or insert if competent, as appropriate for therapy.
2. Insert short peripheral or midline catheter per agency protocol for PPN.
3. Ascertain correct tip placement of CVAD before beginning PN.
4. Adhere to proper hand hygiene, aseptic technique, and standard precautions when caring for VAD and when performing infusions.
5. Maintain VAD patency and site care/dressing changes per agency protocol (at least every 7 days when using a transparent dressing; every 2 days when using gauze dressings).
6. Monitor
   a. VAD-related complications: Pay particular attention to phlebitis/infiltration with peripheral I.V. catheters; risk for bloodstream infection with all VADs
   b. Daily weights
   c. Intake and output
   d. Serum albumin, total protein, electrolyte, glucose, chemistry profile
   e. Vital signs
   f. BG every 6 hours
      - Adult hospitalized patients: Serum glucose should be maintained between 140 and 180 mg/dL (McMahon et al., 2013).

Continued

- Home care patients: Attempt to keep under 150 mg/dL (Krzywda & Meyer, 2014).

7. Check the label of the PN solution and ensure that it matches the orders before hanging each solution container.
8. The hang time of a PN solution container should never exceed 24 hours.
9. Use an EID to administer PN solutions.
10. Change administration sets every 96 hours for fat-free PN solutions and every 24 hours for TNAs. For IVFE administered separately, discard administration set after each infusion.
11. Use a 0.22-micron filter for fat-free PN solutions and a 1.2-micron filter for TNAs.
12. Administer insulin as ordered to maintain BG in the ordered range.
13. Report abnormal signs and symptoms associated with PN to the physician and modify care accordingly.
14. Observe for signs and symptoms of electrolyte imbalance (see Chapter 3 for a review of signs and symptoms).

◼ Complications Associated With Parenteral Nutrition

Complications associated with PN are divided into three categories: (1) vascular access device (VAD)-related complications, (2) metabolic, and (3) nutritional (Table 12-5). (See Chapter 9 for a thorough discussion of VAD-related complications.) When administering PPN, there is risk for phlebitis and infiltration. As with any CVAD, risks include pneumothorax, air embolism (during insertion and during maintenance of the device), venous thrombosis, catheter occlusion, malposition, and infection. Of note, PN administration is a well-known risk factor for bloodstream infection. This chapter focuses on metabolic and nutritional complications associated with nutritional support.

Metabolic Complications

Altered Glucose Metabolism: Rebound Hypoglycemia

Rebound hypoglycemia may occur with the discontinuation of cyclic PN or if continuous PN is interrupted because of continued secretion of insulin by the pancreas in response to the high-dextrose solution. Hypoglycemia is defined as BG less than 70 mg/dL (McMahon et al., 2013). Symptoms include diaphoresis, irritability, nervousness, and shaking and may result in a decrease in level of consciousness. Rebound hypoglycemia

> Table 12-5 COMPLICATIONS ASSOCIATED WITH PN

Complication/ Etiology	Symptoms	Treatment	Prevention
Metabolic Complications (Most Common; Other Electrolyte Imbalances Possible; See Chapter 3)			
Hypoglycemia: Rebound Cause: Abrupt cessation of parenteral nutrition (PN)	Diaphoresis, irritability, nervousness, shakiness, decreased level of consciousness	Administer dextrose or decrease insulin	Maintain steady rate of infusion; wean gradually Taper rate down for last 1–2 hours of cyclic infusions
Hyperglycemia Cause: Carbohydrate intolerance, insulin resistance, rapid PN delivery, diabetes, infection/sepsis, traumatic stress	Increased serum glucose, acetone breath, anxiety, confusion, dehydration, polydipsia, polyuria, malaise	Administer insulin	Decreased dextrose concentration or decreased rate Increase calories with lipids Monitor blood glucose
Hypokalemia Cause: Shift of K into cells, gastrointestinal (GI) losses, diuretic therapy, steroid administration, anorexia	Serum K <3.5 mEq/L, anorexia, fatigue, muscle weakness, decreased gastric motility, postural hypotension, electro-cardiographic (ECG) changes	Adjust PN formula	Monitor serum potassium, intake and output
Hyperkalemia Cause: Renal impairment, iatrogenic-induced, metabolic and respiratory acidosis, tissue damage	Serum K elevated >5.5 mEq/L, ECG changes, cardiac arrest, muscular weakness, flaccid muscles, intestinal colic, diarrhea	Adjust PN formula, dialysis	Monitor serum potassium, intake and output
Hypomagnesemia Cause: GI losses, refeeding after starvation, renal disease	Apprehension, depression, apathy, neuromuscular hyperexcitability, tremors, premature ventricular contractions (PVCs), tachycardia, ventricular fibrillation	Adjust PN formula	Monitor serum magnesium, assess for neuromuscular changes
Hypophosphatemia Cause: Inadequate phosphorus in PN formula, burns, malabsorption, starvation	Apprehension, irritability, seizures, decreased red blood cells (RBCs), muscle weakness, insulin resistance	Adjust PN formula	Monitor serum phosphorus levels

Continued

> Table 12-5   COMPLICATIONS ASSOCIATED WITH PN—cont'd

Complication/ Etiology	Symptoms	Treatment	Prevention
Hypocalcemia Cause: Vitamin D deficiency, insufficient calcium or magnesium intake, malabsorption, pancreatitis	Central nervous system (CNS) irritability, confusion, muscle cramps in extremities, muscle spasms, laryngeal spasms, seizures, tetany	Adjust PN formula	Monitor serum calcium levels, avoid calcium-depleting medications, maintain adequate calcium intake
Infection			
Cause: Microbial contamination at the catheter insertion site, microbial contamination via the catheter hub, homogeneous seeding from other sources, contaminated infusate (rare)	Chills, fever, malaise, elevated white blood cell (WBC) count, tachycardia, tachypnea, flushing hypotension	Blood cultures Catheter removal (catheter tip culture) and replacement may be required Antibiotics Administer oxygen Prepare to treat for septic shock	Hand hygiene Maintain aseptic technique with all aspects of infusion related care Use 0.22-micron filter with nonlipid PN formulas; use 1.2-micron filter with lipid-containing formulas
Nutritional Alterations			
Refeeding Syndrome Cause: Occurs during initial phase of PN Body during its bout of starvation has adapted somewhat to nutritional deprivation and decreased basal energy requirements Causes electrolyte shift	Cardiorespiratory complications (dyspnea, tachycardia advancing to heart failure and cardiac arrest)	Monitor serum electrolytes, especially phosphorus and potassium Treat symptoms; adjust infusion rate	Can be averted by starting PN gradually and then gradually increasing rate Monitor patient response to PN
Essential Fatty Acid Deficiency (EFAD) Cause: Deficient intake	Desquamating dermatitis, alopecia, brittle nails, delayed wound healing, thrombocytopenia, decreased immunity, increased capillary fragility	Intravenous fat emulsion (IVFE)	Accurate calculation of protein, fat, and carbohydrate ratios to maintain a positive nitrogen balance
Altered Mineral Balance Cause: Result of deficiencies caused by malnourishment or starvation	Chromium: Elevated serum lipid levels, insulin resistance, glucose tolerance Copper: Hypochromic microcytic anemia, neutropenia	Supply adequate supplementation in PN	Monitor for abnormal laboratory values

> Table 12-5   COMPLICATIONS ASSOCIATED WITH PN—cont'd

Complication/ Etiology	Symptoms	Treatment	Prevention
	Iron: Fatigue, glossitis, hypochromic microcytic anemia Manganese: CNS changes Selenium: Cardiomyopathies Zinc: Alopecia, apathy, confusion, poor wound healing		
Altered Vitamin Balance Cause: Disease processes can alter vitamin requirements PN must supply the needed fat- and water-soluble vitamin supplements	Vitamin A: Dry, scaly, rough, cracked skin; decreased saliva; impaired digestion; diarrhea Vitamin D: Decreased serum calcium or phosphorus levels Vitamin E: RBC hemolysis Vitamin K: Delayed clotting Vitamin B_1: Increased serum and urine lactate or pyruvate levels, anorexia, confusion, fatigue, painful calf muscle Vitamin B_2: Glossitis, stomatitis, dermatitis, photophobia Vitamin B_3 (niacin): Dermatitis, glossitis, diarrhea, dementia Vitamin B_{12}: Anorexia, depression, dyspnea, memory lapses, delirium, hallucinations Folic acid: Macrocytic anemia, diarrhea, glossitis Vitamin C: Bleeding gums, petechiae, depression	Provide vitamin supplements in PN	Monitor for symptoms and assess for deficits

is prevented by ensuring that there are no interruptions in the infusion. For patients on cyclic infusions, the infusion rate may be tapered down over the last 1 to 2 hours.

Altered Glucose Metabolism: Hyperglycemia

Hyperglycemia is a common and significant complication associated with PN and is caused by poor tolerance of the high dextrose concentrations.

Other factors that put the patient at risk for hyperglycemia are the presence of overt or latent diabetes mellitus, older age, sepsis, hypokalemia, and hypophosphatemia. Hyperglycemia is associated with increased risk for complications such as pneumonia and acute renal failure and with an increased mortality rate (McMahon et al., 2013). Close attention to BG monitoring and management are critical. Current guidelines from A.S.P.E.N. state that the target BG range is between 140 and 180 mg/dL (McMahon et al., 2013).

Conditions of stress result in impaired glucose tolerance and hyperglycemia in up to 25% of patients on PN. Infusion of large amounts of glucose can also unmask latent diabetes, making hyperglycemia one of the most common complications encountered with PN. Another consideration when infusing formulas containing high concentrations of glucose is the potential effect of carbohydrate metabolism on respiration. Metabolism of carbohydrates results in increased production of carbon dioxide that must be compensated for by increased minute ventilation. This could precipitate respiratory failure in patients with pre-existing respiratory disease or interfere with weaning from mechanical ventilation.

Factors that predispose a patient to glucose intolerance include:
- Presence of overt or latent diabetes mellitus
- Older age
- Pancreatitis
- Hypokalemia
- Hypophosphatemia
- Thiamine or B_6 deficiency
- Some antibiotics
- Steroids
- Conditions of stress, such as sepsis or surgery (Krzywda & Meyer, 2014)

Alterations in Hepatic Function

Abnormalities in hepatic function are common in patients receiving PN. They include steatosis, cholestasis, and gallbladder stones (Kumpf & Gervasio, 2012). Although the causes are not clear, factors may include continuous dextrose infusion, EFAD, excessive lipid infusion, amino acid imbalance, toxic effects of PN degradation products, and overgrowth of intestinal flora (Krzywda & Meyer, 2014).

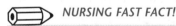 *NURSING FAST FACT!*

In adults, laboratory findings indicative of hepatic function alterations include elevations in alkaline phosphatase and transaminase levels. Cholestasis and gallbladder disease are potential complications of long-term PN.

Electrolyte Imbalances

Major electrolyte imbalances associated with PN can occur if excessive or deficient amounts of electrolytes are supplied in the daily fluid allowance. Electrolyte balance is addressed in Chapter 3. The most common imbalances associated with PN include imbalances of potassium, magnesium, and phosphate (Krzywda & Meyer, 2014). Interventions include frequent monitoring of serum electrolytes and adjustments in the PN solution.

- *Potassium: Hypokalemia.* Potassium is also driven into the intracellular space during PN. Serum potassium can become depleted with an inadequate supply of this electrolyte. Insulin administration further intensifies intracellular potassium.
- *Potassium: Hyperkalemia.* A high potassium blood level can occur with renal impairment, can be iatrogenic induced, or can occur with metabolic and respiratory acidosis when potassium shifts out of the cells. Interventions include reducing the amount of potassium ion in the PN solution.
- *Magnesium: Hypomagnesemia.* The magnesium electrolyte also is driven into the intracellular space during PN administration.
- *Phosphate: Hypophosphatemia.* Adenosine triphosphate (ATP) is required for all cell energy production. Protein synthesis begins when PN is administered and phosphate is driven into the intracellular space as a component of ATP. Therefore, a deficiency of phosphate can occur.

Nutritional Complications

Refeeding Syndrome

Cardiac and pulmonary failure can occur when aggressive nutritional support is initiated in a severely malnourished patient. **Refeeding syndrome** is a rare complication. This occurs when the body, during its bout with starvation, adapts to nutritional deprivation and compensates by decreasing basal energy requirements and diminishing cardiac reserves. This initiation of nutritional support, especially if it is undertaken too aggressively, can lead to an electrolyte shift from the plasma to the intracellular fluid and can result in hypophosphatemia in particular. Cardiorespiratory complications can occur. The result of refeeding syndrome is manifested by dyspnea, tachycardia advancing to heart failure, and cardiac arrest (Krzywda & Meyer, 2014).

Essential Fatty Acid Deficiency

Essential fatty acid deficiency is a risk when the PN formula is lipid free. Clinical signs and symptoms include:

- Alopecia
- Impaired wound healing

- Thrombocytopenia
- Dry and scaly skin

The condition is corrected when an IVFE is added to the formula. Fats may be administered in amounts that supply 30% to 50% of the calories.

Altered Vitamin and Trace Element Balance

Because of the addition of vitamins and trace elements to the formula, deficiencies are not common. Twice yearly serum levels are recommended for long-term PN, and patients should be monitored for signs and symptoms of deficiencies (Winkler et al., 2012). It is important that multivitamins be added to the solution just prior to infusion because vitamin degradation can occur when vitamins are present in the PN admixture for extended periods of time.

■ Discontinuation of Nutritional Support

Before discontinuation of parenteral or enteral nutritional support, one of the following criteria should be applicable:

- Enteral nutrition should not be discontinued until nutrient requirements can be met by oral nutrients.
- PN should not be discontinued until nutrient requirements can be met by enteral or oral nutrients.
- Parenteral or enteral nutrition support should be discontinued based on the patient's medical condition, such as the presence of significant complications.
- Parenteral or central nutrition support is terminated when the LIP judges that the patient no longer benefits from the therapy.

AGE-RELATED CONSIDERATIONS

The Pediatric Patient

Pediatric PN differs from the adult PN in nutritional requirements and formulas, monitoring parameters, and administration methods. PN is indicated in infants and children who are unable to tolerate adequate enteral feedings to sustain their nutritional requirements. Patients who require PN fall into two main categories: those with congenital or acquired abnormalities of the GI tract (e.g., severe inflammatory bowel disease, paralytic ileus, intestinal atresia) and those with intractable diarrhea syndromes (Krzywda & Meyer, 2010). PN may also be required in children who are premature, who suffer from chronic malnutrition (failure to thrive), or who are at high risk for developing malnutrition as a result of acute medical illness or prolonged postoperative recovery.

Assessment

- Nutritional assessment of pediatric patients includes use of standard growth curves. Calculation of the ratio of weight to height indicates wasting, and calculation of the ratio of height to age indicates stunting of growth. Anthropometric measurements are used as gauges of somatic protein and fat stores. Visceral protein stores are evaluated by determining serum albumin, serum transferrin, prealbumin, and retinol-binding protein levels.
- Pediatric requirements for PN follow general guidelines and are based on protein, calorie, and fluid needs per kilogram of body weight. Indirect calorimetry is recommended for estimating energy expenditure and to reduce the risk of over- or underfeeding (Krzywda & Meyer, 2010; Mehta, Compher, & A.S.P.E.N. Board of Directors, 2009).
- Children have a high basal metabolic rate per unit of body weight, an increased evaporative fluid loss, and immature kidneys. Fluid requirements must be carefully assessed to prevent dehydration or overhydration. There are many factors affecting fluid needs, such as thermal blankets, phototherapy, and radiant warmers (Krzywda & Meyer, 2010).
- The protein needs of pediatric patients are higher than adults when compared to body weight (Gargasz, 2012). Furthermore, certain amino acids that are nonessential for adults may be essential for pediatric patients, including histidine, tyrosine, and cysteine. Special amino acid formulas are available to meet these pediatric needs (Krzywda & Meyer, 2010).
- Children develop EFAD more quickly than adults, within 1 week, when lipid-free solutions are administered; however, lipids may be harmful when administered to the jaundiced infant (Krzywda & Meyer, 2010).
- Another area of assessment includes psychological support. Many pediatric patients on PN are infants who are acutely ill and deprived of maternal warmth and comfort. Cuddling and holding the child should be encouraged, along with allowing the parents to participate in their child's care. Allowing "breaks" from PN may be beneficial to a child who is able to enjoy regular activities. Some patients receiving PN are not acutely ill and have the energy of any other child.

Monitoring

PN must be monitored in the pediatric patient to meet the demands of growth and development.

- The nurse must monitor the child's physical status, including reporting abnormal findings of temperature spikes, hyper-/hypoglycemia, chills, rashes, irritability, and changes in level of consciousness. Serum level of various chemistry and hematology tests are checked daily for the first week and then decreased to a weekly schedule for the stable hospitalized or home PN patient.
- Many children require long-term support at home. Monitoring includes many of the same parameters as for adults. Monitoring during initiation of PN includes daily weight, intake and output, daily electrolytes until stable, serum glucose measurements every 8 to 12 hours, serum triglycerides and free fatty acid levels weekly, and hepatic function test biweekly.

Continued

- Children require evaluation of growth determinations, including weight, height, and head circumference for the duration of therapy.
- Cyclic PN should be considered in patients such as those on long-term PN or those with cholestasis.

Practice Guidelines to Prevent Complications in the Pediatric Patient
- Hepatobiliary dysfunction is a common complication in pediatric patients. Cholestasis can appear in pediatric patients after 2 weeks. To manage this complication, interventions include decreasing protein intake, converting to cyclic PN, and providing some nutrients via the enteral tract if possible (Krzywda & Meyer, 2010). The use of DEHP infusion systems (i.e., containers/administration set) was found to increase the risk of cholestasis (von Rettberg, Hannman, Subotic, et al., 2009).
- Hyperglycemia is of particular concern in neonatal patients. It can cause complications including retinopathy, bronchopulmonary dysplasia, necrotizing enterocolitis, infections, longer hospital stays, and death. Insulin administration by continuous infusion is safe and effective in controlling PN-associated hyperglycemia in infants (Gargasz, 2012). Management of hyperglycemia includes avoiding excess dextrose concentrations, providing fat emulsions, and using insulin for persistent hyperglycemia.

The Older Adult

The physiological changes that occur with advancing age affect nutritional requirements, independent of disease or rehabilitation demands. Physiological changes that decrease caloric requirements include a reduction in lean body mass and redistribution of fat around internal organs (DiMaria-Ghalili, 2012). Furthermore, changes in taste, whether caused by atrophy, medications, or nutrient deficiency, may contribute to an altered nutritional status. Based predominantly on an international sample of patients in hospitals and nursing homes, it is estimated that 39% to 47% of hospitalized older adults are either malnourished or at nutritional risk (Kaiser et al., 2010).

Inadequate dietary intake in elderly people is multifaceted. Causes of malnutrition in older adults include presence of chronic illnesses, poor oral health, polypharmacy, social isolation, dementia, obesity, frailty, and changes in functional status affecting their ability to obtain, prepare, and eat food (Mueller & Zelig, 2012).

Data related to use of PN in the older adult are very limited; however, PN may be an option when nutritional requirements cannot be met orally or via the enteral route. The use of PPN via a peripheral I.V. is discouraged because of the fragility of veins (Mueller & Zelig 2012). Because of the presence of the normal changes of aging (e.g., diminished renal function) and the presence of chronic illnesses, metabolic problems including fluid and electrolyte disturbances are more common. Older adults are more likely to have vitamin and trace element deficiencies.

Practice Guidelines

1. Older adult patients should undergo nutrition screening to identify those who require formal nutrition assessment.
2. Age and lifestyle parameters should be used to assess the nutrition status of elderly persons.
3. Potential drug–nutrient interactions should be assessed in all elderly patients receiving medications.
4. Diet and specialized nutritional support for elderly persons should take into consideration altered nutrient requirements observed in this age group.

 Home Care Issues

Provision of PN in the home setting dates back to the 1970s. Home parenteral nutrition (HPN) is well established and should be instituted and supervised by a multidisciplinary team with knowledge and expertise; this is stated in the guidelines developed by the European Society for Parenteral and Enteral Nutrition (ESPEN) (Staun et al., 2009). HPN may be a long-term or even life-time infusion therapy for certain patients. HPN may be administered as a 24 hour/day infusion or, more commonly, as a cyclic infusion. Cyclic HPN is most often administered overnight, allowing patients freedom from the infusion pump during the daytime.

Advantages of home treatment for nutritional support include lower cost and the ability of the patient to remain in familiar, comfortable surroundings, thereby decreasing the confusion associated with age-related environment changes. In many cases, it allows the patient to return to normal activities, and it is associated with a lower risk of acquiring a health-care–associated infection. In addition, a person's control over his or her body and the self-care responsibility increase self-esteem.

Patient Selection

Candidates for PN within the home care environment include patients who have long-term disease in which oral and enteral nutrition have been demonstrated as ineffective in providing nutritional support. Typical diagnoses associated with HPN include intestinal failure, short bowel syndrome, malabsorption, chronic bowel obstruction, Crohn's disease, radiation enteritis, intestinal/pancreatic fistulas, pancreatitis, and severe, life-threatening malnutrition (Winkler et al., 2012).

Discharge Planning

Before initiating the discharge planning process, reimbursement for home care must be verified. Private third-party payers vary in coverage. Certain diagnoses and PN infusions may be covered under the durable medical equipment benefit under Part B of the Medicare program. Patients must meet criteria that include "permanence," interpreted as requiring PN for at least 3 months.

Issues to address during discharge planning include the patient's ability to participate in care, the stability of the clinical condition, caregiver/family

Continued

Home Care Issues—cont'd

support, and home environmental safety. Because, the goal for most patients on HPN is complete independence by the patient and/or caregiver in administration and monitoring of the infusion, the ability to participate in care is a necessary aspect of assessment. Intellectual and functional abilities should be carefully assessed. The ability to adhere to aseptic technique and to manage an EID, the adequacy of eyesight, and manual dexterity are important attributes. Ideally, a formal teaching program should be initiated in the hospital prior to discharge. Before sending a patient home on HPN, the patient must be clinically stable before going home on PN as defined by:

• Weight maintained or increased per goals of PN
• Stable blood chemistry levels
• Stable nutritional laboratory indicators
• No evidence of rebound hypoglycemia with discontinuation of cyclic infusions
• No adverse reactions to HPN infusion

Home safety must be determined before discharge from the hospital. The home environment should be reasonably clean and safe for storage of supplies and preparation for infusion. Electricity, telephone access, and refrigeration are necessary. Ambulatory infusion pumps used in the home setting can be powered by disposable batteries, but for cost effectiveness most use rechargeable batteries. The HPN solution is usually delivered weekly, and a reliable refrigerator is required for storage.

NOTE > In some cases, the home infusion pharmacy may provide a small refrigerator dedicated to PN storage.

Preparing for Home Parenteral Nutrition

The home education process should include but is not limited to:

• Verbal and written instructions on appropriate procedures based on an assessment of how the patient best learns with attention to age, cognition, developmental level, health literacy, culture, and language (INS, 2011, p. S16)
• Demonstration and return demonstration of procedures by the primary caregiver
    • Inspection of HPN containers and contents
    • Aseptic technique required for adding multivitamins to the HPN and for all interventions related to administration via the VAD
    • Proper storage
• Evaluation and documentation of competency
• Self-monitoring
• Limitations of physical activity
• Emergency intervention and problem-solving
• Care of infusion equipment, solutions, and supplies
• Disposal of supplies

Home Care Issues—cont'd

• Expectations of home care and medical and nursing follow-up
• Statement of when and whom to contact when complications occur
Practice criteria for delivery of PN in the home and hospital are the same.

NOTE > Ambulatory pumps have features specific for HPN administration.

Monitoring

Complications have been previously addressed. Of note, the most common
complication for patients receiving HPN is catheter-related bloodstream infection (Winkler et al., 2012). Monitoring for signs and symptoms of infection and
providing patients and families with thorough education aimed at risk reduction are important aspects of home care nursing. Patients should be instructed
on BG monitoring, daily weights, monitoring intake and output, being atten-
tive to changes (e.g., increased or decreased urine/ostomy output), and monitoring for signs of infection (e.g., fever, VAD site redness, swelling).

> EBP A study investigated the incidence and causative factors of compli-
> cations that occur within the first 90 days after discharge from hospital
> to home for patients on new home PN. A complication developed in one-
> third of the patients, and the majority required rehospitalization. Infec-
> tious complications were the most prevalent, followed by mechanical
> and then metabolic. Trends that the authors found included the follow-
> ing: (1) patients with single-lumen catheters experienced more overall
> complications, and (2) more complications occurred among patients
> with ostomies (Burgoa, Seidner, Hamilton, Staffor, & Steiger, 2006).

BG levels should be checked during PN infusions and then compared to
levels when the patient is off the cyclic PN. As a general guideline, glucose
levels should be less than 150 mg/dL (Krzywda & Meyer, 2014). During the
peak of the cyclic PN infusion, some physicians may allow BG levels as high
as 200 mg/dL. It is important to collaborate with the referring nutritional
support program/prescribing physician when obtaining reporting parameters. It is important to recognize that a sudden increase in BG may be an early
sign of infection and that further evaluation is necessary.

Psychosocial Issues

Psychosocial issues include those related to the complexity of managing life on
PN and inability to eat normally. It is important to assess the home situation
and patient adaptations. Results of a patient questionnaire to assess shortcomings in care included satisfaction with attention to medical issues but lack of attention to psychosocial problems (Huisman-deWaal, van Achterberg, Jansen,
Wanten, & Schoonhoven, 2011). Fatigue and diarrhea are symptoms that patients

Continued

Home Care Issues—cont'd

often have that impact daily life (Staun et al., 2009). Lack of sleep due to nighttime infusions, limitations on freedom and social activities, and dependency on others are additional issues these patients face. It is important for the nurse to assess for psychosocial issues and provide the opportunity for patients and their families to discuss them. Referrals to behavioral health professionals may be appropriate.

An excellent resource and support for patients is the Oley Foundation. It is a nonprofit support organization, established in 1983, that provides education, self-help, and research for persons who are on PN or enteral nutrition. Membership is free. There are excellent patient educational tools, a newsletter, and other resources available on the site.

Website

The Oley Foundation: www.Oley.org

Patient Education

The patient receiving PPN or PN will require education, periodic assessment, and retraining as needed. Many of the points listed in patient education for home care issues apply to patients in all settings.

- Inform the patient about the purpose and duration of the projected nutritional support.
- Instruct the patient on the hang time of the product with the composition, intended use, and expected outcomes of the formulation.
- Educate the patient and caregiver about management of the VAD.
- Instruct the patient receiving enteral feedings about clean techniques for handling the tube, maintaining the access site, and flushing the tube to maintain patency.
- Inform the patient about complications associated with PPN administration, including:
  - Metabolic complications such as hypoglycemia and electrolyte imbalances (recognize and respond to these complications)
  - Mechanical or procedural problems (catheter or tube occlusion, leakage, breakage, or dislodgement)
  - Equipment malfunction or breakage
  - Infusion contamination precipitate or inhomogeneity (recognize and report signs and symptoms of localized or systemic infectious process)
- Provide 24-hour phone numbers for home care agency or physician so that patient or caregiver can access professional help.

🔖 Nursing Process

The nursing process is a six-step process for problem solving to guide nursing action (see Chapter 1 for details on the steps of the nursing process). The following table focuses on nursing diagnoses, nursing outcomes classification (NOC), and nursing interventions classification (NIC) for patients receiving nutritional support. Nursing diagnoses should be patient specific and outcomes and interventions individualized. The NOC and NIC presented here are suggested directions for development of specific outcomes and interventions.

Nursing Diagnoses Related to Nutritional Support	Nursing Outcomes Classification (NOC)	Nursing Interventions Classification (NIC)
Fluid volume excess, risk for related to: Rapid administration of PN	Fluid balance, hydration	Fluid management, fluid monitoring
Health maintenance, ineffective related to: Poor dietary habits, with perceptual or cognitive impairment	Health beliefs: Perceived resources, health-promoting behavior, health-seeking behavior	Health education, support system enhancement
Infection, risk for, related to: Concentrated glucose solution, invasive administration of fluids; inadequate intake of calories and protein	Immune status; infection control, risk detection; infection management	Infection control, infection protection
Nutrition, less than body requirements, related to: Inability to ingest or digest food or absorb nutrients as a result of biological or psychological factors	Nutritional status, nutrient intake; food and fluid intake; weight control	Feeding, nutrition management, nutrition therapy, nutrition counseling
Skin integrity, impaired or risk for, related to: Internal: Inadequate intake of protein; imbalanced nutritional state; impaired metabolic state	Tissue integrity: Skin and mucous membranes	Skin care, skin surveillance, wound care
Self-care deficit: related to inability to chew food; inability to get food; inability to handle utensils; inability to ingest food; inability to swallow food	Activities of daily living, eating	Self-care assistance, feeding

Sources: Ackley & Ladwig (2011); Bulechek, Butcher, Dochterman, & Wagner (2013); Moorhead, Johnson, Maas, & Swanson (2013).

Chapter Highlights

- Candidates for nutritional support include those with:
  - Altered catabolic states
  - Chronic weight loss
  - Conditions requiring bowel rest
  - Excessive nitrogen loss
  - Hepatic or renal failure
  - Hypermetabolic states
  - Malabsorption states
  - Malnutrition
  - Multiple trauma
  - Serum albumin levels below 3.5 g/dL
- There are three classifications of malnutrition: marasmus, kwashiorkor, and mixed malnutrition.
- Effects of malnutrition include a decrease in protein stores, albumin depletion, and impaired immune status.
- Nutritional assessment includes:
  - History (medical, social, dietary)
  - Anthropometric measurements (height, weight, skinfold tests, midarm circumference)
  - Laboratory testing (serum albumin, serum transferrin, prealbumin and retinol-binding protein, total lymphocyte counts, serum electrolytes)
  - Energy requirements
  - Physical examination
  - Other indices (nitrogen balance, indirect calorimetry, prognostic nutritional index)
- PN is an I.V. solution that includes carbohydrates, amino acids, lipids, electrolytes, multivitamins, and minerals formulated to meet an individual patient's needs.
- Modalities for delivery of nutritional support include:
  - Enteral nutrition
  - PN, which may be administered via a peripheral vein or a central vein
- PPN, delivered into a peripheral vein, is indicated for patients who are malnourished, or at risk for malnutrition, and are not candidates for enteral nutrition. It consists of a 2% to 5% amino acid solution in combination with 5% to 10% dextrose. Fat emulsions of 10% to 20% may be combined or administered separately. This therapy is delivered for a limited time, usually less than 2 weeks.
- PN delivered via a CVAD is the I.V. administration of hypertonic glucose (20%–70%) and amino acids (3.5%–15%), along with all additional components required for complete support.
- PN must be filtered with a 0.22-micron filter, except when lipids are added to TNAs, which must have a 1.2-micron filter.

- Complications of PN include:
  - VAD-related complications
  - Metabolic complications
  - Nutritional complications

▄▄ Thinking Critically: Case Study

A 45-year-old man is admitted with severe exacerbation of his Crohn's disease. He is 6 feet 1 inches tall, weighs 132 pounds (60 kg), and has experienced a 45-pound weight loss in the past 3 months (25%). He is weak and pale, has dry mucous membranes, a red beefy tongue, and cracks at the sides of his mouth. He has an ileostomy and has developed a draining enterocutaneous fistula. Because of severe malabsorption as a result of the Crohn's disease, PN is ordered. He is to receive a solution of 20% dextrose, 50 g of protein/L with standard electrolytes, and daily multiple vitamin/trace elements. The goal is 2 L of this solution per day. With lipids, this will provide an average of 2260 calories per day, 100 g of protein, and 21/4 L of fluid per day. The solution is initiated at 1 L/day and increases according to patient tolerance. The PN will be infused through a peripherally inserted central catheter.

Case Study Questions

1. What are the points of care in monitoring this patient?
2. Why is the presence of the enterocutaneous fistula significant in terms of this patient's nutritional needs (considering increased fluid requirements and wound healing)?
3. What potential complications related to PN is this patient at risk for?

 Media Link: Answers to the case study and more critical thinking activities are provided on Davis*Plus*.

Post-Test

1. The type of malnutrition that most commonly occurs in the acutely ill hospitalized patient is:

   a. Kwashiorkor
   b. Marasmus
   c. Mixed malnutrition
   d. Anorexia nervosa

2. How many kilocalories/mL does a 20% lipid emulsion provide?

   a. 1.0
   b. 1.1
   c. 2.0
   d. 2.2

3. Which of the following are the three essential substrates included in PN required for anabolism and tissue synthesis?

   a. Trace elements, protein, and fats
   b. Protein, carbohydrates, and fats
   c. Fats, electrolytes, and carbohydrates
   d. Vitamins, electrolytes, and protein

4. Which of the following are considered anthropometric measurements? (*Select all that apply.*)

   a. Mid-arm muscle circumference
   b. Weight
   c. Skinfold thickness
   d. Serum transferrin

5. Which of the following filters should be used with TNA solutions?

   a. 0.22-micron filter
   b. 0.45-micron filter
   c. 1.2-micron filter
   d. 170-micron filter

6. To treat or prevent essential fatty acid deficiency, which of the following should be included in PN?

   a. Trace elements
   b. Transferrin
   c. Crystalline amino acids
   d. Lipids

7. Due to its' short half-life, which of the following visceral proteins is most useful in monitoring protein malnutrition during refeeding?

   a. Albumin
   b. Transferrin
   c. Prealbumin
   d. Total protein

8. Refeeding syndrome is associated with which of the following electrolyte abnormalities?

   a. Hyponatremia
   b. Hypercalcemia
   c. Hypophosphatemia
   d. Hypermagnesemia

9. Which of the following are common components of the nutritional assessment? (*Select all that apply.*)

   a. Social history
   b. Dietary history
   c. Physical examination

  d. Anthropometric measurements
  e. Laboratory diagnostic evaluation

 10. Which of the following are points of care in delivery of PPN? (*Select all that apply.*)

  a. PPN is mildly hypertonic and should be delivered into a large peripheral vein.
  b. A 20% dextrose solution can be delivered via PPN.
  c. Phlebitis is a complication of PPN; the catheter site should be observed with frequent documentation of the condition of the vein and site.
  d. PPN is most commonly used for short-term therapy for fairly stable patients whose normal GI functioning will resume within 3 to 4 weeks.

 Media Link: Answers to the Chapter 12 Post-Test and more test questions together with rationales are provided on Davis*Plus*.

▪ References

Ackley, B. J., & Ladwig, G. B. (2011). *Nursing diagnosis handbook: An evidence-based guide to planning care* (9th ed.). St. Louis, MO: Mosby Elsevier.

American Society for Parenteral and Enteral Nutrition (A.S.P.E.N.) Board of Directors and Clinical Practice Committee. (2012). Definition of terms, style, and conventions used in A.S.P.E.N. Board of Directors-approved documents. Retrieved from https://www.nutritioncare.org/Professional_Resources/Guidelines_and_Standards/Guidelines/2012_Definitions_of_Terms,_Style,_and_Conventions_Used_in_A_S_P_E_N__Board_of_Directors-Approved_Documents/ (Accessed March 1, 2013).

American Society for Parenteral and Enteral Nutrition (A.S.P.E.N.) Board of Directors. (2007). Standards of practice for nutrition support nurses. *Nutrition in Clinical Practice, 22,* 458-465.

Barber, J. R., & Sacks, G. S. (2012). Parenteral nutrition formulations. In C. M. Mueller (Ed.), *The A.S.P.E.N. adult nutrition core curriculum* (2nd ed.) (pp. 245-264). Silver Spring, MD: A.S.P.E.N.

Brantley, S. L., & Mills, M. E. (2012). Overview of enteral nutrition. In C. M. Mueller (Ed.), *The A.S.P.E.N. adult nutrition core curriculum* (2nd ed.) (pp. 170-184). Silver Spring, MD: A.S.P.E.N.

Bulechek, G. M., Butcher, H. K., Dochterman, J. M., & Wagner, C. M. (2013). *Nursing interventions classification (NIC)* (6th ed.). St. Louis, MO: Mosby Elsevier.

Burgoa, L. J., Seidner, D., Hamilton, C., Staffor, J., & Steiger, E. (2006). Examination of factors that lead to complications for new home parenteral nutrition patients. *Journal of Infusion Nursing, 29*(2), 74-80.

Centers for Disease Control and Prevention (CDC). (2011). About BMI for adults. Retrieved from http://www.cdc.gov/healthyweight/assessing/bmi/adult_bmi/index.html (Accessed February 27, 2013).

DiMaria-Ghalili, R. A. (2012). Nutrition in the elderly: nursing standard of practice protocol: nutrition in aging. Retrieved from: http://consultgerirn.org/topics/nutrition_in_the_elderly/want_to_know_more (Accessed March 6, 2013).

Gahart, L., & Nazareno, A. R. (2012). *Intravenous medications* (28th ed.). St. Louis, MO: Mosby Elsevier.

Gargasz, A. (2012). Neonatal and pediatric parenteral nutrition. *AACN Advanced Critical Care, 23*(4), 451-464.

Huang, E. Y., Chen, C., Abdullah, F., Aspelund, G., Barnhart, D. C., Calkins, C. M., . . . Arca, M. J. (2011). Strategies for the prevention of central venous catheter infections: An American Pediatric Surgical Association Outcomes and Clinical Trials Committee systematic review. *Journal of Pediatric Surgery, 46,* 2000-2011.

Huisman-de Waal, G., van Acheterberg, T., Jansen, J., Wanten, G., & Schoonhoven, L. (2011). "High-tech" home care: Overview of professional care in patients on home parenteral nutrition and implications for nursing care. *Journal of Clinical Nursing, 20*(15-16), 2125-2134.

Infusion Nurses Society (INS). (2011). Infusion nursing standards of practice. *Journal of Intravenous Nursing, 34*(1S), S1-S110.

Jensen, G. L., Hsiao, P. Y., & Wheeler, D. (2012). Nutrition screening and assessment. In C. M. Mueller (Ed.), *The A.S.P.E.N. adult nutrition core curriculum* (2nd ed.) (pp. 155-169). Silver Spring, MD: A.S.P.E.N.

Kaiser, M. J., Bauer, J. M., Rämsch, C., Uter, W., Guigoz, Y., Cederholm, T., . . . Siber, C. C. (2010). Frequency of malnutrition in older adults: A multinational perspective using the mini nutritional assessment. *Journal of the American Geriatrics Society, 58,* 1734-1738.

Kumpf, V. J., & Gervasio, J. (2012). Complications of parenteral nutrition. In C. M. Mueller (Ed.), *The A.S.P.E.N. adult nutrition core curriculum* (2nd ed.) (pp. 284-297). Silver Spring, MD: A.S.P.E.N.

Krzydwa, E. A., & Meyer, D. (2010). Parenteral nutrition. In M. Alexander, A. Corrigan, L. Gorski, J. Hankins, & R. Perucca (Eds.), *Infusion nursing: An evidence-based practice* (3rd ed.) (pp. 316-350.) St. Louis: Saunders/Elsevier.

Krzydwa, E. A., & Meyer, D. (2014). Parenteral nutrition. In M. Alexander, A. Corrigan, L. Gorski, & L. Phillips (Eds.), *Core curriculum for infusion nursing* (4th ed). (pp. 309-355). Philadelphia: Lippincott, Williams, & Wilkins.

Maiefski, M., Rupp, M. E., & Hermsen, E. D. (2009). Ethanol lock therapy: Review of the literature. *Infection Control and Hospital Epidemiology, 30*(11), 1096-1108.

McMahon, M. M., Nystrom, E., Braunschweig, C., Miles, J., Compher, C., American Society for Parenteral and Enteral Nutrition (A.S.P.E.N.), & American Society for Parenteral and Enteral Nutrition. (2013). A.S.P.E.N. clinical guidelines: Nutrition support of adult patients with hyperglycemia. *Journal of Parenteral and Enteral Nutrition, 37*(1), 23-36.

Mehta, N. M., Compher, C., & A.S.P.E.N. Board of Directors. (2009). A.S.P.E.N. clinical guidelines: Nutrition support of the critically ill child. *Journal of Parenteral and Enteral Nutrition, 33*(3), 260-276.

Mirtallo, J., Canada T., Johnson D., Kumpf, V., Petersen, C., Sacks, G., . . . Task Force for the Revision of Safe Practices for Parenteral Nutrition. (2004). Safe practices for parenteral nutrition. *JPEN Journal of Parenteral and Enteral Nutrition, 28*(6), S39-S70.

Mirtallo, J. M., & Patel, M. (2012). Overview of parenteral nutrition. In
    C. M. Mueller (Ed.), *The A.S.P.E.N. adult nutrition core curriculum* (2nd ed.)
    (pp. 234-244). Silver Spring, MD: A.S.P.E.N.

Moorhead, S., Johnson, M., Maas, M., & Swanson, E. (2013). *Nursing outcomes
    classification (NOC)* (5th ed.). St. Louis, MO: Mosby Elsevier.

Mueller, C., & Zelig, R. (2012). Nutrition support for older adults. In
    C. M. Mueller (Ed.), *The A.S.P.E.N. adult nutrition core curriculum* (2nd ed.)
    (pp. 620-629). Silver Spring, MD: A.S.P.E.N.

Mueller, C., Compher, C., Druyan, M. E. & A.S.P.E.N. Board of Directors. (2011).
    A.S.P.E.N. clinical guidelines: Nutrition screening, assessment and interven-
    tion in adults. *Journal of Parenteral and Enteral Nutrition, 35*(1), 16-24.

O'Grady, N. P., Alexander, M., Burns, L. A., Dellinger, E. P., Garland, J., Heard,
    S. O., ... Healthcare Infection Control Practices Advisory Committee (HICPAC).
    (2011). Guidelines for the prevention of intravascular catheter related infec-
    tions, 2011. *American Journal of Infection Control, 39*(4 Suppl), S1-S34. Also
    available at http://www.cdc.gov/hicpac/pdf/guidelines/bsi-guidelines-
    2011.pdf (Accessed September 15, 2012).

Oliveira, C., Nasr, A., Brindle, M., & Wales, P. W. (2012). Ethanol locks to
    prevent catheter-related bloodstream infections in parenteral nutrition:
    A meta-analysis. *Pediatrics, 129*(2), 318-329.

Porth, C. M., & Matfin, G. (2010). *Pathophysiology: Concepts of altered health states*
    (6th ed.). Philadelphia, PA: Lippincott Williams & Wilkins.

Rollins, C. J. (2012). Drug-nutrient interactions. In C. M. Mueller (Ed.), *The
    A.S.P.E.N. adult nutrition core curriculum* (2nd ed.) (pp. 298-312). Silver
    Spring, MD: A.S.P.E.N.

Smeltzer, S. C., Bare, B. G., Hinkle, J. L., & Cheever, K. H. (2010). *Brunner &
    Suddarths's textbook of medical-surgical nursing* (12th ed.). Philadelphia:
    Lippincott Williams & Willkins.

Staun, M., Pironi, L., Bozzetti, F., Baxter, J., Forbes, A., Joly, F., ... ESPEN. (2009).
    ESPEN guidelines on parenteral nutrition: home parenteral nutrition in
    adults. *Clinical Nutrition, 28*, 467-479.

Stout, S. M., & Cober, M. P. (2010). Metabolic effects of cyclic parenteral nutrition
    infusion in adults and children. *Nutrition in Clinical Practice, 25*(3), 277-281.

Ukleja, A., Freeman, K. L., Gilbert, K., Kochevar, M., Kraft, M. D., Russell, M. K.,
    & the American Society for Parenteral and Enteral Nutrition Board of
    Directors. (2010). Standards of nutrition support: Adult hospitalized
    patients. *Journal of Parenteral and Enteral Nutrition, 25*(4), 403-414.

United States Pharmacopeia (USP). (2008). Revised general chapter <797>
    Pharmaceutical compounding: Sterile preparations. USP 31-NF 26(Suppl 2).
    The Pharmacists' Pharmacopeia (2nd ed.). Rockville, MD: Author.

von Rettberg, H., Hannman, T., Subotic, U., Brade, J., Schaible, T., Waag, K. L., &
    Loff, S. (2009). Use of di(2-ethylhexyl) phthalate-containing infusion systems
    increases the risk for cholestasis. *Pediatrics, 124*(2), 710-716.

Winkler, M., Hagan, E., & Albina, J. E. (2012). Home nutrition support. In
    C. M. Mueller (Ed.), *The A.S.P.E.N. adult nutrition core curriculum* (2nd ed.)
    (pp. 639-655). Silver Spring, MD: A.S.P.E.N.

Wooley, J. A., & Frankenfield, D. (2012). Energy. In C. M. Mueller (Ed.), *The
    A.S.P.E.N. adult nutrition core curriculum* (2nd ed.) (pp. 22-35). Silver Spring,
    MD: A.S.P.E.N.

Index

Note: Page numbers followed by f refer to figures, page numbers followed by t refer to tables.